Osteoimmunology: Molecular Mechanisms and Clinical Applications

Osteoimmunology: Molecular Mechanisms and Clinical Applications

Editor: Melonie Armstrong

FOSTER
ACADEMICS
www.fosteracademics.com

www.fosteracademics.com

FOSTER ACADEMICS

Cataloging-in-Publication Data

Osteoimmunology : molecular mechanisms and clinical applications / edited by Melonie Armstrong.
p. cm.
Includes bibliographical references and index.
ISBN 978-1-64646-605-4
1. Immunology. 2. Musculoskeletal system--Immunology. 3. Molecular immunology. 4. Clinical immunology.
5. Bones--Immunology. 6. Musculoskeletal system--Diseases--Immunological aspects. 7. Bones--Diseases--Immunological aspects. I. Armstrong, Melonie.
QR181 .O883 2023
616.079--dc23

Foster Academics,
118-35 Queens Blvd., Suite 400,
Forest Hills, NY 11375, USA

ISBN 978-1-64646-605-4 (Hardback)

Contents

Preface

Osteoimmunology refers to an interdisciplinary research field that combines the field of immunology and osteology. It focuses on the potential treatments and mechanisms associated with bone related diseases, such as rheumatoid arthritis, periodontitis and osteoporosis that are caused by or linked with failure of the immune system. Receptor activator of nuclear factor kappaB ligand (RANKL) is the prime regulator of osteoclastogenesis. It is known to be responsible for the increased activation of osteoclasts, such as direct activation of T cells and indirect increase in the expression of RANKL, and consequently promoting osteoclastic activity. Osteoblasts have significance in the maintenance of the hematopoietic stem cell. Furthermore, they are also relevant in the development of lymphocytes, along with immune cell functions in the development of osteoclast and osteoblast. This book elucidates the concepts and innovative models around prospective developments with respect to osteoimmunology. Also included herein is a detailed explanation of the molecular mechanisms and clinical applications of this field. Those with an interest in this field would find this book helpful.

The researches compiled throughout the book are authentic and of high quality, combining several disciplines and from very diverse regions from around the world. Drawing on the contributions of many researchers from diverse countries, the book's objective is to provide the readers with the latest achievements in the area of research. This book will surely be a source of knowledge to all interested and researching the field.

In the end, I would like to express my deep sense of gratitude to all the authors for meeting the set deadlines in completing and submitting their research chapters. I would also like to thank the publisher for the support offered to us throughout the course of the book. Finally, I extend my sincere thanks to my family for being a constant source of inspiration and encouragement.

Editor

1

Updates on Osteoimmunology: What's New on the Cross-Talk Between Bone and Immune System

*Marco Ponzetti and Nadia Rucci**

Department of Biotechnological and Applied Clinical Sciences, University of L'Aquila, L'Aquila, Italy

***Correspondence:**
Nadia Rucci
rucci@univaq.it

The term osteoimmunology was coined many years ago to describe the research field that deals with the cross-regulation between bone cells and the immune system. As a matter of fact, many factors that are classically considered immune-related, such as InterLeukins (i.e., IL-6, -11, -17, and -23), Tumor Necrosis Factor (TNF)-α, Receptor-Activator of Nuclear factor Kappa B (RANK), and its Ligand (RANKL), Nuclear Factor of Activated T-cell, cytoplasmatic-1 (NFATc1), and others have all been found to be crucial in osteoclast and osteoblast biology. Conversely, bone cells, which we used to think would only regulate each other and take care of remodeling bone, actually regulate immune cells, by creating the so-called "endosteal niche." Both osteoblasts and osteoclasts participate to this niche, either by favoring engraftment, or mobilization of Hematopoietic Stem Cells (HSCs). In this review, we will describe the main milestones at the base of the osteoimmunology and present the key cellular players of the bone-immune system cross-talk, including HSCs, osteoblasts, osteoclasts, bone marrow macrophages, osteomacs, T- and B-lymphocytes, dendritic cells, and neutrophils. We will also briefly describe some pathological conditions in which the bone-immune system cross-talk plays a crucial role, with the final aim to portray the state of the art in the mechanisms regulating the bone-immune system interplay, and some of the latest molecular players in the field. This is important to encourage investigation in this field, to identify new targets in the treatment of bone and immune diseases.

Keywords: osteoimmunology, RANKL, osteoclasts, osteoblasts, immune cells, inflammation, rheumatoid arthritis, osteoporosis

INTRODUCTION

Evidence collected over the years draw bone researchers to the conclusion that bone accomplishes several unexpected functions besides its classical role in locomotion, protection of vital organs and in the regulation of calcium and phosphate homeostasis. As a matter of fact, it is now well-accepted that bone has a role in the regulation of glucose metabolism, energy expenditure (1–3), male fertility and cognitive functions, through osteoblasts secretion of osteocalcin (4). Therefore, we can assume that bone is a central organ, capable of regulating several other tissues and to be in turn influenced by them.

An intriguing aspect testifying the versatility of bone and its cells, is its deep cross-talk with the immune system. This led to the establishment of a new interdisciplinary field, named osteoimmunology, thanks to the great contribution of studies by Takayanagi and many others. These pointed out the pivotal role of some classical immunoregulatory factors in osteoclast differentiation (5) as well as the cross-talk between autoimmune diseases, such as Rheumatoid Arthritis (RA), and bone destruction (6). Intriguingly, the cross-talk between the immune system and bone is bidirectional, meaning that bone cells also influence immune cells.

In this review, we will describe the main milestones in the history of osteoimmunology, as well as the latest findings enriching this discipline, with the final aim to have a state-of-the-art reference of the mechanisms regulating the bone-immune system interplay. This is important to encourage investigation in this field, in order to identify new targets in the treatment of bone and immune diseases.

BONE BIOLOGY

In the past, bone was seen as a static tissue, a simple "scaffolding" for all the other organs. Now we know bone is actually extremely dynamic, undergoing continuous cycles of modeling during growth and remodeling during adulthood, which guarantee adequate mechanical properties and proper bone shape (7). Bone modeling and remodeling are guaranteed by the action of three types of bone cells: osteoclasts, which resorb bone, osteoblasts, which depose bone, and osteocytes, which are former osteoblasts buried in bone matrix, controlling bone mechano-physiology, and able to resorb and depose bone. The cycle of bone remodeling happens following these 4 phases: (1) latent phase: bone-lining cells are activated by osteocytes following a stimulus, starting osteoclast differentiation (**Figure 1**) and exposing the bone surface; (2) activation phase: osteoclasts resorb the portion of bone left exposed by the bone-lining cells. When they are done resorbing, they detach from bone and undergo apoptosis; (3) reverse phase: macrophage-like reverse cells migrate to the resorbed lacuna and clean it of the debris left by osteoclasts. Reverse cells also secrete factors that summon osteoblasts in the resorption lacuna; (4) formation phase: this is the longest phase in bone remodeling, lasting up to 6 months. Osteoblasts occupy the resorption lacuna and fill it up with organic osteoid matrix, which they then mineralize (7). In this last phase, osteoblasts may undergo apoptosis, or embed themselves in the bone matrix they produce, eventually becoming osteocytes (8). Bone modeling and remodeling are very similar as far as the mechanisms and the cellular players go. The key difference is that modeling happens during growth and fracture repair, and guarantees bone mass accrual, while remodeling happens in adulthood, does not change bone mass, but keeps mechanical properties at physiological levels, by continuously renewing the bone matrix. Although this is quite an accurate depiction of "normal" bone modeling/remodeling, it has become clear in the last years, that the molecular and cellular players involved in the maintenance and accrual of bone mass are many more than originally expected. A key player in the maintenance of bone mass in bone pathophysiology is undoubtedly the immune system, giving rise to an extremely important field of research: osteoimmunology. This will be discussed in the following paragraphs and chapters.

OSTEOIMMUNOLOGY

The term osteoimmunology was likely adopted for the first time by Arron and Choi (9), to describe the phenomenon of T-cell-mediated regulation of osteoclasts. Most of the research projects related to bone-immune system cross-talk are quite recent and mainly focused on the influence of the immune system on osteoclast physiology. As a matter of fact, these cells share a common origin with immune cells, since they both arise from bone marrow hematopoietic stem cells (10). Moreover, like other hematopoietic cells, osteoclast precursors can be detected as circulating cells in blood and their number increases under inflammatory conditions, characterized by high levels of the potent inflammatory cytokine Tumor Necrosis Factor (TNF)-α (11, 12).

Bone Cells and the Immune System

In the following paragraphs, the many ways through which bone cells are linked to the immune system, and how they regulate immunity, will be discussed.

Osteoblasts

A pivotal work demonstrating a close connection between bone and the hematopoietic compartment came in 2003, when Calvi and colleagues demonstrated that mice genetically engineered to express a constitutively active PTH/PTHrP receptor in osteoblasts, had more Hematopoietic Stem Cells (HSCs). This was due to an increase in osteoblastic Jagged1, which in turn mediated said effect through activation of Notch1 (**Figure 2**). Intriguingly, when Calvi and colleagues myeloablated WT mice, and subsequently performed bone marrow transplantation, treatment with intermitting doses of PTH improved the engraftment rate to 100%. This could be important for human conditions that require similar procedures (13). Likewise, Zhang et al. found a direct correlation between the number of a subset of osteoblasts, called Spindle-shaped-N-cadherin^{+}CD45^{-} Osteoblasts (SNOs) and the number of HSCs. Moreover, long-term HSCs were found bound to SNOs by an N-cadherin/βcatenin-dependent mechanism (14). These data clearly demonstrate that a subpopulation of osteoblasts plays a crucial role in HSCs regulation, thus identifying in the bone marrow the so called "endosteal niche" besides the well-known vascular niche (15).

Later on, Zhu and colleagues definitely demonstrated that osteoblasts contribute to the commitment and differentiation of B lymphocytes from hematopoietic stem cells (16). In particular, in mice subjected to osteoblast conditional ablation, B-lymphocyte differentiation was compromised because of the lack of transition from Rag2^{-} to Rag2^{+} committed lymphoid progenitors. This effect was likely due to osteoblast secretion of InterLeukin (IL)-7 and C-X-C motif chemokine Ligand (CXCL)12 *alias* Stromal cell-Derived Factor (SDF) 1, two cytokines pivotal for B cells differentiation (17, 18). A collection

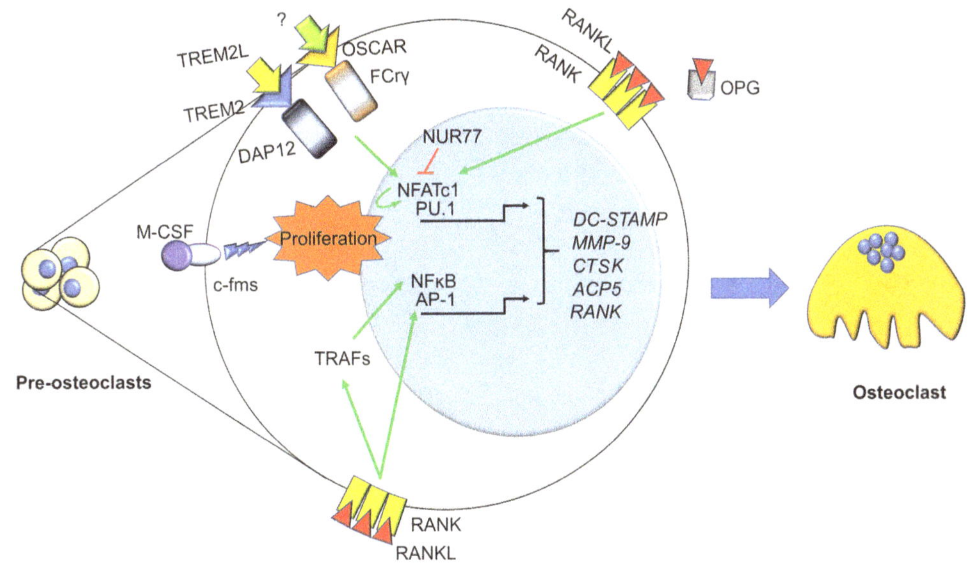

FIGURE 1 | Immune factors in osteoclastogenesis. Osteoclasts differentiation from pre-osteoclasts involves several factors, most of which are derived from the immune system. Signaling from TREM2, OSCAR, c-FMS, and RANK cause the nuclear translocation of several transcription factors activating pre-osteoclasst proliferation and differentiation. These include the master osteoclastogenesis controllers NFATc1, which also self-amplifies, and NFkB, along with the early commitment factor PU.1 and AP1. This is enacted both directly by RANK, and indirectly through TRAFs and PLCγ. Osteoclastogenesis can be hindered by several factors, two key ones are the decoy receptor for RANKL, OPG, and the immune factor NUR77, which can inhibit NFATc1 stopping its self-amplifcation loop. The final outcome of these molecular pathways is the transcription of key osteoclast genes, such as DC-STAMP, MMP9. *CTSK*, ACP5, and RANK, which eventually results in the generation of a mature osteoclast.

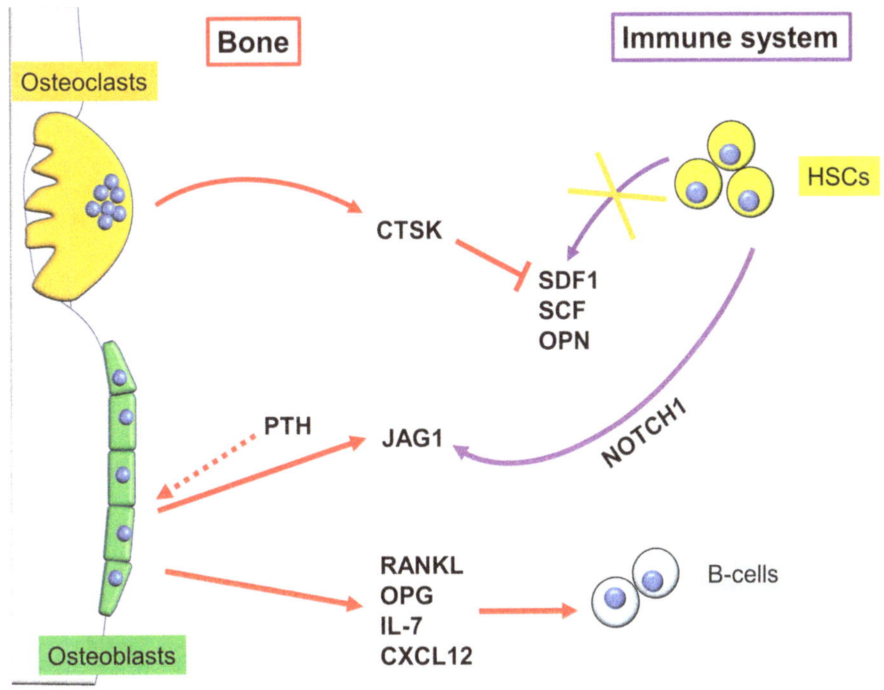

FIGURE 2 | Regulation of immune cells by bone cells. Osteoclasts reduce hematopoietic stem cells (HSCs) homing by secreting cathepsin K (CTSK), which in turn degrades stromal cell-derived factor (SDF)1, stem cell factor (SCF), and osteopontin (OPN) depriving the bone niche of HSC-binding sites, which causes their mobilization. Osteoblasts, after stimulation with pro-osteoblastogenic factors such as intermittent parathyroid hormone (PTH), express Jagged1 (Jag1), which binds NOTCH1 on HSCs, and allows them to engraft and survive into the endosteal niche. B cells and bone cells communicate in multiple ways. For example, osteoblasts produce IL-7 and the chemokine CXCL12, that are fundamental for B-cells survival and activity.

TABLE 1 | Factors produced by immune cells influencing osteoblast activity.

Factor	Source	Action	References
IL-11	Bone marrow stromal cells	Increase osteoblast activity	(19)
IL-6	Bone marrow stromal cells, osteoblasts, macrophages, muscle tissue, fibroblasts	Reduce osteoblast differentiation and activity	(20, 21)
IFN-γ	T-cells, NK-cells	Increase osteoblast activity	(22, 23)
IL-17F	Th17 cells	Increase osteoblast activity	(24, 25)
IL-15	PG-stimulated stromal cells, NK-cells	Reduce viability, increase apoptosis	(26)
OSM	B-cells	Increase osteoblast activity	(27)

of the main immune-derived factors promoting or hindering osteoblast differentiation and activity is present in **Table 1**.

Osteocytes

Osteocytes are the main producers of Receptor Activator of Nuclear factor Kappa B ligand (RANKL) in the bone, therefore since this cytokine is crucial not only for osteoclasts but also for lymphocyte development (see next paragraph) it is conceivable that this cell type could influence the immune system. Indeed, it has been demonstrated that RANKL arising from osteocytes contributes to the increased osteoclastogenesis and bone loss observed in estrogen deficient conditions. Moreover, specific deletion of the Rankl gene in osteocytes also prevented the increase in B cell formation caused by estrogen deficiency (28). In support of the relationship between osteocytes and the immune system, Sato and colleagues found that *in vivo* ablation of osteocytes leads to severe lymphopenia, caused by the loss of lymphoid- supporting stroma in the thymus and in the bone marrow, which is reverted by re-establishing the osteocyte population (29).

Osteoclasts

Osteoclasts have been shown to regulate the HSC niche both directly and indirectly through osteoblasts (**Figure 2**). Firstly, osteoclasts can increase HSC mobilization by secreting cathepsin K, a crucial protein for osteoclast function, which cleaves SDF1, OsteoPontiN (OPN), and Stem Cell Factor (SCF), depriving the bone niche of HSC-binding sites. Consequently, HSCs mobilize to the circulation and are no longer kept quiescent (30). Furthermore, it has been shown that *oc/oc* mice, which have an inactivating mutation in the *T Cell, Immune ReGulator 1, ATPase, H^+ transporting, lysosomal V0 protein A3 (Tcirg1)* gene and therefore almost entirely lack osteoclasts activity (31), have an overrepresented Mesenchymal Stem Cell (MSC) fraction. However, despite the higher number of precursors, MSCs differentiate less into osteoblasts, which impairs osteoblast-mediated HSCs homing to bone (32). Therefore, osteoclasts number and activity need to be tightly regulated, because any alteration could lead to excessive HSCs mobilization. Furthermore, *oc/oc* mice present with improper B lymphopoiesis, which is blocked at the pro-B stage, leading to fewer mature B-cells. T-cell activation is also affected, leading to a form of B-T-cells immunodeficiency (33).

As it is well-known, osteoclast differentiation strictly relies on the RANKL/RANK pathway (34, 35). RANKL interacts with its receptor RANK expressed by osteoclast precursors, thus recruiting TNFR-Associated Factors (TRAFs), which in turn trigger osteoclast differentiation by stimulating nuclear translocation of Nuclear Factor k-light-chain-enhancer of activated B cells (NFkB), Activator Protein 1 (AP1) complex and Nuclear Factor of Activated T-cells, cytoplasmic, calcineurin-dependent 1 (NFATc1) (36). All these factors stimulate transcription of several osteoclast-specific genes, such as Tartrate Resistant Acid Phosphatase (TRAcP), calcitonin receptor, cathepsin K, OSteoClast Associated Receptor (OSCAR), alpha V β3 integrin, Matrix Metalloproteinase (MMP) 9, and Dendritic Cell-Specific Transmembrane Protein (DC-STAMP) the latter involved in osteoclast fusion [**Figure 1**, (7)].

Of note, RANKL is also produced by activated T-lymphocytes as soluble form and is expressed in lymph nodes and thymus. Its importance in the immunological context was demonstrated by the fact that mice lacking RANKL showed not only a bone phenotype, resulting in osteopetrosis due to the lack of osteoclasts, but also presented with immunological defects, with impaired lymphocytes development and lack of lymph node organogenesis (37). Consistently, Dougall et al. demonstrated that RANK is essential for osteoclast and lymph node development, since RANK knockout mice showed an osteopetrotic phenotype along with a lack of peripheral lymph nodes and a marked deficiency in B and T lymphocytes (38). In contrast, OsteoProteGerin (OPG) is a decoy receptor for RANKL, belonging to the TNF Receptor (TNFR) superfamily, which prevents RANKL interaction with its receptor RANK, eventually leading to inhibition of osteoclast formation (35). Not only osteoblasts but also B lymphocytes produce OPG, thus concurring to regulate osteoclastogenesis (39).

The awareness of a close interconnection between bone and immune system was increased by Takayanagi et al. (40), who demonstrated that mice lacking Immunoreceptor Tyrosine-based Activation Motif (ITAM)-harboring adaptors, Fc Receptor common Gamma subunit (FcRγ) and DNAX-Activating Protein (DAP)12, presented with an osteopetrotic phenotype caused by a reduction of osteoclast differentiation. Indeed, they showed that RANKL/RANK pathway requires the ITAM-dependent costimulatory signals to activate osteoclast differentiation (5). Later, they found that FcRgamma and DAP12 associated to OSCAR and receptor expressed on myeloid cells

2 (TREM2), respectively, eventually leading to PhosphoLipase C (PLC)γ activation, which in turn activates calcium signaling, necessary for NFATc1 auto-amplification (41, 42). Osteoclasts also express Bruton's Tyrosine Kinase (Btk) and Tec, which have a physiological role in B cells (43), and mice double knock out for both these kinases manifest osteoclast-poor osteopetrosis, likely due to a suppression of the RANKL induced phosphorylation of PLCγ (44).

Regulation of osteoclast formation is a complex mechanism, calling into questions more and more pathways. One of the last is NR4A1 (alias Nur77), which belongs to the orphan nuclear receptor family, already known to be a key regulator of myeloid and lymphoid differentiation and function (45, 46). Recent findings demonstrated a role for this nuclear orphan receptor in the suppression of osteoclast differentiation (47). Moreover, Scholtysek and colleagues clarified a role for NR4A1 in controlling pre-osteoclast recruitment and migration, with an effect linked to the myeloid lineage. In fact, myeloid-specific but not osteoblast-specific deletion of NR4A1 resulted in osteopenia due to an increase of osteoclast number (48). The immune-related factors influencing osteoclast formation and biology are many more; a list of the most important ones is presented in **Table 2**.

TABLE 2 | Secreted and membrane-bound immune factors promoting osteoclastogenesis.

Factor	Source	References
RANKL	Osteoblasts, osteocytes, neutrophils, sinoviocytes, T-cells	(28, 37, 49)
OPG	Osteoblasts, B-cells	(35, 50)
M-CSF	Osteoblasts, activated T-cells	(6, 51, 52)
TNFα	Activated leucocytes	(11, 12)
IL-1α, −1β	Activated leucocytes, osteoblasts, synoviocytes, endothelial cells	(53)
IL-7	Osteoblasts, bone marrow stromal cells, leucocytes	(53)
IL-8	Activated leucocytes	(53)
IL-11	Bone marrow stromal cells	(19)
IL-23	Dendritic cells, Th17 T-cells	(24, 54)
IL-34	Dendritic cells, Th17 T-cells, synoviocytes, osteoblasts	(24, 53)
Prostaglandins	Bone marrow and bone cells	(55)
SOFAT	T-cells	(56)
IL-6	Bone marrow stromal cells, osteoblasts, macrophages, muscle tissue, fibroblasts	(19–21, 57, 58)
IFN-γ	T-cells, NK-cells	(22, 23)
IL-17A	Th17 cells	(24, 59, 60)
IL-15	PG-stimulated stromal cells, NK-cells	(26)

Immune Cells in Bone Physiology

As described, bone cells can influence the immune system, and employ several immune factors for their physiologic function. The opposite is also true: immune cells can influence bone health in many ways, as will be described in the following paragraphs.

T-Cells

T-cells are a key component of adaptive immunity. These small and relatively rare cells have a key role not only in immunity, but also in osteoimmunology. T-cells are not all created equal, and in this group, we can find cytotoxic $CD8^+$ T-cells, $CD4^+$ T-helpers, further subcategorized in Th1, Th2, Th17, and T-reg cells, the latter having an important role in preventing excessive or improper (e.g. self-directed) immune response (61). The links between T-cells and bone biology are numerous: essentially all the subtypes of T-cells are able to influence bone cells (mostly osteoclasts). However, a particularly important role for Th17 and T-reg cells is emerging. Th17 cells have been proposed to be the most osteoclastogenesis-inducing T-cells. They are characterized by the expression of a cytokine signature: IL-17A, IL-17F (hence the name), IL-22, IL-26, and IFN-γ (62). These cells can induce Macrophage Colony-Stimulating Factor (*M-CSF*) and *RANKL* expression in osteoblasts and stromal cells (6), produce RANKL and TNF-α, while parallelly increasing *RANK* expression in osteoclast precursors (63). These features make them potent osteoclastogenesis inducers, which have been already described as players in human bone diseases, such as RA (64) and multiple myeloma (65). With regards to T-reg cells, their role is clearly anti-osteoclastogenic, and it is enacted through a soluble factors-mediated mechanism, as well as a contact-mediated mechanism (24). In fact, co-culture experiments of whole Peripheral Blood Mononuclear Cells (PBMCs) or T-reg-depleted PBMCs resulted in higher osteoclast formation in the former (66), which seems to be dependent on TGF-β and IL-4, while the latter was found to be Cytotoxic T-Lymphocyte Antigen (CTLA)4-dependent (67). In the aforementioned reports, *in vitro* bone resorption was reduced up to 80% by the action of T-reg cells, which makes them potentially very important in autoimmune osteolysis-inducing disease such as RA. In fact, this has been proposed and demonstrated in mice (68), although human studies are still lacking to date.

Dendritic Cells

Dendritic Cells (DCs) are antigen-presenting cells entrusted with the important role of directing cell-mediated immunity toward the right targets, as quickly as possible and avoiding self-immunity (69). Their role in bone biology has in fact been historically thought as mostly indirect, through T-cells (70). Dendritic cells are in fact not only able to present antigens to T-cells, but also to regulate their activity and subtype balance through cytokine signaling (69, 71). However, another interesting concept that could be important for RA is that DCs can transdifferentiate into osteoclasts through M-CSF and RANKL stimulation, as if they were osteoclast precursors. Since DCs are numerous in and around the inflamed synovium in RA, they could well-contribute to the osteolytic disease in RA (72). However, DCs have not been further investigated in the last years in osteoimmunology in human studies.

Neutrophils

Neutrophils also play a role in bone biology, and particularly in inflammation-induced bone loss (73). In fact, neutrophils are usually the first cell type migrating to damage sites, including bone (74), and they can secrete many chemokines, cytokines and small molecules, which are able to act as immunomodulatory factors. For example, by CCL2 and CCL20 secretion, neutrophils are able to summon Th17 cells (73) which in turn cause bone loss, as discussed in the above paragraphs. However, absence of neutrophils can be even more damaging to bone tissue, as it eventually results in local IL-17-driven inflammatory bone loss (75). Remarkably, activated neutrophils express RANKL in the inflammatory site, and if that site is the synovium, they can actively participate in osteoclastogenesis, which increases RA-related osteolysis (76). In summary, although the role of neutrophils in osteoimmunology is not cut-and-dried, the general consensus is that activated neutrophils are osteoclastogenesis inducers, both directly and indirectly.

B-Cells

B-cell development relies on the production of several factors, including RANKL, OPG, IL-7, and CXCL12, which are produced by bone marrow stromal cells and osteoblasts [**Figure 2**, (50)]. As already mentioned, RANK knockout mice presented with a reduction in the number of mature B220$^+$IgM$^+$ and B220$^+$IgG$^+$ B-cells in lymph nodes (38, 77). Further studies demonstrated that not only RANKL arising from the bone marrow/bone compartment is crucial for B-cell development, but also B-cells themselves produce RANKL, which then acts as an autocrine factor (78). However, when RANK was conditionally deleted in the pro-B cells, B cell development was not affected (79) thus suggesting that RANKL could interact with an alternative receptor.

The evidence that B cells produce RANKL suggests that they could influence osteoclasts, and this is the case. In fact, Onal and colleagues demonstrated that mice lacking RANKL in B lymphocytes were partially protected from ovariectomy-mediated bone loss, through a mechanism counteracting the increase in osteoclasts number that is a hallmark of this mouse model. Conditional knock out of RANKL in T-lymphocytes had no effect on ovariectomy-induced bone loss (78). Interestingly, IL-7 transgenic mice showed focal osteolysis, besides the expected increase of pro-B and pre-B cells, while mice lacking the IL-7 receptor showed suppression in B-lymphocyte development associated to an increased bone mass (80).

In vitro studies have shown that purified B cells can be driven to differentiate into osteoclasts when treated with RANKL, thus acting as a source of osteoclast progenitors *in vitro* (81, 82). In contrast, *in vivo* lineage-tracing studies to investigate whether cells committed to the B cell lineage can act as osteoclast progenitors found that this was not the case, therefore the authors conclude that the role of B cells is not to act as osteoclast progenitors but as cells supporting osteoclasts formation (28).

Natural Killer (NK) Cells

Natural Killer (NK) cells, as all other lymphocytes, play a role in the regulation of bone homeostasis. In fact, several reports emerged stating that they are particularly important in bone destruction induced by RA, and they are also able to induce osteoblast cell death (26, 83, 84). This makes NK cells a potential therapeutic target to reduce RA-induced bone destruction. However, NK cells have also been described as helpful and necessary to slow down RA by recent reports (85), casting doubts over the efficacy of a hypothetical anti-NK-cells treatment in RA.

Osteomacs and Bone Marrow Macrophages

As other organs in the body, bone and bone marrow present with resident macrophages, which include bone marrow macrophages and osteal macrophages (86). The latter, also known as osteomacs, are F4/80 positive and TRAcP negative, and are located close to the bone surface. It has been recently demonstrated that in 2-day-old mouse calvarial osteoblasts a small population of CD45$^+$F4/80$^+$ osteomacs can be detected (87). This subpopulation cooperates with osteoblasts and megakaryocytes to promote hematopoietic progenitor and HSC function (87, 88). The same authors also demonstrated that highly purified CD45$^+$F4/80$^+$ osteomacs from neonatal calvarial osteoblasts can differentiate into TRAcP positive osteoclasts able to resorb bone (88).

Notably, *in vitro* and *in vivo* studies demonstrated a role for these bone macrophages in osteoblast differentiation by producing Bone Morphogenetic Proteins (BMPs) (89) and Oncostatin M (27). Moreover, Chang and colleagues found that depletion of osteal macrophages in primary osteoblasts inhibited their differentiation (90). *In vivo* approaches able to selectively ablate osteal macrophages but not osteoclasts showed that their lack determined a decrease in bone formation, a reduction in bone growth in young mice and osteoporosis (90–92). Therefore, osteomacs are versatile cells, able to regulate bone mass, become osteoclasts, and actively participate in the homeostasis of the immune system.

Inflammation and Inflammatory Factors

Several cells of the immune system (T and B cells, NK cells, monocyte/macrophage and dendritic cells) produce InterFeroN (IFN)-γ, which has a pivotal role in innate and adaptive immune responses as well as in the regulation of inflammation (22, 23). In bone, IFN-γ affects both osteoblasts and osteoclasts. The former, which produce low levels of this cytokine, are indeed positively affected, since IFN-γ increases osteoblast differentiating genes, like Runt related transcription factor 2 (Runx2), Osterix, ALkaline Phosphatase (ALP) and Osteocalcin (93, 94) and mice knock out for the IFN-γ receptor showed reduced osteoblast differentiation (95). Conversely, IFN-γ has an inhibitory effect on adipogenesis (96).

Much data has been collected about the inhibitory effect of IFN-γ on osteoclast differentiation [for a review see (23)]. This protein is known to counteract the effect of M-CSF on osteoclast precursors by reducing the expression of its receptor c-fms, eventually leading to a reduced pool of Rank-positive preosteoclasts (97). Furthermore, IFN-γ promotes TRAF6 degradation (53, 98), thus inhibiting the downstream signaling which involves JNK and NFkB, while it induces osteoclast apoptosis by activating Fas-FasL-mediated death signaling (99). However, other studies show a pro-osteoclastogenic effect of IFN-γ in the late state of differentiation. This depends on the upregulation of NFATc1 and c-fos, which in turn stimulate *DC-STAMP* expression, thus promoting osteoclast fusion (100). Another indirect pro-osteoclastogenic effect of IFN-γ is due to its ability to increase the secretion of CXCL10, also known as Interferon gamma induced Protein 10 (IP-10), by macrophages and this cytokine in turn stimulates the production of RANKL and TNF-α by T cells (101).

Inflammatory diseases, such as RA, periodontal disease (see later), systemic lupus erythematous, inflammatory bowel diseases and cystic fibrosis are all characterized by bone loss (6, 102–106), which is not only secondary to the employ of anti-inflammatory corticosteroid therapies (107), but is also due to a direct effect of inflammatory cytokines on osteoclasts, thus creating a sort of "vicious cycle".

So far, a plethora of inflammatory cytokines have been identified as positive modulators of osteoclasts [for a review see (53)]. Above all the proinflammatory cytokine TNF-α, which directly stimulates osteoclastogenesis by a mechanism independent of RANKL (108) as well as indirectly, by promoting RANK expression on preosteoclasts (109) and increasing RANKL and M-CSF production by osteoblasts and activated T cells (50, 51).

The IL-6 family includes at least three pro-osteoclastogenic cytokines: IL-6, -11 and -23. The first stimulates osteoclastogenesis by a mechanism independent of RANKL, since the presence of OPG does not blunt this effect (57). This is accompanied by a positive stimulation of RANKL production by stromal cells and osteoblasts (19, 58). As for osteoblasts, IL-6 reduces their differentiation *in vivo* (20) and *in vitro* by affecting the MEK2 and Akt2 pathways (21).

Also, IL-11 has a pro-osteoclastogenic effect (19), while on the osteoblast side it seems to be pro-osteogenic (110, 111).

IL-23 is mainly produced by dendritic cells and macrophages, and it indirectly stimulates osteoclastogenesis by increasing RANK and RANKL expression by osteoclast precursors and osteoblasts, respectively (54). Other factors strongly promoting osteoclastogenesis are prostaglandins (55), IL-1α, -1β, -7, -8, and -34 (53).

OSTEOIMMUNOLOGY IN BONE AND IMMUNE DISEASES

As it is easy to imagine, the link between bone and the immune system in physiology is also maintained in pathological conditions: many diseases affecting bone have an immunologic origin, while some immunological disorders, such as acute myeloid leukemia, can originate from bone-derived signals, as will be described in the following paragraphs.

Rheumatoid Arthritis

Rheumatoid arthritis (RA) is a T helper (Th) type 1, degenerative disease with strong genetic predisposition factors (up to 50%), characterized by synovitis, persistent inflammation and the generation of antibodies against endogenous proteins, especially rheumatoid factor (112). Takayanagi's group demonstrated a close connection between RA and osteoclast deregulation (6). Indeed, despite the high levels of IFN-γ, which is known to inhibit osteoclastogenesis, the T-cells' activation observed in this pathology results in an exacerbated osteoclast activation. This is due to the action of a subset of activated T-cells, called Th-17 because they produce IL-17. Of note, in a mouse model of RA, IL-17 ablation reduced bone destruction (59). This cytokine is of interest, because it stimulates the expression of more pro-osteoclastogenic cytokines, including IL-6, IL-8, and TNF-α also in absence of RANKL (113, 114). Moreover, in the synovium of RA patients, IL-17 induces the production of IL-32, which in turn stimulates IL-17 expression (60) creating a feed-forward loop. Therefore, this cytokine plays a crucial role not only in the onset of RA but also in the bone destruction that this disease presents with (6). Furthermore, IL-6 production increases RANKL expression in synoviocytes, leading to further exacerbated osteoclastic bone destruction (49).

Osteoporosis

Estrogen deficiency is the leading cause of osteoporosis in post-menopausal women. Pacifici and colleagues found that this condition results in increased production of inflammatory cytokines. This was a cornerstone discovery, that elucidated a new facet of post-menopausal osteoporosis, describing it as an inflammatory disease (115). The protective effect of estrogen in bone has been well characterized and is mainly due to a direct action on both osteoclasts and osteoblasts. In the former, estrogens significantly increase apoptosis (116, 117) and reduce RANKL-dependent osteoclast formation (118), while in osteoblasts they exert an anabolic effect by at least increasing osteoblast survival and collagen I production (119). Consistently, it has been demonstrated that estrogens suppress RANKL production not only in osteoblasts but also in T and B cells (120), while the lack of estrogens increases the release of pro-osteoclastogenic cytokines (i.e., TNF-α and RANKL) by activated T cells (121–123) thus indirectly identifying immune cells as additional players in the onset of osteoporosis. Estrogens withdrawal also leads to a significant increase of B-cells' number (124).

Regarding the role of immune cells-derived-IFN-γ in osteoporosis, results are conflicting (23). In particular, while Breuil and colleagues found reduced secreted levels of IFN-γ by $CD4^+$ T-cells in osteoporotic patients (121) previous studies did not find any differences (125, 126).

Periodontal Disease

Another pathological phenomenon in which immune cells deregulation causes bone loss is periodontal disease, where activated B and T cells concur to stimulate osteoclast resorption by producing RANKL (127, 128). Consistently, Weitzmann and colleagues identified a T cell-secreted cytokine, named Secreted Osteoclastogenic Factor of Activated T-cells (SOFAT) that promotes osteoclastogenesis independently of RANKL (129, 130). Moreover, increased mRNA expression of SOFAT has been found in human periodontal samples, while SOFAT injection induced osteoclast formation in a mouse model of periodontal disease (56).

Bone Fracture Repair

This physiological process is orchestrated not only by bone cells, but also by immune cells, whose deregulation can delay fracture repair (131, 132). In fact, in conditions of B and T cells depletion, an impairment of bone regeneration, due to a reduction of osteoblast differentiation and bone mineralization, has been observed (25, 133). Consistently, immunocompromised HIV patients present with a delay of fracture healing repair (131).

One of the earliest phases of bone healing is characterized by an inflammatory state, with the release of IL-1, IL-6, and TNF-α, which recruit B and T lymphocytes, the latter having a pro-osteogenic role by releasing IL-17F (25). In fact, at variance with IL-17A, known for its pro-osteoclastogenic role, the pro-inflammatory cytokine IL-17F is expressed during bone healing, where it increases Col1a1, osteocalcin, and bone sialoproteins in treated osteoblasts (25). Neutrophil granulocytes are also present during the early phase of bone repair, and they clean debris and damaged cells in the site of injury (134). Another crucial step for bone fracture repair is the recruitment of MSCs which again involves immune cells (i.e., NK cells and macrophages) since they produce chemoattractant molecules such as CXCL7 (alias NAP2) and Monocyte Inflammatory Protein (MIP)-1α (135, 136). Once recruited, MSCs are fostered to differentiate toward the osteoblast lineage, through macrophage-derived BMPs (137) while activated monocytes stimulate the expression of Runx2 (138). At the same time, once the bone-repair process activates, the inflammatory reaction should be switched off in order to avoid any inflammation-derived damage. To this aim, MSCs exert an immunosuppressive role, by stimulating the differentiation of T-reg lymphocytes, inducing the apoptosis of the pro-inflammatory Th1 and Th17 lymphocytes and inhibiting migration of B-lymphocytes (139–142).

Myelodysplasia and Acute Myeloid Leukemia

Another strong link between bone and the immune system is the fact that osteoblasts can influence the progression of pre-neoplastic and neoplastic transformations in the myeloid lineage. In fact, osteoblasts are able to slow down leukemia progression in mouse, creating an unfavorable microenvironment for leukemic blast growth (143). Consistently, osteoblast number is reduced by more than half in leukemic patients. Simulating this situation by mouse genetics, causes leukemic blasts to grow faster and engraft better (143). The same authors demonstrated that osteoblasts have another tight link to human leukemia: osteoblasts that have been genetically engineered to express a constitutively active form of β-catenin, are able to induce leukemic transformation in myeloid cells, causing MyeloDysplaSia (MDS) and then Acute Myeloid Leukemia (AML) (144).

The concept of bone cells inducing malignant transformation, however, was not new, since already a few years earlier, Raaijmakers and colleagues found that ablating the miRNA processing protein dicer from osteoblast progenitors induces dysfunctional haematopoiesis, eventually leading to MDS and AML development (145). The field of "niche-induced leukemia" has received much attention, and still many groups are working on this topic to date.

LATEST DEVELOPMENTS IN OSTEOIMMUNOLOGY

In the last few years, despite much of the field has already emerged, several groups are still actively discovering new molecules that can be considered part of the osteoimmunology world. This has been the case for a secreted protein named homologous to Lymphotoxin, exhibits Inducible expression and competes with HSV Glycoprotein D for binding to Herpesvirus entry mediator, a receptor expressed on T lymphocytes (LIGHT, a.k.a. Tumor Necrosis Factor SuperFamily member 14, TNFSF14), which has been linked to increased bone resorption in osteoarthritis more than 10 years ago (146, 147), and has known a *renaissance* in the last few years as target for bone loss (148) and biomarker for bone disease in multiple myeloma (149). This molecule seems to have a dual effect in bone: high levels are linked to bone loss, and so is its absence. The mechanisms involving it are therefore quite complex, although agonists and antagonists of the LIGHT pathway are in development and testing. This behavior is also common to another regulator of bone mass that has recently emerged in the last few years: LipoCaliN-2 (Lcn2). This protein is also called Neutrophil Gelatinase-Associated Lipocalin (NGAL), since it can bind and stabilize MMP9, a crucial factor for neutrophil extravasation. Furthermore, Lcn2 is also readily overexpressed during inflammation, and following treatment with TNFα, IL-17, and IL-1β, and its role in inflammatory diseases is only starting to emerge; what is sure is that this molecule can be considered a player in innate immunity. In 2009, we discovered that Lcn2 is strongly overexpressed in osteoblasts following *in vitro* mechanical unloading (150). Furthermore, we confirmed these findings *in vivo*, which led to the concept that Lcn2 is a mechanoresponsive gene that regulates bone homeostasis (151). Surprisingly though, removing this protein genetically, reduces bone mass instead of increasing it (152). This is likely due to the fact that Lcn2 impairs osteoblasts when overexpressed, and impairs energy metabolism when removed, which causes an indirect osteoblast dysfunction (152). The role of Lcn2 in bone is still under investigation by ours and other groups where it has been found to influence hematopoiesis (153), and even appetite through the melatonin receptor MC4R (154).

CONCLUSIONS

The concept of osteoimmunology is aging well, almost 20 years since the term was coined. This way of interpreting bone and the immune system has been steadily providing new insights about how the two of them operate and cooperate. As an example, the role of pro-inflammatory cytokines in promoting osteoclastogenesis, and the many parallelisms between immune cells and osteoclasts have proved crucial to understand the biology of these giant bone-eating cells. Intriguingly, the control mechanisms between bone and the immune system are complex, tightly interconnected, and involve many players. The underlying complexity of this field has made it difficult for researchers to find clear-cut results, the kind that leads to the direct clinical application. Nevertheless, thanks to the effort of many scientists, nowadays clinics can use drugs, classically employed to treat osteoporosis, for immunological diseases [e.g., Denosumab for RA; (155)]. In conclusion, although the study of osteoimmunology has provided many answers, it also raised more questions, which we need to answer in order to improve standards of care for patients of both immune and bone disorders, by exploiting the cross-talk between these two remarkable systems, which are actually starting to look like a single one.

AUTHOR CONTRIBUTIONS

MP prepared the cartoons and the tables. NR drafted the manuscript, MP and NR finalized, reviewed and approved the manuscript in its final form.

REFERENCES

1. Fernandez-Real JM, Izquiredo M, Ortega F, Gorostiaga E, Gomez-Ambrosi J, Moreno-Navarrete JM, et al. The relationship of serum osteocalcin concentration to insulin secretion, sensitivity and disposal with hypocaloric diet and resistance training. *J Clin Endocrinol Metab.* (2009) 94:237–45. doi: 10.1210/jc.2008-0270
2. Hwang YC, Jeong IK, Ahn KJ, Chung HY. The uncarboxylated form of osteocalcin is associated with improved glucose tolerance and enhanced beta-cell function in middle-age male subjects. *Diabetes Met Res Rev.* (2009) 25:768–72. doi: 10.1002/dmrr.1045
3. Yeap BB, Chubb SA, Flicker L, McCul KA, Ebeling PR, Beilby JP, et al. Reduced serum total osteocalcin is associate with metabolic syndrome in older men via waist circumference, hyperglycemia, and triglyceride levels. *Eur J Endocrinol.* (2010) 163:265–72. doi: 10.1530/EJE-10-0414
4. Wei J, Karsenty G. An overview of the metabolic functions of osteocalcin. *Curr Osteopor Rep.* (2015) 13:180–5. doi: 10.1007/s11914-015-0267-y
5. Koga T, Inui M, Inoue K, Kim S, Suematsu A, Kobayashi E, et al. Costimulatory signals mediated by ITAM motif cooperate with RANKL for bone homeostasis. *Nature.* (2004) 428:758–63. doi: 10.1038/nature02444
6. Sato K, Suematsu A, Okamoto K, Yamaguchi A, Morishita Y, Kadono Y, et al. Th17 functions as an osteoclastogenic helper T cell subset that links T cell activation and bone destruction. *J Exp Med.* (2006) 203:2673–82. doi: 10.1084/jem.20061775
7. Cappariello A, Maurizi A, Veeriah V, Teti A. The great beauty of osteoclast. *Arch Biochem Biophys.* (2014) 561:13–21. doi: 10.1016/j.abb.2014.06.017
8. Capulli M, Paone R, Rucci N. Osteoblast and osteocyte: games without frontiers. *Arch Biochem Biophys.* (2014) 561:3–12. doi: 10.1016/j.abb.2014.05.003
9. Arron JR, Choi Y. Bone versus immune system. *Nature.* (2000) 408:535–6. doi: 10.1038/35046196
10. Walker DG. Bone resorption restored in osteopetrotic mice by transplants of normal bone marrow and spleen cells. *Science.* (1975) 190:784–5. doi: 10.1126/science.1105786
11. Li P, Schwarz EM, O'Keefe RJ, Ma L, Looney RJ, Ritchlin CT, et al. Systemic tumor necrosis factor alpha mediates an increase in peripheral CD11bhigh osteoclast precursors in tumor necrosis factor alpha-transgenic mice. *Arthritis Rheum.* (2004) 50:265–76. doi: 10.1002/art.11419
12. Yao Z, Li P, Zhang Q, Schwarz EM, Keng P, Arbini A, et al. Tumor necrosis factor-alpha increases circulating osteoclast precursor numbers by promoting their proliferation and differentiation in the bone marrow through up-regulation of c-Fms expression. *J Biol Chem.* (2006) 281:11846–55. doi: 10.1074/jbc.M512624200
13. Calvi LM, Adams GB, Weibrecht KW, Weber JM, Olson DP, Knight MC, et al. Osteoblastic cells regulate the haematopoietic stem cell niche. *Nature.* (2003) 425:841–6. doi: 10.1038/nature02040
14. Zhang J, Niu C, Ye L, Huang H, He X, Tong WG, et al. Identification of the hematopoietic stem cell niche and control of the niche size. *Nature.* (2003) 425:836–41. doi: 10.1038/nature02041
15. Zhu J, Emerson SG. A new bone to pick: osteoblasts and the haematopoitic stem-cell niche. *Bioessays.* (2004) 26:595–9. doi: 10.1002/bies.20052
16. Zhu J, Garrett R, Jung Y, Kim N, Wang J, Joe GJ, et al. Osteoblasts support B-lymphocyte commitment and differentiation from hematopoietic stem cells. *Blood.* (2007) 109:3706–12. doi: 10.1182/blood-2006-08-041384
17. Egawa T, Kawabata K, Kawamoto H, Amada K, Okamoto R, Fujii N, et al. The earliest stages of B cell development require chemokine stromal cell-derived factor/pre-B cell growth- stimulating factor. *Immunity.* (2001) 15:323–34. doi: 10.1016/S1074-7613(01)00185-6
18. Miller JP, Izon D, DeMuth W, Gerstein R, Bhandoola A, Allman D. The earliest step in B lineage differentiation from common lymphoid progenitors is critically dependent upon interleukin 7. *J Exp Med.* (2002) 196:705–11. doi: 10.1084/jem.20020784
19. Girasole G, Passeri G, Jilka RL, Manolagas SC. Interleukin 11: a new cytokine critical for osteoclast development. *J Clin Invest.* (1994) 93:1516–24. doi: 10.1172/JCI117130
20. De Benedetti F, Rucci N, Del Fattore A, Peruzzi B, Paro R, Longo M, et al. Impaired skeletal development in interleukin-6-transgenic mice: a model for the impact of chronic inflammation on the growing skeletal system. *Arthritis Rheum.* (2006) 54:3551–63. doi: 10.1002/art.22175
21. Kaneshiro S, Ebina K, Shi K, Higuchi C, Hirao M, Okamoto M, et al. IL-6 negatively regulates osteoblast differentiation through the SHP2/MEK2 and SHP2/Akt2 pathways *in vitro*. *J Bone Miner Metab.* (2014) 32:378–92. doi: 10.1007/s00774-013-0514-1
22. Schroder K, Hertzog PJ, Ravasi T, Hume DA. Interferon-gamma: an overview of signals, mechanisms and functions. *J Leukoc Biol.* (2004) 75:163–89. doi: 10.1189/jlb.0603252
23. Tang M, Tian L, Luo G, Yu X. Interferon-gamma-mediated osteoimmunology. *Front Immunol.* 9:13. doi: 10.3389/fimmu.2018.01508
24. Mori G, D'Amelio P, Faccio R, Brunetti G. The Interplay between the bone and the immune system. *Clin Dev Immunol.* 2013:720504. doi: 10.1155/2013/720504
25. Nam D, Mau E, Wang Y, Wright D, Silkstone D, Whetstone H, et al. T-lymphocytes enable osteoblast maturation via IL-17F during early phase of fracture repair. *PLoS ONE.* (2012) 7:e40044. doi: 10.1371/journal.pone.0040044
26. Takeda H, Kikuchi T, Soboku K, Okabe I, Mizutani H, Mitani A, et al. Effect of IL-15 and natural killer cells on osteoclasts and osteoblasts in a mouse coculture. *Inflammation.* (2014) 37:657–69. doi: 10.1007/s10753-013-9782-0
27. Guihard P, Boutet MA, Brounais B, David E, Brion R, Delecrin J, et al. Induction of osteogenesis in mesenchymal stem cells by activated monocytes/macrophages depends on oncostatin M signaling. *Stem Cells.* (2012) 30:762–72. doi: 10.1002/stem.1040
28. Fujiwara Y, Piemontese M, Liu Y, Thostenson JD, Xiong J, O'Brien CA. RANKL (Receptor Activator of NFkB Ligand) produced by osteocytes is required for the increase in B cells and bone loss caused by estrogen deficiency in mice. *J Biol Chem.* (2016) 291:24838–50. doi: 10.1074/jbc.M116.742452
29. Sato M, Asada N, Kawano Y, Wakahashi K, Minagawa K, Kawano H et al. Osteocytes regulate primary lymphoid organs and fat metabolism. *Cell Metab.* (2013) 18:749–58. doi: 10.1016/j.cmet.2013.09.014
30. Kollet O, Dar A, Shivtiel S, Kalinkovich A, Lapid K, Sztainberg Y, et al. Osteoclasts degrade endosteal components and promote

mobilization of hematopoietic progenitor cells. *Nat Med.* (2006) 12:657–64. doi: 10.1038/nm1417
31. Seifert MF, Marks SC Jr. Morphological evidence of reduced bone resorption in the osteosclerotic (oc) mouse. *Am J Anat.* (1985) 172:141–53. doi: 10.1002/aja.1001720204
32. Mansour A, Abou-Ezzi G, Sitnicka E, Jacobsen SE, Wakkach A, Blin-Wakkach C. Osteoclasts promote the formation of hematopoietic stem cell niches in the bone marrow. *J Exp Med.* (2012) 209:537–49. doi: 10.1084/jem.20110994
33. Blin-Wakkach C, Wakkach A, Sexton PM, Rochet N, Carle GF. Hematological defects in the oc/oc mouse, a model of infantile malignant osteopetrosis. *Leukemia.* (2004) 18:1505–11. doi: 10.1038/sj.leu.2403449
34. Lacey DL, Timms E, Tan HL, Kelley MJ, Dunstan CR, Burgess T, et al. Osteoprotegerin ligand is a cytokine that regulates osteoclast differentiation and activation. *Cell.* (1998) 93:165–76. doi: 10.1016/S0092-8674(00)81569-X
35. Simonet WS, Lacey DL, Dunstan CR, Kelley M, Chang MS, Luthy R, et al. Osteoprotegerin: a novl secreted protein involved in the regulation of bone density. *Cell.* (1997) 89:309–19. doi: 10.1016/S0092-8674(00)80209-3
36. Feng X, Teitelbaum SL. Osteoclasts: new insights. *Bone Res.* (2013) 1:11–26. doi: 10.4248/BR201301003
37. Yasuda H, Shima N, Nakagawa N, Yamaguchi K, Kinosaki M, Mochizuki S, et al. Osteoclast differentiation factor is a ligand for osteoprotegerin/osteoclastogenesis-inhibitory factor and is identical to TRANCE/RANKL. *Proc Natl Acad Sci USA.* (1998) 95:3597–3602. doi: 10.1073/pnas.95.7.3597
38. Dougall WC, Glaccum M, Charrier K, Rohrbach K, Brasel K, De Smedt T, et al. RANK is essential for osteoclast and lymph node development. *Genes Dev.* (1999) 13:2412–24. doi: 10.1101/gad.13.18.2412
39. Boyce BF, Yao Z, Xing L. Osteoclasts have multiple roles in bone in addition to bone resorption. *Crit Rev Eukaryot Gene Expr.* (2009) 19:171–80. doi: 10.1615/CritRevEukarGeneExpr.v19.i3.10
40. Takayanagi H. Osteoimmunology: shared mechanisms and crosstalk between the immune and bone systems. *Nature Rev Immunol.* (2007) 7:292–304. doi: 10.1038/nri2062
41. Barrow AD, Raynal N, Andersen TL, Slatter DA, BIhan D, Pugh N, et al. OSCAR is a collagen receptor that costimulates osteoclastogenesis in DAP12-deficient human and mice. *J Clin Invest.* (2011) 121:3505–16. doi: 10.1172/JCI45913
42. Otero K, Shinohara M, Zhao H, Cella M, Gilfillan S, Colucci A, et al. TREM2 and β-catenin regulate bone homeostasis by controlling the rate of osteoclastogenesis. *J Immunol.* (2012) 188:2612–21. doi: 10.4049/jimmunol.1102836
43. Ellmeier W, Jung S, Sunshine MJ, Hatam F, Xu Y, Baltimore D, et al. Severe B cell deficiency in mice lacking the tec kinase family members Tec and Btk. *J Exp Med.* (2000) 192:1611–24. doi: 10.1084/jem.192.11.1611
44. Shinohara M, Koga T, Okamoto K, Sakaguchi S, Arai K, Yasuda H, et al. Tyrosine kinases Btk and Tec regulate osteoclast differentiation by linking RANK and ITAM signals. *Cell.* (2008) 132:794–806. doi: 10.1016/j.cell.2007.12.037
45. Hanna RN, Carlin LM, Hubbelin HG, Nackiewicz D, Green AM, Punt JA, et al. The transcription factor NR4A1 (Nur77) controls bone marrow differentiation and the survival of Ly6C-monocytes. *Nat Immunol.* (2011) 12:778–85. doi: 10.1038/ni.2063
46. Tacke R, Hilgendorf I, Garner H, Waterborg C, Park K, Nowyhed H, et al. The transcription factor NR4A1 is essential for the development of a novel macrophage subset in the thymus. *Sci Rep.* (2015) 5:10055. doi: 10.1038/srep10055
47. Li X, Wei W, Huynh H, Zuo H, Wang X, Wang Y. Nur77 prevents excessive osteoclastogenesis by inducing ubiquitin ligase Cbl-b to mediate NFATc1. *Elife.* 4:e07217. doi: 10.7554/eLife.07217
48. Scholtysek C, Ipseiz N, Böhm C, Krishnacoumar B, Stenzel M, Czerwinski T, et al. NR4A1 regulates motility of osteoclast precursors and serves as target for the modulation of systemic bone turnover. *J Bone Miner Res.* (2018) 33:2035–47. doi: 10.1002/jbmr.3533
49. Hashizume M, Hayakawa N, Mihara M. IL-6 trans-signalling directly induces RANKL on fibroblast-like synovial cells and is involved in RANKL induction by TNF-alpha and IL-17. *Rheumatology (Oxford).* (2008) 47:1635–40. doi: 10.1093/rheumatology/ken363
50. Nagasawa T. Microenvironmental niches in the bone marrow required for B-cell development. *Nat Rev Immunol.* (2006) 6:107–16. doi: 10.1038/nri1780
51. Kitaura H, Zhou P, Kim HJ, Novack DV, Ross FP, Teitelbaum SL. M-CSF mediates TNF-induced inflammatory osteolysis. *J Clin Invest.* (2005) 115:3418–27. doi: 10.1172/JCI26132
52. Weitzmann MN, Cenci S, Rifas L, Brown C, Pacifici R. Interleukin-7 stimulates osteoclast formation by up-regulating the T-cell production of soluble osteoclastogenic cytokines. *Blood.* (2000) 96:1873–8.
53. Amarasekara DS, Yun H, Kim S, Lee N, Kim H, Rho J. Regulation of osteoclast differentiation by cytokine networks. *Immune Netw.* 18:e8. doi: 10.4110/in.2018.18.e8
54. Chen L, Wei XQ, Evans B, Jiang W, Aeschlimann D. IL-23 promotes osteoclast formation by up-regulation of receptor activator of NF-kappaB (RANK) expression in myeloid precursor cells. *Eur J Immunol.* (2008) 38:2845–54. doi: 10.1002/eji.200838192
55. Raisz LG. Prostaglandins and bone: physiology and pathophysiology. *Osteoarthritis Cartilage.* (1999) 7:419–21. doi: 10.1053/joca.1998.0230
56. Jarry CR, Durante PM, Freitas FF, de Macedo CG, Clemente-Napimoga JT, Saba-Chujfi E, et al. Secreted osteoclastogenic factor of activated T cells (SOFAT), a novel osteoclast activator, in chronic periodontitis. *Hum Immunol.* (2013) 74:861866. doi: 10.1016/j.humimm.2013.04.013
57. Kudo O, Sabokbar A, Pocock A, Itonaga I, Fujikawa Y, Athanasou NA. Interleukin-6 and interleukin-11 support human osteoclast formation by a RANKL-independent mechanism. *Bone.* (2003) 32:1–7. doi: 10.1016/S8756-3282(02)00915-8
58. Yoshitake F, Itoh S, Narita H, Ishihara K, Ebisu S. Interleukin-6 directly inhibits osteoclast differentiation by suppressing receptor activator of NF-kappaB signaling pathways. *J Biol Chem.* (2008) 283:11535–40. doi: 10.1074/jbc.M607999200
59. Lubberts E, Koenders MI, van der Berg WB. The role of T-cell interleukin-17 in conducting destructive arthritis: lessons from animal models. *Arthritis Res Ther.* (2005) 7:29–37. doi: 10.1186/ar1478
60. Moon YM, Yoon BY, Her YM, Oh HJ, Lee JS, Kim KW, et al. IL-32 and IL-17 interact and have the potential to aggravate osteoclastogenesis in rheumatoid arthritis. *Arthritis Res Ther.* (2012) 14:R246. doi: 10.1186/ar4089
61. Danks L, Takayanagi H. Immunology and bone. *J Biochem.* (2013) 154:29–39. doi: 10.1093/jb/mvt049
62. Adamopoulos IE, Bowman EP. Immune regulation of bone loss by Th17 cells. *Arthritis Res Ther.* 10:225. doi: 10.1186/ar2502
63. Adamopoulos IE, Chao CC, Geissler R, Laface D, Blumenschein W, Iwakura Y et al. Interleukin-17A upregulates receptor activator of NF-kappaB on osteoclast precursors. *Arthritis Res Ther.* (2010) 12:R29. doi: 10.1186/ar2936
64. Maddur MS, Miossec P, Kaveri SV, Bayry J. Th17 cells: biology, pathogenesis of autoimmune and inflammatory diseases, and therapeutic strategies. *Am J Pathol.* (2012) 181:8–18. doi: 10.1016/j.ajpath.2012.03.044
65. Noonan K, Marchionni L, Anderson J, Pardoll D, Roodman GD, Borrello I. A novel role of IL-17-producing lymphocytes in mediating lytic bone disease in multiple myeloma. *Blood.* (2010) 116:3554–63. doi: 10.1182/blood-2010-05-283895
66. Kim YG, Lee CK, Nah SS, Mun SH, Yoo B, Moon HB. Human CD4+CD25+ regulatory T cells inhibit the differentiation of osteoclasts from peripheral blood mononuclear cells. *Biochem Biophys Res Commun.* (2007) 357:1046–52. doi: 10.1016/j.bbrc.2007.04.042
67. Zaiss MM, Axmann R, Zwerina J, Polzer K, Gückel E, Skapenko A et al. Treg cells suppress osteoclast formation: a new link between the immune system and bone. *Arthritis Rheum.* (2007) 56:4104–12. doi: 10.1002/art.23138
68. Zaiss MM, Frey B, Hess A, Zwerina J, Luther J, Nimmerjahn F et al. Regulatory T cells protect from local and systemic bone destruction in arthritis. *J Immunol.* (2010) 184:7238–46. doi: 10.4049/jimmunol.0903841
69. Steinman RM, Banchereau J. Taking dendritic cells into medicine. *Nature.* (2007) 449:419–26. doi: 10.1038/nature06175
70. Thomas R, MacDonald KP, Pettit AR, Cavanagh LL, Padmanabha J, Zehntner S. Dendritic cells and the pathogenesis of rheumatoid arthritis. *J Leukoc Biol.* (1999) 66:286–92. doi: 10.1002/jlb.66.2.286
71. Santiago-Schwarz F, Anand P, Liu S, Carsons SE. Dendritic cells (DCs) in rheumatoid arthritis (RA): progenitor cells and soluble factors contained in RA synovial fluid yield a subset of myeloid DCs that preferentially

activate Th1 inflammatory-type responses. *J Immunol.* (2001) 167:1758–68. doi: 10.4049/jimmunol.167.3.1758

72. Rivollier A, Mazzorana M, Tebib J, Piperno M, Aitsiselmi T, Rabourdin-Combe C, Jurdic P, Servet-Delprat C. Immature dendritic cell transdifferentiation into osteoclasts: a novel pathway sustained by the rheumatoid arthritis microenvironment. *Blood.* (2004) 104:4029–37. doi: 10.1182/blood-2004-01-0041
73. Hajishengallis G, Moutsopoulos NM, Hajishengallis E, Chavakis T. Immune and regulatory functions of neutrophils in inflammatory bone loss. *Semin Immunol.* (2016) 28:146–58. doi: 10.1016/j.smim.2016.02.002
74. Mortaz E, Alipoor SD, Adcock IM, Mumby S, Koenderman L. Update on neutrophil function in severe inflammation. *Front Immunol.* (2018) 9:2171. doi: 10.3389/fimmu.2018.02171
75. Moutsopoulos NM, Konkel J, Sarmadi M, Eskan MA, Wild T, Dutzan N. Defective neutrophil recruitment in leukocyte adhesion deficiency type I disease causes local IL-17-driven inflammatory bone loss. *Sci Transl Med.* (2014) 6:229ra40. doi: 10.1126/scitranslmed.3007696
76. Poubelle PE, Chakravarti A, Fernandes MJ, Doiron K, Marceau AA. Differential expression of RANK, RANK-L, and osteoprotegerin by synovial fluid neutrophils from patients with rheumatoid arthritis and by healthy human blood neutrophils. *Arthritis Res Ther.* 9:R25. doi: 10.1186/ar2137
77. Kong YY, Yoshida H, Sarosi I, Tan HL, Timms E, Capparelli C, et al. OPGL is a key regulator of osteoclastogenesis, lymphocyte development and lymph-node organogenesis. *Nature.* (1999) 397:315–323. doi: 10.1038/16852
78. Onal M, Xiong J, Chen X, Thosten JD, Almeida JD, Manolagas SC, et al. Receptor activator of nuclear factor kB ligand (RANKL) protein expression by B lymphocytes contributes to ovariectomy-induced bone loss. *J Biol Chem.* (2012) 287:29851–60. doi: 10.1074/jbc.M112.377945
79. Perlot T, Penninger JM. Development and function of murine B cells lacking RANK. *J Immunol.* (2012) 188:1201–5. doi: 10.4049/jimmunol.1102063
80. Miyaura C, Onoe Y, Inada M, Maki K, Ikuta K, Ito M, et al. Increased B-lymphopoiesis by interleukin 7 induces bone loss in mice with intact ovarian functions: similarity to estrogen deficiency. *Proc Natl Acad Sci USA.* (1997) 94:9360–65. doi: 10.1073/pnas.94.17.9360
81. Pugliese LS, Gonçalves TO, Popi AF, Mariano M, Pesquero JB, Lopes JD. B-1 lymphocytes differentiate into functional osteoclast-like cells. *Immunobiology.* (2012) 217:336–44. doi: 10.1016/j.imbio.2011.07.014
82. Manabe N, Kawaguchi H, Chikuda H, Miyaura C, Inada M, Nagai R, et al. Connection between B lymphocyte and osteoclast differentiation pathways. *J Immunol.* (2001) 167:2625–31. doi: 10.4049/jimmunol.167.5.2625
83. Söderström K, Stein E, Colmenero P, Purath U, Müller-Ladner U, de Matos CT, Tarner IH, Robinson WH, Engleman EG. Natural killer cells trigger osteoclastogenesis and bone destruction in arthritis. *Proc Natl Acad Sci USA.* (2010) 107:13028–33. doi: 10.1073/pnas.1000546107
84. Feng S, Madsen SH, Viller NN, Neutzsky-Wulff AV, Geisler C, Karlsson L, et al. Interleukin-15-activated natural killer cells kill autologous osteoclasts via LFA-1, DNAM-1 and TRAIL, and inhibit osteoclast-mediated bone erosion *in vitro*. *Immunology.* (2015) 145:367–79. doi: 10.1111/imm.12449
85. Ahern DJ, Brennan FM. The role of Natural Killer cells in the pathogenesis of rheumatoid arthritis: major contributors or essential homeostatic modulators? *Immunol Lett.* (2011) 136:115–21. doi: 10.1016/j.imlet.2010.11.001
86. Michalski MN, McCauley LK. Macrophages and skeletal health. *Pharmacol Ther.* (2017) 174:43–54. doi: 10.1016/j.pharmthera.2017.02.017
87. Chitteti BR, Cheng YH, Poteat B, Rodriguez-Rodriguez S, Goebel WS, Carlesso N, et al. Impact of interactions of cellular components of the bone marrow microenvironment on hematopoietic stem and progenitor cell function. *Blood.* (2010) 115:3239–48. doi: 10.1182/blood-2009-09-246173
88. Mohamad SF, Xu L, Ghosh J, Childress PJ, Abeysekera I, Himes ER, et al. Osteomacs interact with megakaryocytes and osteoblasts to regulate murine hematopoietic stem cell function. *Blood Adv.* (2017) 1:2520–28. doi: 10.1182/bloodadvances.2017011304
89. Champagne CM, Takebe J, Offenbacher S, Cooper LF. Macrophage cell lines produce osteoinductive signals that include bone morphogenetic protein-2. *Bone.* (2002) 30:26–31. doi: 10.1016/S8756-3282(01)00638-X
90. Chang MK, Raggatt IJ, Alexander KA, Kuliwaba JS, Fazzalari NL, Schroder K, et al. Osteal tissue macrophages are intercalated throughout human and mouse bone lining tissues and regulate osteoblast function *in vitro* and *in vivo*. *J Immunol.* (2008) 181:1232–44. doi: 10.4049/jimmunol.181.2.1232
91. Cho SW, Soki FN, Koh AJ, Eber MR, Entezami P, Park S, et al. Osteal macrophages support physiologic skeletal remodeling and anabolic actions of parathyroid hormone in bone. *Proc Natl Acad Sci USA.* (2014) 111:1545–50. doi: 10.1073/pnas.1315153111
92. Vi L, Baht GS, Whetstone H, Mg A, Wei Q, Poon R, et al. Macrophages promote osteoblastic differentiation *in-vivo*: implications in fracture repair and bone homeostasis. *J Bone Miner Res.* (2015) 30:1090–102. doi: 10.1002/jbmr.2422
93. Gowen M, MacDonald BR, Russel RG. Actions of recombinant human gamma-interferon and tumor necrosis factor alpha on the proliferation and osteoblastic characteristics of human trabecular bone cells *in vitro*. *Arthritis Rheum.* (1988) 31:1500–7. doi: 10.1002/art.1780311206
94. Maruhashi T, Kaifu T, Yabe R, Seno A, Chung SH, Fujikado N, et al. DCIR maintains bone homeostasis by regulating IFN-gamma production in T cells. *J Immunol.* (2015) 194:5681–91. doi: 10.4049/jimmunol.1500273
95. Duque G, Huang DC, Dion N, Macoritto M, Rivas D, Li W, et al. Interferon-gamma plays a role in bone formation *in vivo* and rescues osteoporosis in ovariectomized mice. *J Bone Miner Res.* (2011) 26:1472–83. doi: 10.1002/jbmr.350
96. Vidal C, Bermeo S, Li W, Huang D, Kremer R, Duque G. Interferon gamma inhibits adipogenesis *in vitro* and prevents marrow fat infiltration in oophorectomized mice. *Stem Cells.* 30:10428. doi: 10.1002/stem.1063
97. Ji JD, Park-Min KH, Shen Z, Fajardo RJ, Goldring SR, McHugh KP, et al. Inhibition of RANK expression and osteoclastogenesis by TLRs and IFN-gamma in human osteoclast precursors. *J Immunol.* (2009) 183:7223–33. doi: 10.4049/jimmunol.0900072
98. Xiong Q, Zhang I, Ge W, Tang P. The roles of interferons in osteoclasts and osteoclastogenesis. *Joint Bone Spine.* (2016) 83:276–81. doi: 10.1016/j.jbspin.2015.07.010
99. Kohara H, Kitaura H, Fujimura Y, Yoshimatsu M, Morita Y, Eguchi T, et al. IFN-gamma directly inhibits TNF-alpha-induced osteoclastogenesis *in vitro* and *in vivo* and induces apoptosis mediated by Fas/Fas ligand interactions. *Immunol Lett.* (2011) 137:53–61. doi: 10.1016/j.imlet.2011.02.017
100. Kim JW, Lee MS, Lee CH, Kim HY, Chae SU, Kwak HB, et al. Effect of interferon-gamma on the fusion of mononuclear osteoclasts into bone-resorbing osteoclasts. *BMB Rep.* (2012) 45:281–6. doi: 10.5483/BMBRep.2012.45.5.281
101. Kwak HB, Ha H, Kim HN, Lee JH, Kim HS, Lee S, et al. Reciprocal cross-talk between RANKL and interferon-gamma-inducible protein 10 is responsible for bone-erosive experimental arthritis. *Arthritis Rheum.* (2008) 58:1332–42. doi: 10.1002/art.23372
102. Yoshihara A, Seida Y, Hanada N, Miyazaki H. A longitudinal study of the relationship between periodontal disease and bone mineral density in community-dwelling older adults. *J Clin Periodontol.* (2004) 31:680–4. doi: 10.1111/j.1600-051X.2004.00548.x
103. Garcia-Carrasco M, Mendoza-Pinto C, Escarcega RO, Jimenez-Hernandez M, Etchegaray Morales I, Munguia Realpozo P, et al. Osteoporosis in patients with systemic lupus erythematosus. *Isr Med Assoc J.* (2009) 11:486–91.
104. Paganelli M, Albanse C, Borrelli O, Civitelli F, Canitano N, Viola F, et al. Inflammation is the main determinant of low bone mineral density in pediatric inflammatory bowel disease. *Inflamm Bowel Dis.* (2007) 13:416–23. doi: 10.1002/ibd.20039
105. Ali T, Lam D, Bronze MS, Humphrey MB. Osteoporosis in inflammatory bowel disease. *Am J Med.* (2009) 122:599–604. doi: 10.1016/j.amjmed.2009.01.022
106. Shead EF, Haworth CS, Barker H, Bilton D, Compston JE. Osteoclast function, bone turnover and inflammatory cytokines during infective exacerbations of cystic fibrosis. *J Cyst Fibros.* (2010) 9:93–8. doi: 10.1016/j.jcf.2009.11.007
107. Buckley L, Humphrey MB. Glucocorticoid-induced osteoporosis. *N Engl J Med.* (2018) 379:2547–56. doi: 10.1056/NEJMcp1800214
108. Azuma Y, Kaji K, Katogi R, Takeshita S, Kudo A. Tumor necrosis factor-alpha induces differentiation of and bone resorption by osteoclasts. *J Biol Chem.* (2000) 275:4858–64. doi: 10.1074/jbc.275.7.4858
109. Komine M, Kukita A, Kukita T, Ogata Y, Hotokebuchi T, Kohashi O. Tumor necrosis factor-alpha cooperates with receptor activator of

nuclear factor kappaB ligand in generation of osteoclasts in stromal cell-depleted rat bone marrow cell culture. *Bone*. (2001) 28:474–83. doi: 10.1016/S8756-3282(01)00420-3

110. Matsumoto T, Kuriwaka-Kido R, Kondo I, Kido S. Regulation of osteoblast differentiation by interleukin-11 via AP-1 and Smad signaling. *Endocr J*. (2012) 59:91–101. doi: 10.1507/endocrj.EJ11-0219
111. Suga K, Saitoh M, Fukushima S, Takahashi K, Nara H, Yasuda S, et al. Interleukin-11 induces osteoblast differentiation and acts synergistically with bone morphogenetic protein-2 in C3H10T1/2 cells. *J Interferon Cytokine Res*. (2001) 21:695–707. doi: 10.1089/107999001753124435
112. Scott DL, Wolfe F, Hizinga TW. Rheumatoid arthritis. *Lancet*. (2010) 376:1094–108. doi: 10.1016/S0140-6736(10)60826-4
113. Hwang SY, Kim JY, Kim KW, Park MK, Moon Y, Kim WU, et al. IL-17 induces production of IL-6 and IL-8 in rheumatoid arthritis synovial fibroblasts via NF-kappaB- and PI3-kinase/Akt-dependent pathways. *Arthritis Res Ther*. (2004) 6:R120-8. doi: 10.1186/ar1038
114. Ivanovic DV, Di Battista JA, Martel-Pelletier J, Jolicoeur PC, He Y, Zhang M, et al. IL-17 stimulates the production and expression of proinflammatory cytokines, IL-beta and TNF-alpha, by human macrophages. *J Immunol*. (1998) 160:3513–21.
115. Pacifici R, Brown C, Puscheck E, Friedrich E, Slatopolsky E, Maggio D, et al. Effect of surgical menopause and estrogen replacement on cytokine release from human blood mononuclear cells. *Proc Natl Acad Sci USA*. (1991) 88:5134–8. doi: 10.1073/pnas.88.12.5134
116. Hughes DE, Dai A, Tiffee JC, Li HH, Mundy GR, Boyce BF. Estrogen promotes apoptosis of murine osteoclasts mediated by TGF-beta. *Nat Med*. (1996) 2:1132–6. doi: 10.1038/nm1096-1132
117. Piva R, Penolazzi L, Lambertini E, Giordano S, Gambari R. Induction of apoptosis of human primary osteoclasts treated with a transcription factor decoy mimicking a promoter region of estrogen receptor alpha. *Apoptosis*. (2005) 10:1079–94. doi: 10.1007/s10495-005-0618-8
118. Srivastava S, Toraldo G, Weitzmann MN, Cenci S, Ross FP, Pacifici R. Estrogen decreases osteoclast formation by down-regulating receptor activator of NF-kappa B ligand (RANKL) induced JNK activation. *J Biol Chem*. (2001) 276:8836–40. doi: 10.1074/jbc.M010764200
119. Manolagas SC, O'Brien CA, Almeida M. The role of estrogen and androgen receptors in bone health and disease. *Nat Rev Endocrinol*. (2013) 9:699–712. doi: 10.1038/nrendo.2013.179
120. Eghbali-Fatourechi G, Khosla S, Sanyal A, Boyle WJ, Lacey DL, Riggs BL. Role of RANK ligand in mediating increased bone resorption in early postmenopausal women. *J Clin Invest*. (2003) 111:1221–30. doi: 10.1172/JCI200317215
121. Breuil Y, Ticchioni M, Testa J, Roux CH, Ferrari P, Breittmayer JP, et al. Immune changes in post-menopausal osteoporosis: the immunos study. *Osteoporos Int*. (2010) 21:805–14. doi: 10.1007/s00198-009-1018-7
122. D'Amelio P, Grimaldi A, Di Bella S, Brianza SZM, Cristofaro MA, Tamone C, et al. Estrogen deficiency increases osteoclastogenesis up-regulating T cells activity: a key mechanism in osteoporosis. *Bone*. (2008) 43:92–100. doi: 10.1016/j.bone.2008.02.017
123. Adeel S, Singh K, Vydareny KH, Kumari M, Shah E, Weitzmann MN, et al. Bone loss in surgically ovariectomized premenopausal women is associated with T Lymphocyte activation and thymic hypertrophy. *J Investig Med*. (2013) 61:1178–83. doi: 10.2310/JIM.0000000000000016
124. Masuzawa T, Miyamura C, Onoe Y, Kusano K, Ohta H, Nozawa S, et al. Estrogen deficiency stimulates B lymphopoiesis in mouse bone marrow. *J Clin Invest*. (1994) 94:1090–97. doi: 10.1172/JCI117424
125. Zheng SX, Vrindts Y, Lopez M, De Groote D, Zangerle PF, Collette J, et al. Increase in cytokine production (IL-1 beta, IL-6, TNF-alpha but not IFN-gamma, GM-CSF or LIF) by stimulated whole blood cells in postmenopausal osteoporosis. *Maturitas*. (1997) 26:63–71. doi: 10.1016/S0378-5122(96)01080-8
126. Hustmyer FG, Walker E, Yu XP, Girasole G, Sakagami Y, Peacock M, et al. Cytokine production and surface antigen expression by peripheral blood mononuclear cells in postmenopausal osteoporosis. *J Bone Miner Res*. (1993) 8:51–9. doi: 10.1002/jbmr.5650080108
127. Brunetti G, Colucci S, Pignataro P, Coricciati M, Mori G, Cirulli N, et al. T cells support osteoclastogenesis in an *in vitro* model derived from human periodontitis patients. *J Periodontol*. (2005) 76:1675–80. doi: 10.1902/jop.2005.76.10.1675
128. Kawai T, Matsuyama T, Hosokawa Y. B and T lymphocytes are the primary sources of RANKL in the bone resorptive lesion of periodontal disease. *Am J Pathol*. (2006) 169:987–98. doi: 10.2353/ajpath.2006.060180
129. Rifas L, Weitzmann MN. A novel T cell cytokine, secreted osteoclastogenic factor of activated T cells, induces osteoclast formation in a RANKL-independent manner. *Arthritis Rheumatol*. (2009) 60:3324–35. doi: 10.1002/art.24877
130. Weitzmann MN. T-cells and B-cells in osteoporosis. *Curr Opin Endocrinol Diabetes Obes*. (2014) 21:461–7. doi: 10.1097/MED.0000000000000103
131. Richardson J, Hill AM, Johnston CJ, McGregor A, Norrish AR, Eastwood D, et al. Fracture healing in HIV-positive populations. *J Bone Joint Surg Br*. (2008) 90:988–94. doi: 10.1302/0301-620X.90B8.20861
132. El-Jawhari JJ, Jones E, Giannoudis PV. The role of immune cells in bone haling; what we know, do not know and future perspectives. *Injury*. (2016) 47:2399–406. doi: 10.1016/j.injury.2016.10.008
133. Askalonov AA. Changes in some indices of cellular immunity in patients with uncomplicated and complicated healing of bone fractures. *J Hyg Epidemiol Microbiol Immunol*. (1981) 25:307–10.
134. Timlin M, Toomey D, Condron C, Power C, Street J, Murray P, et al. Fracture hematoma is a potent proinflammatory mediator of neutrophil function. *J Trauma*. (2005) 58:1223–9. doi: 10.1097/01.TA.0000169866.88781.F1
135. Almeida CR, Caires HR, Vasconcelos DP, Barbosa MA. NAP-2 secreted by human NL cells can stimulate mesenchymal stem/stromal cell recruitment. *Stem Cell Rep*. (2016) 6:466–73. doi: 10.1016/j.stemcr.2016.02.012
136. Ito H. Chemokines in mesenchymal stem cell therapy for bone repair: a novel concept of recruiting mesenchymal stem cells and possible cell sources. *Mod Rheumatol*. (2011) 21:113–21. doi: 10.3109/s10165-010-0357-8
137. Nakase T, Yoshikawa H. Potential roles of bone morphogenetic proteins (BMPs) in skeletal repair and regeneration. *J Bone Miner Metab*. (2006) 24:425–33. doi: 10.1007/s00774-006-0718-8
138. Omar OM, Granéli C, Ekström K, Karlsson C, Johansson A, Lausmaa J, et al. The stimulation of an osteogenic response by classical monocyte activation. *Biomaterials*. (2011) 32:8190–204. doi: 10.1016/j.biomaterials.2011.07.055
139. Luz-Crawford P, Kurte M, Bravo-Alegría J, Contreras R, Nova-Lamperti E, Tejedor G, et al. Mesenchymal stem cells regenerate a $CD4^{+}CD25^{+}Foxp3^{+}$ regulatory T cell population during the differentiation process of Th1 and Th17 cells. *Stem Cell Res Ther*. (2013) 4:65. doi: 10.1186/scrt216
140. Akiyama K, Chen C, Wang D, Xu X, Qu C, Yamaza T, et al. Mesenchymal-stem-cell-induced immunoregulation involves FAS-ligand-/FAS-mediated T cell apoptosis. *Cell Stem Cell*. (2012) 10:544–55. doi: 10.1016/j.stem.2012.03.007
141. Klyushnenkova E, Mosca JD, McIntosh KR. Human mesenchymal stem cells suppress allogeneic T cell response *in vitro*: implications for allogenic transplantation. *Blood*. (1998) 92:642a–642a.
142. Corcione A, Benvenuto F, Ferretti E, Giunti D, Cappiello V, Cazzanti F, et al. Human mesenchymal stem cells modulate B-cell functions. *Blood*. (2006) 107:367–72. doi: 10.1182/blood-2005-07-2657
143. Krevvata M, Silva BC, Manavalan JS, Galan-Diez M, Kode A, Matthews BG, et al. Inhibition of leukemia cell engraftment and disease progression in mice by osteoblasts. *Blood*. (2014) 124:2834–46. doi: 10.1182/blood-2013-07-517219
144. Kode A, Manavalan JS, Mosialou I, Bhagat G, Rathinam CV, Luo N, et al. Leukaemogenesis induced by an activating β-catenin mutation in osteoblasts. *Nature*. (2014) 506:240–4. doi: 10.1038/nature12883
145. Raaijmakers MH, Mukherjee S, Guo S, Zhang S, Kobayashi T, Schoonmaker JA, et al. Bone progenitor dysfunction induces myelodysplasia and secondary leukaemia. *Nature*. (2010) 464:852–7. doi: 10.1038/nature08851
146. Edwards JR, Sun SG, Locklin R, Shipman CM, Adamopoulos IE, Athanasou NA, et al. LIGHT (TNFSF14), a novel mediator of bone resorption, is elevated in rheumatoid arthritis. *Arthritis Rheum*. (2006) 54:1451–62. doi: 10.1002/art.21821
147. Ishida S, Yamane S, Nakano S, Yanagimoto T, Hanamoto Y, Maeda-Tanimura M, et al. The interaction of monocytes with rheumatoid synovial cells is a key step in LIGHT-mediated inflammatory bone destruction. *Immunology*. (2009) 128:e315–e324. doi: 10.1111/j.1365-2567.2008.02965.x

148. Brunetti G, Faienza MF, Colaianni G, Gigante I, Oranger A, Pignataro P, et al. Impairment of bone remodeling in LIGHT/TNFSF14-deficient mice. *J Bone Miner Res.* (2018a) 33:704–19. doi: 10.1002/jbmr.3345
149. Brunetti G, Rizzi R, Storlino G, Bortolotti S, Colaianni G, Sanesi L, et al. LIGHT/TNFSF14 as a new biomarker of bone disease in multiple myeloma patients experiencing therapeutic regimens. *Front Immunol.* 23:2459. doi: 10.3389/fimmu.2018.02459
150. Capulli M, Rufo A, Teti A, Rucci N. Global transcriptome analysis in mouse calvarial osteoblasts highlights sets of genes regulated by modeled microgravity and identifies a "mechanoresponsive osteoblast gene signature". *J Cell Biochem.* (2009) 15:240–52. doi: 10.1002/jcb.22120
151. Rucci N, Capulli M, Piperni SG, Cappariello A, Lau P, Frings-Meuthen P, Heer M, Teti A. Lipocalin 2: a new mechanoresponding gene regulating bone homeostasis. *J Bone Miner Res.* 2015 30:357-68. doi: 10.1002/jbmr.2341
152. Capulli M, Ponzetti M, Maurizi A, Gemini-Piperni S, Berger T, Mak TW, et al. A complex role for Lipocalin 2 in bone metabolism: global ablation in mice induces osteopenia caused by an altered energy metabolism. *J Bone Miner Res.* (2018) 33:1141–53. doi: 10.1002/jbmr.3406
153. Costa D, Principi E, Lazzarini E, Descalzi F, Cancedda R, Castagnola P, et al. LCN2 overexpression in bone enhances the hematopoietic compartment via modulation of the bone marrow microenvironment. *J Cell Physiol.* (2017) 232:3077–87. doi: 10.1002/jcp.25755
154. Mosialou I, Shikhel S, Liu JM, Maurizi A, Luo N, He Z, et al. MC4R-dependent suppression of appetite by bone-derived lipocalin 2. *Nature.* (2017) 16;543:385-390. doi: 10.1038/nature 21697
155. Chiu YG, Ritchlin CT. Denosumab: targeting the RANKL pathway to treat rheumatoid arthritis. *Expert Opin Biol Ther.* (2017) 17:119–28. doi: 10.1080/14712598.2017.1263614

2

Chronic Implant-Related Bone Infections—Can Immune Modulation be a Therapeutic Strategy?

Elisabeth Seebach* and Katharina F. Kubatzky*

Department of Infectious Diseases, Medical Microbiology and Hygiene, Heidelberg University Hospital, Heidelberg, Germany

***Correspondence:**
Elisabeth Seebach
elisabeth.seebach@med.uni-heidelberg.de
Katharina F. Kubatzky
kubatzky@uni-heidelberg.de

Chronic implant-related bone infections are a major problem in orthopedic and trauma-related surgery with severe consequences for the affected patients. As antibiotic resistance increases in general and because most antibiotics have poor effectiveness against biofilm-embedded bacteria in particular, there is a need for alternative and innovative treatment approaches. Recently, the immune system has moved into focus as the key player in infection defense and bone homeostasis, and the targeted modulation of the host response is becoming an emerging field of interest. The aim of this review was to summarize the current knowledge of impaired endogenous defense mechanisms that are unable to prevent chronicity of bone infections associated with a prosthetic or osteosynthetic device. The presence of foreign material adversely affects the immune system by generating a local immune-compromised environment where spontaneous clearance of planktonic bacteria does not take place. Furthermore, the surface structure of the implant facilitates the transition of bacteria from the planktonic to the biofilm stage. Biofilm formation on the implant surface is closely linked to the development of a chronic infection, and a misled adaption of the immune system makes it impossible to effectively eliminate biofilm infections. The interaction between the immune system and bone cells, especially osteoclasts, is extensively studied in the field of osteoimmunology and this crosstalk further aggravates the course of bone infection by shifting bone homeostasis in favor of bone resorption. T cells play a major role in various chronic diseases and in this review a special focus was therefore set on what is known about an ineffective T cell response. Myeloid-derived suppressor cells (MDSCs), anti-inflammatory macrophages, regulatory T cells (T_{reg}s) as well as osteoclasts all suppress immune defense mechanisms and negatively regulate T cell-mediated immunity. Thus, these cells are considered to be potential targets for immune therapy. The success of immune checkpoint inhibition in cancer treatment encourages the transfer of such immunological approaches into treatment strategies of other chronic diseases. Here, we discuss whether immune modulation can be a therapeutic tool for the treatment of chronic implant-related bone infections.

Keywords: chronic implant-related bone infection, osteomyelitis, bacterial infection, biofilm, immune modulation, MDSCs, T cells, immune checkpoint molecules

INTRODUCTION

Primary hip and knee arthroplasties belong to the most successful surgeries of this century (>1,000,000/year in the U.S.) and the numbers of surgeries are rising due to demographical changes (1). Concomitantly, the number of revision surgeries and associated complications is increasing. Prosthetic joint infections (PJIs) are one of the most feared complications that often result in revision of the artificial joint with serious consequences for the patients and high costs for the respective health systems (1, 2). For primary arthroplasty the incidence of infection ranges between 1 and 2% depending on the register (1, 3). A current study states the risk of re-infection after PJI-induced revision surgery at around 8% for hips (4) and knees (5), but also much higher values (up to 57.1%) are published (6, 7). In trauma-related bone reconstructions (2,000,000/year in the U.S.), fracture-related infections (FRIs) associated with osteosynthetic stabilization are a major problem as the surgery field is often contaminated due to bacterial access through open wounds and broken bone that penetrates the skin (open fractures). This leads to an infection risk ranging from 10% (8, 9) to 50% depending on the fracture type (10). Thus, chronic implant-related bone infections are a serious burden in current and future health care.

Homeostasis of Bone

Bone is a dynamic organ undergoing constant remodeling in order to maintain homeostasis of bone formation and degradation, and to preserve bone mass. Bone remodeling is organized by the interplay between bone forming osteoblasts (OBs) and bone resorbing osteoclasts (OCs). OBs differentiate from mesenchymal stromal cells (MSCs) that reside within the bone marrow, whereas OCs develop from myeloid precursor cells. Osteoclastogenesis is regulated through the osteoprotegerin (OPG)/receptor activator of NF-κB (RANK)/RANK-Ligand (RANKL) pathway. OPG serves as a negative regulator of osteoclastogenesis that inhibits the RANK—RANKL interaction via binding of RANKL [reviewed in (11, 12)]. Bone homeostasis depends on the local cytokine milieu. While inflammation is necessary to induce physiological bone healing (13), it can lead to increased bone resorption under pathological situations such as bone infections (14).

Definition of Bone Infections

Osteomyelitis is an infection of the bone that is characterized by an inflammatory reaction and destruction of bone due to bacterial colonization of the bone itself, the bone marrow and the surrounding tissue. Osteomyelitis can occur by local spread of bacteria from an adjacent, contaminating source caused by trauma or bone surgery; or secondary to a vascular undersupply as it is mostly the case in diabetic foot ulcers. Hematogenous osteomyelitis is caused by bacteria, which come from a source of infection localized somewhere else in the body (e.g., a dental infection) and enter the bone via the blood stream (15, 16). PJIs caused by hematogenous seeding of the prosthesis often appear a long time after bone surgery (late bone infection: >2 years after surgery), whereas contamination during implantation of the medical device or during hospitalization before the wound has closed usually leads to early (<3 months after surgery) or delayed post-operative infections (3 months—2 years after surgery) (2). Zimmerli and Sendi further suggest a clinically more relevant classification that is used as a guide for surgical management. Here, PJIs are defined as early post-operative when symptoms occur within 1 month and are called chronic when diagnosed later than 1 month after surgery. Hematogenous PJIs are classified as acute when symptoms occur <3 weeks after a former uneventful post-operative period and chronic when symptoms persist for over 3 weeks (17). The predominantly isolated bacteria are part of the physiological skin microflora, such as *Staphylococcus aureus* (*S. aureus*), coagulase-negative staphylococci and enterococci (1, 18). Early and acute symptoms of infection, such as pain, warming and swelling of the site of infection and fever, are mostly associated with highly virulent bacteria like *S. aureus*; whereas less virulent bacteria, such as *Staphylococcus epidermidis* (*S. epidermidis*), cause more subtle symptoms typical for a low-grade inflammation that often are not diagnosed before infection chronicity (2). FRIs are mostly caused by inoculation of bacteria through an open wound/penetrated skin or through the surgical access needed for osteosynthetic bone reconstruction with *S. aureus* being the primary causative agent (19). At present, they are defined as early when occurring <2 weeks, delayed at 3–10 weeks and late >10 weeks after implantation of the osteosynthetic device (17, 20). However, the criteria for FRIs that can be used as guidelines for clinical management as they are established for PJIs are still under discussion (21). The early and acute states of osteomyelitis are characterized by bacterial colonization of the bone, pus formation, vascular undersupply and a strong inflammatory immune response associated with fever, pain and swelling (15, 16). The resulting increased levels of pro-inflammatory cytokines, such as tumor necrosis factor alpha (TNF-α), interleukin-1 beta (IL-1β) and IL-6, induce tissue destruction and a shift toward osteoclastogenesis and bone resorption (14). At this stage, a prompt and aggressive antibiotic and surgical treatment is generally sufficient to clear the infection. Unsuccessful treatment however results in the manifestation of a chronic bone infection, which is characterized by persistence of bacteria, areas of dead bone, so-called sequestra, periosteal new bone formation, fistula and low-grade inflammation. The recurrence of infection with fever is a clear sign for a chronic progression of the disease (15, 16) and depends on different bacteria reservoirs. *S. aureus* is known to survive intracellularly within non-professional phagocytes such as osteoblasts (22), an immune evasion mechanism still controversially discussed for *S. epidermidis* (23–25). A current study showed that *S. aureus* colonizes the canaliculi and osteocyte lacunae of living cortical bone (26). Furthermore, many bacteria are able to form sessile communities; referred to as biofilms, which preferentially colonize dead bone and foreign devices (17, 27). Biofilms evade bacterial clearance through the immune system and antibiotic treatment and therefore are one key characteristic of chronic implant-related bone infections and a major cause for bacterial persistence (28, 29). Current treatment strategies aim to eradicate biofilms to reduce the risk of re-infection.

Current Treatment Concepts

Current treatment concepts are based on the surgical removal of the infected tissue and strict antibiotic treatment to reduce bacterial burden as much as possible (17). Antibiotic regimens depend on the result of susceptibility testing of isolated cultures and should be administered for a total duration of 6–12 weeks. In the case of Staphylococcus subspecies, treatment guidelines recommend the use of rifampin, which is effective against biofilm-embedded bacteria, in combination with an intravenously administrable antibiotic for 2 weeks followed by an oral antibiotic therapy. For Methicillin-resistant strains, the combination of rifampin with vancomycin is recommended (20, 30). Surgical treatment of PJIs includes debridement with implant retention and one- or two-stage exchanges with placement of an antibiotic-laden spacer between the explantation and re-implantation of the prosthesis for up to 8 weeks. The procedure applied mainly relies on the time-point, when an implant-related bone infection is diagnosed. In early/acute infections the biofilm is still immature and the infection can be eradicated with retention of the implant. The success rate of this procedure is >80% when the implant is stable and the causative pathogen is susceptible to antibiotic treatment. Otherwise, in the case of Methicillin-resistant *S. aureus* (MRSA) or after chronic manifestation of infection associated with mature biofilm, for example, the foreign device has to be exchanged (30, 31). In FRIs, the decision for retention, exchange or removal of the implant mainly depends on the onset of infection (early-delayed-late), the type of fixation device and fracture consolidation. Here, infection clearance can be achieved because the foreign material can be removed after bone bridging has occurred. Until then, the stability of the bone fracture needs to be preserved meaning that after extensive debridement, external fixation and bone reconstruction may be required. Local delivery of antibiotics either by non-resorbable bone cement or degradable bone graft materials can be beneficial (19, 20). All of these approaches are associated with tremendous consequences for the patients with long hospital stays, repeated surgeries and an impairment of limb function between explantation and re-implantation of the devices. Due to the enhanced tolerance of biofilm-embedded bacteria against most antibiotics and the existence of dormant cells within biofilms, bone niches and/or host cells, treatment approaches often do not end in complete clearance of the pathogen and re-infection occurs frequently (32, 33). As a last consequence, this can lead to non-healing bone defects (non-union), stiffening of the affected joint or even amputation of the infected limb (20, 34).

Role of the Implant and Biofilm Formation

The implant itself represents a major risk factor for the initial development and chronic progression of osteomyelitis and recurrence of infection. In a tissue cage model in guinea pigs, the presence of a foreign material decreased the required infection dose from $>10^8$ CFUs *S. aureus* to 10^2 CFUs (35). Also in rats, infection doses as low as 10^2 CFUs *S. aureus* were sufficient to induce implant-associated bone infections without any further promoter such as soft tissue trauma or bone injury (36). One reason for this increased susceptibility is that the implant adversely affects the immune system by activating neutrophils, phagocytic cells, and the complement system. This results in an inflammatory and cytotoxic local environment that causes cell death and tissue damage (37). In this immune-compromised environment, successful clearance of bacteria by the host defense does not take place. Bacteria additionally profit from the foreign material as their surface structures serve as an attractive source for bacterial attachment that facilitate the transition from the planktonic to the biofilm stage (38). The concept of "race to the surface" describes the balance between tissue integration and bacterial colonization of an implant. The success of its implantation depends on the immediate interaction with host cells and the integration within the respective tissue (osseointegration in case of orthopedic devices), which prevents bacterial adhesion and biofilm formation. If bacterial colonization occurs first, tissue integration is impaired and bacteria can persist by forming biofilms (39, 40).

In the presence of a medical device, biofilm formation starts with the adhesion of planktonic bacteria to the implant surface, a process mediated by hydrophobic, electrostatic and van der Waals interactions that allows unspecific attachment (**Figure 1**). Directly after insertion into the body, the implant is coated with serum and tissue proteins. This allows specific attachment of bacteria by bacterial adhesion molecules (microbial surface components recognizing adhesive matrix molecules, MSCRAMMs) that bind to host proteins such as collagen and fibronectin (41). After the initial colonization, bacteria begin to produce a biofilm consisting of exopolysaccharides, proteins, lipids and nucleic acids that form a protective, slimy layer around them (extracellular polymeric substance, EPS). This effectively shields the included bacteria from immune cells and antibiotics (28, 38). Polysaccharide intercellular adhesin (PIA), for example, is a glycosaminoglycan of the EPS that mediates cell-cell adhesion and aggregation of bacteria in staphylococci biofilms (42). Immature biofilms are found in early post-operative and acute hematogenous infections (30). Biofilm maturation is characterized by biofilm growth, bacterial multiplication and production of additional virulence factors (28). Mature biofilms have a high bacterial density and are a constant source of bacterial spreading (43). They are associated with chronic infections (30). Biofilm formation and maturation, production of virulence factors and release of bacteria by mature biofilm are mediated by quorum sensing (QS) signaling systems (28, 44, 45). QS allows cell-to-cell communication between bacteria due to the release of small molecules called "autoinducers". By this, bacteria are able to determine their population density and react on environmental changes in a population-wide manner (46, 47). Within the hostile environment of mature biofilms, bacteria differentiate into a non-growing phenotype called "persister cells". This dormant cell population is highly tolerant to antibiotics and contributes to the chronicity and the risk of re-infection of implants (41, 48). Another bacteria

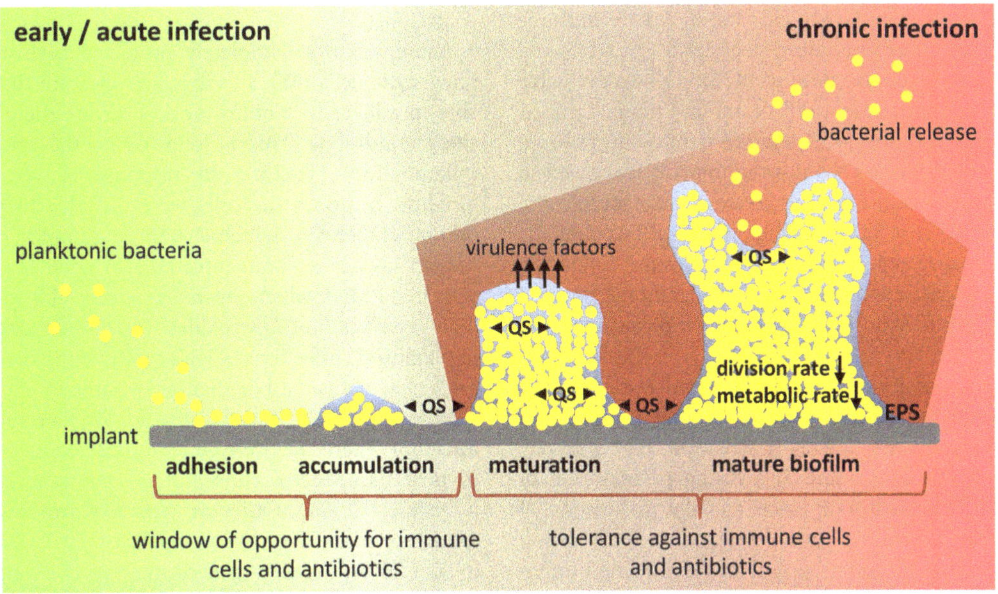

FIGURE 1 | Biofilm formation and window of opportunity for an effective clearance of bacteria. Implant-related bone infections are defined as early and chronic post-operative or acute and chronic hematogenous depending on the time interval between implantation of the medical device and onset of symptoms. Early and acute infections are associated with immature biofilms, whereas mature biofilms play a role in chronic situations. Biofilm formation starts when planktonic bacteria adhere to the implant surface. Attached bacteria then accumulate and start to produce biofilm. During biofilm maturation bacteria strongly multiply, build up further biofilm, and release virulence factors. Mature biofilm shows a high bacterial density with low division rate and decreased metabolic activity (persister cells). Release of planktonic bacteria by biofilm disassembly can lead to recurrence of infection. All these steps are mediated by an intercellular signaling system referred to as quorum sensing (QS). There is only a small window of opportunity for immune cells and antibiotic treatment to successfully clear bacteria and prevent biofilm formation and infection persistence. Biofilm maturation however is characterized by increasing tolerance against immune cells and antibiotics and leads to chronicity of infection. EPS, extracellular polymeric substance; QS, quorum sensing.

phenotype associated with recurrent bone infections are small colony variants (SCVs). SCVs are a metabolically inactive and slow-growing form of bacteria that forms due to defects in electron transport and thymidine biosynthesis (49). Mainly, SCVs are related to intracellular persistence of bacteria as they survive within host cells, but their contribution to biofilm formation and antibiotic tolerance is also discussed (50, 51). In addition to its function as a physical barrier and environment for SCV and persister cell formation, it is hypothesized that biofilm and embedded bacteria affect the local immunological environment in favor of decreased bacterial killing and enhanced persistence (37, 52, 53). The interaction between the foreign device, bacteria and biofilm dampens the host immune response and is one major reason for the ineffective elimination and chronicity of implant-related bone infections (37). Thus, the investigation of endogenous defense mechanisms has moved into focus and the possibility to modulate a misdirected host immune response might provide an attractive target for innovative therapeutic strategies against chronic implant-related bone infections.

The aim of this review is 2-fold: First to summarize the immune response against implant-related bone infections highlighting the transition from acute to chronic infection defined by the presence of biofilm. Secondly, to examine immune modulatory interventions that have been applied for the treatment of other chronic diseases and discuss their feasibility and application for treating chronic implant-related osteomyelitis.

IMMUNE RESPONSE AGAINST CHRONIC IMPLANT-RELATED BONE INFECTIONS

In the presence of planktonic bacteria, polymorphonuclear neutrophils (PMNs) and macrophages (Mϕs) infiltrate the site of infection. Here, they are activated via binding of pathogen-associated molecular patterns (PAMPs) to the respective pattern recognition receptors (PRRs) such as toll-like receptors (TLRs), which results in the activation of transcription factors such as the nuclear factor "kappa-light-chain-enhancer" of activated B-cells (NF-κB) [reviewed in (54, 55)]. As a consequence, the cells generate an inflammatory environment by secretion of pro-inflammatory cytokines and contribute to bacterial killing by release of antimicrobial peptides, generation of reactive oxygen (ROS) and nitrogen species (NOS) and phagocytosis. Furthermore, PMNs form extracellular fibril matrices consisting of granule proteins and DNA that helps to trap bacteria for further degradation (neutrophil extracellular traps, NETs) [reviewed in (52)]. Thus, in the absence of foreign materials, the innate immune system is usually able to control infection at the planktonic stage leading to bacterial clearance and effective prevention of infection progression.

In the case of implant-related infections, the implant is recognized as a foreign body that induces an innate immune reaction. The release of anti-microbial peptides, ROS, NOS, and NETs and "frustrated" phagocytosis of the non-phagocytosable material leads to cell exhaustion, cell death, and tissue damage. Thus, an immune compromised environment with reduced bacterial killing is established around the implant [reviewed in (37, 41, 56)]. Additionally, the implant creates a niche for bacteria to evade the host defense by hiding in structural pores of the surface that are inaccessible for the larger immune cells (41). So, the foreign material makes clearance of planktonic bacteria ineffective, which ultimately results in bacterial persistence and chronicity of infection.

In a mouse model of chronic implant-associated *S. aureus* osteomyelitis, it was shown that biofilm formation on contaminated implants already started on the first day after surgery. Between days 3 and 7, a strong proliferation of bacteria and biofilm growth took place, and the maturation of biofilm reached its maximum around day 14, when proliferation declined, and bacterial dispersal became apparent. The biofilm then stayed stable over the remaining study period for up to 56 days (57). This means that the planktonic window in which an effective bacterial clearance could take place is rather small and that during the course of implant-related bone infections, the immune system is almost entirely confronted with biofilm (**Figure 1**). The following findings explain at least in part the immune privileged nature of mature biofilms (**Figure 2**).

The biofilm itself plays an important role in shielding the embedded bacteria against the immune cells and protects the bacteria from immune cell recognition. Mature biofilm consists of a dense extracellular polymeric matrix, which is difficult to penetrate and engulf by phagocytes (58). On the other hand, the EPS contains PAMPs, which normally induce a pro-inflammatory immune response through TLR signaling. However, in the context of biofilms, exopolysaccharides such as PIA, which represent the main matrix component, are associated with immune evasion and protection against innate defense mechanisms (52, 59). Extracellular DNA (eDNA) is an EPS component that consists of eukaryotic DNA from host cells (e.g., through NET formation by PMNs) as well as prokaryotic DNA released by QS-controlled autolysis of bacteria. eDNA has an important role in stabilizing the biofilm matrix and in horizontal gene transfer (52, 60). Bacterial DNA is highly immunogenic and can be recognized by TLR9 (61). For *S. aureus* biofilms however, it was shown that biofilms evade TLR2 and TLR9 recognition. Possible explanations are that the exposure of PAMPs due to the biofilm-shielded bacteria is reduced, and polysaccharides of the biofilm EPS may interfere with TLR-ligand engagement (58, 62). In *Pseudomonas aeruginosa* biofilms, eDNA seems to induce a pro-inflammatory and anti-microbial neutrophil response, as neutrophil activity against *in vitro* biofilms is reduced after DNase treatment (63). However, eDNA also induces increased tolerance against anti-microbial peptides (64). Besides physical and chemical protection, biofilm formation leads to an acidic, hypoxic and nutrient-deprived local environment, which alters immune cell metabolism and activation (65). The release of toxins by the biofilm embedded bacteria further impairs immune cell function and induces cell death (66, 67).

Biofilm is not completely protected against recognition by phagocytic cells (68). *In vitro* data indicate that leukocytes are able to adhere to biofilms and penetrate them under laminar-shear conditions. This is followed by the production of pro-inflammatory cytokines in response to young and mature biofilms; however, the cells were not able to phagocytose the biofilm-embedded bacteria (69). In samples of patients with implant-associated bone infections, Wagner et al. isolated highly activated PMNs, which showed a reduced ability to migrate and a high production of superoxides. The authors concluded that like in planktonic infections, PMNs infiltrate the site of infection and get locally activated but then are unable to effectively clear the biofilm embedded bacteria. Instead, PMNs remain at the site of infection where they release cytotoxic products that contribute to host tissue destruction but do not effectively control the infection (70, 71). Other *in vitro* experiments confirmed the release of granule proteins and DNA by PMNs as a response to biofilm exposure, but in contrast to the study of Leid et al., they could also observe phagocytosis of biofilm bacteria (72). Effective phagocytosis normally depends on the opsonization of bacteria by antibodies and complement factors (73). In contrast to planktonic bacteria, phagocytosis of biofilm by PMNs seems to be independent of opsonization as serum treatment of biofilms did not enhance bacterial uptake. However, reduced deposition of IgG and C3b on biofilm-embedded bacteria contributes to their ineffective killing by PMNs, which may be due to other mechanisms such as a decreased ROS production (74, 75). The biofilm destruction by PMNs was dependent on its maturation stage: whereas immature biofilm (day 2 and 6) was infiltrated and cleared by PMNs at least *in vitro*, mature biofilm (day 15) was shown to be more tolerant against the host immune response (76). This can be explained by the increased biofilm mass making it more difficult for the immune cells to penetrate and engulf the biofilm, but also by an altered gene expression profile of the biofilm embedded bacteria as a reaction to attacking phagocytic cells. Up-regulation for example of the accessory gene regulator (*agr*) locus, which encodes for a staphylococci QS system that activates multiple pathogenicity factors, leads to increased tolerance against immune cell killing and phagocytosis (77, 78). Data from a mouse post-arthroplasty infection model revealed that the recruitment of neutrophils to the site of infection depends on IL-1β. Moreover, the respective knock-out mice showed decreased numbers of neutrophils with more biofilm formation indicating that neutrophils reduce biofilm burden at least to some extent (62). Consistent with these findings, IL-1β expression was decreased during biofilm infection in a mouse catheter-biofilm model (58). Macrophages can either be activated via the classical route which results in a more pro-inflammatory subtype (M1) related to bacterial killing, or via the alternative route which induces a more anti-inflammatory/regulatory and pro-fibrotic subtype (M2) (79). In the mouse catheter-biofilm model, it was shown that biofilm skews infiltrating macrophages from the M1 toward the M2 subtype, as evidenced by a decrease in inducible nitric oxide synthases (iNOS) and an increase in arginase-1 (Arg-1) production. Ultimately, this induced an

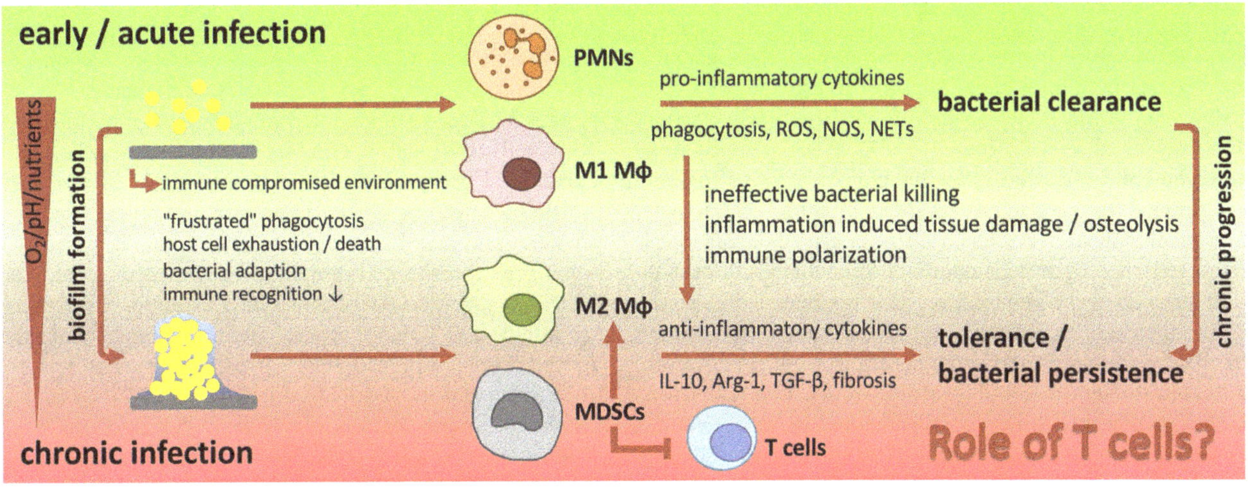

FIGURE 2 | Changing immune response during biofilm formation and chronic progression of implant-related bone infections. Planktonic infections are usually spontaneously cleared by the innate immune system. Neutrophils and classically activated (M1) macrophages are the pre-dominant cell populations that induce a pro-inflammatory cytokine milieu, release antimicrobial products, and phagocytose bacteria. In implant-associated infections the foreign material itself induces an immune reaction. As a result, an immune compromised environment around the implanted device is established that is characterized by an ineffective immune response against the non-phagocytosable material, dysfunction of immune cells and immune cell death. Bacteria take advantage of the foreign material and the impaired immune reaction and start to colonize the implant and form a biofilm. Biofilm-embedded bacteria can adapt to the host defense mechanisms, which results in a decreased immune recognition and enhanced bacterial survival and persistence. The unresolved inflammation is then associated with tissue damage and in the case of bone infections with osteolysis. Additionally, biofilm formation influences the local environment and induces a hypoxic, nutrient-deprived and acidic milieu that further impairs immune cell function. As a consequence, biofilms skew the immune system toward an anti-inflammatory response with a pre-dominantly alternative (M2) macrophage polarization and a high number of immune suppressive MDSCs that are known to inhibit T cell immunity and to induce immune tolerance. Ultimately, this leads to chronicity of infection. The role of T cells in the defense against chronic implant-associated infections is not fully understood and only a few studies focus on this topic. PMNs, polymorphonuclear neutrophils; Mϕ, macrophage; MDSCs, myeloid-derived suppressor cells; ROS, reactive oxygen species; NOS, nitrogen species; NETs, neutrophil extracellular traps; IL-10, interleukin-10; Arg-1, arginase-1; TGF-β, transforming growth factor-beta.

anti-inflammatory and more pro-fibrotic response preventing effective phagocytosis and bacterial killing (58). The deposition of a fibrotic matrix around the biofilm associated with an alternative macrophage response prevented immune cells from infiltrating the site of infection, which further promoted bacterial persistence. This biofilm-mediated immune suppression was overcome by an early administration of classically activated (M1) macrophages or the treatment with the C5a receptor agonist EP67, which induces a pro-inflammatory macrophage phenotype and indeed resulted in reduced biofilm formation (80). The mechanistic details of how biofilms can polarize macrophages are not completely understood, but one explanation can be an altered immunometabolism. Planktonic bacteria pre-dominantly induce aerobic glycolysis, which provides necessary intermediates for anabolic processing of pro-inflammatory effector molecules such as ROS and NO. Biofilms instead lead to a more anti-inflammatory response, which is generally associated with oxidative phosphorylation (OxPhos). Biofilm formation changes the environmental conditions, which alters the metabolic profiles of macrophages toward OxPhos and anti-inflammation [reviewed in (65)].

Myeloid-derived suppressor cells (MDSCs) are described as a heterogeneous cell population consisting of immature monocytes (M-MDSCs) and granulocytes (G-MDSCs) initially found to suppress T cell activation (81). Typically, these cells differentiate into neutrophils, Mϕs and dendritic cells (DCs) at the site of inflammation, but under chronic conditions such as cancer or chronic infections, respectively, MDSCs arrest in an immature state and promote a negative regulation of the immune system (82). By this, MDSCs have an important role in keeping the balance between long-lasting inflammation and tissue damage, but also contribute to disease chronicity. The mechanisms behind biofilm-mediated MDSC accumulation and arrest have not been determined yet and are important aspects of future research. The group of Tammy Kielian found a remarkable presence of MDSCs in a mouse orthopedic biofilm model (83) as well as in samples from patients with prosthetic joint infections that underwent revision surgery (84, 85). MDSC levels increased continuously after the onset of biofilm formation and then stabilized after chronic progression of infection (85). MDSCs are known to inhibit the pro-inflammatory activation of macrophages. Antibody-mediated depletion of MDSCs within the mouse model therefore resulted in improved bacterial clearance (83). Enhanced numbers of MDSCs and M2 macrophages were also found in a rat PJI model. Additionally, *in vitro* experiments showed that the biofilm was able to induce the differentiation of M-MDSCs into anti-inflammatory M2-like macrophages (86). Using knock-out models for IL-12 or IL-10, the group of Tammy Kielian showed that the presence of IL-12 was required for the recruitment of MDSCs to the site of infection (85), but that the immune suppressive action of MDSCs was mediated by release of IL-10, a cytokine known to shift macrophage polarization toward an anti-inflammatory phenotype (87). The loss of IL-12 or IL-10 resulted in lower numbers of MDSCs, enhanced presence of pro-inflammatory monocytes, increased bacterial clearance and decreased biofilm burden. Adoptive transfer of wild-type MDSCs restored MDSC influx and immune suppressive action with aggravated disease outcome (85, 87). MDSC-derived Arg-1 only showed a minimal effect on biofilm growth. Instead, Arg-1 seemed to play a role in host immune cell activity against planktonic bacteria, which again confirmed the divergent immune responses against planktonic and biofilm infections (88).

The last step of the biofilm lifecycle is the release of bacteria back into their planktonic stage. By this, the bacteria become re-accessible for antibiotics and host defense mechanisms; however, this can also be linked to the spreading of infection and sepsis (43, 89). Furthermore, there is evidence that bacteria released from mature biofilms induce an increased pro-inflammatory reaction when compared to their planktonic counterparts that further supports inflammation-associated tissue destruction and infection relapse (90).

Role of T Cells

T cells belong to the adaptive immunity and mediate the specific immune response. They can be divided into cluster of differentiation (CD)4-positive helper T cells and CD8-positive cytotoxic T cells. Cytotoxic CD8 T cells directly eliminate infected cells through the release of cytotoxic proteins. CD4 helper T cells need to get activated by professional antigen presenting cells (APCs) in order to support a cellular and humoral immune response. T cell activation occurs after binding of an antigen- major histocompatibility complex (MHC)-complex to a T cell receptor (TCR) and further requires costimulation by binding of CD28 present on T cells to CD80/86. Depending on the cytokine environment, CD4 helper T cells differentiate into Th1, Th2, and Th17 subtypes as well as regulatory T cells (T_{reg}s) (91). The contribution of T cells during the immune response against chronic implant-related bone infections is not fully determined and there are some contradictory data about the presence, effector function and inhibition of T cells at the site of biofilm infections that will be addressed in the following section (**Tables 1A,B**).

Studies using human tissue samples indicate that CD4 and CD8 T cells are present at the site of implant-related biofilm infections (92, 93). T cells isolated from the infectious samples showed a high proportion of $CD28^-/CD11b^+$ cells that indicates terminally differentiated T effector cells. These cells further produced high levels of perforin and IFN-γ typical for cytotoxic T cells which are classically associated with virus infections (**Table 1A**) (93–95). Whether this T cell response participates in infection defense or contributes to bone destruction by promoting osteoclastogenesis is yet unknown and has to be addressed in future studies. Mouse models showed that chronic implant-related bone infections can have a pronounced pro-inflammatory Th1 and Th17 response that is unable to clear infections at an early stage (**Table 1B**) (97, 99). Indeed, an early induction of a Th2/T_{reg} based response was able to prevent chronicity of infection (98). Heim et al. found only low numbers of T cells at the site of orthopedic biofilm infections in human samples (**Table 1A**) (84, 85) as well as in the corresponding mouse model (**Table 1B**) (83). The authors explain this with a high presence of MDSCs in their samples (see section above) (83) and they showed that the MDSCs, in particular G-MDSCs, suppressed T cell proliferation throughout the course of infection (83, 96). This fits with the finding of Kumar et al. who reported a reduced T cell proliferation in patient samples from chronic prosthesis infection (93). Along with inhibiting local T cell proliferation, MDSCs were associated with decreased T cell homing to the site of infection by down-regulated L-selectin (CD62L) expression (100), which might additionally explain the low numbers of T cell infiltrates. The mediators behind MDSC-derived T cell suppression are not clear yet, but this seems to be independent of IL-10 and IL-12 (85, 87). Besides that, Heim et al. found that the effects of MDSC-mediated immune suppression were more obvious on phagocytic cells (monocytes and neutrophils) than on T cells. The absence of MDSC action in the orthopedic biofilm mouse model led to an increased influx of monocytes and neutrophils and restored pro-inflammatory activity of these cells and resulted in decreased bacterial burden (83, 85, 87). Interestingly, in the same mouse model, PMNs as well as monocytes also exhibited suppressive activity on T cell proliferation after biofilm had developed (96). Besides playing a major role in innate immunity against pathogens, PMNs are discussed to directly interact with T cells. They are assumed to be able to activate T cells through MHC class II–mediated antigen-presentation as well as to exert an immune suppressive action on T cells by depletion of L-arginine via Arg-1 thereby exhibiting a more MDSC-like phenotype (101). This indicates that biofilm maturation potentially changes the initial pro-inflammatory PMN function toward a more anti-inflammatory action, which might then have an additional impact on the T cell response during infection progression.

Brady et al. compared the immune response in subcutaneous mouse models of acute and chronic implant-related biofilm *S. aureus* infection. By analyzing cytokine and chemokine levels of respective tissues using proteomic arrays, they found increased cytokine levels indicating a promoted pro-inflammatory Th1/Th17 response in their biofilm model. This was associated with down-regulated chemokine levels and decreased T cell homing to the site of infection, creating a strong pro-inflammatory reaction with low T cell infiltration (102). Interestingly, by comparing early (day 7) with late (day 21) biofilm infection in their chronic infection model, they found a similar cytokine response during the course of infection, which did not show any remarkable changes, but simply decreased when the infection become chronic. This is explained partly by the fact that at this time most bacteria are metabolically inactive and production of virulence factors and pro-inflammatory mediators has declined. Further research is needed to investigate possible additional factors that play a role in the dampened response after biofilm formation and chronicity of infection.

The activation of naïve T cells by APCs is an essential step of the T cell response. It is therefore conceivable that an altered APC function can lead to an ineffective T cell immunity against biofilms. Likely, APCs are already impaired by the implant and contribute to the immune

TABLE 1A | T cell response against implant-related bone infections—human studies.

Research question	Approach	Major findings	References
Characterization of leukocyte infiltrates and cytokine expression in PJI samples compared to aseptic loosening.	• Samples from endoprosthesis patients with PJI or aseptic loosening were analyzed for leukocyte counts and subtypes (FACS) and cytokines (Multiplex Assay).	➢ Higher leukocyte numbers in infected vs. aseptic samples. ➢ Higher numbers of G-MDSCs in infected vs. aseptic samples (no difference in neutrophils or monocytes). ➢ Reduced T cell numbers in infected vs. aseptic samples (non-significant). ➢ Increased levels of IL-10, IL-6 and CXCL-1 in infected vs. aseptic samples. ➢ **Accumulation of immune suppressive G-MDSCs in PJIs prevents activation of antimicrobial effector mechanisms by this leading to infection persistence.**	(84)
Characterization of leukocyte infiltrates and cytokine expression in PJI and aseptic human samples for comparison with data from a mouse orthopedic infection model.	• Samples from endoprosthesis patients with PJI or aseptic loosening were analyzed for leukocyte counts and subtypes (FACS) and cytokines (qPCR, Multiplex Assay).	➢ Increased MDSC-like and reduced T cell numbers with elevated pro-inflammatory cytokine levels in infected compared to aseptic human samples. ➢ **Comparable immune response during orthopedic biofilm infection between mouse and human system.**	(85)
Analysis of T cell activity in human tissue samples after infectious vs. aseptic implant loosening.	• FACS, histological and gene expression analysis of T cell infiltrates in tissue samples from patients undergoing infectious or aseptic revision surgery.	➢ Increased numbers of $CD28^{-}CD11b^{+}$ (activated) CD4 or CD8 T cells in infected samples vs. aseptic samples. ➢ Increased expression of T cell marker CD3 and no differences of monocyte marker CD14 and osteoclast marker cathepsin K in infected vs. aseptic samples. ➢ **Enhanced numbers of activated T cells in implant-associated infection.**	(92)
Characterization of T cell phenotype in chronically infected vs. non-infected bone samples.	• Analysis of cortical bone samples from patients undergoing primary prosthetic surgery (non-infected) and samples from patients undergoing revision surgery (chronically infected) by multiparametric FACS.	➢ Presence of CD4 and CD8 T cells in both samples, increased HLA-DR expression on T cells and reduced T cell proliferation in infected vs. non-infected samples, no T_{reg}s or T cell apoptosis in infected samples. ➢ Increase of $CD28^{-}$ CD4 T cells and $CD80^{+}$, $CD40^{+}$ and $CD40L^{+}$ CD4 and CD8 T cells in infected vs. non infected samples. ➢ Increased perforin and CD11b and decreased CD7 expression in $CD28^{-}$ T cells. ➢ Increased number of (long-term activated) cytotoxic $CD28^{-}$ CD4 T cells with reduced proliferation capacity in chronically infected bones.	(93)
Analysis of systemic and local T cell activation in patients with implant-associated bone infections.	• Blood and lavage from site of infection were taken from patients with implant-associated bone infections and analyzed by FACS for T cell activation markers.	➢ Upregulation of CD11b and loss of CD28 on CD4 T cells in blood samples of infected patients compared to healthy donors. ➢ Increased expression of TLR1,2,4 associated with $CD11b^{+}CD28^{-}$ CD4 T cells in blood samples of infected patients. ➢ Accumulation of $CD11b^{+}CD28^{-}$ CD4 T cells and $CD57^{+}$ CD8 T cells at site of infection. ➢ Increased IFN-γ expression by T cells from site of infection. ➢ **Recruitment and activation of CD4 and CD8 effector T cells in patients with implant-associated bone infections.**	(94)
Analysis of T cell infiltration in patients with implant-associated bone infections compared to patients with sterile joint inflammation.	• Blood and lavage from site of infection were taken from patients with implant-associated bone infections and analyzed by FACS for T cell markers. • As control synovial fluid from patients with rheumatoid arthritis (RA) was used.	➢ Loss of CD62L expression by T cells isolated from the infection or inflammation site compared to respective blood sample. ➢ Shift of local CD4/CD8 ratio toward CD8 in infected and CD4 in RA patients. ➢ Perforin and granzyme B expression by CD8 T cells at site of infection. ➢ Detection of $CD28^{+}$ and $CD28^{-}$ subpopulation in lavage with increased CD11b and CD57 expression on $CD28^{-}$ CD8 T cells. ➢ **Expansion and infiltration of cytotoxic CD8 effector T cells in patients with implant-associated bone infections.**	(95)

Bold text indicates key finding of the respective study.

TABLE 1B | T cell response against implant-related bone infections—mouse models.

Research question	Approach	Major findings	References
Characterization of invading MDSC subpopulations in a mouse orthopedic biofilm infection model.	• Insertion of a K-wire in femora of C57BL/6 mice and inoculation of 10^3 CFU *S. aureus* (SA) at the implant tip. • Analysis of infiltrating leukocyte populations by FACS, cytospin, *in vivo* proliferation assay, *in vitro* T cell activation capacity and RNA sequencing on days 3, 7, 14, and 28.	➢ Identification of $CD11b^{high}$ granulocytic MDSCs and $CD11b^{low}$ PMNs. ➢ **G-MDSCs proliferate at the site of biofilm infection and suppress T cell response over the whole course of infection (planktonic and biofilm phase), whereas PMNs show immune suppressive activity only after biofilm development.**	(96)
Monitoring of the immune reaction during sterile or infected bone healing in an implant-stabilized mouse fracture model.	• Fixation of a SA pre-incubated osteosynthetic device (9 × 10^5 CFU/implant) and creation of an osteotomy in femora of C57BL/6 mice. • Quantitative microbiology and analysis of immune response by histology, FACS, qPCR, and Multiplex Cytokine Assay over 35 days.	➢ Positive cultures over whole period with highest bacterial loads on days 1–3. ➢ Complete bone healing in non-infected controls by day 35, non-union with osteolysis in infected animals. ➢ Minimal inflammatory cell infiltration in controls on day 3 with signs of tissue healing on day 7, increased invasion of inflammatory cells in infected animals on day 3 with strong inflammation/osteolysis on day 7. ➢ Increased cell numbers in lymph nodes and spleen of infected animals. ➢ Increased IL-4 and late IFN-γ expression in controls and increased IL-17, TNF-α, IL-1β, and IL-10 expression in infected animals. ➢ **Bone healing is associated with sustained Th2 and late Th1 and bone infection with a central Th17 and pro-inflammatory response unable to control infection (with decrease in bone healing markers TGF-β and PDGF).**	(97)
Role of MDSC-derived IL-10 in MDSC-mediated immune suppression in orthopedic biofilm infections.	• Insertion of a K-wire in femora of C57BL/6 wt and IL-10 ko mice and inoculation of 10^3 CFU SA at the implant tip. • Adoptive transfer experiments of wt MDSCs in IL-10 ko mice. • Analysis of bacterial burden by SA recovery, MDSC and monocyte/Mϕ invasion and cytokine profile by ELISA, FACS, cytokine array and qPCR on days 3, 7, and 14 and analysis of *in vitro*-derived wt and IL-10 ko MDSC activity by T cell proliferation assay.	➢ Infiltrating MDSCs are the main source of increased IL-10 levels in orthopedic implant biofilm infections. ➢ Decreased MDSCs and increased monocyte/Mϕ recruitment in IL-10 ko mice on day 14 with enhanced pro-inflammatory activity of monocytes/Mϕ and decreased bacterial burden. Partly reversible by adoptive transfer of wt MDSCs. No changes in neutrophil and T cell infiltrates in IL-10 ko mice. ➢ Inhibition of T cell proliferation by biofilm-associated MDSCs is independent of IL-10. ➢ **MDSC-derived IL-10 induces an anti-inflammatory monocyte phenotype at the site of biofilm infection that promotes bacterial persistence, but has no direct effect on T cell proliferation.**	(87)
Role of IL-12 in MDSC recruitment and MDSC-mediated immune suppression in orthopedic biofilm infections.	• Insertion of a K-wire in femora of C57BL/6 wt and IL-12 ko mice and inoculation of 10^3 CFU SA at the implant tip. • Adoptive transfer experiments of wt MDSCs in IL-12 ko mice. • Analysis of bacterial burden by SA recovery, MDSC and monocyte/Mϕ invasion and cytokine profile by ELISA, FACS, cytokine array and qPCR on days 7, 14, 21, and 28, CT and histology and analysis of MDSC activity isolated from site of infection of wt and IL-12 ko mice by T cell proliferation assay. • Comparison of data with human samples of PJIs.	➢ Detection of bacteria during the whole period with strong inflammation of infected tissue and bone destruction. ➢ Increased cytokine (IL-12, IL-1β, TNF-α, and G-CSF) and chemokine levels in infected animals, associated with increased MDSC and neutrophil and reduced monocyte/Mϕ and early T cell invasion compared to aseptic samples. ➢ IL-12 ko mice show decreased MDSC recruitment and decreased cytokine levels with enhanced monocyte and neutrophil infiltration and decreased bacterial burden compared to wt mice. ➢ Adoptive transfer of wt MDSCs in IL-12 ko mice reduces monocyte and neutrophil invasion and leads to increased bacterial burden compared to wt mice. ➢ MDSC isolated from site of infection in IL-12 ko mice are able to inhibit T cell proliferation like MDSC from wt mice. ➢ **IL-12 promotes MDSC accumulation at the site of infection, causing a MDCS-mediated reduction of monocyte and neutrophil invasion. No direct role of IL-12 in activation of immune suppressive MDSC function and T cell proliferation.**	(85)

(Continued)

TABLE 1B | Continued

Research question	Approach	Major findings	References
Role of MDSCs and MDSC-mediated T cell suppression in orthopedic biofilm infections.	• Insertion of a K-wire in femora of C57BL/6 mice and inoculation of 10^3 CFU SA at the implant tip. • Antibody-mediated depletion of MDSC *in vivo*. • Histological, Multiplex cytokine array, FACS and qPCR analysis of tissue samples, T cell proliferation assay and monocyte co-culture experiments.	➢ Increased numbers of MDSCs in samples of infected animals vs. non-infected controls on day 7. ➢ MDSCs isolated from infected tissue inhibit T cell proliferation and cytokine secretion. ➢ MDSC depletion reduce biofilm burden (mainly by restoring pro-inflammatory activity of monocyte). ➢ **Biofilm-associated MDSCs inhibit T cell response.**	(83)
Prevention of chronicity of an implant-associated biofilm infection through a Th1↓/Th2↑ polarized immune reaction.	• Implantation of SA pre-treated pins (3×10^5 CFU/pin) in tibiae of Th1-biased C57BL/6, Th2-biased Balb/c and STAT6 ko Balb/c mice. • Treg depletion in Balb/c with anti-CD25 and Th1 suppression in C57BL/6 with anti-IL12p40 treatment. • Analysis of bacterial clearance, Treg frequency and local cytokine profile on days 7 and 21.	➢ Spontaneous bacterial clearance in ~75% of Balb/c mice. ➢ Higher levels of IL-4 and IL-10 and T_{reg} frequency in Balb/c and increased neutrophil infiltration in C57BL/6 mice. ➢ STAT6 ko and T_{reg} depletion lead to loss of protection in Balb/c mice. ➢ Anti-IL12p40 treatment induces bacterial clearance in ~40% of C57BL/6 mice. ➢ **Early induction of Th2/T_{reg} and suppression of Th1/Th17 response protects from chronicity.**	(98)
Investigation of immune response during chronic progression of an implant-associated biofilm infection.	• Implantation of SA pre-treated pins (2×10^5 CFU/pin) in tibiae of C57BL/6 mice. • Analysis of activated immune cells, antibody production and local cytokine up to day 28.	➢ Activation of a CD4 T cell response, early production of Th1-IgG subtype IgG2b and local pro-inflammatory cytokine profile in infected animals. ➢ **An early Th1 and Th17 and reduced T_{reg} immune response is ineffective to prevent infection and leads to chronicity.**	(99)

Bold text indicates key finding of the respective study.

compromised environment and increased bacterial colonization. Two biodegradable and biocompatible materials that are known to provoke a normal foreign body response were tested for DC activation and subsequent DC-mediated T cell proliferation and polarization in the presence or absence of *S. aureus* and *S. epidermidis*, respectively (103). The authors found that the biomaterials alone did not induce DC activation and subsequent DC-mediated T cell activation, but in combination with bacteria, DCs had a slightly changed cytokine secretion profile. However, these changes were too small to affect subsequent T cell activation. Thus, the presence of a foreign material does not impair APC-mediated T-cell activation upon bacterial exposure. The altered cytokine secretion by DCs stimulated by bacteria in the presence of a biomaterial could still have an impact on other immune cells like PMNs and macrophages which can promote bacterial survival. In this study only planktonic bacteria were used to stimulate DCs in the presence of a biomaterial. Therefore, the influence of biofilm formed on the biomaterial and potential changes in DC and subsequent T cell activation remain to be investigated.

So far, there are only a few studies that address the T cell response in chronic implant-associated bone infections and results argue for the presence of activated cytotoxic T cells at the site of biofilm formation and an early pro-inflammatory Th1/Th17 response. However, the decreased homing to the site of biofilm infection and a reduced T cell proliferation and potentially impaired function might trigger the formation of biofilm-associated suppressive immune cells.

It has to be taken into consideration that mouse studies that investigate the immune response against implant-related bone infections usually use *S. aureus* to induce biofilm-infections (**Table 1B**). However, *S. aureus* is a highly virulent pathogen that causes a strong pro-inflammatory Th1 immune response in planktonic infections (102) and early and acute bone infections (30). It needs to be investigated whether the findings also apply for less virulent bacteria like *S. epidermidis* that is associated with less symptomatic but chronic implant-infections. A recent study compared *S. aureus* and *S. epidermidis* -induced implant-associated osteomyelitis in mice (104). This study revealed that *S. aureus* caused osteolysis, reactive bone formation and abscess formation, whereas this was not apparent in *S. epidermidis* infection. Both bacteria colonized the implant and formed biofilm. The findings underline the different roles of *S. aureus* and *S. epidermidis* in chronic implant-related bone infections. In human studies, the cohorts include patients with implant-related bone infections caused by different bacteria and the time point of revision surgery and immune analysis might depend on the virulence of the respective bacteria. So, it is possible that different stages of biofilm infection are within the same cohort. This might explain the apparently conflicting findings in T cell quantities between the different studies (84, 92). Investigations of T cells in implant-related bone infections have been restricted to the evaluation of numbers and types of T cells present at the site of biofilms. The functionality of biofilm-associated T cells and the mechanisms behind the T cell response have not been examined yet. Apparently, there is a need for further research to investigate the insufficient T cell response during biofilm formation and chronic progression of implant-related bone infections in more detail.

Humoral Immune Response

The identification of a protective humoral immunity (105) and biofilm-associated antigens raised the hope for vaccination strategies (106). Indeed, administration of a multicomponent and protein-based vaccine before bacterial challenge with subsequent antibiotic treatment significantly reduced the risk for infection in a biofilm model of osteomyelitis in rabbits (107). Passive immunization against implant-related osteomyelitis in mice with neutralizing antibodies associated with protective immunity in orthopedic infections led to reduced bacterial burden, osteolysis, and abscess formation, respectively, due to increased opsonophagocytosis of bacterial megaclusters by recruited macrophages (108, 109). A current study showed that a combinatory approach using passive immunization together with antibiotic and surgical treatment was capable of reducing re-infection in a mouse model of MRSA-induced implant-related osteomyelitis, thereby enabling osseointegration and bone healing (110). Despite this promising animal data, unfortunately, attempts to develop an effective vaccination strategy for humans have been unsuccessful so far (111).

Role of the Bone Environment

Due to the crosstalk between bone and immune cells, cells of the bone environment (OBs, OCs, MSCs) are also involved in the course of bone infection. A pro-inflammatory immune cell environment induces a shift in bone homeostasis toward increased osteoclastogenesis and bone resorption, which is further supported by local osteoblasts that can release pro-inflammatory proteins in response to bacteria (112, 113). Dapunt et al. showed that expression of pro-inflammatory proteins by osteoblasts is not only induced by planktonic bacteria but also by biofilm components. This indicates that OBs not only play a role in the host response against biofilm-associated infections, but also enhance osteolysis associated with these infections (114, 115). Besides an increased osteoclastogenesis, new bone deposition by osteoblasts is reduced as the infectious environment and bacterial internalization lead to decreased mineralization and increased apoptosis of osteoblastic cells (116). Release of internalized bacteria and dying osteoblasts might further impair the immune response against the bacteria.

In the case of osteosynthetically stabilized fractures, implant-associated bone infections impair the healing process and can lead to non-unions. During bone regeneration, the host response against bacteria and biofilm seems to interfere with the naturally occurring immune reaction required to induce the healing cascade. This unresolved pro-inflammatory environment is ineffective to clear the infection and at the same time is detrimental to bone regeneration (97, 117). MSCs as osteogenic precursor cells have an important role in bone healing (118). They are also known to have immune modulatory activity and exert an immune suppressive effect on T cells (119), which might impact the development and progression of bone infections. Indeed, in a rat plate-stabilized ostectomy-model, local implantation of MSCs to improve bone regeneration aggravated implant-associated bone infections (120).

These data indicate that implant-associated bone infections and septic non-unions are characterized by a complex interplay between bacteria, cells of the immune system, and cells of the bone environment.

Osteoclasts as Immune Competent Cells

Besides being the main players in bone resorption, osteoclasts are part of the immune system and interact with immune cells, especially with T cells [reviewed in (121, 122)]. Interactions are ambilateral with T cells influencing osteoclastogenesis and OCs having an impact on T cell activity. Activated T cells express RANKL which stimulates the differentiation of human monocytes into mature osteoclasts (123). Th17 helper cells and their cytokine IL-17 are shown to enhance osteoclastogenesis, while the Th1 and Th2 cytokines IFN-γ and IL-4 are associated with an anti-osteoclastogenic potential (124, 125). T_{reg}s were proven to have an inhibitory effect on osteoclast generation [reviewed in (126)]. In addition to the anti-osteoclastogenic effects of T_{reg}-derived cytokines IL-10 and TGF-β, direct cell-cell contact through binding of cytotoxic T-lymphocyte-associated protein-4 (CTLA-4) to CD80/86 on osteoclast precursors inhibits osteoclastogenesis (127) (more information on this are provided in the following section about immune modulation). OCs can function as antigen presenting cells that can activate T cells upon antigen exposure (128). However, a suppressive effect of OCs on the *in vitro* T cell response via the induction of indoleamine 2,3-dioxygenase (IDO) was also described (129, 130). Furthermore, OCs can prime CD8 T cells toward a regulatory phenotype (OC-iTc_{reg}) which then again has a suppressive effect on T cell activation and inhibit osteoclastogenesis [reviewed in (131)]. Taken together, it can be said that osteoclast precursors share many of the immune suppressive characteristics that have been associated with MDSCs (121, 132).

So far, research investigating the immunological function of osteoclasts has been done under sterile conditions either in *in vitro* experiments or in animal models of sterile bone loss, such as inflammatory arthritis or osteoporosis. Whether similar findings can be obtained in an infectious setting such as implant-associated bone infections need further investigations.

In summary, the implant as a foreign material as well as the bacteria, especially in form of a biofilm, lead to a dysregulation of the immune response and misbalance of bone homeostasis in favor of bacterial persistence, bone destruction and infection chronicity. We suggest that this impaired osteoimmunological environment represents an attractive target for modulation, making immune therapy an interesting approach for the treatment of chronic implant-related bone infections.

MODULATION OF THE IMMUNE RESPONSE DURING CHRONIC IMPLANT-RELATED BONE INFECTIONS

Enormous effort has been put into the development of new antibiotics, anti-microbial coatings of the implant, vaccination strategies as well as interruption of the QS system to avoid biofilm formation and chronicity of implant-related bone infections, yet with limited success (32). Modulation of the immune system is a promising field in treating chronic diseases and offers the potential to combine current therapeutic and surgical strategies while strengthening endogenous defense mechanisms. Especially the success of immune therapy in cancer treatment encourages to take a broader view and transfer novel approaches into other diseases. The following section will address what is known about immune therapy in other chronic diseases and discuss whether there are targets for immune modulation that might allow treating chronic implant-related bone infections (**Figure 3** and **Table 2**).

Immune Regulation During Chronic Diseases

Immune responses are tightly regulated to prevent an unresolved immune reaction, which would lead to long-lasting inflammation and tissue damage. The regulation of this process is mediated by cells of the innate and adaptive immune system including immune suppressive MDSCs, anti-inflammatory (M2) Mϕ and regulatory T_{reg}s that help to generate an immune microenvironment characterized by high levels of IL-10, Arg-1 and TGF-β (133). In general, this limits the pro-inflammatory effector phase, which ends with antigen clearance, resolution of inflammation and the induction of an immunological memory. In contrast, disease continuation and long-term exposure to antigens, as it occurs in tumors or chronic infections, induce an enhanced up-regulation of inhibitory molecules by immune cells. Ultimately, this leads to immune cell dysfunction associated with ineffective control and persistence of disease. Upon long-term stimulation, T cells increasingly express inhibitory receptors, known as "immune checkpoint molecules," of which CTLA-4 and programmed cell death protein-1 (PD-1) are the most prominent members. Binding of their respective ligands expressed on immune and non-immune cells leads to T cells with low or diminished effector functions that are called anergic or exhausted T cells. T cell dysfunction has moved into the focus of interest as it can be reversed by the use of immune checkpoint inhibitors (ICIs), which makes them an attractive target for re-stimulation of the immune response [reviewed in (134)]. Blockade of immune checkpoints has been successfully introduced into certain cancer treatments (135) and is discussed as a treatment option for infectious diseases such as malaria, HIV (136) and sepsis (137). Furthermore, Fc-fusion proteins of immune checkpoint molecules are currently being investigated for their use as immune suppressive therapy e.g., in autoimmune disorders (138). Immune therapy therefore includes immune activating and immune suppressing approaches, both of which represent attractive targets for treatment of chronic infections depending on the local immune environment.

Immune Activation or Suppression in Chronic Implant-Related Bone Infections

Long-lasting interactions of bacteria, biofilm components, and host cells that occur in chronic implant-related bone infections severely impair the immune response. Thus, immune therapy can be an interesting tool to restore appropriate immune function. As suggested by the literature, chronic implant-related bone infections initially provoke a more pro-inflammatory immunity. This is then dampened to a more anti-inflammatory and immune tolerant response during the chronic course of infection, which prevents tissue damage but also contributes to bacterial persistence. However, pro- and anti-inflammation cannot be simply attributed to different stages of the disease as they occur simultaneously throughout the course of infection. Favoring one above the other would risk to further aggravate immune pathology. The immune reaction during the early planktonic phase is additionally impaired by the presence of the implant, whose influence has to be considered in immune therapeutic intervention. Furthermore, the type of bacteria plays an important role in the induced immune response; highly virulent strains like *S. aureus* cause strong pro-inflammatory immune reactions, whereas more benign strains such as *S. epidermidis* induce rather moderate and subtle immune responses. All this has to be considered when an immune therapeutic approach is suggested because non-specific boosting of the immune system might end in hyper-inflammation causing tissue damage, while immune inhibition might lead to increased bacterial burden, bacteremia and/or secondary infections. To avoid such conceivable scenarios, we should learn from the lessons already made in sepsis immune-stimulatory therapy which has so far failed to reliably and safely improve patient outcome (139, 140), before introducing immune modulation in the treatment of chronic implant-related bone infections: (1) The immune response is changing throughout the infection, therefore correct timing of therapeutic intervention is indispensable to ensure immune stimulation or inhibition. (2) The immune status of leukocytes can differ depending on the location (lymphoid organs, peripheral blood or site of infection). Systemic immune stimulation/inhibition might not be appropriate and a more tissue/infection site-specific approach should be preferred. Specification can be provided by targeting immune molecules depending on the cell subsets they are preferentially expressed, anatomic prevalence of their expression and/or their distinguished function (141). (3) The immune profile can be highly heterogeneous between patients. Personalized immune therapy should be provided to optimize individual outcome and predictive immune biomarkers should be included in the decision-making for the respective therapeutic target to guarantee responsiveness and minimize adverse effects (135). As the targets of immune modulation have unique functions, combinatory approaches can improve efficacy of immune therapeutic treatment (142). The combination of modulators of innate immune defense with classical ICI targeting adaptive immunity and/or cell-based therapeutic vaccination would allow treatment at multiple levels. However, to ensure optimum patient outcome and safety, immune therapeutics can only be used as medication in addition to current antibiotic and surgical treatment options.

Targeting Immune Checkpoint Molecules

The first ICI approved for therapy of advanced melanoma was an antibody against CTLA-4 (ipilimumab) in 2011 (143, 144). CTLA-4 is a homologous but antagonistic and competitive receptor for CD28 that has a higher affinity for binding

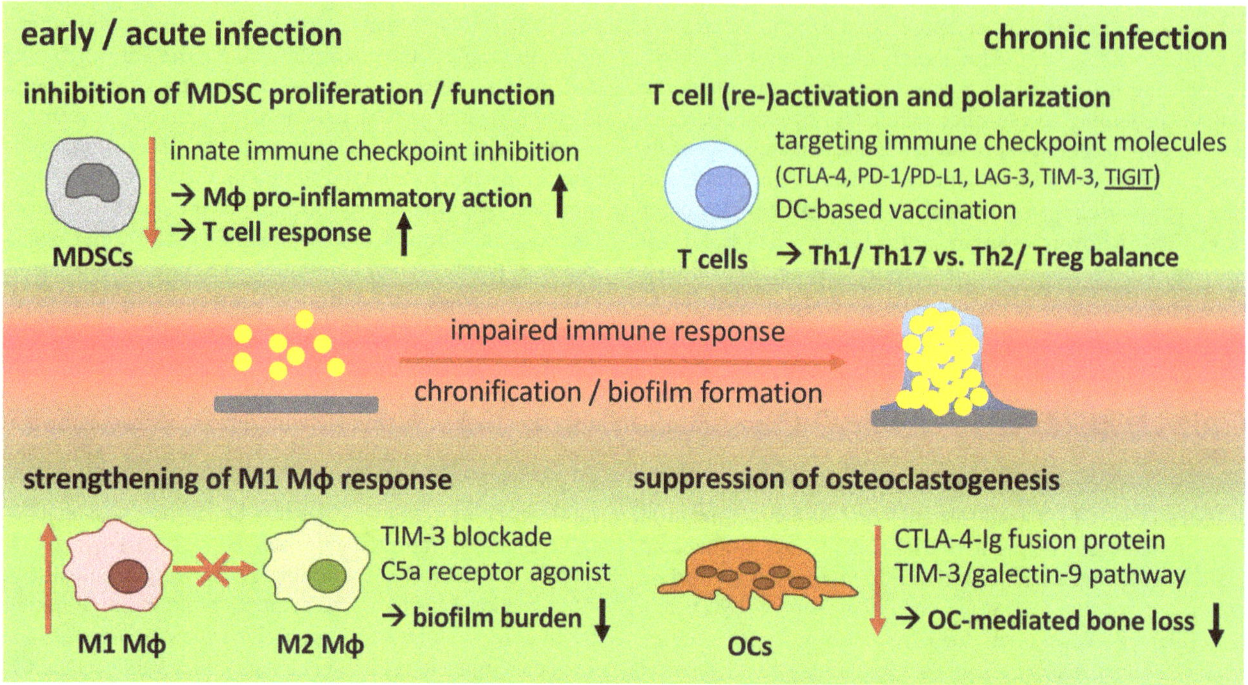

FIGURE 3 | Potential targets for immune modulation during chronic progression of implant-related bone infections. Biofilm formation skews the immune response toward an anti-inflammatory, immune inhibitory and tolerant environment that is associated with high numbers of MDSCs, M2 macrophages, and an ineffective T cell response. Immune modulation by therapeutic intervention offers the possibility to generate a more effective immune response that supports bacterial killing and the reduction of biofilm burden. An early inhibition of MDSC activity and the induction of a more pro-inflammatory (M1) Mϕ response are potential targets to strengthen innate defense mechanisms. Re-stimulation of T cell effector functions by targeting immune checkpoint molecules can overcome T cell dysfunction caused by chronic disease progression and might prevent re-infection after revision surgery. Targeting TIGIT as well as using DC-based vaccination strategies may provide the opportunity to direct T cell polarization toward Th1 or Th2 -dominated responses. When boosting the immune system, its impact on inflammatory tissue destruction has to be considered as a balance between anti-bacterial activity and cytotoxicity is required. CTLA-4 and the TIM-3/galectin-9 pathway are important immune regulators that can also be used as checkpoints to control osteoclast numbers as a means to reduce bone resorption. MDSCs, myeloid-derived suppressor cells; Mϕ, macrophage; DC, dendritic cell; OCs, osteoclasts; ICI, immune checkpoint inhibitor; CTLA-4, cytotoxic T-lymphocyte-associated protein-4; PD-1/PD-L1, programmed cell death protein-1/PD ligand-1; LAG-3, lymphocyte activation gene-3; TIM-3, T cell immunoglobulin and mucin-domain containing protein-3; TIGIT, T cell immunoglobulin and ITIM domain.

CD80/86 than CD28. Binding of CTL-4 to CD80/86 results in transendocytosis of CD80/86 and inhibition of T cell co-stimulation. Under physiological conditions, CTLA-4 plays an important role in ensuring self-tolerance. The administration of anti-CTLA-4 antibodies proved to be efficient in tumor control but at the same time showed a high incidence of adverse effects and autoimmunity. Activation of this pathway can therefore be a promising approach to treat autoimmune disorders [reviewed in (145)]. Treatment with a soluble CTLA-4-Ig fusion protein (abatacept), which links the extracellular domain of human CTLA-4 to a fragment of the Fc part of human IgG1 (146), was successful in reducing the symptoms of rheumatoid arthritis (RA) (147). However, it aggravated the course of septic arthritis in a mouse model (148). To our knowledge, nothing is known about a potential role of CTLA-4-mediated inhibition of CD28 in chronic implant-related bone infections. Most T cells isolated from blood and tissue of patients undergoing infection-induced revision surgery were shown to be CD28^{-} (92, 93), which might indicate that in chronicity, the majority of effector T cells would not respond to CTLA-4 based therapy. Interestingly, it was shown that binding of CTLA-4 to CD80/86 expressed on the surface of murine bone marrow leukocytes and human blood monocytes directly inhibited RANKL and TNF-mediated differentiation of these cells into osteoclasts *in vitro* and reduced osteoclast formation and bone resorption in an arthritic joint model in mice (149). This suggests that CTLA-4 can be considered as an anti-osteoclastogenic molecule. The inhibitory effect of CD80/86 engagement by CTLA-4 on osteoclastogenesis was further investigated by Bozec et al., who found that induction of apoptosis in osteoclast precursor cells via the IDO/tryptophan pathway was responsible for the reduced osteoclast formation. As expected, the CTLA-4-Ig fusion protein abatacept led to reduced numbers of osteoclast precursor cells and osteoclasts in RA patients and in cell culture experiments. Blocking CTLA-4 with the neutralizing antibody ipilimumab increased the osteoclastogenic potential in humans (150). These data indicate that targeting checkpoint molecules like CTLA-4 provide the opportunity to control osteoclast numbers and bone homeostasis. Still, it has to be considered that in an

TABLE 2 | Potential targets for immune modulation during chronic implant-related bone infections.

		Target	Mechanism	Potential benefit for chronic implant-related bone infections
T cell immunity		CTLA-4	Competitive binding of CD80/86 and inhibition of T cell co-stimulation. Anti-CTLA-4 antibodies restore T cell activation.	Isolated T cells from chronic implant-related bone infections are mostly $CD28^{-}$. Usefulness of CTLA-4 to re-activate T cells after chronicity of infection is therefore questionable.
		PD-1/PD-L1	Induction of effector T cell exhaustion. Blocking this pathway by antibodies restores T cell function.	Role of exhausted T cells in chronicity of bone infections is unclear. Cells of the bone environment (MSCs, OCs) express PD-L1 upon inflammation, therefore inhibition of this pathway might decrease bone cell-mediated T cell suppression.
		LAG-3/TIM-3/TIGIT	Inhibition of APC-mediated T cell activation and Th1/Th17 -mediated T cell response.	Blood T cells from patients with chronic osteomyelitis show increased expression of LAG-3 and impaired proliferation/function. Hence, LAG-3 blockade can increase T cell activation in chronic implant-related bone infections. An early Th2/T_{reg} immunity was shown to prevent biofilm formation and chronicity in a murine orthopedic implant infection model. TIGIT treatment at an early time point can be supportive to clear infections via induction of a Th2-based T cell response.
Innate immunity	MDSCs	Innate IC molecules	Controlling MDSC proliferation and function.	MDSCs are associated with an anti-inflammatory environment in chronic implant-related bone infections. Eliminating MDSCs can prevent unwanted immune suppression and strengthen pro-inflammatory immune reactions.
	Mϕ	TIM-3	Inhibitory receptor on Mϕs, by this suppressing a pro-inflammatory response.	Chronic implant-related bone infections are associated with a shift toward an anti-inflammatory (M2) Mϕ phenotype which supports bacterial persistence. Blockade of TIM-3 can strengthen a pro-inflammatory (M1) Mϕ response and enhance bacterial killing.
		C5a receptor	Binding of C5a receptor influences Mϕ polarization.	Targeting Mϕ polarization via C5a receptor ligands can prevent formation of anti-inflammatory (M2) Mϕs associated with chronic infection. Early treatment with a C5a receptor agonist induces a pro-inflammatory (M1) Mϕ response which leads to reduced biofilm burden in a mouse implant-infection model (80).
	DCs	Antigen presentation	Induction of an antigen-specific T cell immunity and desired T cell differentiation.	The role of DCs in chronic implant-related bone infections is unclear, but DC therapy could allow the generation of biofilm-specific DCs and the induction of a more effective host immune response.
Osteoclastogenesis		CTLA-4	Inhibition of osteoclastogenesis through binding to CD80/86 on monocytes. Administration of a CTLA-4-Ig fusion protein reduces osteoclast numbers.	Bone infections are associated with high numbers of osteoclasts and increased bone resorption, CTLA-4 treatment can reduce inflammation-induced bone destruction.
		TIM-3/galectin-9	Binding of galectin-9 to TIM-3 expressed on osteoclast precursors suppresses osteoclastogenesis.	Targeting the TIM-3/galectin-9 pathway can reduce osteoclast formation and bone loss in chronic implant-related bone infections.

auto-inflammatory environment, treatment with CTLA-4 is beneficial in reducing osteoclastogenesis, but under infectious conditions it might suppress necessary immune activity and by this potentially aggravate disease progression. Thus, immune checkpoint-mediated inhibition of osteoclastogenesis can be a promising target to decrease inflammation-induced bone resorption and reduce bacterial colonization of damaged tissue, but additional impairment of the immune response has to be excluded.

The best studied immune checkpoint molecule is PD-1 and its ligands PD-L1 and PD-L2, which are targeted to treat T cell dysfunction in cancer and chronic infectious diseases. Compared to CTLA-4, which acts at the level of T cell activation, PD-1 is up-regulated on effector T cells after continuous stimulation. Thus, the PD-1/PD-L1 pathway suppresses activity and function of effector T cells and induces T cell exhaustion (144). Several antibodies targeting the PD-1/PD-L1 pathway have been approved for the treatment of specific cancers and new therapeutics as well as new applications are currently investigated in clinical trials (135). Antibodies against PD-1/PD-L1 have also been transferred into treatment approaches for chronic virus diseases and malaria to improve CD4 and CD8 effector T cell function (136). Additionally, they were shown to have the potential to reverse sepsis-induced immune suppression (137). Negative side effects of PD-1/PD-L1 blockade seem to be less frequent when compared to CTLA-4 treatment. However, nearly half of the patients do not respond to PD-1 blockade alone (136) and combinatory therapy was shown to be more effective, albeit more toxic (151). The role of PD-L2 has not yet been fully clarified: initially, PD-L2 was described as a second ligand for PD-1 that negatively influences T cell immunity (152, 153). A costimulatory function of PD-L2 and the initiation of a Th1 response is also discussed (154). PD-L2 is furthermore suggested to counteract PD-1/PD-L1-mediated T cell exhaustion making a soluble PD-L2 fusion protein an attractive candidate to block the PD-1/PD-L1 pathway (136, 155). In an *in vitro* setting with *S. epidermidis* strains isolated from patients with orthopedic implant loosening, it was shown that after phagocytic uptake SCVs trigger an anti-inflammatory macrophage response with up-regulated PD-L1/L2 expression so that they are able to survive intracellularly without damaging the host cell (156). Whether this also applies to biofilm embedded bacteria has not been investigated yet. Furthermore, MSCs, which are in close contact to the site of bone infections, up-regulate PD-L1/L2 expression and secretion upon stimulation with pro-inflammatory cytokines (157, 158) or induce PD-L1 expression in DCs after exposure to LPS (159). By this, they directly and indirectly inhibit T cell proliferation and function. It can be speculated that the PD-1/PD-L1 pathway might play a role in the persistence of implant-related bone infections. Until now, to our knowledge there is nothing described about an up-regulation of PD-1 on T cells and PD-L1/L2 on host cells associated with biofilm formation during chronic progression of implant-related bone infections. As chronic implant-related bone infections were linked to high numbers of $CD28^-$ T cells (92–94) and as it was shown recently that CD28 is indispensable for effectiveness of PD-1 blockade (160, 161), it remains to be seen whether these patients would indeed profit from a PD-1/PD-L1 targeted therapy. OCs were found to mediate their immune suppressive action through galectin-9 and PD-L1 expression and induction of PD-L1 expression on tumor cells in multiple myeloma (162, 163). As OCs are highly present at the site of bone infection, PD-L1 antibodies that can decrease OC-mediated T cell inhibition might enhance T cell immunity in chronic implant-related bone infections.

Lymphocyte activation gene-3 (LAG-3), T cell immunoglobulin and mucin-domain containing protein-3 (TIM-3) and T cell immunoglobulin and ITIM domain (TIGIT) are other immune checkpoint molecules that are currently explored as targets for immune therapy. LAG-3 is up-regulated on CD4 and CD8 T cells as well as on natural killer cells (NK cells). It affects effector T cell function and T_{reg} suppressive activity by binding to MHC class II with higher affinity than CD4 or LSECtin (liver and lymph node sinusoidal endothelial cell C-type lectin). Since LSECtin is involved in antigen uptake (164) and MHC class II is essential for antigen presentation, LAG-3 is suggested to impair the antigen-specific signal in T cell activation [reviewed in (141, 142)]. Indeed, an increased expression of LAG-3 was found on T cells in blood samples of patients suffering from chronic osteomyelitis and was associated with impaired T cell proliferation and function (165). This gives a hint that LAG-3 blockade could be a potential approach for treating chronic implant-associated bone infections. Furthermore, a soluble Lag-3-Ig fusion protein (IMP321) has been shown to lead to APC activation via MHC class II, thus being a candidate to support APC-mediated immunity (166, 167). TIM-3 is expressed on DCs and Mϕs as well as on activated CD4 T cells, predominantly of the Th1 type, CD8 T cells and NK cells [reviewed in (142)]. Via interaction with galectin-9, TIM-3 plays a protective role in autoimmunity by regulating the Th1 response and subsequent macrophage activation (168), triggering cell death (169), and increasing MDSC expansion (170). In cancer and chronic virus infections, high TIM-3 expression was linked to T cell dysfunction. Co-blockade of PD-1 and TIM-3 is superior at improving anti-tumor and anti-viral effector function than PD-1 inhibition alone [reviewed in (141)]. In line with this, TIM-3 expressing T_{reg}s showed an increased expression of suppressive molecules and were highly effective in inhibiting Th1/Th17 immune responses (171). Furthermore, high expression levels of TIM-3 on Mϕs are associated either with a quiescent state or an anti-inflammatory (M2) phenotype. Blockade of the TIM-3 pathway therefore may result in a more efficient pro-inflammatory (M1) macrophage response (172) which was shown to reduce biofilm burden in a catheter-associated biofilm infection model in mice (80). Binding of galectin-9 to TIM-3 expressed on osteoclast precursor cells suppressed osteoclast formation and thereby attenuated inflammatory bone loss in adjuvant-induced arthritis (173) indicating a further therapeutic application of the TIM-3/galectin-9 system next to modulating the immune response. TIGIT is a co-inhibitory receptor present on activated T cells, NK cells and T_{reg}s and competes with its stimulatory counterpart CD226 for binding of CD155 expressed on APCs, T cells and non-immune cells. CD226 predominantly promotes a Th1/Th17 response with high levels of IFN-γ and IL-17, whereas binding of TIGIT induces a shift toward a Th2 and IL-10 dominated immunity. Therefore, TIGIT interacts with APCs, effector T cells as well as T_{reg}s to dampen pro-inflammatory immune responses at multiple levels in favor of a more tolerogenic immune environment [reviewed in (141)]. Prabhakara et al. showed that an early shift from a Th1/Th17 response toward a Th2/T_{reg} immunity was capable of preventing biofilm formation and chronicity of an orthopedic implant infection in mice (98). TIGIT treatment to strengthen a Th2 dominated response might therefore be a supportive strategy in clearing implant-related bone infections at an early stage.

Lag-3, TIM-3, and TIGIT are suggested to regulate immune function at the site of tissue inflammation to inhibit immune pathology, whereas CTLA-4 and PD-1 act more systemically. Because their primary role is to maintain immune homeostasis and self-tolerance in the healthy organism, the first three are predicted to be less toxic (141). Furthermore, due to their specialized roles either at the stage of T cell activation or T cell effector function, molecules from these two groups might exert synergistic effects and provide a more efficient therapeutic outcome when used in combination (142).

Targeting Innate Immunity

Next to directly improving T cell immunity, another approach is to target innate immune cells and modulate the immune response in a more general way. High MDSC activation and accumulation are found in various cancers where they inhibit T cell proliferation and function, leading to tumor tolerance (174). MDSCs are associated with inflammation-induced tumor progression, as they are activated by pro-inflammatory IL-1β that subsequently induces a tumor-promoting IL-10-dominated environment and an anti-inflammatory (M2) macrophage response (175, 176). Heim et al. showed that MDSC-derived IL-10 is responsible for the anti-inflammatory monocyte response and bacterial persistence in an orthopedic biofilm infection model (87). This indicates that there are some common characteristics between these two chronic diseases. Furthermore, MDSCs express ICI ligands that can directly impair T cell function (177) and also reduce the efficacy of immune checkpoint inhibitors in cancer therapy (178). Therefore, targeting MDSCs in combination with ICI is a promising approach to improve patient outcome (179). Next to the application of approved therapeutics that are effective in reducing MDSC numbers and/or function (e.g., all-trans retinoic acid), the investigation of new drugs that eliminate MDSCs is of high interest. An innate immune checkpoint inhibitor that targets MDSC proliferation and function is currently being investigated in a phase 1 clinical trial (INB_{03}) (180). MDSCs contribute to the immune compromised environment in implant-related bone infections and to the chronicity of infection. An early inhibition of MDSC function could be a possible approach to circumvent unwanted immune suppression directly at the onset of infection. In combination with a strict antibiotic treatment this might be able to clear the infection before biofilm manifestation and might prevent bacterial persistence.

Another approach is to directly target macrophage polarization. As tumors and chronic infections are associated with an environment favoring an anti-inflammatory (M2) macrophage response and immune suppression, shifting the balance toward the more pro-inflammatory (M1) macrophage subtype might increase the ability to kill tumor cells and bacteria (181).

Hanke et al. used a cell transfer of exogenously M1-activated Mϕs or administration of a C5a receptor agonist (EP67) in a catheter-associated infection model in mice, which resulted in a pronounced pro-inflammatory Mϕ response and in a reduction of biofilm burden (80). M1 Mϕ not only prevented biofilm formation when injected at an early time point of infection, but were also capable of reducing established biofilms, whereas antibiotic treatment had no effect. This indicates that redirection toward a pro-inflammatory milieu can attenuate mature biofilms. DCs are antigen-presenting cells that activate T cells and induce adaptive defense mechanisms (91). This makes them an attractive tool for immune stimulatory treatment of chronic diseases. Different strategies have been reported and include vaccination strategies with autologous and *ex vivo*-generated DCs that had been stimulated with tumor antigens. After re-injection, these cells can induce an effective anti-cancer immunity through priming of a Th1 and specific cytotoxic T cell response. However, *ex vivo* manipulation is expensive and includes a high risk of infection. The *in vivo* targeting of DCs by antibodies coupled with the respective antigens specifically binding to DC receptors involved in antigen presentation is an attractive alternative [reviewed in (182)]. The role of DCs in the unsuccessful immune response against implant-related bone infections and a potential contribution to biofilm formation has not been investigated so far. Targeting DCs offers the possibility to control the type of T cell response and to induce a biofilm-specific T cell immunity by loading them with biofilm-antigens. Therefore, DC therapy might be an attractive approach to improve a specific host immune defense against implant-related bone infections.

In summary, immune modulation can be a promising approach to restore a desired immune microenvironment during the course of chronic implant-related bone infections: an early immune modulatory intervention might be able to inhibit biofilm formation and inflammation-associated tissue destruction, and might allow the elimination of infection at its onset. After chronic progression of the infection, a comprehensive approach combining surgical removal of infectious tissue, antibiotic treatment and strengthening of the host immune response might improve therapeutic outcome. The combination of rifampin and immune re-activation might be a strategy to eliminate mature biofilms that can increase the chance for surgical regimes with implant retention. After implant exchange, strengthening the specific immunity against the initial infection can help provide an immune response that is able to eliminate potentially remaining bacteria (persister cells) and prevent re-infection. It needs to be clarified in future studies whether the activation of a biofilm-specific immune response by immune therapy is sufficient to combat mature biofilm and other sources of bacterial persistence (SCVs, canalicular propagation) independent of surgical and antibiotic treatment. However, more basic research is needed to address whether an immune modulatory intervention can be a useful treatment strategy in implant-related osteomyelitis. As immune therapy is associated with adverse immune reactions, a safe and beneficial application has to be ensured before applying immune therapeutic approaches into patients with chronic implant-related bone infections.

CONCLUDING REMARKS

Chronic implant-related bone infections are a major problem in orthopedic and trauma surgery. As numbers of joint replacements are rising, complications such as bone infections also increase. Current treatment options are associated with severe consequences for patients and often fail to eliminate the infection. The high risk of chronicity for such infections is due to successful evasion strategies of bacteria with biofilm formation being one major mechanism behind bacterial persistence. The presence of a foreign material facilitates biofilm formation and further supports the persistence of an infection. Thus, there is a high interest to clear infections already at the planktonic stage before biofilm transition occurs and to prevent reinfection after antibiotic and surgical treatment. For this, however, novel therapeutic strategies are required. Immune therapy shows promising results in the treatment of different chronic diseases and strengthening endogenous defense mechanisms could be an attractive new approach for chronic implant-related bone infections. So far, investigations of the immune response against chronic implant-related bone infections demonstrate a discrepancy between a strong pro-inflammatory immune reaction that is associated with osteoclastogenesis and bone destruction, and an immune suppression that potentially impairs successful bacterial killing. Future treatment strategies involving the immune system have to consider this two-sided immune response to avoid adverse reactions. Since the amount of information is limited, the success of immune therapeutic intervention in chronic implant-related bone infections mostly remains speculative and further research is needed to investigate appropriate and safe targets. Furthermore, it has to be clarified if an immune modulatory approach is also capable of targeting bacterial persistence e.g., within biofilms. Immune modulation can serve as an additional and required medical treatment option to restore an effective host response. It is to be hoped that the combination of antibiotic and surgical treatment with immune therapeutic intervention may lead to the successful management of chronic implant-related bone infections in the future.

AUTHOR CONTRIBUTIONS

ES reviewed the relevant literature and wrote the manuscript. KK critically revised the manuscript. Both authors have read and approved the manuscript.

FUNDING

ES was funded by the Physician Scientist Program of the Medical Faculty of Heidelberg. We acknowledge the financial support of the Deutsche Forschungsgemeinschaft (DFG) and the Ruprecht-Karls-Universität Heidelberg within the funding program Open Access Publishing.

ACKNOWLEDGMENTS

We thank Nikolas Stevens for technical support and Christy Yu for critically proofreading the manuscript.

REFERENCES

1. Tande AJ, Patel R. Prosthetic joint infection. *Clin Microbiol Rev.* (2014) 27:302–45. doi: 10.1128/CMR.00111-13
2. Zimmerli W, Trampuz A, Ochsner PE. Prosthetic-joint infections. *N Engl J Med.* (2004) 351:1645–54. doi: 10.1056/NEJMra040181
3. Kurtz SM, Lau E, Watson H, Schmier JK, Parvizi J. Economic burden of periprosthetic joint infection in the United States. *J Arthroplasty.* (2012) 27:61–5 e1. doi: 10.1016/j.arth.2012.02.022
4. Kunutsor SK, Whitehouse MR, Blom AW, Beswick AD, Team I. Re-infection outcomes following one- and two-stage surgical revision of infected hip prosthesis: a systematic review and meta-analysis. *PLoS ONE.* (2015) 10:e0139166. doi: 10.1371/journal.pone.0139166
5. Kunutsor SK, Whitehouse MR, Lenguerrand E, Blom AW, Beswick AD, Team I. Re-infection outcomes following one- and two-stage surgical revision of infected knee prosthesis: a systematic review and meta-analysis. *PLoS ONE.* (2016) 11:e0151537. doi: 10.1371/journal.pone.0151537
6. Marculescu CE, Berbari EF, Hanssen AD, Steckelberg JM, Harmsen SW, Mandrekar JN, et al. Outcome of prosthetic joint infections treated with debridement and retention of components. *Clin Infect Dis.* (2006) 42:471–8. doi: 10.1086/499234
7. Lee J, Kang CI, Lee JH, Joung M, Moon S, Wi YM, et al. Risk factors for treatment failure in patients with prosthetic joint infections. *J Hosp Infect.* (2010) 75:273–6. doi: 10.1016/j.jhin.2010.03.012
8. Spencer J, Smith A, Woods D. The effect of time delay on infection in open long-bone fractures: a 5-year prospective audit from a district general hospital. *Ann R Coll Surg Engl.* (2004) 86:108–12. doi: 10.1308/003588404322827491
9. Darouiche RO. Treatment of infections associated with surgical implants. *N Engl J Med.* (2004) 350:1422–9. doi: 10.1056/NEJMra035415
10. Okike K, Bhattacharyya T. Trends in the management of open fractures. A critical analysis. *J Bone Joint Surg Am.* (2006) 88:2739–48. doi: 10.2106/00004623-200612000-00025
11. Khosla S. Minireview: the OPG/RANKL/RANK system. *Endocrinology.* (2001) 142:5050–5. doi: 10.1210/endo.142.12.8536
12. Raggatt LJ, Partridge NC. Cellular and molecular mechanisms of bone remodeling. *J Biol Chem.* (2010) 285:25103–8. doi: 10.1074/jbc.R109.041087
13. Kolar P, Schmidt-Bleek K, Schell H, Gaber T, Toben D, Schmidmaier G, et al. The early fracture hematoma and its potential role in fracture healing. *Tissue Eng Part B Rev.* (2010) 16:427–34. doi: 10.1089/ten.teb.2009.0687
14. Wright JA, Nair SP. Interaction of staphylococci with bone. *Int J Med Microbiol.* (2010) 300:193–204. doi: 10.1016/j.ijmm.2009.10.003
15. Lazzarini L, Mader JT, Calhoun JH. Osteomyelitis in long bones. *J Bone Joint Surg Am.* (2004) 86-A:2305–18. doi: 10.2106/00004623-200410000-00028
16. Lew DP, Waldvogel FA. Osteomyelitis. *Lancet.* (2004) 364:369–79. doi: 10.1016/S0140-6736(04)16727-5
17. Zimmerli W, Sendi P. Orthopaedic biofilm infections. *APMIS.* (2017) 125:353–64. doi: 10.1111/apm.12687
18. Schierholz JM, Beuth J. Implant infections: a haven for opportunistic bacteria. *J Hosp Infect.* (2001) 49:87–93. doi: 10.1053/jhin.2001.1052
19. Trampuz A, Zimmerli W. Diagnosis and treatment of infections associated with fracture-fixation devices. *Injury.* (2006) 37(Suppl 2):S59–66. doi: 10.1016/j.injury.2006.04.010
20. Metsemakers WJ, Kuehl R, Moriarty TF, Richards RG, Verhofstad MHJ, Borens O, et al. Infection after fracture fixation: current surgical and microbiological concepts. *Injury.* (2018) 49:511–22. doi: 10.1016/j.injury.2016.09.019
21. Metsemakers WJ, Morgenstern M, McNally MA, Moriarty TF, McFadyen I, Scarborough M, et al. Fracture-related infection: a consensus on definition from an international expert group. *Injury.* (2018) 49:505–10. doi: 10.1016/j.injury.2017.08.040
22. Loffler B, Tuchscherr L, Niemann S, Peters G. Staphylococcus aureus persistence in non-professional phagocytes. *Int J Med Microbiol.* (2014) 304:170–6. doi: 10.1016/j.ijmm.2013.11.011
23. Khalil H, Williams RJ, Stenbeck G, Henderson B, Meghji S, Nair SP. Invasion of bone cells by Staphylococcus epidermidis. *Microbes Infect.* (2007) 9:460–5. doi: 10.1016/j.micinf.2007.01.002
24. Valour F, Trouillet-Assant S, Rasigade JP, Lustig S, Chanard E, Meugnier H, et al. Staphylococcus epidermidis in orthopedic device infections: the role of bacterial internalization in human osteoblasts and biofilm formation. *PLoS ONE.* (2013) 8:e67240. doi: 10.1371/journal.pone.0067240
25. Campoccia D, Testoni F, Ravaioli S, Cangini I, Maso A, Speziale P, et al. Orthopedic implant infections: incompetence of *Staphylococcus epidermidis*, *Staphylococcus lugdunensis*, and *Enterococcus faecalis* to invade osteoblasts. *J Biomed Mater Res A.* (2016) 104:788–801. doi: 10.1002/jbm.a.35564

26. de Mesy Bentley KL, Trombetta R, Nishitani K, Bello-Irizarry SN, Ninomiya M, Zhang L, et al. Evidence of *Staphylococcus aureus* deformation, proliferation, and migration in canaliculi of live cortical bone in murine models of osteomyelitis. *J Bone Miner Res.* (2017) 32:985–90. doi: 10.1002/jbmr.3055
27. Costerton JW, Stewart PS, Greenberg EP. Bacterial biofilms: a common cause of persistent infections. *Science.* (1999) 284:1318–22. doi: 10.1126/science.284.5418.1318
28. Hoiby N, Ciofu O, Johansen HK, Song ZJ, Moser C, Jensen PO, et al. The clinical impact of bacterial biofilms. *Int J Oral Sci.* (2011) 3:55–65. doi: 10.4248/IJOS11026
29. Leid JG. Bacterial biofilms resist key host defenses. *Microbe.* (2009) 4:66–70.
30. Li C, Renz N, Trampuz A. Management of periprosthetic joint infection. *Hip Pelvis.* (2018) 30:138–46. doi: 10.5371/hp.2018.30.3.138
31. Zimmerli W, Moser C. Pathogenesis and treatment concepts of orthopaedic biofilm infections. *FEMS Immunol Med Microbiol.* (2012) 65:158–68. doi: 10.1111/j.1574-695X.2012.00938.x
32. Moriarty TF, Kuehl R, Coenye T, Metsemakers WJ, Morgenstern M, Schwarz EM, et al. Orthopaedic device-related infection: current and future interventions for improved prevention and treatment. *EFORT Open Rev.* (2016) 1:89–99. doi: 10.1302/2058-5241.1.000037
33. Lebeaux D, Ghigo JM, Beloin C. Biofilm-related infections: bridging the gap between clinical management and fundamental aspects of recalcitrance toward antibiotics. *Microbiol Mol Biol Rev.* (2014) 78:510–43. doi: 10.1128/MMBR.00013-14
34. Jones RE, Russell RD, Huo MH. Alternatives to revision total knee arthroplasty. *J Bone Joint Surg Br.* (2012) 94:137–40. doi: 10.1302/0301-620X.94B11.30620
35. Zimmerli W, Waldvogel FA, Vaudaux P, Nydegger UE. Pathogenesis of foreign body infection: description and characteristics of an animal model. *J Infect Dis.* (1982) 146:487–97. doi: 10.1093/infdis/146.4.487
36. Lucke M, Schmidmaier G, Sadoni S, Wildemann B, Schiller R, Stemberger A, et al. A new model of implant-related osteomyelitis in rats. *J Biomed Mater Res B Appl Biomater.* (2003) 67:593–602. doi: 10.1002/jbm.b.10051
37. Zimmerli W, Sendi P. Pathogenesis of implant-associated infection: the role of the host. *Semin Immunopathol.* (2011) 33:295–306. doi: 10.1007/s00281-011-0275-7
38. Arciola CR, Campoccia D, Speziale P, Montanaro L, Costerton JW. Biofilm formation in Staphylococcus implant infections. A review of molecular mechanisms and implications for biofilm-resistant materials. *Biomaterials.* (2012) 33:5967–82. doi: 10.1016/j.biomaterials.2012.05.031
39. Gristina AG. Biomaterial-centered infection: microbial adhesion versus tissue integration. *Science.* (1987) 237:1588–95. doi: 10.1126/science.3629258
40. Busscher HJ, van der Mei HC, Subbiahdoss G, Jutte PC, van den Dungen JJ, Zaat SA, et al. Biomaterial-associated infection: locating the finish line in the race for the surface. *Sci Transl Med.* (2012) 4:153rv10. doi: 10.1126/scitranslmed.3004528
41. Arciola CR, Campoccia D, Montanaro L. Implant infections: adhesion, biofilm formation and immune evasion. *Nat Rev Microbiol.* (2018) 16:397–409. doi: 10.1038/s41579-018-0019-y
42. Otto M. Staphylococcal biofilms. *Curr Top Microbiol Immunol.* (2008) 322:207–28. doi: 10.1007/978-3-540-75418-3_10
43. Boles BR, Horswill AR. Staphylococcal biofilm disassembly. *Trends Microbiol.* (2011) 19:449–55. doi: 10.1016/j.tim.2011.06.004
44. Kong KF, Vuong C, Otto M. Staphylococcus quorum sensing in biofilm formation and infection. *Int J Med Microbiol.* (2006) 296:133–9. doi: 10.1016/j.ijmm.2006.01.042
45. Yarwood JM, Schlievert PM. Quorum sensing in Staphylococcus infections. *J Clin Invest.* (2003) 112:1620–5. doi: 10.1172/JCI20442
46. Henke JM, Bassler BL. Bacterial social engagements. *Trends Cell Biol.* (2004) 14:648–56. doi: 10.1016/j.tcb.2004.09.012
47. Kaufmann GF, Park J, Janda KD. Bacterial quorum sensing: a new target for anti-infective immunotherapy. *Expert Opin Biol Ther.* (2008) 8:719–24. doi: 10.1517/14712598.8.6.719
48. del Pozo JL, Patel R. The challenge of treating biofilm-associated bacterial infections. *Clin Pharmacol Ther.* (2007) 82:204–9. doi: 10.1038/sj.clpt.6100247
49. Proctor RA, von Eiff C, Kahl BC, Becker K, McNamara P, Herrmann M, et al. Small colony variants: a pathogenic form of bacteria that facilitates persistent and recurrent infections. *Nat Rev Microbiol.* (2006) 4:295–305. doi: 10.1038/nrmicro1384
50. Singh R, Ray P, Das A, Sharma M. Role of persisters and small-colony variants in antibiotic resistance of planktonic and biofilm-associated *Staphylococcus aureus*: an *in vitro* study. *J Med Microbiol.* (2009) 58:1067–73. doi: 10.1099/jmm.0.009720-0
51. Garcia LG, Lemaire S, Kahl BC, Becker K, Proctor RA, Denis O, et al. Antibiotic activity against small-colony variants of *Staphylococcus aureus*: review of *in vitro*, animal and clinical data. *J Antimicrob Chemother.* (2013) 68:1455–64. doi: 10.1093/jac/dkt072
52. Watters C, Fleming D, Bishop D, Rumbaugh KP. Host responses to biofilm. *Prog Mol Biol Transl Sci.* (2016) 142:193–239. doi: 10.1016/bs.pmbts.2016.05.007
53. Gries CM, Kielian T. Staphylococcal biofilms and immune polarization during prosthetic joint infection. *J Am Acad Orthop Surg.* (2017) 25(Suppl. 1):S20–4. doi: 10.5435/JAAOS-D-16-00636
54. Janeway CA Jr, Medzhitov R. Innate immune recognition. *Annu Rev Immunol.* (2002) 20:197–216. doi: 10.1146/annurev.immunol.20.083001.084359
55. Kawai T, Akira S. The role of pattern-recognition receptors in innate immunity: update on Toll-like receptors. *Nat Immunol.* (2010) 11:373–84. doi: 10.1038/ni.1863
56. Franz S, Rammelt S, Scharnweber D, Simon JC. Immune responses to implants - a review of the implications for the design of immunomodulatory biomaterials. *Biomaterials.* (2011) 32:6692–709. doi: 10.1016/j.biomaterials.2011.05.078
57. Nishitani K, Sutipornpalangkul W, de Mesy Bentley KL, Varrone JJ, Bello-Irizarry SN, Ito H, et al. Quantifying the natural history of biofilm formation *in vivo* during the establishment of chronic implant-associated *Staphylococcus aureus* osteomyelitis in mice to identify critical pathogen and host factors. *J Orthop Res.* (2015) 33:1311–9. doi: 10.1002/jor.22907
58. Thurlow LR, Hanke ML, Fritz T, Angle A, Aldrich A, Williams SH, et al. *Staphylococcus aureus* biofilms prevent macrophage phagocytosis and attenuate inflammation *in vivo*. *J Immunol.* (2011) 186:6585–96. doi: 10.4049/jimmunol.1002794
59. Vuong C, Voyich JM, Fischer ER, Braughton KR, Whitney AR, DeLeo FR, et al. Polysaccharide intercellular adhesin (PIA) protects Staphylococcus epidermidis against major components of the human innate immune system. *Cell Microbiol.* (2004) 6:269–75. doi: 10.1046/j.1462-5822.2004.00367.x
60. Montanaro L, Poggi A, Visai L, Ravaioli S, Campoccia D, Speziale P, et al. Extracellular DNA in biofilms. *Int J Artif Organs.* (2011) 34:824–31. doi: 10.5301/ijao.5000051
61. Dalpke A, Zimmermann S, Heeg K. CpG DNA in the prevention and treatment of infections. *Biodrugs.* (2002) 16:419–31. doi: 10.2165/00063030-200216060-00003
62. Bernthal NM, Pribaz JR, Stavrakis AI, Billi F, Cho JS, Ramos RI, et al. Protective role of IL-1beta against post-arthroplasty Staphylococcus aureus infection. *J Orthop Res.* (2011) 29:1621–6. doi: 10.1002/jor.21414
63. Fuxman Bass JI, Russo DM, Gabelloni ML, Geffner JR, Giordano M, Catalano M, et al. Extracellular DNA: a major proinflammatory component of *Pseudomonas aeruginosa* biofilms. *J Immunol.* (2010) 184:6386–95. doi: 10.4049/jimmunol.0901640
64. Lewenza S. Extracellular DNA-induced antimicrobial peptide resistance mechanisms in *Pseudomonas aeruginosa*. *Front Microbiol.* (2013) 4:21. doi: 10.3389/fmicb.2013.00021
65. Yamada KJ, Kielian T. Biofilm-leukocyte cross-talk: impact on immune polarization and immunometabolism. *J Innate Immun.* (2018): 11:280–8. doi: 10.1159/000492680
66. Scherr TD, Hanke ML, Huang O, James DB, Horswill AR, Bayles KW, et al. *Staphylococcus aureus* biofilms induce macrophage dysfunction through leukocidin AB and alpha-toxin. *MBio.* (2015) 6:e01021-15. doi: 10.1128/mBio.01021-15
67. Scherr TD, Heim CE, Morrison JM, Kielian T. Hiding in plain sight: interplay between staphylococcal biofilms and host immunity. *Front Immunol.* (2014) 5:37. doi: 10.3389/fimmu.2014.00037
68. Dapunt U, Hansch GM, Arciola CR. Innate immune response in implant-associated infections: neutrophils against biofilms. *Materials.* (2016) 9:E387. doi: 10.3390/ma9050387

69. Leid JG, Shirtliff ME, Costerton JW, Stoodley P. Human leukocytes adhere to, penetrate, and respond to *Staphylococcus aureus* biofilms. *Infect Immun.* (2002) 70:6339–45. doi: 10.1128/IAI.70.11.6339-6345.2002
70. Wagner C, Kaksa A, Muller W, Denefleh B, Heppert V, Wentzensen A, et al. Polymorphonuclear neutrophils in posttraumatic osteomyelitis: cells recovered from the inflamed site lack chemotactic activity but generate superoxides. *Shock.* (2004) 22:108–15. doi: 10.1097/01.shk.0000132488.71875.15
71. Wagner C, Kondella K, Bernschneider T, Heppert V, Wentzensen A, Hansch GM. Post-traumatic osteomyelitis: analysis of inflammatory cells recruited into the site of infection. *Shock.* (2003) 20:503–10. doi: 10.1097/01.shk.0000093542.78705.e3
72. Meyle E, Stroh P, Gunther F, Hoppy-Tichy T, Wagner C, Hansch GM. Destruction of bacterial biofilms by polymorphonuclear neutrophils: relative contribution of phagocytosis, DNA release, and degranulation. *Int J Artif Organs.* (2010) 33:608–20. doi: 10.1177/039139881003300906
73. van Kessel KP, Bestebroer J, van Strijp JA. Neutrophil-mediated phagocytosis of *Staphylococcus aureus*. *Front Immunol.* (2014) 5:467. doi: 10.3389/fimmu.2014.00467
74. Stroh P, Gunther F, Meyle E, Prior B, Wagner C, Hansch GM. Host defence against Staphylococcus aureus biofilms by polymorphonuclear neutrophils: oxygen radical production but not phagocytosis depends on opsonisation with immunoglobulin G. *Immunobiology.* (2011) 216:351–7. doi: 10.1016/j.imbio.2010.07.009
75. Kristian SA, Birkenstock TA, Sauder U, Mack D, Gotz F, Landmann R. Biofilm formation induces C3a release and protects *Staphylococcus epidermidis* from IgG and complement deposition and from neutrophil-dependent killing. *J Infect Dis.* (2008) 197:1028–35. doi: 10.1086/528992
76. Gunther F, Wabnitz GH, Stroh P, Prior B, Obst U, Samstag Y, et al. Host defence against Staphylococcus aureus biofilms infection: phagocytosis of biofilms by polymorphonuclear neutrophils (PMN). *Mol Immunol.* (2009) 46:1805–13. doi: 10.1016/j.molimm.2009.01.020
77. Scherr TD, Roux CM, Hanke ML, Angle A, Dunman PM, Kielian T. Global transcriptome analysis of Staphylococcus aureus biofilms in response to innate immune cells. *Infect Immun.* (2013) 81:4363–76. doi: 10.1128/IAI.00819-13
78. Ricciardi BF, Muthukrishnan G, Masters E, Ninomiya M, Lee CC, Schwarz EM. *Staphylococcus aureus* evasion of host immunity in the setting of prosthetic joint infection: biofilm and beyond. *Curr Rev Musculoskelet Med.* (2018) 11:389–400. doi: 10.1007/s12178-018-9501-4
79. Benoit M, Desnues B, Mege JL. Macrophage polarization in bacterial infections. *J Immunol.* (2008) 181:3733–9. doi: 10.4049/jimmunol.181.6.3733
80. Hanke ML, Heim CE, Angle A, Sanderson SD, Kielian T. Targeting macrophage activation for the prevention and treatment of Staphylococcus aureus biofilm infections. *J Immunol.* (2013) 190:2159–68. doi: 10.4049/jimmunol.1202348
81. Gabrilovich DI, Nagaraj S. Myeloid-derived suppressor cells as regulators of the immune system. *Nat Rev Immunol.* (2009) 9:162–74. doi: 10.1038/nri2506
82. Veglia F, Perego M, Gabrilovich D. Myeloid-derived suppressor cells coming of age. *Nat Immunol.* (2018) 19:108–19. doi: 10.1038/s41590-017-0022-x
83. Heim CE, Vidlak D, Scherr TD, Kozel JA, Holzapfel M, Muirhead DE, et al. Myeloid-derived suppressor cells contribute to *Staphylococcus aureus* orthopedic biofilm infection. *J Immunol.* (2014) 192:3778–92. doi: 10.4049/jimmunol.1303408
84. Heim CE, Vidlak D, Odvody J, Hartman CW, Garvin KL, Kielian T. Human prosthetic joint infections are associated with myeloid-derived suppressor cells (MDSCs): implications for infection persistence. *J Orthop Res.* (2018) 36:1605–13. doi: 10.1002/jor.23806
85. Heim CE, Vidlak D, Scherr TD, Hartman CW, Garvin KL, Kielian T. IL-12 promotes myeloid-derived suppressor cell recruitment and bacterial persistence during *Staphylococcus aureus* orthopedic implant infection. *J Immunol.* (2015) 194:3861–72. doi: 10.4049/jimmunol.1402689
86. Peng KT, Hsieh CC, Huang TY, Chen PC, Shih HN, Lee MS, et al. *Staphylococcus aureus* biofilm elicits the expansion, activation and polarization of myeloid-derived suppressor cells *in vivo* and *in vitro*. *PLoS ONE.* (2017) 12:e0183271. doi: 10.1371/journal.pone.0183271
87. Heim CE, Vidlak D, Kielian T. Interleukin-10 production by myeloid-derived suppressor cells contributes to bacterial persistence during Staphylococcus aureus orthopedic biofilm infection. *J Leukoc Biol.* (2015) 98:1003–13. doi: 10.1189/jlb.4VMA0315-125RR
88. Yamada KJ, Heim CE, Aldrich AL, Gries CM, Staudacher AG, Kielian T. Arginase-1 expression in myeloid cells regulates *Staphylococcus aureus* planktonic but not biofilm infection. *Infect Immun.* (2018) 86:IAI.00206-18. doi: 10.1128/IAI.00206-18
89. Otto M. Staphylococcal infections: mechanisms of biofilm maturation and detachment as critical determinants of pathogenicity. *Annu Rev Med.* (2013) 64:175–88. doi: 10.1146/annurev-med-042711-140023
90. Franca A, Perez-Cabezas B, Correia A, Pier GB, Cerca N, Vilanova M. *Staphylococcus epidermidis* biofilm-released cells induce a prompt and more marked *in vivo* inflammatory-type response than planktonic or biofilm cells. *Front Microbiol.* (2016) 7:1530. doi: 10.3389/fmicb.2016.01530
91. Pennock ND, White JT, Cross EW, Cheney EE, Tamburini BA, Kedl RM. T cell responses: naive to memory and everything in between. *Adv Physiol Educ.* (2013) 37:273–83. doi: 10.1152/advan.00066.2013
92. Dapunt U, Giese T, Prior B, Gaida MM, Hansch GM. Infectious versus non-infectious loosening of implants: activation of T lymphocytes differentiates between the two entities. *Int Orthop.* (2014) 38:1291–6. doi: 10.1007/s00264-014-2310-5
93. Kumar G, Roger PM, Ticchioni M, Trojani C, Bernard de Dompsur R, Bronsard N, et al. T cells from chronic bone infection show reduced proliferation and a high proportion of CD28(-) CD4 T cells. *Clin Exp Immunol.* (2014) 176:49–57. doi: 10.1111/cei.12245
94. Kotsougiani D, Pioch M, Prior B, Heppert V, Hansch GM, Wagner C. Activation of T lymphocytes in response to persistent bacterial infection: induction of CD11b and of toll-like receptors on T cells. *Int J Inflam.* (2010) 2010:526740. doi: 10.4061/2010/526740
95. Wagner C, Heck D, Lautenschlager K, Iking-Konert C, Heppert V, Wentzensen A, et al. T lymphocytes in implant-associated posttraumatic osteomyelitis: identification of cytotoxic T effector cells at the site of infection. *Shock.* (2006) 25:241–6. doi: 10.1097/01.shk.0000192119.68295.14
96. Heim CE, West SC, Ali H, Kielian T. Heterogeneity of Ly6G(+) Ly6C(+) myeloid-derived suppressor cell infiltrates during *Staphylococcus aureus* biofilm infection. *Infect Immun.* (2018) 86:e00684-18. doi: 10.1128/IAI.00684-18
97. Rochford ETJ, Sabate Bresco M, Zeiter S, Kluge K, Poulsson A, Ziegler M, et al. Monitoring immune responses in a mouse model of fracture fixation with and without Staphylococcus aureus osteomyelitis. *Bone.* (2016) 83:82–92. doi: 10.1016/j.bone.2015.10.014
98. Prabhakara R, Harro JM, Leid JG, Keegan AD, Prior ML, Shirtliff ME. Suppression of the inflammatory immune response prevents the development of chronic biofilm infection due to methicillin-resistant *Staphylococcus aureus*. *Infect Immun.* (2011) 79:5010–8. doi: 10.1128/IAI.05571-11
99. Prabhakara R, Harro JM, Leid JG, Harris M, Shirtliff ME. Murine immune response to a chronic *Staphylococcus aureus* biofilm infection. *Infect Immun.* (2011) 79:1789–96. doi: 10.1128/IAI.01386-10
100. Hanson EM, Clements VK, Sinha P, Ilkovitch D, Ostrand-Rosenberg S. Myeloid-derived suppressor cells down-regulate L-selectin expression on CD4+ and CD8+ T cells. *J Immunol.* (2009) 183:937–44. doi: 10.4049/jimmunol.0804253
101. Muller I, Munder M, Kropf P, Hansch GM. Polymorphonuclear neutrophils and T lymphocytes: strange bedfellows or brothers in arms? *Trends Immunol.* (2009) 30:522–30. doi: 10.1016/j.it.2009.07.007
102. Brady RA, Mocca CP, Plaut RD, Takeda K, Burns DL. Comparison of the immune response during acute and chronic *Staphylococcus aureus* infection. *PLoS ONE.* (2018) 13:e0195342. doi: 10.1371/journal.pone.0195342
103. Balraadjsing PP, de Jong EC, Grijpma DW, Tanck MW, Zaat SA. Poly(trimethylene carbonate) and poly(D,L-lactic acid) modify human dendritic cell responses to staphylococci but do not affect Th1 and Th2 cell development. *Eur Cell Mater.* (2018) 35:103–16. doi: 10.22203/eCM.v035a08
104. Nishitani K, Ishikawa M, de Mesy Bentley K, Ito H, Matsuda S, Daiss J, et al. Evidence of *Staphylococcus epidermidis* biofilm infection in the absence of abscess formation or osteolysis in a murine implant-associated osteomyelitis model. *Orthopaed Proc.* (2018) 100-B(SuppL. 3):56.

105. Li D, Gromov K, Soballe K, Puzas JE, O'Keefe RJ, Awad H, et al. Quantitative mouse model of implant-associated osteomyelitis and the kinetics of microbial growth, osteolysis, and humoral immunity. *J Orthop Res.* (2008) 26:96–105. doi: 10.1002/jor.20452
106. Brady RA, Leid JG, Camper AK, Costerton JW, Shirtliff ME. Identification of Staphylococcus aureus proteins recognized by the antibody-mediated immune response to a biofilm infection. *Infect Immun.* (2006) 74:3415–26. doi: 10.1128/IAI.00392-06
107. Brady RA, O'May GA, Leid JG, Prior ML, Costerton JW, Shirtliff ME. Resolution of Staphylococcus aureus biofilm infection using vaccination and antibiotic treatment. *Infect Immun.* (2011) 79:1797–803. doi: 10.1128/IAI.00451-10
108. Gedbjerg N, LaRosa R, Hunter JG, Varrone JJ, Kates SL, Schwarz EM, et al. Anti-glucosaminidase IgG in sera as a biomarker of host immunity against Staphylococcus aureus in orthopaedic surgery patients. *J Bone Joint Surg Am.* (2013) 95:e171. doi: 10.2106/JBJS.L.01654
109. Varrone JJ, de Mesy Bentley KL, Bello-Irizarry SN, Nishitani K, Mack S, Hunter JG, et al. Passive immunization with anti-glucosaminidase monoclonal antibodies protects mice from implant-associated osteomyelitis by mediating opsonophagocytosis of Staphylococcus aureus megaclusters. *J Orthop Res.* (2014) 32:1389–96. doi: 10.1002/jor.22672
110. Yokogawa N, Ishikawa M, Nishitani K, Beck CA, Tsuchiya H, Mesfin A, et al. Immunotherapy synergizes with debridement and antibiotic therapy in a murine 1-stage exchange model of MRSA implant-associated osteomyelitis. *J Orthop Res.* (2018) 36:1590–8. doi: 10.1002/jor.23801
111. Proctor RA. Recent developments for Staphylococcus aureus vaccines: clinical and basic science challenges. *Eur Cell Mater.* (2015) 30:315–26. doi: 10.22203/eCM.v030a22
112. Kubatzky KF, Uhle F, Eigenbrod T. From macrophage to osteoclast - How metabolism determines function and activity. *Cytokine.* (2018) 112:102–15. doi: 10.1016/j.cyto.2018.06.013
113. Josse J, Velard F, Gangloff SC. *Staphylococcus aureus* vs. osteoblast: relationship and consequences in osteomyelitis. *Front Cell Infect Microbiol.* (2015) 5:85. doi: 10.3389/fcimb.2015.00085
114. Dapunt U, Giese T, Stegmaier S, Moghaddam A, Hansch GM. The osteoblast as an inflammatory cell: production of cytokines in response to bacteria and components of bacterial biofilms. *BMC Musculoskelet Disord.* (2016) 17:243. doi: 10.1186/s12891-016-1091-y
115. Dapunt U, Maurer S, Giese T, Gaida MM, Hansch GM. The macrophage inflammatory proteins MIP1alpha (CCL3) and MIP2alpha (CXCL2) in implant-associated osteomyelitis: linking inflammation to bone degradation. *Mediat Inflamm.* (2014) 2014:728619. doi: 10.1155/2014/728619
116. Marriott I. Apoptosis-associated uncoupling of bone formation and resorption in osteomyelitis. *Front Cell Infect Microbiol.* (2013) 3:101. doi: 10.3389/fcimb.2013.00101
117. Blanchette KA, Prabhakara R, Shirtliff ME, Wenke JC. Inhibition of fracture healing in the presence of contamination by Staphylococcus aureus: effects of growth state and immune response. *J Orthop Res.* (2017) 35:1845–54. doi: 10.1002/jor.23573
118. Bruder SP, Fink DJ, Caplan AI. Mesenchymal stem cells in bone development, bone repair, and skeletal regeneration therapy. *J Cell Biochem.* (1994) 56:283–94. doi: 10.1002/jcb.240560303
119. Bunnell BA, Betancourt AM, Sullivan DE. New concepts on the immune modulation mediated by mesenchymal stem cells. *Stem Cell Res Ther.* (2010) 1:34. doi: 10.1186/scrt34
120. Seebach E, Holschbach J, Buchta N, Bitsch RG, Kleinschmidt K, Richter W. Mesenchymal stromal cell implantation for stimulation of long bone healing aggravates Staphylococcus aureus induced osteomyelitis. *Acta Biomater.* (2015) 21:165–77. doi: 10.1016/j.actbio.2015.03.019
121. Charles JF, Aliprantis AO. Osteoclasts: more than 'bone eaters'. *Trends Mol Med.* (2014) 20:449–59. doi: 10.1016/j.molmed.2014.06.001
122. Takayanagi H. New immune connections in osteoclast formation. *Ann N Y Acad Sci.* (2010) 1192:117–23. doi: 10.1111/j.1749-6632.2009.05303.x
123. Kotake S, Udagawa N, Hakoda M, Mogi M, Yano K, Tsuda E, et al. Activated human T cells directly induce osteoclastogenesis from human monocytes: possible role of T cells in bone destruction in rheumatoid arthritis patients. *Arthritis Rheum.* (2001) 44:1003–12. doi: 10.1002/1529-0131(200105)44:5<1003::AID-ANR179>3.3.CO;2-R
124. Sato K, Suematsu A, Okamoto K, Yamaguchi A, Morishita Y, Kadono Y, et al. Th17 functions as an osteoclastogenic helper T cell subset that links T cell activation and bone destruction. *J Exp Med.* (2006) 203:2673–82. doi: 10.1084/jem.20061775
125. Takayanagi H, Ogasawara K, Hida S, Chiba T, Murata S, Sato K, et al. T-cell-mediated regulation of osteoclastogenesis by signalling cross-talk between RANKL and IFN-gamma. *Nature.* (2000) 408:600–5. doi: 10.1038/35046102
126. Bozec A, Zaiss MM. T regulatory cells in bone remodelling. *Curr Osteoporos Rep.* (2017) 15:121–5. doi: 10.1007/s11914-017-0356-1
127. Zaiss MM, Axmann R, Zwerina J, Polzer K, Guckel E, Skapenko A, et al. Treg cells suppress osteoclast formation: a new link between the immune system and bone. *Arthritis Rheum.* (2007) 56:4104–12. doi: 10.1002/art.23138
128. Li H, Hong S, Qian J, Zheng Y, Yang J, Yi Q. Cross talk between the bone and immune systems: osteoclasts function as antigen-presenting cells and activate CD4+ and CD8+ T cells. *Blood.* (2010) 116:210–7. doi: 10.1182/blood-2009-11-255026
129. Grassi F, Manferdini C, Cattini L, Piacentini A, Gabusi E, Facchini A, et al. T cell suppression by osteoclasts *in vitro*. *J Cell Physiol.* (2011) 226:982–90. doi: 10.1002/jcp.22411
130. Li H, Lu Y, Qian J, Zheng Y, Zhang M, Bi E, et al. Human osteoclasts are inducible immunosuppressive cells in response to T cell-derived IFN-gamma and CD40 ligand *in vitro*. *J Bone Miner Res.* (2014) 29:2666–75. doi: 10.1002/jbmr.2294
131. Buchwald ZS, Aurora R. Osteoclasts and CD8 T cells form a negative feedback loop that contributes to homeostasis of both the skeletal and immune systems. *Clin Dev Immunol.* (2013) 2013:429373. doi: 10.1155/2013/429373
132. Charles JF, Hsu LY, Niemi EC, Weiss A, Aliprantis AO, Nakamura MC. Inflammatory arthritis increases mouse osteoclast precursors with myeloid suppressor function. *J Clin Invest.* (2012) 122:4592–605. doi: 10.1172/JCI60920
133. Ortega-Gomez A, Perretti M, Soehnlein O. Resolution of inflammation: an integrated view. *EMBO Mol Med.* (2013) 5:661–74. doi: 10.1002/emmm.201202382
134. Wherry EJ, Kurachi M. Molecular and cellular insights into T cell exhaustion. *Nat Rev Immunol.* (2015) 15:486–99. doi: 10.1038/nri3862
135. Darvin P, Toor SM, Sasidharan Nair V, Elkord E. Immune checkpoint inhibitors: recent progress and potential biomarkers. *Exp Mol Med.* (2018) 50:165. doi: 10.1038/s12276-018-0191-1
136. Wykes MN, Lewin SR. Immune checkpoint blockade in infectious diseases. *Nat Rev Immunol.* (2018) 18:91–104. doi: 10.1038/nri.2017.112
137. Patil NK, Guo Y, Luan L, Sherwood ER. Targeting immune cell checkpoints during sepsis. *Int J Mol Sci.* (2017) 18:2413. doi: 10.3390/ijms18112413
138. Paluch C, Santos AM, Anzilotti C, Cornall RJ, Davis SJ. Immune checkpoints as therapeutic targets in autoimmunity. *Front Immunol.* (2018) 9:2306. doi: 10.3389/fimmu.2018.02306
139. Cavaillon JM, Eisen D, Annane D. Is boosting the immune system in sepsis appropriate? *Crit Care.* (2014) 18:216. doi: 10.1186/cc13787
140. Davies R, O'Dea K, Gordon A. Immune therapy in sepsis: are we ready to try again? *J Intensive Care Soc.* (2018) 19:326–44. doi: 10.1177/1751143718765407
141. Anderson AC, Joller N, Kuchroo VK. Lag-3, Tim-3, and TIGIT: co-inhibitory receptors with specialized functions in immune regulation. *Immunity.* (2016) 44:989–1004. doi: 10.1016/j.immuni.2016.05.001
142. De Sousa Linhares A, Leitner J, Grabmeier-Pfistershammer K, Steinberger P. Not all immune checkpoints are created equal. *Front Immunol.* (2018) 9:1909. doi: 10.3389/fimmu.2018.01909
143. Hodi FS, O'Day SJ, McDermott DF, Weber RW, Sosman JA, Haanen JB, et al. Improved survival with ipilimumab in patients with metastatic melanoma. *N Engl J Med.* (2010) 363:711–23. doi: 10.1056/NEJMoa1003466
144. Dyck L, Mills KHG. Immune checkpoints and their inhibition in cancer and infectious diseases. *Eur J Immunol.* (2017) 47:765–79. doi: 10.1002/eji.201646875
145. Rowshanravan B, Halliday N, Sansom DM. CTLA-4: a moving target in immunotherapy. *Blood.* (2018) 131:58–67. doi: 10.1182/blood-2017-06-741033

146. Linsley PS, Brady W, Urnes M, Grosmaire LS, Damle NK, Ledbetter JA. CTLA-4 is a second receptor for the B cell activation antigen B7. *J Exp Med.* (1991) 174:561–9. doi: 10.1084/jem.174.3.561
147. Genovese MC, Becker JC, Schiff M, Luggen M, Sherrer Y, Kremer J, et al. Abatacept for rheumatoid arthritis refractory to tumor necrosis factor alpha inhibition. *N Engl J Med.* (2005) 353:1114–23. doi: 10.1056/NEJMoa050524
148. Ali A, Welin A, Schwarze JC, Svensson MN, Na M, Jarneborn A, et al. CTLA4 immunoglobulin but not anti-tumor necrosis factor therapy promotes staphylococcal septic arthritis in mice. *J Infect Dis.* (2015) 212:1308–16. doi: 10.1093/infdis/jiv212
149. Axmann R, Herman S, Zaiss M, Franz S, Polzer K, Zwerina J, et al. CTLA-4 directly inhibits osteoclast formation. *Ann Rheum Dis.* (2008) 67:1603–9. doi: 10.1136/ard.2007.080713
150. Bozec A, Zaiss MM, Kagwiria R, Voll R, Rauh M, Chen Z, et al. T cell costimulation molecules CD80/86 inhibit osteoclast differentiation by inducing the IDO/tryptophan pathway. *Sci Transl Med.* (2014) 6:235ra60. doi: 10.1126/scitranslmed.3007764
151. Boutros C, Tarhini A, Routier E, Lambotte O, Ladurie FL, Carbonnel F, et al. Safety profiles of anti-CTLA-4 and anti-PD-1 antibodies alone and in combination. *Nat Rev Clin Oncol.* (2016) 13:473–86. doi: 10.1038/nrclinonc.2016.58
152. Latchman Y, Wood CR, Chernova T, Chaudhary D, Borde M, Chernova I, et al. PD-L2 is a second ligand for PD-1 and inhibits T cell activation. *Nat Immunol.* (2001) 2:261–8. doi: 10.1038/85330
153. Zhang Y, Chung Y, Bishop C, Daugherty B, Chute H, Holst P, et al. Regulation of T cell activation and tolerance by PDL2. *Proc Natl Acad Sci USA.* (2006) 103:11695–700. doi: 10.1073/pnas.0601347103
154. Tseng SY, Otsuji M, Gorski K, Huang X, Slansky JE, Pai SI, et al. B7-DC, a new dendritic cell molecule with potent costimulatory properties for T cells. *J Exp Med.* (2001) 193:839–46. doi: 10.1084/jem.193.7.839
155. Karunarathne DS, Horne-Debets JM, Huang JX, Faleiro R, Leow CY, Amante F, et al. Programmed death-1 ligand 2-mediated regulation of the PD-L1 to PD-1 axis is essential for establishing CD4(+) T cell immunity. *Immunity.* (2016) 45:333–45. doi: 10.1016/j.immuni.2016.07.017
156. Magrys A, Paluch-Oles J, Bogut A, Kielbus M, Plewik D, Koziol-Montewka M. The role of programmed death ligand 1 pathway in persistent biomaterial-associated infections. *J Microbiol.* (2015) 53:544–52. doi: 10.1007/s12275-015-5022-7
157. Davies LC, Heldring N, Kadri N, Le Blanc K. Mesenchymal stromal cell secretion of programmed death-1 ligands regulates T cell mediated immunosuppression. *Stem Cells.* (2017) 35:766–76. doi: 10.1002/stem.2509
158. Pennesi G. PD1-mediated mesenchymal stem cells immunemodulation: the two sides of the coin. *Int Clin Pathol J.* (2018) 6:164–5 doi: 10.15406/icpjl.2018.06.00179
159. Moravej A, Karimi MH, Geramizadeh B, Azarpira N, Zarnani AH, Yaghobi R, et al. Mesenchymal stem cells upregulate the expression of PD-L1 but not VDR in dendritic cells. *Immunol Invest.* (2017) 46:80–96. doi: 10.1080/08820139.2016.1225757
160. Hui E, Cheung J, Zhu J, Su X, Taylor MJ, Wallweber HA, et al. T cell costimulatory receptor CD28 is a primary target for PD-1-mediated inhibition. *Science.* (2017) 355:1428–33. doi: 10.1126/science.aaf1292
161. Kamphorst AO, Wieland A, Nasti T, Yang S, Zhang R, Barber DL, et al. Rescue of exhausted CD8 T cells by PD-1-targeted therapies is CD28-dependent. *Science.* (2017) 355:1423–7. doi: 10.1126/science.aaf0683
162. An G, Acharya C, Feng X, Wen K, Zhong M, Zhang L, et al. Osteoclasts promote immune suppressive microenvironment in multiple myeloma: therapeutic implication. *Blood.* (2016) 128:1590–603. doi: 10.1182/blood-2016-03-707547
163. Tai YT, Cho SF, Anderson KC. Osteoclast immunosuppressive effects in multiple myeloma: role of programmed cell death ligand 1. *Front Immunol.* (2018) 9:1822. doi: 10.3389/fimmu.2018.01822
164. Dominguez-Soto A, Aragoneses-Fenoll L, Martin-Gayo E, Martinez-Prats L, Colmenares M, Naranjo-Gomez M, et al. The DC-SIGN-related lectin LSECtin mediates antigen capture and pathogen binding by human myeloid cells. *Blood.* (2007) 109:5337–45. doi: 10.1182/blood-2006-09-048058
165. Wang Y, Wang J, Meng J, Jiang H, Zhao J, Qian H, et al. Epigenetic modification mediates the increase of LAG-3(+) T cells in chronic osteomyelitis. *Inflammation.* (2017) 40:414–21. doi: 10.1007/s10753-016-0486-0
166. Triebel F. LAG-3: a regulator of T-cell and DC responses and its use in therapeutic vaccination. *Trends Immunol.* (2003) 24:619–22. doi: 10.1016/j.it.2003.10.001
167. Sierro S, Romero P, Speiser DE. The CD4-like molecule LAG-3, biology and therapeutic applications. *Expert Opin Ther Targets.* (2011) 15:91–101. doi: 10.1517/14712598.2011.540563
168. Monney L, Sabatos CA, Gaglia JL, Ryu A, Waldner H, Chernova T, et al. Th1-specific cell surface protein Tim-3 regulates macrophage activation and severity of an autoimmune disease. *Nature.* (2002) 415:536–41. doi: 10.1038/415536a
169. Zhu C, Anderson AC, Schubart A, Xiong H, Imitola J, Khoury SJ, et al. The Tim-3 ligand galectin-9 negatively regulates T helper type 1 immunity. *Nat Immunol.* (2005) 6:1245–52. doi: 10.1038/ni1271
170. Dardalhon V, Anderson AC, Karman J, Apetoh L, Chandwaskar R, Lee DH, et al. Tim-3/galectin-9 pathway: regulation of Th1 immunity through promotion of CD11b+Ly-6G+ myeloid cells. *J Immunol.* (2010) 185:1383–92. doi: 10.4049/jimmunol.0903275
171. Gautron AS, Dominguez-Villar M, de Marcken M, Hafler DA. Enhanced suppressor function of TIM-3+ FoxP3+ regulatory T cells. *Eur J Immunol.* (2014) 44:2703–11. doi: 10.1002/eji.201344392
172. Ocana-Guzman R, Torre-Bouscoulet L, Sada-Ovalle I. TIM-3 regulates distinct functions in macrophages. *Front Immunol.* (2016) 7:229. doi: 10.3389/fimmu.2016.00229
173. Moriyama K, Kukita A, Li YJ, Uehara N, Zhang JQ, Takahashi I, et al. Regulation of osteoclastogenesis through Tim-3: possible involvement of the Tim-3/galectin-9 system in the modulation of inflammatory bone destruction. *Lab Invest.* (2014) 94:1200–11. doi: 10.1038/labinvest.2014.107
174. Tamadaho RSE, Hoerauf A, Layland LE. Immunomodulatory effects of myeloid-derived suppressor cells in diseases: role in cancer and infections. *Immunobiology.* (2018) 223:432–42. doi: 10.1016/j.imbio.2017.07.001
175. Bunt SK, Clements VK, Hanson EM, Sinha P, Ostrand-Rosenberg S. Inflammation enhances myeloid-derived suppressor cell cross-talk by signaling through Toll-like receptor 4. *J Leukoc Biol.* (2009) 85:996–1004. doi: 10.1189/jlb.0708446
176. Ostrand-Rosenberg S, Sinha P, Beury DW, Clements VK. Cross-talk between myeloid-derived suppressor cells (MDSC), macrophages, and dendritic cells enhances tumor-induced immune suppression. *Semin Cancer Biol.* (2012) 22:275–81. doi: 10.1016/j.semcancer.2012.01.011
177. Ballbach M, Dannert A, Singh A, Siegmund DM, Handgretinger R, Piali L, et al. Expression of checkpoint molecules on myeloid-derived suppressor cells. *Immunol Lett.* (2017) 192:1–6. doi: 10.1016/j.imlet.2017.10.001
178. Weber R, Fleming V, Hu X, Nagibin V, Groth C, Altevogt P, et al. Myeloid-derived suppressor cells hinder the anti-cancer activity of immune checkpoint inhibitors. *Front Immunol.* (2018) 9:1310. doi: 10.3389/fimmu.2018.01310
179. Toor SM, Elkord E. Therapeutic prospects of targeting myeloid-derived suppressor cells and immune checkpoints in cancer. *Immunol Cell Biol.* (2018) 96:888–97. doi: 10.1111/imcb.12054
180. Tesi RJ. MDSC; the most important cell you have never heard of. *Trends Pharmacol Sci.* (2019) 40:4–7. doi: 10.1016/j.tips.2018.10.008
181. Labonte AC, Tosello-Trampont AC, Hahn YS. The role of macrophage polarization in infectious and inflammatory diseases. *Mol Cells.* (2014) 37:275–85. doi: 10.14348/molcells.2014.2374
182. Freitas-Silva R, Brelaz-de-Castro MC, Pereira VR. Dendritic cell-based approaches in the fight against diseases. *Front Immunol.* (2014) 5:78. doi: 10.3389/fimmu.2014.00078

3

Spatial Distribution of Macrophages During Callus Formation and Maturation Reveals Close Crosstalk Between Macrophages and Newly Forming Vessels

Jonathan Stefanowski[1,2†], Annemarie Lang[1,2,3†], Ariana Rauch[2], Linus Aulich[2], Markus Köhler[2], Alexander F. Fiedler[2], Frank Buttgereit[1,2,3], Katharina Schmidt-Bleek[3,4], Georg N. Duda[3,4], Timo Gaber[1,2,3], Raluca A. Niesner[2,5] and Anja E. Hauser[1,2]*

[1] Department of Rheumatology and Clinical Immunology, Charité—Universitätsmedizin Berlin, Corporate Member of Freie Universität Berlin, Humboldt-Universität zu Berlin, and Berlin Institute of Health, Berlin, Germany, [2] German Rheumatism Research Centre (DRFZ) Berlin, a Leibniz Institute, Berlin, Germany, [3] Berlin-Brandenburg Center for Regenerative Therapies, Charité—Universitätsmedizin Berlin, Corporate Member of Freie Universität Berlin, Humboldt-Universität zu Berlin, and Berlin Institute of Health, Berlin, Germany, [4] Julius Wolff Institute for Biomechanics and Musculoskeletal Regeneration, Charité—Universitätsmedizin Berlin, Corporate Member of Freie Universität Berlin, Humboldt-Universität zu Berlin, and Berlin Institute of Health, Berlin, Germany, [5] Dynamic and Functional in vivo Imaging, Department of Veterinary Medicine, Freie Universität Berlin, Berlin, Germany

***Correspondence:**
Anja E. Hauser
hauser@drfz.de;
anja.hauser-hankeln@charite.de*

† These authors have contributed equally to this work

Macrophages are essential players in the process of fracture healing, acting by remodeling of the extracellular matrix and enabling vascularization. Whilst activated macrophages of M1-like phenotype are present in the initial pro-inflammatory phase of hours to days of fracture healing, an anti-inflammatory M2-like macrophage phenotype is supposed to be crucial for the induction of downstream cascades of healing, especially the initiation of vascularization. In a mouse-osteotomy model, we provide a comprehensive characterization of vessel ($CD31^+$, $Emcn^+$) and macrophage phenotypes (F4/80, CD206, CD80, Mac-2) during the process of fracture healing. To this end, we phenotype the phases of vascular regeneration—the expansion phase (d1–d7 after injury) and the remodeling phase of the endothelial network, until tissue integrity is restored (d14–d21 after injury). Vessels which appear during the bone formation process resemble type H endothelium ($CD31^{hi}Emcn^{hi}$), and are closely connected to osteoprogenitors ($Runx2^+$, Osx^+) and $F4/80^+$ macrophages. M1-like macrophages are present in the initial phase of vascularization until day 3 post osteotomy, but they are rare during later regeneration phases. M2-like macrophages localize mainly extramedullary, and $CD206^+$ macrophages are found to express $Mac\text{-}2^+$ during the expansion phase. VEGFA expression is initiated by $CD80^+$ cells, including $F4/80^+$ macrophages, until day 3, while subsequently osteoblasts and chondrocytes are main contributors to VEGFA production at the fracture site. Using Longitudinal Intravital Microendoscopy of the Bone (LIMB) we observe changes in the motility and organization of $CX3CR1^+$ cells, which infiltrate the injury site after an osteotomy. A transient accumulation, resulting in spatial polarization of both, endothelial cells and macrophages, in regions distal to the fracture site, is evident. Immunofluorescence histology followed by histocytometric analysis reveals that F4/80$^+$CX3CR1$^+$ myeloid cells precede vascularization.

Keywords: bone regeneration, macrophage, endothelial cell, H-type vessel, intravital microscopy, LIMB, CX3CR1 myeloid cells

INTRODUCTION

Bone healing is a spatiotemporally regulated regeneration process, ideally leading to complete restoration of the broken bone without fibrous scar formation (1). Naturally, this regeneration process undergoes endochondral bone formation, if interfragmentary movements strain the fracture gap (2). In the majority of clinical cases, fracture healing follows the endochondral route and may be sub-divided into five phases, namely an (i) initial pro-inflammatory phase, (ii) anti-inflammatory phase, (iii) fibrocartilaginous or soft callus phase, (iv) mineralization or hard callus phase and (v) remodeling phase in which bone tissue regains its physiological shape with a restored bone marrow cavity. While fracture healing occurs in most cases without delay, still 5–10% of patients suffer from delayed healing or non-union. To avoid delayed healing and overcome non-unions, it is important to understand the finely orchestrated processes of bone regeneration (3, 4).

Upon a fracture, the vessels get disrupted and nutrient supply is lacking at the injury site. However, the vascular system is essential for healing, by supplying cells with oxygen and nutrients, removing debris and allowing the recruitment of circulating cells. Endothelial progenitors (CD31$^+$) migrate to the fracture site from the bone marrow or from pre-existing vessels of the periosteum (5–9). In earlier work, we could show that revascularization peaks during two phases of fracture healing: around day 7 (end of the inflammatory phase) and around day 21 (woven bone formation) in sheep (6). Drastic vascular structural plasticity has also been shown during bone marrow regeneration between 7 and 21 days by our group using a longitudinal microendoscopic method at cellular resolution (10). Angiogenic factors, such as vascular endothelial growth factor (VEGF) are of great importance in order to induce vascularization. Street et al. showed that the circulating plasma levels of VEGF are highly increased in patients with fractures and that the fibrin matrix within the fracture hematoma acts like a VEGF reservoir (11). In addition, we reported in a previous study that cells within the fracture hematoma exhibit upregulated VEGF expression and secretion (12, 13). Osteoprogenitor cells also produce VEGF as a consequence of the hypoxic environment, leading to enhanced transcriptional activity of hypoxia-inducible factor 1-alpha (HIF-1α) (14, 15). Buettmann et al. most recently showed that especially the release of VEGFA by Osterix (Osx)$^+$ osteoprogenitors/pre-osteoblasts is critical for vessel formation during fracture healing (16). It is well-known that the crosstalk between endothelium and bone cells is essential for the integrity and formation of bone. Osteoblasts support the vasculature by producing VEGF and basic fibroblast growth factor (bFGF) while endothelial cells (ECs) provide factors that further osteoblast differentiation and activity (17). Furthermore, pre-osteoclasts and non-bone-resorbing osteoclasts have been described to enhance vascularization and osteogenesis in the growth plate area by releasing platelet-derived growth factor-BB (PDGF-BB) or supporting vessel anastomosis (18, 19). While the production of angiogenic factors by osteoprogenitors is well-known, there is evidence accumulating that, conversely, endothelial cells can also impact on bone formation, at least during bone development (7). Bone development is initiated by blood vessel invasion, and the arrival of osteoprogenitors. Subsequently, specialized type H blood vessels secrete osteogenic factors, required for the induction of bone formation and growth (20). Although the presence of type H vessels has been reported at sites of bone regeneration (10, 21), early events inducing the formation of these vessels in those situations have not yet been investigated.

Next to the adaptive immunity, the importance of the innate immune system for regenerative processes has been shown by several studies (22–26). Macrophages have been identified as key players for the recovery of tissue integrity and function. Several different types of myeloid-lineage cells can be distinguished in bone regeneration (23). Tissue-resident macrophages (also termed osteomacs) which express F4/80, can be found closely to bone-lining cells, and support intramembranous bone formation as well as endochondral ossification (22, 25, 26). Recruited immune macrophages (M1-like/M2-like) are more pivotal in endochondral ossification, which has been shown by Schlundt et al., who deleted macrophages in osteotomized mice by treatment with clodronate liposomes, and Alexander et al. who examined macrophage subsets close to the periosteum during regeneration (24, 25). Furthermore, osteoclasts are multinucleated tartrate-resistant acid phosphatase (TRAP)$^+$F4/80$^-$ myeloid cells, which derive from fusion events (22).

In other tissues or scenarios, macrophages are essential for vascularization and angiogenesis. They are able to degrade extracellular matrix (ECM) and release pro-angiogenic factors. Degradation of the ECM enables the migration of endothelial progenitors and activates the angiogenic potential of some ECM molecules, as has been shown for fragments of hyaluronic acid (27). In addition, macrophages also release factors that attract, activate or even inhibit angiogenic cells depending on the phase of vascularization (28). Studies during mouse development revealed the tight association of macrophages with capillaries and the subsequent enhancement of angiogenesis (29, 30). Macrophages have also been shown to regulate vessel permeability comparable to pericytes (31). *Vice versa,* endothelial cells (ECs) also promote the selective growth and differentiation of macrophages, especially the switch towards an M2-like phenotype, which requires direct contact with the endothelium and the regulation via macrophage colony-stimulating factor (M-CSF) signaling (32). However, a potential crosstalk between macrophages and ECs and the details of such interactions during bone regeneration have not been studied so far.

Within this study, we aim to analyze the initial phases of angiogenesis in bone healing with vascular regeneration and their dependence on the presence of macrophages. We focus on the early regeneration events, until the shift from pro- to anti-inflammatory phase, where a close crosstalk of blood vessels with macrophages is most prominent (d1–d7 after injury) and compare this to the bone remodeling phase driven by osteoprogenitors and mineralized tissue formation (d14–d21 after injury).

METHODS

Animal Husbandry, Housing, and Surgery

Mouse-Osteotomy-Model

All animal experiments were approved by the local animal protection authority (LaGeSo; permit numbers: G0039/16 and G0111/13) following the German Animal Welfare Act.

Female C57BL/6N mice aged 10 weeks were ordered from Charles River Laboratories (Sulzfeld, Germany) and underwent surgery at the age of 12 weeks with an average body weight of 22 g. Housing took place in a conventional, semi-barrier (non-SPF) facility and randomly split in groups with at least 2 mice per cage housed in Eurostandard Type II clear-transparent plastic cages with a wire lid and filter top. Fine wood chips (Lignocel FS 14, J. Rettenmaier & Söhne GmbH + Co. KG, Germany) and nesting material (Envirodri®, Shepherd Specialty Papers, USA) was provided. Houses and pipes were removed after surgery to avoid injuries due to the external fixator. Food (Standard mouse diet, Ssniff Spezialdiäten, Germany) and tap water was provided *ad libitum*, and room temperature was between 20 and 22°C with a humidity of 45–50%. The light/dark cycle was a 12/12-h cycle. Animals were tail and cup handled. Anesthesia was induced at 2.5% isoflurane (CP-Pharma, Germany) and maintained at 1.5%. In order to cover pain after the surgery prior to surgery, all animals received Buprenorphine (0.03 mg/kg; Temgesic, Indivior Eu Ltd., UK) s.c. as analgesic, an eye ointment and clindamycin (0.02 ml; Ratiopharm, Germany). After shaving and disinfecting the left femur area animals were placed on a heating mat and osteotomy was performed under aseptic conditions as described earlier (21, 24). In short, the femur was prepared bluntly, after a lateral longitudinal incision of the skin between hip and knee. The external fixator (MouseExFix, RISystem, Switzerland) was placed parallel to the femur by serial drilling of the pins (0.45 mm diameter). With a Gigli wire saw (RISystem, Davos, Switzerland), a 0.70 mm osteotomy gap was created in the middle of the femur and flushed with NaCl. Following skin closure, mice received pre-warmed NaCl (0.2 ml) s.c., permeable wound dressing spray and could recover from anesthesia in their home cage under infrared light and close monitoring. Tramadol was applied via the drinking water (0.1 mg/ml; Grünenthal, Germany) for 3 days after osteotomy (33). Given the short time period of treatment, we expect no negative influence of the analgetics on the fracture healing outcome (33). Surgery was performed by two trained veterinarians. For general scoring and humane endpoints, optimized protocols were used which has been summarized in Lang et al. (34).

Combined Osteotomy and Intravital Imaging Model

All animal experiments were approved by the local animal protection authority (LaGeSo; permit numbers: G0302/17) following the German Animal Welfare Act.

$Cx3cr1^{tm1Litt}$ (CX3CR1:GFP), a fractalkine receptor (CX3CR1) reporter mouse, and C57BL/6J animals were bred in our colony. Heterozygous female mice were 14 weeks of age when osteotomy was performed. Housing took place in a conventional SPF barrier facility. Prior to surgery, all animals received Buprenorphine (0.03 mg/kg; Temgesic, Indivior Eu Ltd., UK) s.c. as analgesic and eye ointment. After shaving and disinfecting the left femur area animals were placed on a heating mat and osteotomy was performed under aseptic conditions. Surgery was performed as previously described (10), using four bi-cortical screws, and combined with osteotomy. In short, the internal fixator's Gradient Refractive INdex (GRIN) lens tubing was modified to be screwed into the fixator plate after implantation and osteotomy. Osteotomy was performed using a 0.22 mm Gigli wire saw (RISystem, Switzerland) and two cuts for an osteotomy gap size of ~816 μm (CI: 787–844 μm; $SD = 85$ μm; $n = 37$). After removing the generated bone piece, the lens tube was positioned into the osteotomy gap and screwed into the fixator plate. Analgetics (Tramadol, Buprenorphine) were applied as described above. For antibiotic treatment mice received one injection of 0.04% Enrofloxacin (Baytril, 10 mg/kg body weight Bayer AG, Germany) before surgery.

Bone Sample Preparation

Femoral bones were explanted, muscles largely removed in a way that osteotomized bone parts maintained one entity. Tissue was fixed using 4% electron microscopy-grade PFA in PBS for 4 h at 4°C, washed in PBS, and ran through a sucrose gradient (10%, 20%, 30%; á 12–24 h). The fixators were removed from the fixed samples, underwent μCT measurement, bones were frozen in SCEM medium (Sectionlab, Japan), cut into slices of 7 μm using Kawamoto's film method (35), and stored at −80°C.

Histology

Movat's Pentachrome staining was conducted as descried previously (21, 24). TRAP staining for quantification was performed using a kit following the manufacturer's instructions (Thermo Scientific, 386A-1KT, MA, US). Individual slides were stained using small volumes of staining solutions on a heating plate at 37°C. For immunofluorescence, individual sections were thawed, rehydrated in PBS, blocked with 10% donkey serum, and stained with antibodies in PBS/0.1% Tween 20/5% donkey serum containing DAPI for 1–2 h. Target proteins were identified using antibodies against CD31/PECAM-1 (goat polyclonal unconjugated, AF2628, R&D Systems, 1:100), CD206/MMR (C068C2 conjugated to AF594, BLD-141726, 1:100), CD80 (goat polyclonal unconjugated, AF740-SP, 1:100), Endomucin (Emcn) (V.7C7 unconjugated, sc-65495, 1:100), F4/80 (Cl:A3-1 unconjugated, MCA497G, 1:400), GFP (goat polyclonal conjugated to AF488, 600-101-215, 1:100), Ly-6C (ER-MP20 biotinylated, MA5-16666, 1:20), Ly-6G (1A8 biotinylated, BLD-127603, 1:200), Mac-2/Galectin-3 (M3/38 unconjugated, BLD-125401, 1:100), Osx (rabbit polyclonal, sc-22536-R, 1:200), Runx2 (EPR14334 conjugated AF647, ab215955, 1:100), Sox9 (EPR14335 unconjugated, ab185230, 1:200), VEGFA (rabbit polyclonal unconjugated, ab46154, 1:100). Primary antibodies were stained with secondary antibodies when unconjugated (1:500, Thermo Fisher, anti-rat conjugated AF488, A21208; anti-rat conjugated AF546, A11081; anti-rat conjugated AF594, A21209; anti-rabbit conjugated AF488, A21206; anti-rabbit conjugated AF546, A10040; anti-rabbit conjugated AF647, A31573; anti-goat conjugated AF647, A21447; or streptavidin conjugated AF546, S11225). Samples were washed between steps and after staining with PBS/0.1 % Tween 20 for 3 × 5 min. Stained samples were kept in PBS for 5 min and embedded using aqueous mounting medium (Fluoromount, Thermo Fisher, MA, US) and analyzed microscopically within 6 days. Simultaneous detection of Ly6C and Ly6G was considered to indicate presence of the Gr-1 protein.

Movat's Pentachrome images were taken with a light microscope in a 2.5 × magnification and the program AxioVision (both Carl Zeiss Microscopy GmbH, Germany). For **Figure 2**, images (CD31 & Emcn) were taken with a Keyence microscope (BZ 9000) using a 10x or 4x objective. All other images were acquired at a Zeiss LSM880 in tile scan mode at a resolution of 2048 × 2048 using a 20x objective, unless specified otherwise. For display, pictures were background subtracted and contrast adjusted using ImageJ 1.52i.

Image Analysis

Image analysis of cell and tissue distribution (**Figure 2**) was performed with ImageJ and an own developed pipeline which has been published and described in detail previously (21). Mean intensity was determined with ImageJ within the marked ROIs distinguishing between the gap, the adjacent to the gap and the bone marrow area. Mean intensities were normalized to the maximum intensity of the image.

Quantification was performed in *CellProfiler 3.1.8.* (36) (**Supplementary Figure 1**). Macrophage subsets were described via the co-localization of identified CX3CR1$^+$, Gr-1$^+$, and F4/80$^+$ objects. CX3CR1$^+$F4/80$^+$Gr1$^+$ objects, representing cells were divided by roundness based on object shape features (FormFactor, Perimeter, Min Feret Diameter, **Supplementary Figure 5**). Objects were only considered cells when they overlapped with a nucleus (DAPI) signal. In a second pipeline localization of F4/80$^+$ macrophages towards the Emcn$^+$ endothelium was analyzed by examination of the direct ($\leq$3.5 µm) and distant (>7 µm) neighborhood of the subset. Localization of the identified subsets was analyzed by counting the identified objects in regions of interests (ROIs). ROIs for the osteotomy gap were determined as shown in **Figure 5E**. For neighborhood analysis and frequency determination (**Figures 3E,F**) either Emcn^{hi} or Emcn^{lo} areas within the osteotomy gap or distant thereof were encircled freehand using ImageJ 1.52i, respectively (**Figure 3D**). Areas close to Sox9$^+$ chondrocytes were excluded as they did contain few, if any macrophages. Emcn^{hi} areas largely overlapped with F4/80^{hi} areas.

Object Identification and Neighborhood Analysis

For the segmentation, the model-based approach was applied (37). *Otsu* was used as a segmentation algorithm calculating the thresholds for the object edge identification. Mid-level pixels were assigned to the background. The threshold calculation was performed adaptively, which allows adaptation of the threshold to different image sub-regions. For each channel, the parameters were manually optimized by visually inspecting the segmentation results. To aid the segmentation, channel specific object ranges were estimated (e.g., nuclei = 3.1–12.5 µm). Clumped cells were separated based on their intensity distribution. Only partly visible cells touching the border of the image were removed from the segmentation process. Nuclei, CX3CR1, F4/80, and Emcn primary objects were identified based exclusively on the image. Due to the dense packing of Gr-1$^+$ cells, segmentation was performed via secondary object identification with prior segmented nuclei as cellular reference. The segmentation was channel dependently refined based on various object features (**Supplementary Figure 1B**). Objects features were extracted on the boundaries of the objects for shape (e.g., perimeter, area, radius; **Supplementary Figure 5**), and intensity, computed from the signal intensity values of the object area within a defined image channel. Filter and thresholds were determined by visual evaluation of specific phenotypic measurements of individual objects within the image and the global distribution of the phenotypic measurement within the whole image.

Spatial Polarization Scoring

Bone orientation was determined using Movat's Pentachrome overview images. Scores were determined for individual channels (DAPI, F4/80, or CD31). Scores were determined considering the staining intensity and abundance of the signal in parts of the bone marrow not affected by the injury (homeostatic control), on the same slide in at least 400 µm distance from the injury site. Scores were: −2 for the absence of staining in the area or reduced signal abundance and intensity throughout the entire area.; −1 for signal either reduced in intensity but displaying comparable abundance, or reduced abundance and comparable intensity; 0 for appearance that resembles homeostasis (unaffected bone marrow in the same section); 1 for higher intensity at comparable or increased abundance that localized only partially along the line between the gap and the adjacent tissue. Adjacent tissue is tissue along the contour between bone marrow and hematoma, bone fragments, and callus; 2 for higher intensity at comparable or increased abundance along the entire length of the line between the gap and the adjacent tissue or in large areas extending >400 µm distance from the gap in the bone marrow tissue. Regions often showed enlarged and unstructured vessel organization, with very bright F4/80 cells between the endothelial lines. Samples were considered spatially polarized when the scored values for F4/80 and vessel marker of proximal and distal to the fracture gap resulted in a difference >2 favoring one side (proximal, distal). Samples which scored a difference of <2 were considered neutral. In total $n = 20$ samples were analyzed, 9 samples scored values other than 0 of which 2 samples were considered neutral, 1 polarized proximally and 6 polarized distally (**Supplementary Figure 4A**).

Longitudinal Intravital Microendoscopy of Murine Osteotomy

As a GRIN lens system, we used custom singlet GRIN needle microendoscope (length ca. 5.07 mm, diameter = 0.60 mm; NEM-060-10-10-850-S-1.0p, GRINTECH Jena, Germany). The GRIN lens was glued into the lens tubing to a final penetration depth of 650 μm when screwed into the fixator plate. CX3CR1:GFP mice were anesthetized and mounted to the microscope as previously described (10). Qtracker 655 Vascular Label (Thermo Fisher, MA, US) were injected and images were acquired (505 × 505 px, 500 × 500 μm, unidirectional, line average 4, step size 4.5–6.5 μm, ca. 18 steps, stack time 60 sec). Image stacks were loaded into Imaris 9.3.0 software (Bitplane Zürich, Switzerland), median filter (3 × 3 × 3) was applied. Videos were exported (1024 × 1024, 4 fps) and images were angled maximum intensity projections. Individual mice were measured at 940–950 nm on day 2, 3, 4, 5 after osteotomy.

Statistical Analysis

Statistical analysis was carried out with GraphPad Prism V.5 or V.8 software. All values are expressed as the mean ± SD if not stated otherwise. Mann-Whitney *U*-test, Wilcoxon-signed rank test and Friedman test with Dunn's *post-hoc* test were mainly used, since Gaussian distribution was not expected due to inter-individual variations. A $p < 0.05$ was considered statistically significant. Image analysis was blinded for time points.

RESULTS

Emcn^{hi}CD31^{hi} Endothelium Is Present During Endochondral Bone Formation in the Osteotomy Gap

Fracture healing consists of consecutive phases. Progression into each phase depends on the undisturbed and error-free course of the respective previous phase (38). In the mouse-osteotomy model used in this study, residuals of cells in the fracture hematoma are visible in Movat's Pentachrome staining at day 3, while the osteotomy gap is filled with a mixture of bone marrow cells including hematopoietic cells at day 7, and endochondral bone formation occurs between day 14 and day 21 (**Figure 1A**). Using immunofluorescence histology, a positive signal for CD31 (Platelet endothelial cell adhesion molecule 1) is seen in elongated cells inside the fracture hematoma, which include no detectable nuclei (**Supplementary Figures 2A–C**), probably indicating that these residuals represent endothelial cells that may have lost their integrity. In order to further characterize the cellular composition within the fracture area, immunofluorescence staining for key transcription factors of mesenchymal differentiation was performed on serial sections of the same bones (**Figure 1B**). Already at day 3, osteoblast progenitors characterized by nuclear expression of Runt-related transcription factor 2 (Runx2) are dispersed in the fracture gap. By day 7, their number has increased, leading to a dense population of the gap, whilst sparing a region in the center. The peripheral borders of the gap and adjacent periosteal regions are populated by cells co-expressing Runx2 and SRY-box transcription factor 9 (Sox9) in the nucleus, indicating their potential for either osteogenic or chondrogenic differentiation (**Figure 1B**). This is in accordance with the blue-greenish color in corresponding regions of Movat's Pentachrome staining, indicative of cartilaginous tissue (Alcian blue positive). At day 14, Runx2$^+$ cells are found to localize on both sides of the gap. Single Runx2$^+$ cells are surrounded by areas characterized by the presence of only a few nuclei, in line with the presence of mineralized bone in those areas, as visualized by Movat's Pentachrome staining (compare: **Figures 1A,B**). Sox9$^+$ cells are exclusively present in the center of the gap at this time point. Notably, the majority of these cells do not co-express Runx2. In contrast, at day 21, a time point when mineralization of the gap is complete, the progenitors identified in this area are almost exclusively Runx2$^+$. In a next step, Osterix (Osx) and CD31 stainings were performed on serial slides from the same individuals. Direct comparison reveals that at day 3, only some Runx2$^+$ cells are also Osx$^+$, indicating various degrees of osteogenic differentiation. From day 7 on, Runx2$^+$ cells are also positive for Osx$^+$, consistent with ongoing maturation of osteoblasts. Osx$^+$ osteoblasts localize in the fracture gap alongside existing and newly formed bone, as indicated by differential interference contrast (DIC) signal. Sox9$^+$ cells can be found at day 14 and 21 in areas with cartilage and close to Osx$^+$ cells, indicating ongoing further differentiation and mineralization, which is accompanied by vascularization. For further quantitative analysis of the vasculature sprouting into the gap, we defined the gap as a rectangular region between the cortical ends and analyzed CD31$^+$ vessels and Osx$^+$ bone cells in this region (**Figure 1C**). At day 3, CD31$^+$ matrix (residuals of the fracture hematoma) and some CD31$^+$ cells are present (compare to **Supplementary Figures 2A–C**), while Osx$^+$ cells enter the osteotomy gap at later time points, between day 7–21 (**Figures 1C,E**). At later phases of fracture healing, endothelial cells displaying the phenotype of type H vessels (Emcn^{hi}CD31^{hi}) closely associate with Osx$^+$ osteoprogenitors/pre-osteoblasts (**Figure 1C**). Investigating the co-localization of Runx2$^+$ and Sox9$^+$ cells with respect to CD31$^+$ endothelium reveals a close localization of Runx2$^+$ cells around vascularized areas, while Sox9$^+$ cells are only found in less vascularized areas (**Figure 1D**). Our results confirm a close relationship between vessel formation and osteoprogenitors/osteoblasts and extend previous reports of this phenomenon, which focused on bone development (7), to a regenerative scenario.

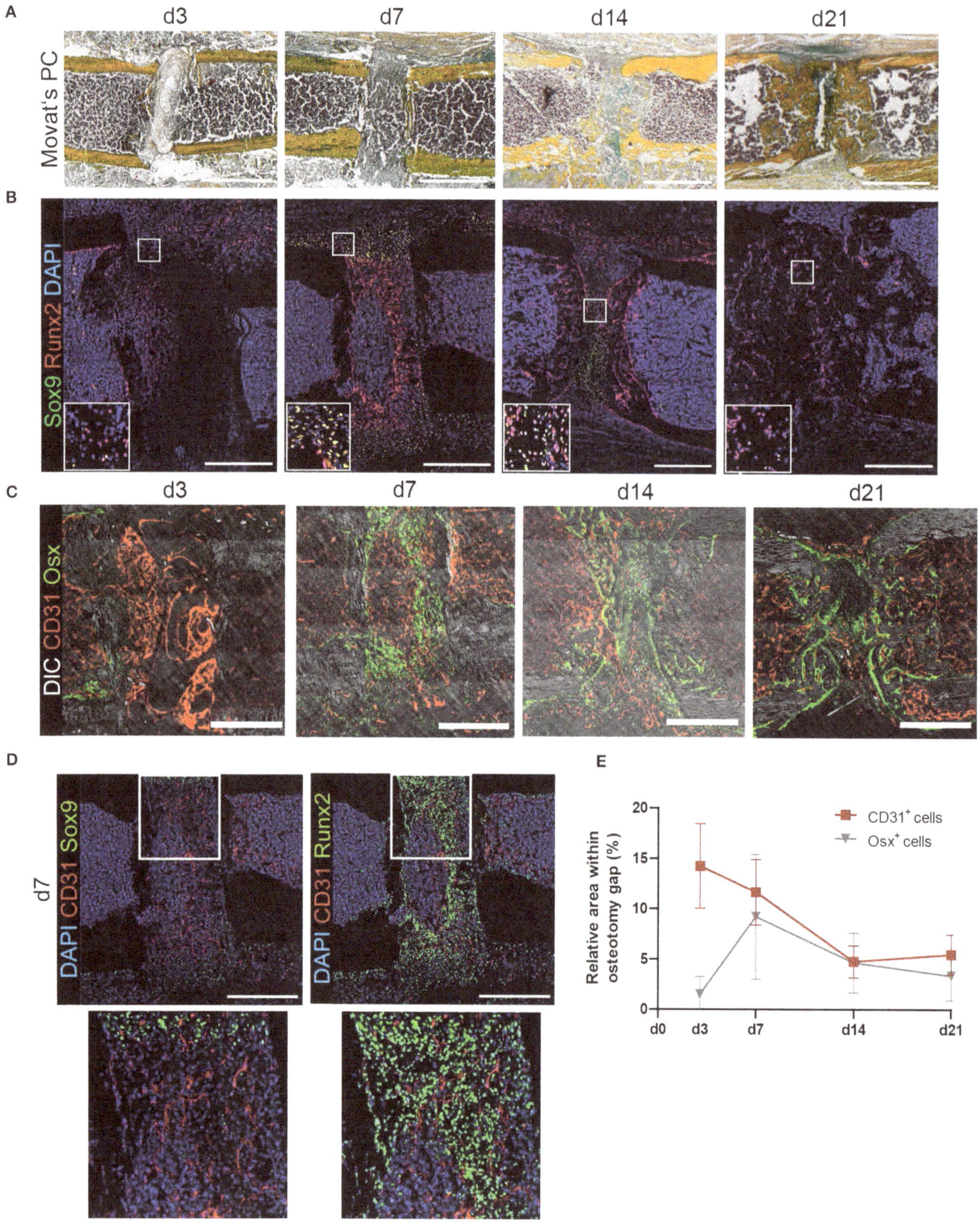

FIGURE 1 | Histological characterization of tissue formation and distribution of mesenchymal progenitor cells, osteoblasts and endothelial cells during bone regeneration in a mouse-osteotomy model. **(A)** Movat's Pentachrome staining indicates the phases of bone regeneration over 21 days. Scale bars = 500 μm. **(B)** Sox9 and Runx2 immunofluorescence staining for progenitor cells undergoing differentiation at day 3, 7, 14, and 21 indicating double-positive cells at day 7 and high numbers of Runx2^{+} cells within the fracture gap at day 14 and 21. Exemplary images of $n = 3$–6 per time point. Scale bars = 200 μm. Insets show enlarged

(Continued)

FIGURE 1 | representative areas marked by white frames. **(C)** Exemplary images at day 3, 7, 14, and 21 displaying the distribution of CD31$^+$ ECs and Osx$^+$ osteoprogenitors/pre-osteoblasts revealing close proximity between CD31$^+$ endothelium and Osx$^+$ cells. Scale bars = 200 μm. **(D)** Exemplary images for Sox9 or Runx2 and CD31 staining at day 7. Insets show enlarged representative areas marked by white frames. While Runx2$^+$ cells can be found closed to endothelial cells, Sox9$^+$ cells can be found in not yet vascularized areas. **(E)** Quantification of cellular compartments present in the fracture gap during regeneration. Endothelial cells (ECs; CD31$^+$) and osteoprogenitors/pre-osteoblasts (Osx$^+$) were quantified based on the relative presence of positive pixels with the respective markers in immunofluorescence images supporting the descriptive analysis on the spatiotemporal distribution of progenitor cells, osteoblasts and endothelial cells over time. Data show mean ± SD for *n* = 3–6.

Localization and Morphologic Characterization of Emcn^{hi}CD31^{hi} Type H Endothelium

While Emcn^{hi}CD31^{hi} endothelium can be found directly in the osteotomy gap and in the adjacent tissue, Emcn^{lo}CD31^{lo} endothelium is prominent in bone marrow regions not affected by the injury. Pixel intensity analysis confirms the differences between the Emcn$^+$ and/or CD31$^+$ cells in and adjacent to the osteotomy gap, compared to the bone marrow (**Figures 2A,B**).

We further characterized the type H vessels in the fracture gap (**Figures 2C,D**). During vascularization of cartilaginous tissue, invading vessel buds (distal loops), previously described as a morphological criterion for type H endothelium (7), can be identified (**Figure 2E**, first row marked by arrows). Furthermore, CD31$^+$ arterioles, which are negative for Emcn, are found within the osteotomy gap. However, a second morphological criterion described to be typical for type H vessels in the growth plate areas, namely their columnar structure, does not appear during regeneration, suggesting that this ordered arrangement is a specific feature of bones undergoing longitudinal growth. Taken together, our data reveal the appearance of Emcn^{hi}CD31^{hi} in the fracture gap, which share additional distinct morphological features with the previously described type H vessels, although they are not organized in columnar structures. This finding suggests an important role of this osteogenic vessel type not only during bone development, but also during regenerative processes of the bone.

M2-Like Macrophages Localize Preferentially Extramedullary

In order to determine the role of macrophages in the context of vascularization during bone regeneration, we analyzed macrophage subsets and their spatial localization relative to type H vessels. Based on the pan-macrophage marker F4/80, which includes also osteomacs, we defined M1- and M2-like macrophages labeled by CD80 and CD206 (Mannose receptor), respectively, as well as Mac-2 (Galectin-3), a marker associated with pro-inflammatory macrophages (22). Over the course of endochondral bone regeneration, F4/80$^+$ cells localize throughout the bone marrow, as well as on the border to bone surfaces, accumulating in various areas (**Figure 3A**). At day 3 post-osteotomy, high numbers of F4/80^{hi} cells localize in periosteal regions adjacent to the osteotomy gap. They can be found periosteal in varying numbers throughout the regeneration process, until the bone remodeling phase at day 21. At day 14, F4/80^{hi} cells are found exclusively in periosteal regions, whereas they are found in both the medulla and the periost at day 21. Extra-medullar F4/80$^+$ macrophages are positive for the anti-inflammatory M2(a) macrophage marker CD206 (**Figure 3A**, blue framed inset). Those M2-like cells are not abundant in the marrow or at sites of vascularization, where expression of CD206 is generally lower and macrophage morphology rather ramified (**Figure 3A**, yellow and orange framed insets). CD206 expression is also found in cells resembling the morphology of endothelia (Emcn$^+$), which are F4/80$^-$ throughout the regeneration process as well as under homeostatic conditions (**Figure 3A**, yellow framed inset; **Supplementary Figures 3C,D**). M1-like macrophages, defined by expression of CD80, are extremely rare and only few are found at day 3, with their abundance comparable to control tissue (**Supplementary Figures 3B,D**). Using the marker Mac-2 in addition, almost all CD206$^+$ macrophages are found to be positive for Mac-2 at day 3, however, not all Mac-2$^+$ cells are CD206$^+$ (**Figure 3B**). Mac-2 positive cells localize in the fracture gap and in proximity to the bone surfaces. Over the course of regeneration, double-positive Mac-2$^+$ and CD206$^+$ cells vanish and cells which are single positive for each of the two markers are detected at day 21, a time point when remodeling is ongoing (**Figure 3B**). Quantitative pixel-based area analysis of F4/80 macrophages, CD31 and TRAP shows that CD31$^+$ and F4/80$^+$ cells are reduced over time, while the number of TRAP$^+$ cells (osteoclasts or activated macrophages) increases (**Figure 3C**; **Supplementary Figure 3A**).

CD206$^+$ macrophages are present throughout the healing process with no apparent preferential localization towards the vasculature, and they are mainly Mac-2$^+$ in the early phase of regeneration. Over the course of regeneration, F4/80-expression decreases in regions adjacent to the callus, and at later time points only few areas, which contain cells expressing F4/80 at intermediate levels, are observed.

F4/80$^+$ and CD80$^+$ Cells Produce VEGFA During Early Regeneration and Osteoblasts and Chondrocytes Are the Main Producers at Later Time Points

Since we could not find substantial amounts of CD80$^+$ cells at day 3 post-osteotomy, we analyzed the regeneration at day 1 and day 2. Some CD80$^+$ cells were found at day 1, and they were abundant in higher numbers at day 2 post-osteotomy (**Figure 4A**). Some of those are F4/80$^+$CD80$^+$ macrophages, which localize in areas adjacent to the osteotomy gap. CD80$^+$ cells are located directly at the injury site (**Figure 4A**, day 2). Macrophages are known to support vascularization via VEGFA during tissue regeneration, which is why next, we analyzed VEGFA using immunofluorescence histology over the time

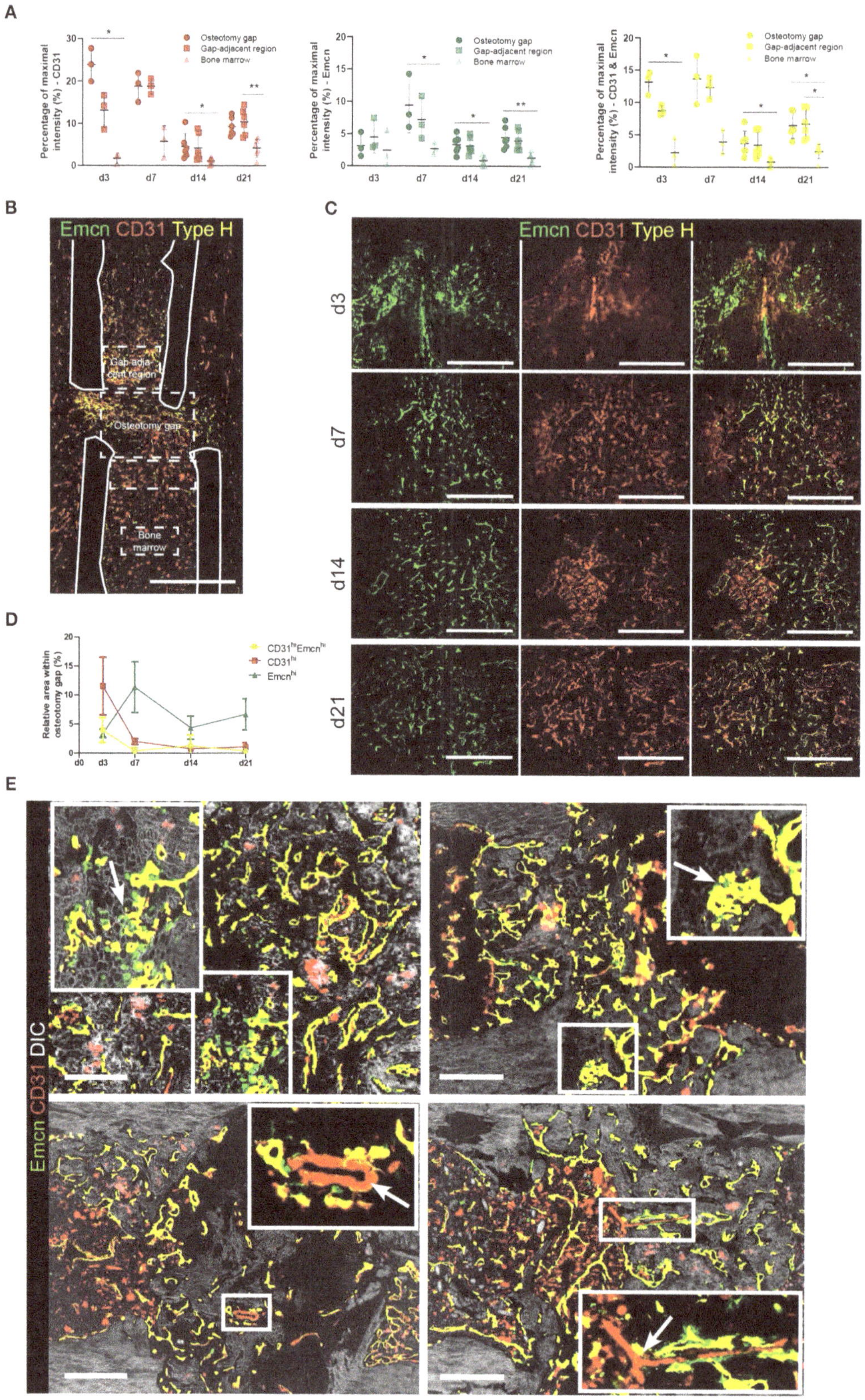

FIGURE 2 | Vessels formed during fracture healing show characteristics of type H endothelium and are embedded in mineralized tissue. **(A)** Intensity analysis of Emcn and/or CD31 in the fracture gap. Mean intensities were normalized to the maximum intensity present in each image. Mean intensities were normalized to 780 the maximum intensity present in each image. Data are shown as scatter dot plot with mean ± SD while one dot is representative for one slide of one individual animal.

(Continued)

FIGURE 2 | Friedman test with Dunn's *post-hoc* test were performed to determine statistical differences; *p*-values are indicated with **p* < 0.05, ***p* < 0.01. **(B)** $Emcn^{hi}$ $CD31^{hi}$ endothelium shows spatial differences in abundance throughout the bone. Exemplary image showing the definition for the osteotomy gap, the gap adjacent regions and the bone marrow area, as used in our analyses. Scale bar = 200 μm. **(C)** Images of $Emcn^{hi}$ $CD31^{hi}$ endothelium at day 3, 7, 14, and 21. Data are representative for $n = 3$ (d3/7) and $n = 6$ (d14/21). **(D)** Quantification of areas occupied by $Emcn^{hi}$ $CD31^{hi}$ type H endothelium during the time course of bone healing. Data are shown as Mean ± SD. **(E)** Emcn and CD31 staining combined with phase contrast images (DIC) in the soft to hard callus transition of fracture healing highlight morphological characteristics also present in growth plate bone growth. Upper panels: invasion of vessels in cartilaginous tissue and type H vessel-like budding is indicated by arrows. Lower panels: $CD31^+$ only vessels are assumed to be arterioles (arrows) (7). Scale bars = 200 μm.

course of bone regeneration (**Figures 4B–D**). VEGFA is not expressed by $F4/80^+CD80^-$ macrophages throughout the entire process, but $CD80^+F4/80^-$ and a fraction of $CD80^+F4/80^+$ cells express VEGFA. This expression was restricted to very early time points, namely day 1 and day 2 (**Figures 4B,C**). From day 3 on, VEGFA is found to be expressed in the fracture gap and along bone surfaces (endosteal, periosteal) and in the bone forming areas (**Figure 4D**). The signal for VEGFA at day 14 is pronounced in areas, which also contain $Sox9^+$ and $Runx2^+$ cells (**Figures 1B, 4D**). Taken together, VEGFA expression is observed in $CD80^+$ cells, including a fraction of $F4/80^+$ cells, in the early phase until day 3, after that, VEGFA is expressed predominantly by osteoblasts and chondrocytes in bone forming areas.

Cells Within the Osteotomy Gap Localize in Proximity to the Endothelium

High abundance and expression of the vascular markers CD31 and Emcn is observed in both, the damaged tissue in the early regeneration, and in bone forming tissue over the subsequent course of regeneration in the osteotomy gap (**Figure 2C**). These areas rich in type H vessels, simultaneously contain $F4/80^{hi}$ cells (**Figures 3A,D**). In order to evaluate the proximity in localization between macrophages and type H endothelium, we defined two regions for each sample, the $Emcn^{hi}$ region and the $Emcn^{lo}$ region (**Figure 3E**). Objects in these regions were segmented based on marker expression of Emcn, F4/80 and DAPI. Over the course of regeneration, similar frequencies of 25.0 ± 11.6 % $F4/80^+$ cells are present in both, the $Emcn^{hi}$ and $Emcn^{lo}$ regions. The frequencies of $F4/80^+$ cells decrease significantly from day 3 until day 21 post-injury (**Figure 3E**), confirming the qualitative results from **Figure 3C**. Next, we analyzed the position of macrophages relative to the endothelium, and found that, a two- to three-fold higher number of objects ($F4/80^+$ objects or identified nuclei, which serve as a control for all cells) localize in proximity to the endothelium in the $Emcn^{hi}$ region as compared to the $Emcn^{lo}$ region (**Figure 3F**). Cells are defined as "in proximity" when they are located less than half a nuclear diameter in distance (<3.5 um) away from the endothelium.

During analysis of immunofluorescence staining in samples of osteotomized, LIMB-implanted bones, we noticed a transient, strongly polarized distribution of newly formed vessels to the distal area of the osteotomy gap (**Figure 5A; Supplementary Figure 4A**). A similar polarization occurs in samples of the osteotomy-model (**Supplementary Figure 4B**). In some cases, this phenomenon is accompanied by a variation in cell density in the respective area, as shown by differences in the abundance of the DAPI signal. Scoring according to the criteria described in the methods section for the abundance and intensity of the markers in the gap-adjacent regions reveals that $CD31^+$ vessels are significantly brighter and more abundant adjacent distally to the gap, as compared to the proximal site (**Figure 5B**). This spatial polarization with respect to bright $CD31^+$ vessels is pronounced at day 4 and decreases quickly afterwards (**Figure 5B**). A similar trend is observed for $F4/80^+$ cells in the same regions (**Figure 5B**). Taken together, these analyses reveal a transient, directional spatial polarization (regarding the localization from the fracture gap) of $CD31^{hi}$ vessels, adjacent to the fracture gap.

$CX3CR1^+$ $F4/80^+$ Macrophages Precede Vascularization

In order to understand the dynamics of macrophages during bone regeneration, we took advantage of the fractalkine receptor (CX3CR1) reporter mouse strain CX3CR1:GFP. These mice were implanted with a Gradient Refractive INdex (GRIN) lens, enabling longitudinal imaging of the bone marrow during regeneration (10). At the same time, these mice underwent osteotomy surgery. Since the first wave of vascularization occurs during resolution of the fracture hematoma, bones that had been treated using the procedure described were fixed and analyzed at day 4, 6, and 8 using immunofluorescence histology. In order to be able to exclude monocytes and granulocytes from the macrophage analysis, we stained sections using antibodies against Ly-6C/Ly-6G (Gr-1). We find that almost all $F4/80^+$ macrophages in the osteotomy gap are also $CX3CR1^+$ (**Figures 5C,D**, yellow), confirming that the reporter mice are suitable for tracking macrophage dynamics during bone regeneration. GFP^+ cells are present within the osteotomy gap at early time points and become less abundant over time. They locate in close proximity to $CD31^{hi}$ endothelium, do not express Gr-1 (**Figure 5D**), excluding the possibility that some of them are granulocytes, which are also described to be $CX3CR1^+$. We analyzed the osteotomy gap between the cortices and the bone marrow as described in **Figure 5E**. At day 6, of all identified cells in the osteotomy gap, the $CX3CR1^+$ cells display the highest increase in cell number, as compared to homeostasis. A minor increase is detected in $F4/80^+$ cells and a strong reduction of $Gr\text{-}1^+$ cells is observed compared to homeostasis (**Figure 5F**). The space is largely occupied by $F4/80^+$ myeloid cells, which are not monocytes ($Gr\text{-}1^-$). The strongest increase in cell number is observed in the $CX3CR1^+Gr\text{-}1\text{-}F4/80^+$ subset, which make up to 12% in ratio to all nuclei at day 6 (**Figure 5G**). Almost 6% of $CX3CR1^+$ objects are $F4/80^-$ and only few are $Gr\text{-}1^+$. Morphologically, the cell phenotype is of non-round shape (**Figure 5E, Supplementary Figure 5**). We then longitudinally sampled time-lapse videos with two-photon microscopy from individual mice over the course of the early regeneration process. On the first and second day, almost no signal is detected inside

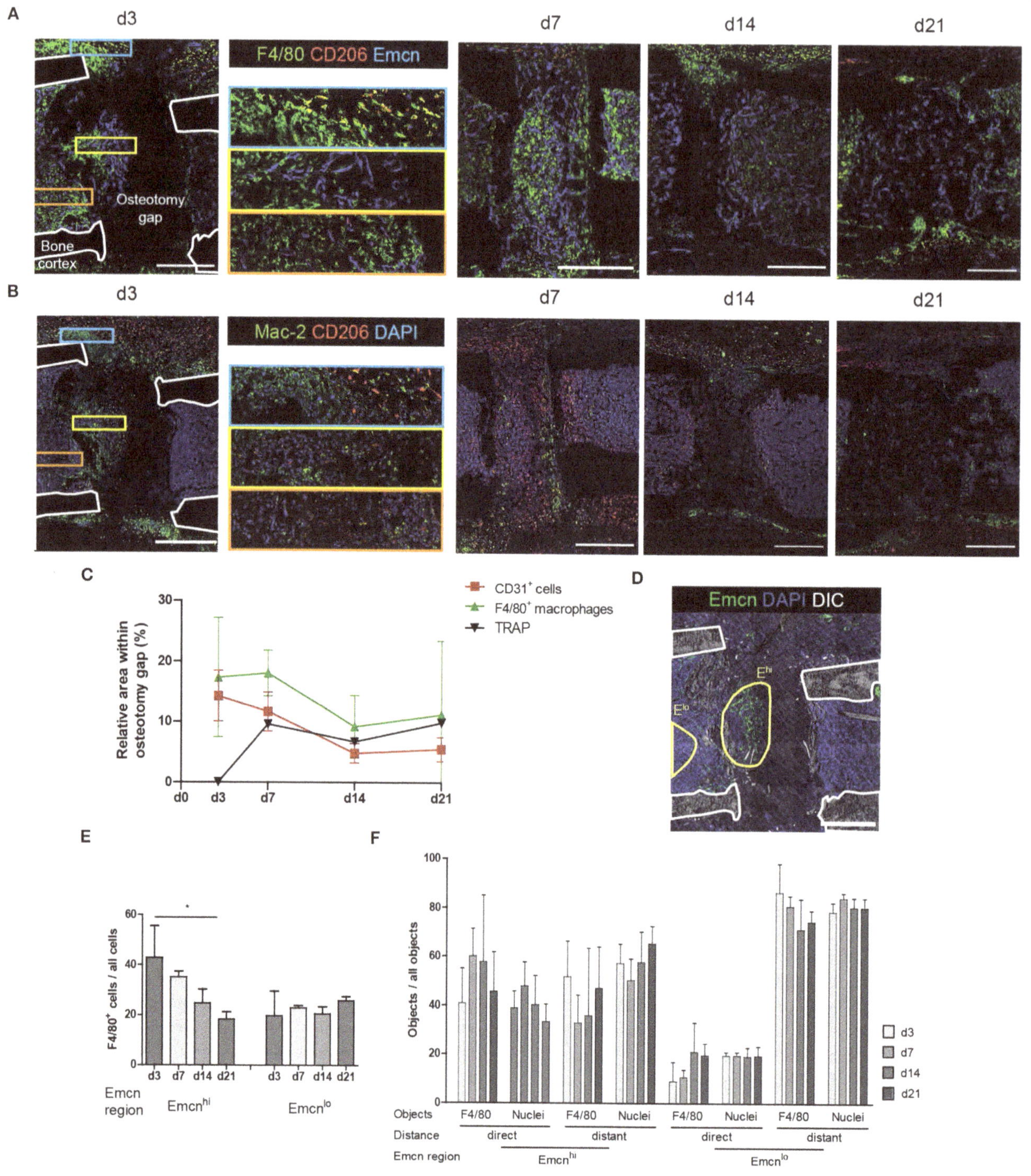

FIGURE 3 | Distinct localization of macrophage subsets during bone regeneration indicates location-dependence of their functions. **(A)** Immunofluorescence staining of F4/80, CD206, and Emcn shows the abundance of F4/80+ cells in the osteotomy gap. They localize close to Emcn^{hi} endothelium. F4/80+CD206+ M2-like macrophages primarily localize in extramedullar areas (blue inset). F4/80^{hi} cells localize in proximity to Emcn^{hi} endothelium (yellow inset). Endothelium shows CD206-positivity in proximity to the gap (orange inset). Scale bars = 500 μm. **(B)** Immunofluorescence staining reveals spatiotemporal distribution of CD206+ and Mac-2+ cells. CD206+ M2-like macrophages were Mac-2+ at d3 and single-positive by d21. Scale bars = 500 μm. **(C)** Pixel-based area analysis of immunofluorescence images of CD31, F4/80, and TRAP show a reduction of CD31 and F4/80 signals over time and an increase in osteoclasts. **(D)** Object-based analysis for **(E,F)**, based on regions within the osteotomy gap which show high or low expression of Emcn (Emcn^{hi} vs. Emcn^{lo}). Scale bar = 500 μm. **(E)** F4/80+ cell frequency in the Emcn^{hi} region decreases between d3 and d21 to levels of the Emcn^{lo} region. Mann Whitney test, two-tailed, $^{*}p = 0.0476$. **(F)** Proximity analysis

(Continued)

FIGURE 3 | performed by object-based quantification in two distances from the endothelium. Data was normalized to the overall number of the object population in the respective region. Compared to the $Emcn^{lo}$ region, more objects ($F4/80^+$ or nuclei) localize in proximity to the endothelium in the $Emcn^{hi}$ region. Cells were considered in proximity to each other when their distance amounted to that equivalent to less than half of a nucleus diameter (<3.5 μm), in order to include cells which are either in contact with or in the direct vicinity of vessels. Cells were considered distant were located further than one cell layer (>7 μm) apart from each other. Data are representative for $n = 3$ (d3/7) and $n = 6$ (d14/21).

the osteotomy gap (data not shown). On day 3, individual $CX3CR1^+$ cells enter the hematoma (**Figure 5H**d3). Those cells display a non-round, but non-ramified shape and move through the tissue (**Supplementary Movie 1**). A front of $CX3CR1^+$ cells forms at the edge of the field of view at day 4, containing both round and non-round cellular phenotypes, forming a dense, partially resident population which expands into the entire field of view (**Figure 5H**, **Supplementary Movies 2, 3**). This invasion is accompanied by the occurrence of perfused vessels that expand, following the $CX3CR1^+$ cell front until the field of view appears vascularized (**Supplementary Movie 4**). Under full vascularization, sessile $CX3CR1^+$ cells localize towards the vasculature and motile cells can be observed to move along the endothelium (**Supplementary Movie 3**). Generally, the abundance of $CX3CR1^+$ in the gap increases with progression of the regeneration process (**Figure 5F**, **Supplementary Movies 3, 4**).

These results indicate that most cells in the fracture gap are myeloid, non-monocytic, non-granulocytic, non-round $CX3CR1^+$ which invade the osteotomy hematoma starting day 2–3, become gradually sessile in the fracture gap at day 3–4, where they precede the vasculature until it becomes fully perfused. After vascularization, $CX3CR1^+F4/80^+$ cells persist until the onset of the remodeling phase.

DISCUSSION

Vascularization is pivotal to the success of complete, scar-free bone regeneration. Here, we show that after bone injury, type H endothelium evolves in the bone formation region and persists throughout the entire bone regeneration process. Our findings show that the phenotype of type H endothelial cell structures described in endochondral long bone growth, is also reflected in bone regeneration. $Emcn^{hi}CD31^{hi}$ endothelium shows association with Osx^+ osteoblasts and displays typical features that can be observed in the growth plate during longitudinal growth, such as invading vessel buds and arch-like structures described before (7). Other than their counterparts in the growth plate, type H vessels generated during regeneration are not columnar. However, this feature is probably not inherent to type H vessels, but merely the result of the highly ordered structure of chondrocytes in the metaphyseal areas. These chondrocytes are organized into columns that are produced in the growth plate, and probably impose their structure on the type H vessels in these areas. In contrast, the tissue structure surrounding type H vessels in a fracture gap appears more disorganized. We have previously shown that the amount of type H vessels can be used as a measure of fracture healing progression (21). Ramasamy et al. reported the effect of shear stress in the vascular formation during bone development, therefore it would be interesting to analyze whether interfragmentary, compressional mechanical cues also act on the formation and structure of type H vessels in fracture healing (39).

We found an extensive staining of CD31 in the gap, which dominates the initial hematoma phase (until day 3–4). This staining seems not to be associated with intact cells, since no nuclei are present. It is possible that $CD31^+$ cells are present in the early fracture hematoma during the first hours after injury and undergo cell death due the hypoxic microenvironment, including a low pH and high lactate level in the tissue, and that the staining pattern observed represents dead endothelial cells.

Based on our results, and similar to a previously reported model in sheep (6), we propose that two phases of vascularization occur during bone regeneration also in mice. The first wave of vascularization occurs during disintegration of the fracture hematoma, where vascular sprouts from existing endothelial cells enter into a hypoxic environment. It occurs between the initial injury and day 6, until the entire volume is fully vascularized for soft callus formation. We observe this phase histologically and by intravital microscopy. After the first wave, and once the callus becomes calcified, we assume that the vascular network within hard callus and bone is remodeled in a second phase, based on the changes that happen during tissue reorganization. It has been described that most of the progenitor cells that contribute to fracture repair immigrate from the periosteum (40). In addition, these progenitor cells either express Sox9 or Runx2, which are regulated by direct repression of the opposing pathway (via β-catenin expression) and define further differentiation into chondrocytes or osteoblasts, respectively (41). However, several studies show the importance of Sox9 expressing progenitor cells that support mineralization and osteogenesis within the fracture gap (42–44). At day 7, we observe a co-localization of Sox9 and Runx2 (**Figure 1B**), it can be speculated that co-expression of both transcription factors marks a switch in the genetic program, from uncommitted pre-osteoblasts to chondrocyte differentiation, similar to what has been shown in bone development (45). Alternatively, Sox9 expressing cells might differentiate into osteoblasts, as described previously (42–44). Our results show close proximity between osteoprogenitors ($Runx2^+$) or osteoblasts (Osx^+) and $CD31^+$ endothelium (**Figures 1C,D**). Endothelial cells, which display the phenotype of type H vessels ($Emcn^{hi}CD31^{hi}$) closely associate with Osx^+ cells in this osteotomy (= cortical defect) model. Type H endothelia have been previously described to be present in the metaphyseal areas of young animals, where they promote bone growth (7). The results presented here indicate a similar crosstalk to occur in endochondral osteogenesis during regeneration.

The large extent of angiogenesis, which occurs in the fracture gap, raises the question for factors and cell types which trigger this event. In the growth plate, hypertrophic chondrocytes

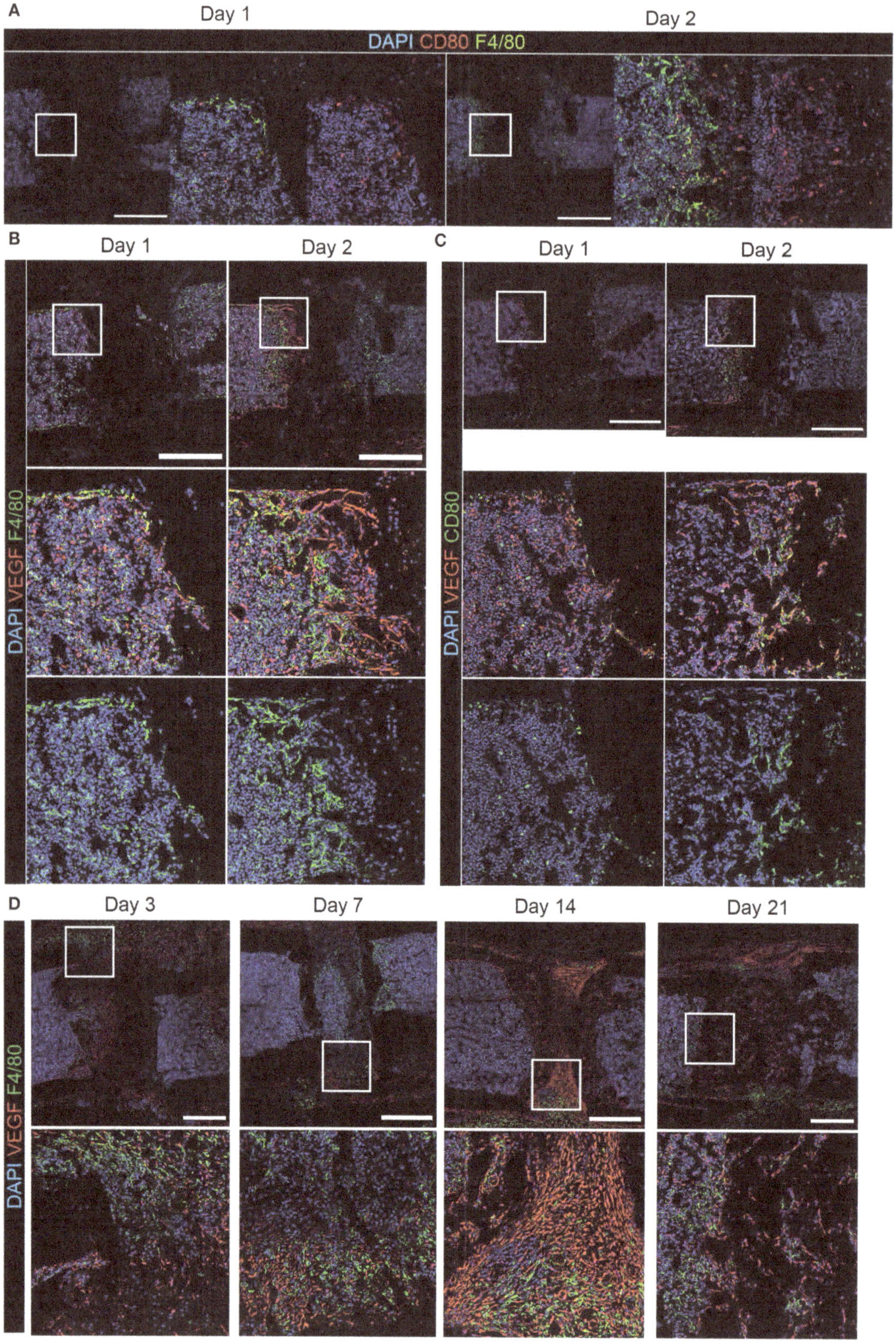

FIGURE 4 | Expression of VEGFA in CD80$^+$ cells and bone forming areas at the osteotomy site. Immunofluorescence staining over the course of regeneration shows **(A)** pro-inflammatory CD80$^+$ cells adjacent to the osteotomy gap, which are in part F4/80$^+$ in the early phase (at day 1 and 2). **(B)** F4/80$^+$ cells were predominantly VEGFA$^-$. **(C)** CD80$^+$VEGFA$^+$ cells localize at the interface between the hematoma and surrounding tissue. **(D)** In areas of bone formation VEGFA expression is high, but F4/80$^+$ cells re VEGFA$^-$ during progressing bone regeneration until day 21. Scale bars = 500 μm. *n*(day 1) = 3, *n*(day 2) = 1.

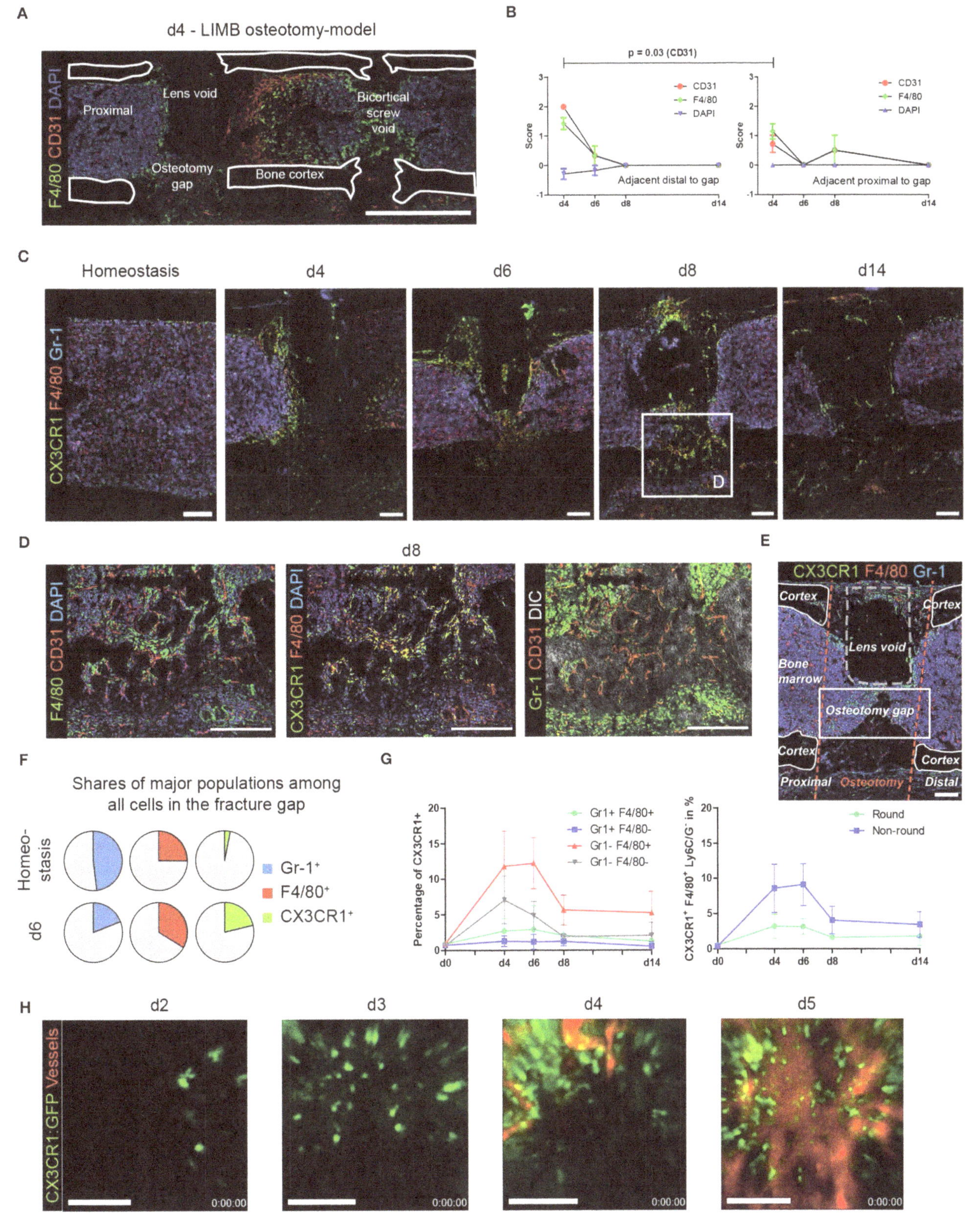

FIGURE 5 | Quantitative analysis and LIMB imaging demonstrate high abundance of the myeloid CX3CR1^{+} F4/80^{+} cell subset preceding vascularization. **(A)** Overview image of a section from a whole bone taken at day 4 after LIMB osteotomy. The LIMB osteotomy-model model uses a gradient refractive index lens which is removed before bone sectioning thus a *lens void* remains. Vessels and macrophages polarize distally in this example. **(B)** Scoring of CD31 and F4/80 allows

(Continued)

FIGURE 5 | quantification of polarization in proximal or distal orientation with respect to the fracture gap. Scoring of DAPI staining was used as internal control. Wilcoxon matched-pairs signed rank test. Data are representative for $n = 7$ (d4), $n = 6$ (d6), $n = 4$ (d8), and $n = 3$ (d14). **(C)** Immunofluorescence images of sections from bones showing the presence of myeloid subsets at various time points after LIMB osteotomy. CX3CR1:GFP$^+$ and F4/80$^+$ cells negative for Ly6C/Ly6G (Gr-1), accumulate at and invade into the fracture gap. Scale bars = 200 μm. **(D)** Inset of the area of d8. The majority of myeloid cells are CX3CR1$^+$F4/80$^+$ and localize in distance from Gr-1$^+$ cells. Scale bars = 200 μm. **(E)** Quantitative analysis is performed in the rectangular region of the fracture gap between corticalis, osteotomy cuts, and lens void (osteotomy gap). Scale bar = 100 μm. **(F)** Quantitative, object-based analysis of the osteotomy gap for Gr-1, F4/80, CX3CR1:GFP show a decrease of Gr-1$^+$, an increase of F4/80$^+$ and massive increase of CX3CR1$^+$ cells. Results of 20 pooled samples. **(G)** Object-analysis among the CX3CR1$^+$ cells reveals that Gr-1$^-$F4/80$^+$ account for the majority of cells present in the gap over the whole time course of regeneration (left panel). Of those, the majority were non-round cells (right panel). **(H)** Intravital two-photon LIMB-microscopy of the osteotomy gap in an individual CX3CR1:GFP mouse. CX3CR1:GFP$^+$ cells invade the osteotomy gap in the displayed field of view (250 × 250 μm) at day 2–3 and fully populate the region by day 3–4. Simultaneously, numerous CX3CR1$^+$ cells precede the vascularization in space and time. Vasculature was made visible using intravenous injection of Qtracker 655. Scale bars = 100 μm. Data are representative of 5 mice analyzed.

produce high amounts of VEGFA, due to the hypoxic microenvironment in those areas, in which HIF stimulates VEGFA expression (7). In a recent publication, Buettmann et al. deleted VEGFA from early osteolineage (Osx$^+$) cells, mature osteoblasts and osteocytes (Dmp1$^+$) as well as ubiquitously in models of cortical fractures (full and stress fractures) and a cortical defect model (drilling). Bone regeneration and periosteal angiogenesis after a cortical defect was impaired only when VEGFA was deleted either ubiquitously or from Osx$^+$ cells, indicating a predominant role of osteolineage cells. After drill hole injury, however, the deletion did not lead to delayed healing, indicating that another cell type than Osx$^+$ is responsible for VEGFA production and the progression of vascularization.

Macrophages have been identified to play a role in bone regeneration, as their deletion either via clodronate (24, 25) or genetically delays healing. Data available in the literature indicate multiple functions for macrophages during bone regeneration. Recently, the supportive function of F4/80$^+$ macrophages during bone regeneration via enhanced osteogenesis when transplanted to aged individuals was demonstrated (46). In addition, it is known that F4/80$^+$ osteomacs support osteoblast function (47). Osteoblast differentiation and mineralization have also been shown to be modulated by macrophages (48, 49). However, the role of macrophages in the vascularization of the fracture is largely unknown. Here, for the first time, we quantitatively and qualitatively map out the vascular network, relate it to the presence of macrophages at relevant time points during bone regeneration in mice and analyze presence and proximity with different approaches. We find that F4/80$^+$ macrophages and type H endothelium localize at the front of damaged tissue in the first phase until soft callus formation, when their presence is reduced. In detail, our proximity analysis reveals that all cells, including F4/80$^+$ macrophages in the regenerating tissue, localize much closer to the endothelium than in unaffected areas in both, the first (d3–d7 after injury) and second (d14–d21 after injury) phase of revascularization. We find CX3CR1$^+$F4/80$^+$ macrophages to be a predominant subset in this process. Phenotypically, these cells are for the most part non-round and ramified. They localize predominantly in a one-cell layer around the endothelium. Future work is needed to study the fate of this subset. It is possible that those cells differentiate or merge with osteoclasts and therefore promote remodeling of the bone.

Using longitudinal intravital microendoscopy of the osteotomized region, we find that CX3CR1$^+$ macrophages precede the occurrence of perfused vessels into the hematoma in the first phase and remain associated to the endothelium. We show the type H endothelium to be closely associated with CX3CR1$^+$F4/80$^+$ macrophages, suggesting that this myeloid population is responsible for vascularization and progression of bone regeneration.

In the fracture hematoma, no chondrocytes are present, so macrophages may be a source of VEGFA in that situation. Here, we identify two major cell populations, which produce VEGFA over the course of regeneration. In the earliest phase, at day 1 and 2 post injury, CD80$^+$ cells are found to be positive for VEFGA by immunofluorescence. From day 3 on, cells inside the area of bone formation and on bone surfaces show a strong VEGFA signal. Based on their localization, the proximity to bone surfaces, we assume that these cells are precursors of, and committed osteoblasts, as well as chondrocytes in cartilage (16; compare **Figures 1A–C**). Until day 3, among the CD80$^+$ cells, we find F4/80$^+$, which we consider M1-like cells, as well as F4/80$^-$, which could either be a subpopulation of mature F4/80$^-$ macrophages or precursors of macrophages, such as F4/80^{low} monocytes (50). In addition, other antigen-presenting cells such as B cells and dendritic cells can be CD80$^+$ (51, 52). It has been previously described that VEGFA-expression of macrophages depends on the stimulation state (53, 54). Additionally, tissue resident F4/80$^+$ macrophages are not known to express VEGFA constantly, but rather they interact with VEGFA-producing cells on promoting vascularization and supporting sprout fusion (29, 55). Our results support previous literature by showing VEGFA-expression from immune cells (56). Here, CD80$^+$ cells were expressing VEGFA in the early phase until day 3, while the majority was F4/80$^-$. CD80$^+$ M1-like macrophages have not been reported to express VEGFA. It can be speculated from our data that CD80$^+$ cells contribute to the presence of VEGFA within the fracture gap until bone cells differentiate and become the dominant producers of VEGFA during the bone formation and remodeling phase.

The presence of M1-like macrophages until day 3, the subsequent decrease, and the absence at later time points in our study indicates that the transition from the pro-inflammatory phase to the anti-inflammatory phase in the myeloid compartment has already taken place at day 3 in the osteotomy models analyzed here. It has been described that a switch from M1-like macrophages to an M2-like phenotype is essential for successful healing. Under chronic inflammatory conditions it is impaired and accompanied by the prolonged presence of M1-like macrophages (57). Consequently, recent research focuses on this switch to improve healing (58, 59). Interestingly, M1- and M2-like macrophages do not localize inside the fracture gap, and rather $CX3CR1^{+}F4/80^{+}$ cells participate in the initial and crucial vascularization process. Our spatial analyses reveal that $CD206^{+}$ macrophages localize in extramedullary areas and, moreover, that they remain positive for the pro-inflammatory maker Mac-2 until d14. After that, cells that are positive for either CD206 or Mac-2 remain present until the remodeling phase. The extramedullary localization of $CD206^{+}$ macrophages may indicate that M2-like macrophages serve functions beyond bone regeneration, for example skeletal muscle regeneration (60).

Of note, during the regeneration process, the immunofluorescence signal for $Emcn^{+}$ in the endothelium partially co-localizes with the signal for the mannose receptor CD206. CD206 expression in endothelial cells has been previously reported to be linked to the phagocytic activity of this cell type (61). In addition, Awert et al. describe CD206 as a marker for perivascular macrophages and show that they locate closely to $Emcn^{+}$ cells in tumors (62). $CD206^{+}$ endothelial cells can be found in different tissues such as the liver (63, 64) or placenta (61). Future experiments need to be performed to investigate the cellular origin of the CD206 signal we observe.

In tissue areas adjacent of the fracture gap, an inhomogeneous distribution of macrophages, as well as endothelia toward the distal end of the femur (spatial polarization), is evident. We suspect that the osteotomy, which interrupts all vessels in the tissue, in combination with placement of the neighboring, distal screw (one of four screws) creates damage to the blood supply occurring from both sides of the fracture (**Supplementary Figure 6**). Large veins and the main sinus exit the bone at few points. However, trans-cortical vessels are predominantly responsible for the arterial blood supply in long bones, as described recently (65). Since the cortical integrity is disrupted by the osteotomy and the screw placement, the blood supply is disturbed to a high degree in a complete osteotomy model. We assume that this results in extensive tissue damage, which in turn initiates the recruitment of macrophages followed by vascularization, leading to the observed phenomenon of transient distal polarization.

Taken together, we demonstrate here that type H endothelium is present throughout the regeneration in standardized osteotomy models in mice. Osx^{+} osteoblasts as well as macrophages are present in close proximity to the vasculature, indicating an important crosstalk. M2-like macrophages are mainly found in extramedullar regions, with no obvious interconnection to the vasculature. In addition, we describe $CX3CR1^{+}F4/80^{+}$ cells to be the predominant macrophage population, which progressively infiltrates the hematoma. These macrophages precede perfused vascularization in the first phase of vascularization and reside there until remodeling takes place. A strong polarization of type H endothelium as well as of macrophages distally to the fracture gap is found in the fracture models. Our findings underline the importance of the innate immune system within the bone regeneration process by linking myeloid cells present in the fracture gap to local angiogenesis.

AUTHOR CONTRIBUTIONS

JS, AL, TG, RN, and AH: study design. JS, AL, AR, LA, MK, KS-B, and AF: data collection and analysis. JS, AL, and AH: data interpretation and writing of the manuscript. KS-B, FB, RN, TG, and GD: revising manuscript.

FUNDING

This study was supported by funding from the Deutsche Forschungsgemeinschaft, FOR2165 (HA5354/6-2 to AH, NI-1167/4-2 to RN), and TRR130, project C01 (to AH and RN). This study was financially supported by the Berlin Institute of Health Center for Regenerative Therapies and the Berlin-Brandenburg School for Regenerative Therapies (BCRT, BSRT). The work of TG was funded by the Deutsche Forschungsgemeinschaft (353142848). AL, FB, and TG acknowledge the support of this work by a grant from the German Federal Institute for Risk Assessment (grant no. 1328-542). We acknowledge support from the German Research Foundation (DFG) and the Open Access Publication Fund of Charité - Universitätsmedizin Berlin.

ACKNOWLEDGMENTS

The authors would like to thank Robert Günther and Mattea Durst for assistance during osteotomy surgeries. JS and AL are members of the Berlin-Brandenburg School for Regenerative Therapies (BSRT).

REFERENCES

1. Manjubala I, Liu Y, Epari DR, Roschger P, Schell H, Fratzl P, et al. Spatial and temporal variations of mechanical properties and mineral content of the external callus during bone healing. *Bone.* (2009) 45:185–92. doi: 10.1016/j.bone.2009.04.249
2. Borgiani E, Figge C, Kruck B, Willie BM, Duda GN, Checa S. Age-related changes in the mechanical regulation of bone healing are explained by altered cellular mechanoresponse. *J Bone Miner Res.* (2019) 34:1923–37. doi: 10.1002/jbmr.3801
3. Schmidt-Bleek K, Petersen A, Dienelt A, Schwarz C, Duda GN. Initiation and early control of tissue regeneration - bone healing as a model system for tissue regeneration. *Expert Opin Biol Ther.* (2014) 14:247–59. doi: 10.1517/14712598.2014.857653
4. Winkler T, Sass FA, Duda GN, Schmidt-Bleek K. A review of biomaterials in bone defect healing, remaining shortcomings and future opportunities for bone tissue engineering: the unsolved challenge. *Bone Joint Res.* (2018) 7:232–43. doi: 10.1302/2046-3758.73.BJR-2017-0270.R1
5. Waddington RJ, Roberts HC, Sugars RV, Schonherr E. Differential roles for small leucine-rich proteoglycans in bone formation. *Eur Cell Mater.* (2003) 6:12–21. doi: 10.22203/eCM.v006a02

6. Lienau J, Schmidt-Bleek K, Peters A, Haschke F, Duda GN, Perka C, et al. Differential regulation of blood vessel formation between standard and delayed bone healing. *J Orthop Res.* (2009) 27:1133–40. doi: 10.1002/jor.20870
7. Kusumbe AP, Ramasamy SK, Adams RH. Coupling of angiogenesis and osteogenesis by a specific vessel subtype in bone. *Nature.* (2014) 507:323–8. doi: 10.1038/nature13145
8. Ramasamy SK, Kusumbe AP, Wang L, Adams RH. Endothelial Notch activity promotes angiogenesis and osteogenesis in bone. *Nature.* (2014) 507:376–80. doi: 10.1038/nature13146
9. Filipowska J, Tomaszewski KA, Niedzwiedzki L, Walocha JA, Niedzwiedzki T. The role of vasculature in bone development, regeneration and proper systemic functioning. *Angiogenesis.* (2017) 20:291–302. doi: 10.1007/s10456-017-9541-1
10. Reismann D, Stefanowski J, Gunther R, Rakhymzhan A, Matthys R, Nutzi R, et al. Longitudinal intravital imaging of the femoral bone marrow reveals plasticity within marrow vasculature. *Nat Commun.* (2017) 8:2153. doi: 10.1038/s41467-017-01538-9
11. Street J, Winter D, Wang JH, Wakai A, Mcguinness A, Redmond HP. Is human fracture hematoma inherently angiogenic? *Clin Orthop Relat Res.* (2000) 378:224–37. doi: 10.1097/00003086-200009000-00033
12. Kolar P, Gaber T, Perka C, Duda GN, Buttgereit F. Human early fracture hematoma is characterized by inflammation and hypoxia. *Clin Orthop Relat Res.* (2011) 469:3118–26. doi: 10.1007/s11999-011-1865-3
13. Hoff P, Gaber T, Strehl C, Schmidt-Bleek K, Lang A, Huscher D, et al. Immunological characterization of the early human fracture hematoma. *Immunol Res.* (2016) 64:1195–206. doi: 10.1007/s12026-016-8868-9
14. Olson S, Hahn D. Surgical treatment of non-unions: a case for internal fixation. *Injury.* (2006) 37:681–90. doi: 10.1016/j.injury.2004.11.039
15. Hu K, Olsen BR. The roles of vascular endothelial growth factor in bone repair and regeneration. *Bone.* (2016) 91:30–8. doi: 10.1016/j.bone.2016.06.013
16. Buettmann EG, Mckenzie JA, Migotsky N, Sykes DA, Hu P, Yoneda S, et al. VEGFA from early osteoblast lineage cells (Osterix+) is required in mice for fracture healing. *J Bone Miner Res.* (2019) 34:1690–706. doi: 10.1002/jbmr.3755
17. Pirosa A, Gottardi R, Alexander PG, Tuan RS. Engineering *in-vitro* stem cell-based vascularized bone models for drug screening and predictive toxicology. *Stem Cell Res Ther.* (2018) 9:112. doi: 10.1186/s13287-018-0847-8
18. Xie H, Cui Z, Wang L, Xia Z, Hu Y, Xian L, et al. PDGF-BB secreted by preosteoclasts induces angiogenesis during coupling with osteogenesis. *Nat Med.* (2014) 20:1270–8. doi: 10.1038/nm.3668
19. Romeo SG, Alawi KM, Rodrigues J, Singh A, Kusumbe AP, Ramasamy SK. Endothelial proteolytic activity and interaction with non-resorbing osteoclasts mediate bone elongation. *Nat Cell Biol.* (2019) 21:430–41. doi: 10.1038/s41556-019-0304-7
20. Sivan U, De Angelis J, Kusumbe AP. Role of angiocrine signals in bone development, homeostasis and disease. *Open Biol.* (2019) 9:190144. doi: 10.1098/rsob.190144
21. Lang A, Kirchner M, Stefanowski J, Durst M, Weber MC, Pfeiffenberger M, et al. Collagen I-based scaffolds negatively impact fracture healing in a mouse-osteotomy-model although used routinely in research and clinical application. *Acta Biomater.* (2019) 86:171–84. doi: 10.1016/j.actbio.2018.12.043
22. Alexander KA, Chang MK, Maylin ER, Kohler T, Muller R, Wu AC, et al. Osteal macrophages promote in vivo intramembranous bone healing in a mouse tibial injury model. *J Bone Miner Res.* (2011) 26:1517–32. doi: 10.1002/jbmr.354
23. Raggatt LJ, Wullschleger ME, Alexander KA, Wu AC, Millard SM, Kaur S, et al. Fracture healing via periosteal callus formation requires macrophages for both initiation and progression of early endochondral ossification. *Am J Pathol.* (2014) 184:3192–204. doi: 10.1016/j.ajpath.2014.08.017
24. Schlundt C, El Khassawna T, Serra A, Dienelt A, Wendler S, Schell H, et al. Macrophages in bone fracture healing: their essential role in endochondral ossification. *Bone.* (2015) 106:78–89. doi: 10.1016/j.bone.2015.10.019
25. Alexander KA, Raggatt LJ, Millard S, Batoon L, Chiu-Ku Wu A, Chang MK, et al. Resting and injury-induced inflamed periosteum contain multiple macrophage subsets that are located at sites of bone growth and regeneration. *Immunol Cell Biol.* (2017) 95:7–16. doi: 10.1038/icb.2016.74
26. Batoon L, Millard SM, Raggatt LJ, Pettit AR. Osteomacs and bone regeneration. *Curr Osteoporos Rep.* (2017) 15:385–95. doi: 10.1007/s11914-017-0384-x
27. Spinelli FM, Vitale DL, Demarchi G, Cristina C, Alaniz L. The immunological effect of hyaluronan in tumor angiogenesis. *Clin Transl Immunol.* (2015) 4:e52. doi: 10.1038/cti.2015.35
28. David Dong ZM, Aplin AC, Nicosia RF. Regulation of angiogenesis by macrophages, dendritic cells, and circulating myelomonocytic cells. *Curr Pharm Des.* (2009) 15:365–79. doi: 10.2174/138161209787315783
29. Fantin A, Vieira JM, Gestri G, Denti L, Schwarz Q, Prykhozhij S, et al. Tissue macrophages act as cellular chaperones for vascular anastomosis downstream of VEGF-mediated endothelial tip cell induction. *Blood.* (2010) 116:829–40. doi: 10.1182/blood-2009-12-257832
30. Al-Roubaie S, Hughes JH, Filla MB, Lansford R, Lehoux S, Jones EA. Time-lapse microscopy of macrophages during embryonic vascular development. *Dev Dyn.* (2012) 241:1423–31. doi: 10.1002/dvdy.23835
31. He H, Mack JJ, Güç E, Warren CM, Squadrito ML, Kilarski WW, et al. Perivascular macrophages limit permeability. *Arterioscler Thromb Vasc Biol.* (2016) 36:2203–12. doi: 10.1161/ATVBAHA.116.307592
32. He H, Xu J, Warren CM, Duan D, Li X, Wu L, et al. Endothelial cells provide an instructive niche for the differentiation and functional polarization of M2-like macrophages. *Blood.* (2012) 120:3152–62. doi: 10.1182/blood-2012-04-422758
33. Jirkof P, Durst M, Klopfleisch R, Palme R, Thone-Reineke C, Buttgereit F, et al. Administration of Tramadol or Buprenorphine via the drinking water for post-operative analgesia in a mouse-osteotomy model. *Sci Rep.* (2019) 9:10749. doi: 10.1038/s41598-019-47186-5
34. Lang A, Schulz A, Ellinghaus A, Schmidt-Bleek K. Osteotomy models - the current status on pain scoring and management in small rodents. *Lab Anim.* (2016) 50:433–41. doi: 10.1177/0023677216675007
35. Kawamoto T, Kawamoto K. Preparation of thin frozen sections from nonfixed and undecalcified hard tissues using Kawamot's film method (2012). *Methods Mol Biol.* (2014) 1130:149–64. doi: 10.1007/978-1-62703-989-5_11
36. Carpenter AE, Kamentsky L, Eliceiri KW. A call for bioimaging software usability. *Nat Methods.* (2012) 9:666–70. doi: 10.1038/nmeth.2073
37. Caicedo JC, Cooper S, Heigwer F, Warchal S, Qiu P, Molnar C, et al. Data-analysis strategies for image-based cell profiling. *Nat Methods.* (2017) 14:849–63. doi: 10.1038/nmeth.4397
38. Einhorn TA, Gerstenfeld LC. Fracture healing: mechanisms and interventions. *Nat Rev Rheumatol.* (2015) 11:45–54. doi: 10.1038/nrrheum.2014.164
39. Ramasamy SK, Kusumbe AP, Schiller M, Zeuschner D, Bixel MG, Milia C, et al. Blood flow controls bone vascular function and osteogenesis. *Nat Commun.* (2016) 7:13601. doi: 10.1038/ncomms13601
40. Colnot C. Skeletal cell fate decisions within periosteum and bone marrow during bone regeneration. *J Bone Miner Res.* (2009) 24:274–82. doi: 10.1359/jbmr.081003
41. Bragdon BC, Bahney CS. Origin of reparative stem cells in fracture healing. *Curr Osteoporos Rep.* (2018) 16:490–503. doi: 10.1007/s11914-018-0458-4
42. Akiyama H, Kim JE, Nakashima K, Balmes G, Iwai N, Deng JM, et al. Osteo-chondroprogenitor cells are derived from Sox9 expressing precursors. *Proc. Natl. Acad. Sci. USA.* (2005) 102:14665–70. doi: 10.1073/pnas.0504750102
43. He X, Bougioukli S, Ortega B, Arevalo E, Lieberman JR, Mcmahon AP. Sox9 positive periosteal cells in fracture repair of the adult mammalian long bone. *Bone.* (2017) 103:12–9. doi: 10.1016/j.bone.2017.06.008
44. Kuwahara ST, Serowoky MA, Vakhshori V, Tripuraneni N, Hegde NV, Lieberman JR, et al. Sox9+ messenger cells orchestrate large-scale skeletal regeneration in the mammalian rib. *Elife.* (2019) 8:e40715. doi: 10.7554/eLife.40715
45. Zhou G, Zheng Q, Engin F, Munivez E, Chen Y, Sebald E, et al. Dominance of SOX9 function over RUNX2 during skeletogenesis. *Proc Natl Acad Sci USA.* (2006) 103:19004–9. doi: 10.1073/pnas.0605170103
46. Vi L, Baht GS, Soderblom EJ, Whetstone H, Wei Q, Furman B, et al. Macrophage cells secrete factors including LRP1 that orchestrate the rejuvenation of bone repair in mice. *Nat Commun.* (2018) 9:5191. doi: 10.1038/s41467-018-07666-0
47. Chang MK, Raggatt LJ, Alexander KA, Kuliwaba JS, Fazzalari NL, Schroder K, et al. Osteal tissue macrophages are intercalated throughout human and mouse bone lining tissues and regulate osteoblast function *in vitro* and *in vivo*. *J Immunol.* (2008) 181:1232–44. doi: 10.4049/jimmunol.181.2.1232

48. Vi L, Baht GS, Whetstone H, Ng A, Wei Q, Poon R, et al. Macrophages promote osteoblastic differentiation *in-vivo*: implications in fracture repair and bone homeostasis. *J Bone Miner Res.* (2015) 30:1090–102. doi: 10.1002/jbmr.2422
49. Hoff P, Gaber T, Strehl C, Jakstadt M, Hoff H, Schmidt-Bleek K, et al. A pronounced inflammatory activity characterizes the early fracture healing phase in immunologically restricted patients. *Int J Mol Sci.* (2017) 18:E583. doi: 10.3390/ijms18030583
50. Gordon S, Plüddemann A, Martinez Estrada F. Macrophage heterogeneity in tissues: phenotypic diversity and functions. *Immunol Rev.* (2014) 262:36–55. doi: 10.1111/imr.12223
51. Mclellan AD, Starling GC, Williams LA, Hock BD, Hart DN. Activation of human peripheral blood dendritic cells induces the CD86 co-stimulatory molecule. *Eur J Immunol.* (1995) 25:2064–8. doi: 10.1002/eji.1830250739
52. Subauste CS, De Waal Malefyt R, Fuh F. Role of CD80 (B7.1) and CD86 (B7.2) in the immune response to an intracellular pathogen. *J Immunol.* (1998) 160:1831–40.
53. Wu WK, Llewellyn OP, Bates DO, Nicholson LB, Dick AD. IL-10 regulation of macrophage VEGF production is dependent on macrophage polarisation and hypoxia. *Immunobiology.* (2010) 215:796–803. doi: 10.1016/j.imbio.2010.05.025
54. Gurevich DB, Severn CE, Twomey C, Greenhough A, Cash J, Toye AM, et al. Live imaging of wound angiogenesis reveals macrophage orchestrated vessel sprouting and regression. *EMBO J.* (2018) 37:e97786. doi: 10.15252/embj.201797786
55. Britto DD, Wyroba B, Chen W, Lockwood RA, Tran KB, Shepherd PR, et al. Macrophages enhance Vegfa-driven angiogenesis in an embryonic zebrafish tumour xenograft model. *Dis Model Mech.* (2018) 11:dmm035998. doi: 10.1242/dmm.035998
56. Bahney CS, Zondervan RL, Allison P, Theologis A, Ashley JW, Ahn J, et al. Cellular biology of fracture healing. *J Orthop Res.* (2019) 37:35–50. doi: 10.1002/jor.24170
57. Claes L, Recknagel S, Ignatius A. Fracture healing under healthy and inflammatory conditions. *Nat Rev Rheumatol.* (2012) 8:133–43. doi: 10.1038/nrrheum.2012.1
58. Lin T, Kohno Y, Huang JF, Romero-Lopez M, Pajarinen J, Maruyama M, et al. NFkappaB sensing IL-4 secreting mesenchymal stem cells mitigate the proinflammatory response of macrophages exposed to polyethylene wear particles. *J Biomed Mater Res A.* (2018) 106:2744–52. doi: 10.1002/jbm.a.36504
59. Lin T, Pajarinen J, Kohno Y, Maruyama M, Romero-Lopez M, Huang JF, et al. Transplanted interleukin-4-secreting mesenchymal stromal cells show extended survival and increased bone mineral density in the murine femur. *Cytotherapy.* (2018) 20:1028–36. doi: 10.1016/j.jcyt.2018.06.009
60. Saclier M, Cuvellier S, Magnan M, Mounier R, Chazaud B. Monocyte/macrophage interactions with myogenic precursor cells during skeletal muscle regeneration. *FEBS J.* (2013) 280:4118–30. doi: 10.1111/febs.12166
61. Sheikh H, Yarwood H, Ashworth A, Isacke CM. Endo180, an endocytic recycling glycoprotein related to the macrophage mannose receptor is expressed on fibroblasts, endothelial cells and macrophages and functions as a lectin receptor. *J Cell Sci.* (2000) 113:1021–32.
62. Arwert EN, Harney AS, Entenberg D, Wang Y, Sahai E, Pollard JW, et al. A unidirectional transition from migratory to perivascular macrophage is required for tumor cell intravasation. *Cell Rep.* (2018) 23:1239–48. doi: 10.1016/j.celrep.2018.04.007
63. Azad AK, Rajaram MVS, Schlesinger LS. Exploitation of the macrophage mannose receptor (CD206) in infectious disease diagnostics and therapeutics. *J Cytol Mol Biol.* (2014) 1:1000003. doi: 10.13188/12325-14653.1000003
64. Beljaars L, Schippers M, Reker-Smit C, Martinez FO, Helming L, Poelstra K, et al. Hepatic localization of macrophage phenotypes during fibrogenesis and resolution of fibrosis in mice and humans. *Front Immunol.* (2014) 5:430. doi: 10.3389/fimmu.2014.00430
65. Grüneboom A, Hawwari I, Weidner D, Culemann S, Müller S, Henneberg S, et al. A network of trans-cortical capillaries as mainstay for blood circulation in long bones. *Nat Metab.* (2019) 1:236–50. doi: 10.1038/s42255-018-0016-5

4

Lack of Adipocytes Alters Hematopoiesis in Lipodystrophic Mice

Anne Wilson[1], He Fu[2], Mariano Schiffrin[2], Carine Winkler[2], Meriem Koufany[3], Jean-Yves Jouzeau[3], Nicolas Bonnet[4], Federica Gilardi[2†], François Renevey[5], Sanjiv A. Luther[5], David Moulin[3,6] and Béatrice Desvergne[2*]*

[1] Department of Oncology, University of Lausanne, Epalinges, Switzerland, [2] Faculty of Biology and Medicine, Center for Integrative Genomics, Genopode, University of Lausanne, Lausanne, Switzerland, [3] IMoPA, UMR7365 CNRS-Université de Lorraine, Vandœuvre-lès-Nancy, France, [4] Division of Bone Diseases, Department of Internal Medicine Specialties, Faculty of Medicine, Geneva University Hospital, Geneva, Switzerland, [5] Department of Biochemistry, Center for Immunity and Infection, University of Lausanne, Epalinges, Switzerland, [6] CHRU de Nancy, Contrat d'interface, Vandœuvre-lès-Nancy, France

***Correspondence:**
Anne Wilson
anne.wilson@unil.ch
Béatrice Desvergne
beatrice.desvergne@unil.ch

†Present Address:
Federica Gilardi,
Forensic Toxicology and Chemistry Unit, University Center of Legal Medicine, Lausanne University Hospital - Geneva University Hospitals, Geneva, Switzerland

Adult hematopoiesis takes place in the perivascular zone of the bone cavity, where endothelial cells, mesenchymal stromal/stem cells and their derivatives such as osteoblasts are key components of bone marrow (BM) niches. Defining the contribution of BM adipocytes to the hematopoietic stem cell niche remains controversial. While an excess of medullar adiposity is generally considered deleterious for hematopoiesis, an active role for adipocytes in shaping the niche has also been proposed. We thus investigated the consequences of total adipocyte deletion, including in the BM niche, on adult hematopoiesis using mice carrying a constitutive deletion of the gene coding for the nuclear receptor peroxisome proliferator-activated receptor-γ (PPARγ). We show that *Pparg*$^{\Delta/\Delta}$ lipodystrophic mice exhibit severe extramedullary hematopoiesis (EMH), which we found to be non-cell autonomous, as it is reproduced when wild-type donor BM cells are transferred into *Pparg*$^{\Delta/\Delta}$ recipients. This phenotype is not due to a specific alteration linked to *Pparg* deletion, such as chronic inflammation, since it is also found in AZIP$^{tg/+}$ mice, another lipodystrophic mouse model with normal PPARγ expression, that display only very moderate levels of inflammation. In both models, the lack of adipocytes alters subpopulations of both myeloid and lymphoid cells. The CXCL12/CXCR4 axis in the BM is also dysregulated in an adipocyte deprived environment supporting the hypothesis that adipocytes are required for normal hematopoietic stem cell mobilization or retention. Altogether, these data suggest an important role for adipocytes, and possibly for the molecular interactions they provide within the BM, in maintaining the appropriate microenvironment for hematopoietic homeostasis.

Keywords: lipodystrophy, PPARγ null mice, AZIPtg/+ mice, bone marrow adipocytes, hematopoiesis, extramedullary hematopoiesis, inflammation, non-cell autonomous alteration of hematopoiesis in PPARγ null mice

INTRODUCTION

Bones and hematopoiesis are intimately linked. Adult hematopoiesis takes place in the bone cavity, where a variety of cells and molecular contacts create a niche allowing hematopoietic stem cells (HSCs) to undergo cell division and differentiation in a highly regulated manner. The concept of a stem cell niche was first coined by Schofield, who hypothesized that the cellular environment in the bone compartment creates multiple cell-cell contacts that are crucial for HSC function (1). Depending on the location in the bone cavity, the different cell types involved and different functions proposed, BM niches are described as endosteal, reticular, sinusoidal or perivascular, mainly involving osteoclast precursors, osteoblast and spindle-shaped osteoblast precursors (SNO), CXCL12-abundant-reticular (CAR) cells, Nestin+ mesenchymal stromal cells (MSCs), E-selectin+ endothelial cells, LeptinR+ perivascular stromal cells, and non-myelinating Schwann cells, respectively [reviewed in (2–4)].

The role of adipocytes, present in large numbers in the BM cavity, remains disputed. Adipocytes, which are the specialized cells of adipose tissue, store energy in the form of lipids, and release it when required by the organism. Adipocytes also secrete cytokines known as adipokines that participate in endocrine-mediated homeostasis (5). Both gain of adipose tissue, as in obesity, and the generalized lack of adipose tissue (generalized lipodystrophy), such as is seen in Berardinelli-Seip syndrome, causes metabolic disorders such as hypertriglyceridemia, metabolic syndrome, and type 2 diabetes (6, 7). While most adipocytes are found within depots forming the diverse adipose tissues, some of them are also found in substantial numbers in a less organized manner, particularly within the BM where their (local) role is less well characterized (8). The first link between adipocytes and the bone microenvironment is the fact that both adipocytes and osteoblasts are derived from a common mesenchymal progenitor, and their respective production is due to a balance between adipogenesis and osteoblastogenesis. A more direct contribution of adipocytes to the stem cell niche in the BM has been previously explored, albeit with contradictory results. First, using leptin deficient mice (*ob/ob* mice), Claycombe et al. showed that supplementation with leptin, a major adipokine secreted by adipocytes, rescued appropriate levels of lymphopoiesis and myelopoiesis in the BM (9). Second, a combination of *in vitro* and *in vivo* experiments has suggested that adiponectin, another adipokine expressed by adipocytes in the BM, is required for optimal HSC growth (10, 11). Third, BM adipocytes also secrete Stem Cell Factor, which contributes to restoring hematopoiesis after irradiation in the long bones but not in the vertebral bones (12). Finally, experiments performed in AZIP-F1 (AZIP$^{tg/+}$) transgenic mice carrying a C/EBP dominant negative transgene that induces deletion of mature adipocytes, showed improved marrow engraftment after irradiation, suggesting that in this specific context adipocytes are negative regulators of hematopoiesis (10, 13). A similar negative effect is also proposed when adipocytes overfill the medullary space upon BM failure in Fanconi Anemia (14).

In the present report, we reveal a novel aspect of the cross-talk between hematopoiesis and adipocytes, by exploiting a generalized lipodystrophic mouse model carrying a constitutive total-body deletion of the nuclear receptor peroxisome proliferator-activated receptor-γ (PPARγ) (15, 16). *Pparg*$^{\Delta/\Delta}$ mice show a complex phenotype including total lipoatrophy, increased lean mass, and hypermetabolism. They develop severe type 2 diabetes, characterized by hyperglycemia, hyperinsulinemia, polyuria, and polydipsia (personal communication, manuscript in preparation). Herein, we demonstrate that the total lack of adipocytes is accompanied by extramedullary hematopoiesis (EMH), which is defined as the production of blood cells occurring outside of the BM, mainly in the liver and spleen (17). We further evaluate the causes of this EMH and provide new insights in the role of adipocyte signaling in hematopoiesis.

MATERIALS AND METHODS

Mice

Genotype designations in this work follow the rules recommended by the Mouse Genome Database Nomenclature Committee. Procedures using mice were authorized by the Cantonal Commission for Animal Experimentation of the Canton of Vaud and carried out in accordance with the International Guiding Principles for Biomedical Research Involving Animals. *Sox2-Cre* transgenic mice (*Sox2-Cre* $^{tg/+}$; Tg(Sox2-cre)1Amc/J), CD45.1+ (B6.SJL-*Ptprc*^{a}*Pepc*^{b}/BoyJ) mice (Jackson Laboratory, Bar Harbour, MA), and *ob/ob* mice were kept in the University of Lausanne Animal Facility. Construction of the *Pparg* floxed (hereafter referred to as *Pparg*^{fl}) and *Pparg*-null alleles resulting from Cre recombination (hereafter referred to as *Pparg*$^{\Delta}$), as well as the mating strategy for the generation of *Sox2-Cre*$^{tg/+}$Pparg$^{em\Delta/\Delta}$ (*Pparg*$^{\Delta/\Delta}$) mice and their control littermates (CTL) with no *Sox2-Cre* transgene but two functional *Pparg* alleles (*Pparg*$^{fl/+}$) have been previously described (16, 18). This strategy ended up with a conditional epiblast-specific deletion of *Pparg* mediated by the *Sox2-Cre* transgene. The preservation of *Pparg* expression in the trophoblast (16) circumvented the embryonic-lethality of homozygous PPARγ knockout mice due to a placental defect (15, 16). Normal placental development allows *Sox2-Cre*$^{tg/+}$*Pparg*$^{em\Delta/\Delta}$ pups to be born, and as expected, these mice are totally deprived of any form of adipose tissue. Both male and female mice 12–22 weeks of age were used. AZIP/F1 mice on an FVB background [Tg(AZIP/F)1Vsn; hereafter referred to as AZIP$^{tg/+}$] and corresponding wild-type FVB controls were obtained from Charles Vinson and the colony was raised as previously described (19).

No *Pparg* expression could be detected in the long bones of *Pparg*$^{\Delta/\Delta}$ mice and the total lack of adipocytes in the BM in these two models, was confirmed by using Resistin, an adipokine specifically expressed by adipocytes and, herein, used as a surrogate marker for the presence of mature adipocytes. Expression of Resistin was indeed barely measurable above the detection threshold in mRNA extracted from *Pparg*$^{\Delta/\Delta}$ bones, and at very low levels in AZIP$^{tg/+}$ bones (**Supplementary Figure S1**).

Flow Cytometry

BM cell suspensions from all mouse strains described above were prepared by crushing the long bones (2 femurs and 2 tibias per mouse) into DMEM/3% FCS. Bone fragments were removed by filtration through 40-μm filters. Splenocyte suspensions were obtained by mashing the organs through sieves into DMEM/3% FCS, washing by centrifugation and filtering through a 40-μm filter cap. Liver hematopoietic mononuclear cells were obtained by mashing entire livers through sieves, after which the cells were washed in DMEM/3% FCS and centrifuged using a Percoll (GE Healthcare) gradient (40% Percoll layered over 80% Percoll) for 30 mins at 2,000 rpm to remove hepatocytes and other non-hematopoietic cells. Cells localized at the interface were recovered, diluted in DMEM/3% FCS, centrifuged and filtered through 40-μm filter caps. Single-cell suspensions were stained as previously described (20). Monoclonal antibody conjugates used for flow cytometry are listed in **Supplementary Table S1**. Cells were analyzed on a 5-laser LSR II cytometer equipped with 355, 405, 488, 561, and 640-nm lasers (Becton Dickinson, San Jose, CA), and the data were analyzed with FlowJo V9 software (TreeStar, Ashland, OR).

Colony Forming Cell (CFC) Assay

Splenocyte cell suspensions were obtained by mashing the spleen through sieves into DMEM/3% FCS, washing by centrifugation then filtering through 70-μm filter caps. BM cells suspensions were obtained as described above. Splenocytes (3×10^5) and BM cells (2×10^4) were seeded into 35 mm dishes in Mouse Methylcellulose Complete Media containing cytokines/growth factors such as EPO, IL-3, IL-6, SCF, or the combination thereof according to the manufacturer's instructions (R&D Systems). After 10–12 days of culture at 37°C in 5% CO_2, Colonies were identified by eye with phase-contrast microscopy.

BM Transplantation

BM chimeras were prepared as previously described (21). Briefly, 12-week old host mice (CD45.1+) were lethally irradiated (1000 rads) and reconstituted with 10^7 T-depleted BM cells (CD45.2+) from either *Pparg*$^{\Delta/\Delta}$ mice or their littermate controls (CTL). For reverse chimeras, 12-week old host mice (*Pparg*$^{\Delta/\Delta}$ or CTL) were reconstituted with 10^7 T-depleted BM cells from CD45.1+ wild-type controls. Hematopoietic reconstitution was assessed by FACS staining of ficoll-purified peripheral blood cells 6 weeks after transfer as described above. Mice were euthanized and analyzed 12 weeks after transfer. Owing to variable reconstitution efficiency between animals, the BM chimera results were expressed as the percentage of donor-derived cells.

Quantitative RT-PCR

Total RNA was isolated from long bones (bone fragments and BM combined), liver, and spleen, using TRIzol LS reagent (ThermoFisher, Waltham, MA) and purified with the RNeasy kit (Qiagen, Hilden, Germany). RNA quality was verified by chip electrophoresis (Agilent 2100 Bioanalyzer; Santa Clara, CA), and the concentration was determined using Nanodrop (Wilmington, DE). Total RNA (500 ng to 1 μg) was reverse-transcribed using the iScript™ cDNA Synthesis Kit (Bio-Rad Laboratories, Hercules, CA) according to the manufacturer's instructions. Real-time PCR was performed with SYBR® Green PCR mastermix using an ABI PRISM® 7900 PCR machine (ThermoFisher). The results were normalized to the levels of Actin beta (*Actb*). For primer sequences, see **Supplementary Table S2**.

Histology

Spleen were fixed in 4% paraformaldehyde and paraffin embedded. Four micro meter paraffin sections were stained with hematoxylin and spleen area as well as white pulp (WP) area were calculated by measuring spleen or WP surface area, using ImageJ software (http://rsbweb.nih.gov/ij/). Red pulp (RP) area was calculated as total spleen area minus WP areas. One representative section per spleen and 3 spleens were analyzed per genotype.

Immunohistochemistry was performed on 8 μm-thick frozen sections of OCT-embedded spleen, which were fixed using acetone followed by primary and secondary antibodies or streptavidin (found in **Supplementary Table 1**), as described previously (22). Images were acquired with a Zeiss Axioplan microscope and treated with Photoshop (Adobe) or Image J opensource software.

Serum Levels of Parathyroid Hormone (PTH) and Inflammatory Markers

Blood was obtained by cardiac puncture immediately after euthanasia. After clotting and centrifugation, serum was collected and stored at −80°C until use. Parathyroid hormone (PTH) was measured by ELISA according to the manufacturer's protocol (Stoughton, MA; LifeSpan Biosciences, Inc., Seattle,WA). Serum levels of Serum Amyloid A (SAA), IL-1β and IL-6 were measured using commercial ELISA kits (Bio-techne, Abingdon, UK). Assays were run in duplicate using adequate dilution buffer (for SAA, sera were diluted between 1:200 and 1:2,000; for IL-1β and IL-6, sera were used pure or diluted 1:2), according to the manufacturer's protocol. A four-parameter logistic formula was used to calculate the sample concentrations from the standard curves. Limit of quantification was 0.022 ng/ml for SAA (manufacturer's data).

Statistical Analyses

The statistical analysis was performed using GraphPad Prism 6 software. Two-group comparisons were performed using Student's *t*-tests or Mann-Withney *U*-test for non-parametric data, as indicated. All data are presented as mean ± SEM.

RESULTS

Significant Increase in Hematopoietic Cells in the Spleen and Liver of Lipodystrophic *Pparg*$^{\Delta/\Delta}$ Mice

To explore both the systemic and local involvement of adipose tissue, we characterized the hematopoietic phenotype of mice carrying a constitutive deletion of the two *Pparg* alleles. We have previously shown that the ablation of PPARγ expression leads to the total absence of both white and brown adipose tissue (18) and the development of various metabolic disorders, which include the early onset of a type 2 diabetes [(23) and unpublished observations]. Adult *Pparg*$^{\Delta/\Delta}$ mice had significantly enlarged spleens and livers, both in volume and weight (**Figures 1A,B**). Histological analyses revealed an alteration of the red pulp of the spleen, with an increase in the red pulp compartment size (**Supplementary Figures S2A,B**) and the presence of numerous and large polynuclear cells corresponding to megakaryocytes (**Figure 1C**). The total surface occupied by the white pulp was similar in the spleen sections from control and *Pparg*$^{\Delta/\Delta}$ mice while the average white pulp cords were smaller (**Supplementary Figures S2A,B**). However, the overall perturbation might lead to an underestimation of the white pulp. Immunohistochemical characterization of the spleen further showed that the segregation of various immune cells into the red and white pulp compartment as well as into the B and T zone of the white pulp was not significantly altered in spleens of *Pparg*$^{\Delta/\Delta}$ mice. Similarly, only a mild reduction in splenic germinal centers was observed (**Supplementary Figures S2C–E**). During fetal life the liver and spleen are the major sites of hematopoiesis, and the perturbations observed, particularly the presence of numerous megakaryocytes, are suggestive of altered hematopoiesis.

Consistent with a perturbation of hematopoiesis, significant increases in total hematopoietic mononuclear cell numbers were observed in the liver and spleen of Pparg$^{\Delta/\Delta}$ mice (**Figure 1D**). Flow cytometric analysis of the major hematopoietic subsets in these organs showed significant increases (10-fold or more) in the numbers of granulocytes, macrophages and erythroblasts.

In contrast to these peripheral organs, the total numbers of hematopoietic cells in the BM of Pparg$^{\Delta/\Delta}$ mice were marginally decreased compared to the controls (**Figure 1D**). While the numbers of granulocytes and macrophages in the BM did not differ in Pparg$^{\Delta/\Delta}$ mice compared to the controls, lymphopoiesis was affected with numbers of B cells and T cells reduced 1.5-fold in Pparg$^{\Delta/\Delta}$ mice, and erythroblasts decreased ~two-fold (**Figures 1E,F**). However, this hematopoietic cell dysregulation was associated with only minor changes in the peripheral blood counts (**Supplementary Figure S3**). Thus, while BM hematopoiesis is mildly altered in the absence of PPARγ, substantial increases in numbers of myeloid (granulocytes and macrophages) and erythroid (erythroblasts and RBCs) lineage cells are observed in peripheral hematopoietic organs such as the liver and spleen.

Lipodystrophic *Pparg*$^{\Delta/\Delta}$ Mice Exhibit Active Extra-Medullary Hematopoiesis

To determine whether the massive increase in hematopoietic cells observed in the peripheral organs was due to a local increase in their production, we assessed the number of HSCs and progenitor cells in these organs as well as in the BM. Under homeostatic conditions, adult hematopoiesis occurs almost exclusively in the BM, where mature hematopoietic lineages are normally produced from HSCs and progenitor cells (**Supplementary Figure S4**) located in specialized BM niches (24). However, under certain conditions (such as BM failure, myelostimulation, or inflammation), substantial numbers of HSCs and multi-potent progenitor cells (MPPs), as well as developing myeloid and erythroid lineages, can be found in peripheral organs such as the spleen and liver, contributing to an extramedullary hematopoiesis (EMH) [reviewed in (17)].

To evaluate and identify cells belonging to the different hematopoietic precursor populations, we analyzed by flow cytometry the LSK (Lin$^-$, Sca-1$^+$, cKit-r$^+$) and LK (Lin$^-$, Sca-1$^-$, cKit-r$^+$) populations. The LSK subset contains long-term (LT-) and short-term (ST-) HSCs, and several Multi-Potent Progenitors (MPPs) populations, while the LK subset contains the Common Myeloid Progenitors (CMPs), and gives rise to both Megakaryocyte Erythroid Progenitors (MEPs) and Granulocyte Monocyte Progenitors (GMPs; see also **Supplementary Figure S4**). Significant increases in both the relative proportion and total numbers of LSK and LK cells were observed in the spleen and liver of *Pparg*$^{\Delta/\Delta}$ mice compared to control mice. In contrast, the absolute and relative number of LSK and LK cells in the BM of *Pparg*$^{\Delta/\Delta}$ mice were modestly affected (**Figures 2A–C**).

To further identify subsets present in the LSK population, we analyzed the distribution of the markers CD34, CD48, and CD150, which define LT- and ST-HSCs as previously described [(20); **Supplementary Figure S4**]. Although LT-HSC (CD34$^-$ CD48$^-$ CD150$^+$) and MPP1 (ST-HSC; CD34$^+$ CD48$^+$ CD150$^+$) subsets were marginally decreased in the BM, the MPP2 (CD34$^+$ CD48$^-$ CD150$^+$) and MPP3/MPP4 (CD34$^+$ CD48$^+$ CD150$^-$ CD135$^{+/-}$) subsets were unchanged (**Figure 2C**). Thus, the HSC and MPP subsets were largely unaffected in the BM of mice lacking PPARγ. In contrast, a global 10- to 100-fold increase in LT-HSC and all MPP subsets (MPP1-4) was observed in the spleen and liver of *Pparg*$^{\Delta/\Delta}$ mice with no changes in their relative proportions compared to those seen in the BM of wild-type controls. These important increases were still observed when calculated as a % of the total cell number in these two organs (**Figures 2D,E**). The clonogenic potential of these hematopoietic precursor populations found in the spleen was also confirmed by performing a Colony Forming Unit assay on BM and spleen cells (**Supplementary Table S3**).

As B cells and T cells are derived from hematopoietic progenitors via a Common Lymphoid Precursor (CLP), which is defined as Lin$^-$, Sca-1^{lo}, cKit-r^{lo} and CD27$^+$, CD127$^+$, CD135$^+$(25), we quantified the proportion and number of CLPs in the BM and spleen of control and *Pparg*$^{\Delta/\Delta}$ mice. No significant changes were observed in the proportion or in the

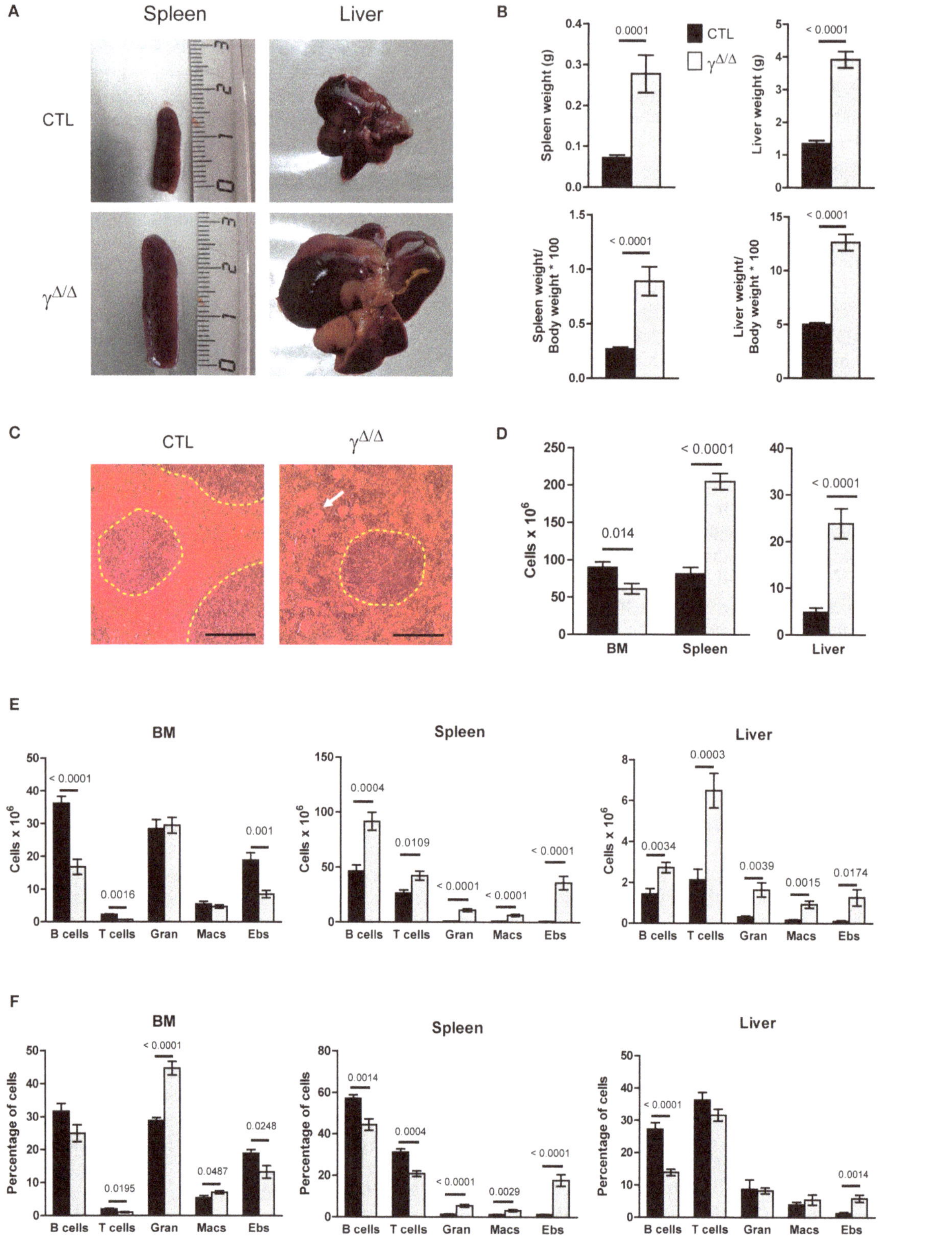

FIGURE 1 | Evaluation of hematopoiesis-derived cell populations in the bone marrow (BM) and peripheral organs of Pparg$^{\Delta/\Delta}$ mice. **(A)** Representative photographs of the spleens and livers of *Pparg*$^{\Delta/\Delta}$ ($\gamma^{\Delta/\Delta}$) mice (lower panels) and littermate control (CTL) mice (upper panels). **(B)** Spleen and liver weight in grams (top panels) and expressed as % of the body weight (bottom panels). **(C)** Hematoxylin & eosin staining of spleen sections; White pulp areas are circled by a dotted line. The white arrow indicates one of the numerous megakaryocytes present in the red pulp in *Pparg*$^{\Delta/\Delta}$ mice. The black bar indicates 200 micrometers. **(D)** Total hematopoietic cell

(Continued)

FIGURE 1 | numbers in the BM (2 tibias and 2 femurs from each mouse), spleen, and liver of control and *Pparg*$^{\Delta/\Delta}$ mice. Mean ± SEM, n = 7–8 mice per genotype. **(E)** Total numbers of mature hematopoietic cell subsets in the BM (left panel), spleen (middle panel) and liver (right panel) of control (dark bars) and *Pparg*$^{\Delta/\Delta}$ (light bars) mice. **(F)** Same as in **(E)**, with cell numbers expressed as a % of the total cell number in the corresponding organ. T cells (CD3$^+$); B cells (B220$^+$); Gran: granulocytes (Gr1$^+$CD11b$^+$), Macs: macrophages (Gr1$^-$CD11b$^+$), Ebs: erythroblasts (Ter119$^+$CD71$^+$); Mean ± SEM n = 7–8 mice per genotype. All significant p-values are indicated above the corresponding bars.

number of CLPs in the BM and spleen of Pparg$^{\Delta/\Delta}$ compared to control mice (data not shown).

Taken together, the increases observed in these HSC and progenitor cell subsets along with the increase in mature myeloid and erythroid subsets in peripheral organs are consistent with a significant EMH occurring in *Pparg*$^{\Delta/\Delta}$ mice.

The EMH Observed in *Pparg*$^{\Delta/\Delta}$ Mice Is Non-cell Autonomous

To determine whether the EMH observed in *Pparg*$^{\Delta/\Delta}$ mice was driven by a hematopoietic cell-autonomous mechanism or by a perturbation of the BM microenvironment, BM transplantation was performed. Lethally γ-irradiated CD45.1$^+$ wild-type recipient mice were reconstituted with either Pparg$^{\Delta/\Delta}$ or control littermate T-depleted BM cells (CD45.2$^+$). After 3 months, reconstitution from the donor was verified by staining peripheral blood lymphocytes (PBLs) for the allelic markers CD45.2 and CD45.1, and the mice were sacrificed for organ analyses. When wild-type recipients were reconstituted with donor BM from *Pparg*$^{\Delta/\Delta}$ or control mice, no significant difference was observed in either the number or proportions of most mature hematopoietic cell types (**Supplementary Figure S5A**). Furthermore, there was no evidence of EMH in these chimeras, as no increases in LSK or LK cells were observed in the spleen or the liver (**Figure 3A**).

We then performed the reciprocal experiment in which lethally irradiated *Pparg*$^{\Delta/\Delta}$ (CD45.2$^+$) recipients were reconstituted with wild-type BM from CD45.1$^+$ mice (reverse chimeras). In contrast to what we observed when using WT recipients, the EMH observed in the peripheral organs of *Pparg*$^{\Delta/\Delta}$ recipient mice was largely recapitulated (**Figure 3B**). Increased numbers and proportions of erythroblasts, granulocytes, lymphocytes, and macrophages were observed in the spleen (**Supplementary Figure S5B**), and liver (data not shown) in these reverse chimeras. Further evidence of EMH was provided by the increase in proportions of LSK and LK cells in the peripheral organs of *Pparg*$^{\Delta/\Delta}$ recipients, but not of control recipients, reconstituted with wild-type donor BM (**Figure 3B**).

Taken together, these results indicate that the EMH observed in *Pparg*$^{\Delta/\Delta}$ mice is non-cell autonomous. Although LT-HSCs (and other stem/progenitor subsets) appeared to home to and seed normally in the BM cavity in lethally irradiated *Pparg*$^{\Delta/\Delta}$ mice, they were also able to efficiently seed peripheral organs such as the spleen and liver and to mobilize to these organs. This suggests that the resulting EMH, rather than a defect of the hematopoietic cells themselves, was driven either by systemic cues or by changes in the microenvironment or factors produced by cells within the local microenvironment.

Respective Contributions of Inflammation and Lipodystrophy to EMH Onset

One important known systemic cause of EMH is inflammation. In a previous report, we showed that *Pparg*$^{\Delta/\Delta}$ mice have altered skin hair follicles, which with aging provoke an inflammatory response in the skin (18). To evaluate the contribution of these systemic disorders in the occurrence of EMH in *Pparg*$^{\Delta/\Delta}$ mice, we analyzed another mouse model that shares a similar phenotype with respect to lipodystrophy, but does not exhibit overt inflammation.

The AZIP$^{tg/+}$ mouse is a hemizygous transgenic mouse strain in which a dominant negative protein (A-ZIP) expressed under the control of the adipose tissue-specific aP2 enhancer/promoter inhibits expression of members of the C/EBP and Jun families of transcription factors. AZIP$^{tg/+}$ mice are born with no WAT and with severely decreased brown adipose tissue (19). One difference between *Pparg*$^{\Delta/\Delta}$ mice and AZIP$^{tg/+}$ mice is the presence of systemic inflammation, suggested in *Pparg*$^{\Delta/\Delta}$ mice by the high levels of Serum Amyloid A (SAA) protein, which is a highly sensitive marker for inflammation particularly in the acute phase, and moderate increased levels of IL-1β. In contrast, SAA, IL-1β, and IL-6 levels were not significantly increased in AZIP$^{tg/+}$ mice, indicating that the inflammation in these mice is very low, if not null (**Figure 4A** and data not shown).

We thus further analyzed the liver and the spleen of the lipodystrophic AZIP$^{tg/+}$ mice. While these animals also displayed enlarged spleens and a significant increase in total numbers of hematopoietic mononuclear cells, these increases were predominantly due to increased numbers of myeloid and erythroid cells (**Supplementary Figure S6**). Importantly, the EMH observed in the absence of PPARγ was recapitulated in AZIP$^{tg/+}$ mutants (**Figure 4B**), with a significant increase in the numbers of LSK cells in the spleen and the liver, and an increase of LK cells in the spleen and to a lesser extent in the liver (**Figure 4C**).

This observation demonstrated that even though inflammation likely contributes to the EMH observed in *Pparg*$^{\Delta/\Delta}$ mice, the lipodystrophy *per se* is responsible for the EMH.

Distinct Features of the EMH in *Pparg*$^{\Delta/\Delta}$ and in AZIP$^{tg/+}$ Mice

In the BM, inflammation provokes an increased demand on the granulocyte/macrophage lineage. This lineage is derived from one of the two cell populations that arise from the CMPs (defined as CD34$^+$, CD16/32$^-$): the MEPs (CD34$^-$, CD16/32$^+$) and the GMPs (CD34$^+$, CD16/32$^+$). We thus further analyzed the relative proportions of MEPs, GMPs, and CMPs found within the BM, according to these markers (see

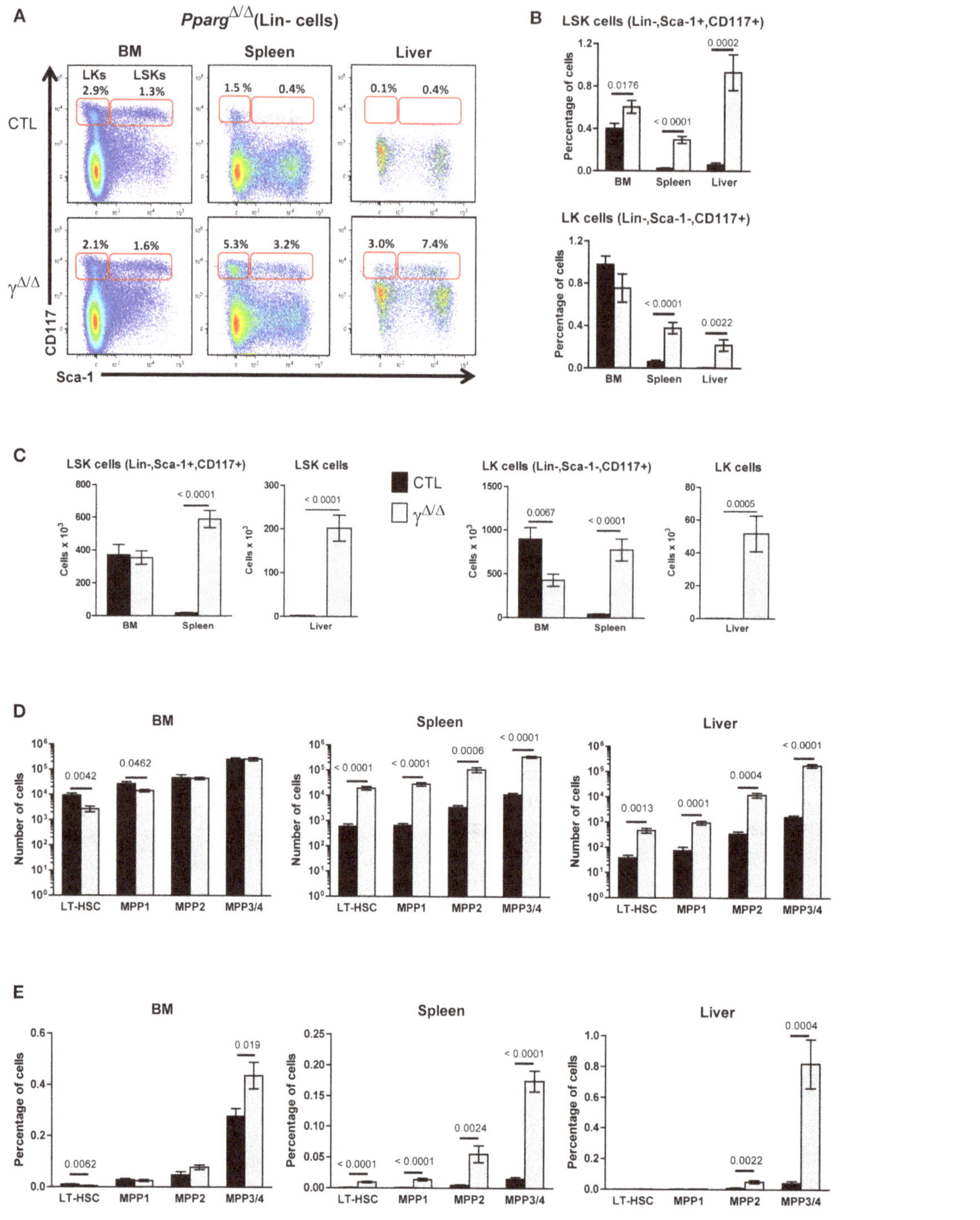

FIGURE 2 | Hematopoietic cell populations in the bone marrow (BM) and peripheral organs of Pparg$^{\Delta/\Delta}$ mice. **(A)** Representative FACS plots showing Sca-1 vs. CD117 staining on lineage-negative BM (left panels), spleen (middle panels), and liver (right panels) cells from littermate control (CTL, upper panels) or *Pparg*$^{\Delta/\Delta}$ (lower panels) mice. The red frames on the left and right of each plot indicate the gating and numbers of LK (Lineage-negative, Sca-1^{-}CD117^{+}) and LSK (Lineage-negative, Sca-1^{+}CD117^{+}) cells, respectively, as a percentage of lineage-negative cells from each organ. **(B)** Histograms showing the percentage of LSK (top panel) and LK (bottom panel) cells, with respect to the total cell numbers in the BM, spleen and liver of control (dark bars) and *Pparg*$^{\Delta/\Delta}$ (light bars) mice. Mean ± SEM, $n = 7$–8 mice per genotype. **(C)** Same as in **(B)**, expressed as absolute numbers of LSK (left panels) and LK cells (right panels). **(D)** Quantification of LT-HSC (CD34^{-}CD150^{+}CD48^{-}), MPP1 (CD34^{+}CD150^{+}CD48^{-}), MPP2 (CD34^{+}CD150^{+}CD48^{+}), and MPP3/4 (CD34^{+}CD150^{-}CD48^{+}) subsets in the LSK population of the BM, spleen, and liver from control (dark bars) and *Pparg*$^{\Delta/\Delta}$ (light bars) mice. Mean ± SEM, $n = 7$–8 mice per genotype. **(E)** Same as in **(D)**, expressed as a percentage of the total cell number in the corresponding organ. All significant *p*-values are indicated above the corresponding bars.

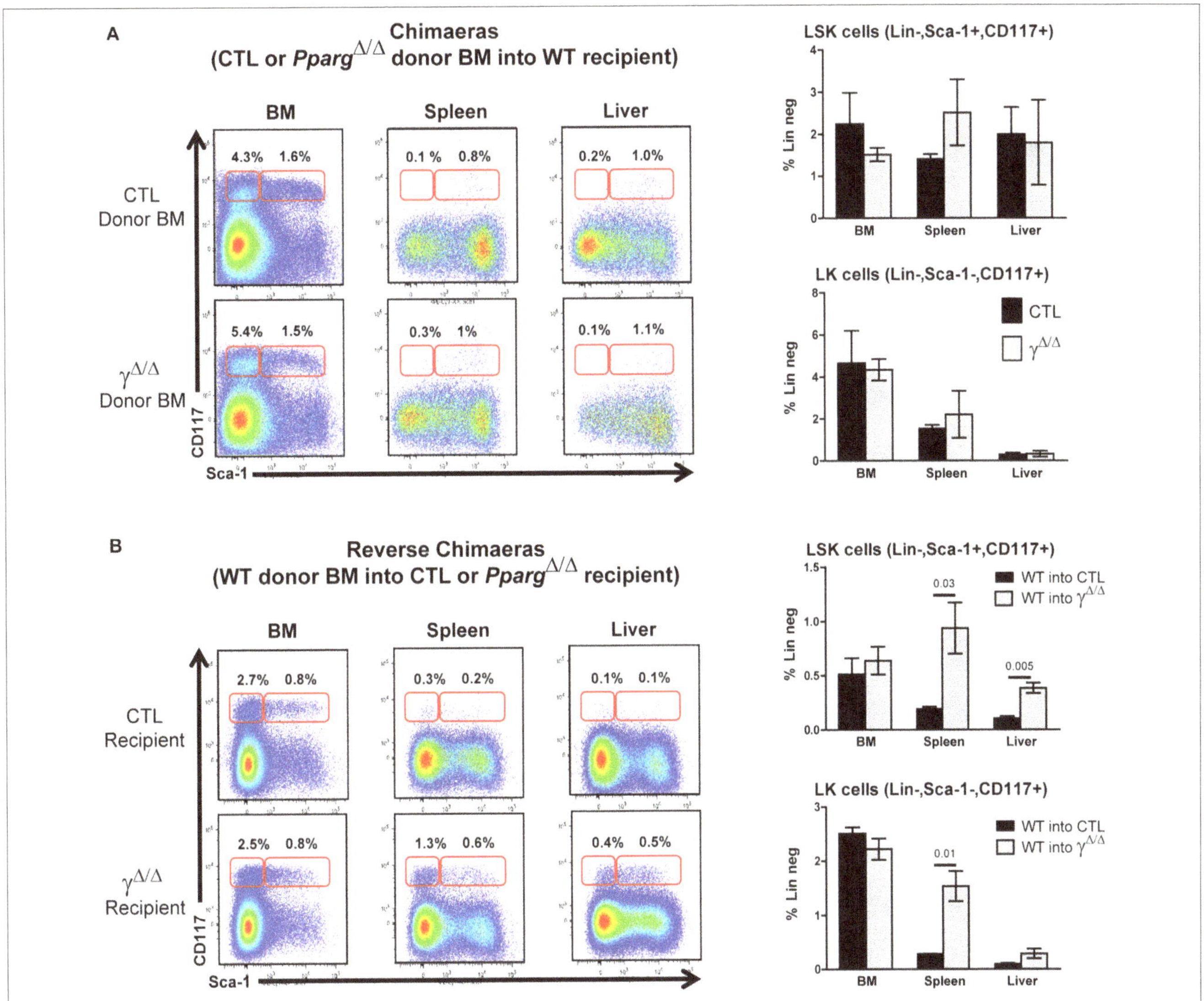

FIGURE 3 | Extramedullary hematopoiesis is non-cell autonomous. **(A)** Chimeras using wild-type recipient: Control or *Pparg*$^{\Delta/\Delta}$ donor BM (both CD45.2^{+}) was transferred into wild-type (WT) recipient CD45.1^{+} mice. Hematopoietic reconstitution was evaluated by FACS analysis 3 months after lethal γ-radiation and i.v. transfer of T-depleted BM. Left panels: representative FACS plots of Sca-1 vs. CD117 (cKit-r) on lineage-negative donor (CD45.2^{+}) BM (left), spleen (middle) or liver (right) cells from mice reconstituted with control BM (top row) or *Pparg*$^{\Delta/\Delta}$ BM (lower row). The red frames on the left and right of each plot indicate the gating and percentage of LK (Lineage-negative, Sca-1^{-}CD117^{+}) and LSK (Lineage-negative, Sca-1^{+}CD117^{+}) cells, respectively. Right panels: Relative proportions (in %) of LSK cells (top panel) and LK cells (bottom panel) over the total cell population of the BM, spleen, and liver. Dark bars represent donor control BM, and light bars represent donor *Pparg*$^{\Delta/\Delta}$ BM, both transplanted into WT host mice. Mean ± SEM, $n = 3$ mice per genotype. There are no significant *p*-values. **(B)** Reverse chimeras: Wild-type (WT) control donor BM (CD45.1^{+}) was transferred into CTL or *Pparg*$^{\Delta/\Delta}$ recipient CD45.2^{+} mice. Left panels: representative FACS plots of Sca-1 vs. CD117 (cKit-r) on lineage-negative donor (CD45.1^{+}) BM (left), spleen (middle), or liver (right) cells transferred into either CTL (upper row) or *Pparg*$^{\Delta/\Delta}$ (lower row) recipient mice. The red frames on the left and right of each plot indicate the gating and percentage of LK (Lineage-negative, Sca-1^{-}CD117^{+}) and LSK (Lineage-negative, Sca-1^{+}CD117^{+}) cells, respectively. Right panels: Relative proportions (in %) of LSK cells (top panel) and LK cells (bottom panel) over the total cell population of the BM, spleen, and liver. Dark bars represent donor control BM into CTL mice, and light bars represent donor control BM into *Pparg*$^{\Delta/\Delta}$ mice. Mean ± SEM, $n = 3$ mice per genotype. All significant *p*-values are indicated above the corresponding bars.

Supplementary Figure S4). In the BM, MEPs were decreased and GMPs increased, whereas CMPs were unchanged, resulting in a relatively lower proportion of MEPs and a higher proportion of granulocyte/macrophage progenitors in the BM of mice lacking PPARγ compared to wild-type controls (**Figures 5A,B**). These results were consistent with the gene expression profiles of their key regulators, with elevated levels of both *Sfpi/PU1* and *Gata2* in the long bones of *Pparg*$^{\Delta/\Delta}$ mice compared to control mice, whereas *Gata1* remained unchanged (**Figure 5D**). Thus, a bias in favor of myeloid over erythroid development in the BM was observed in the absence of PPARγ.

Importantly, the observed shift in the ratio of GMPs to MEPs within the LK subset in *Pparg*$^{\Delta/\Delta}$ mice was also recapitulated

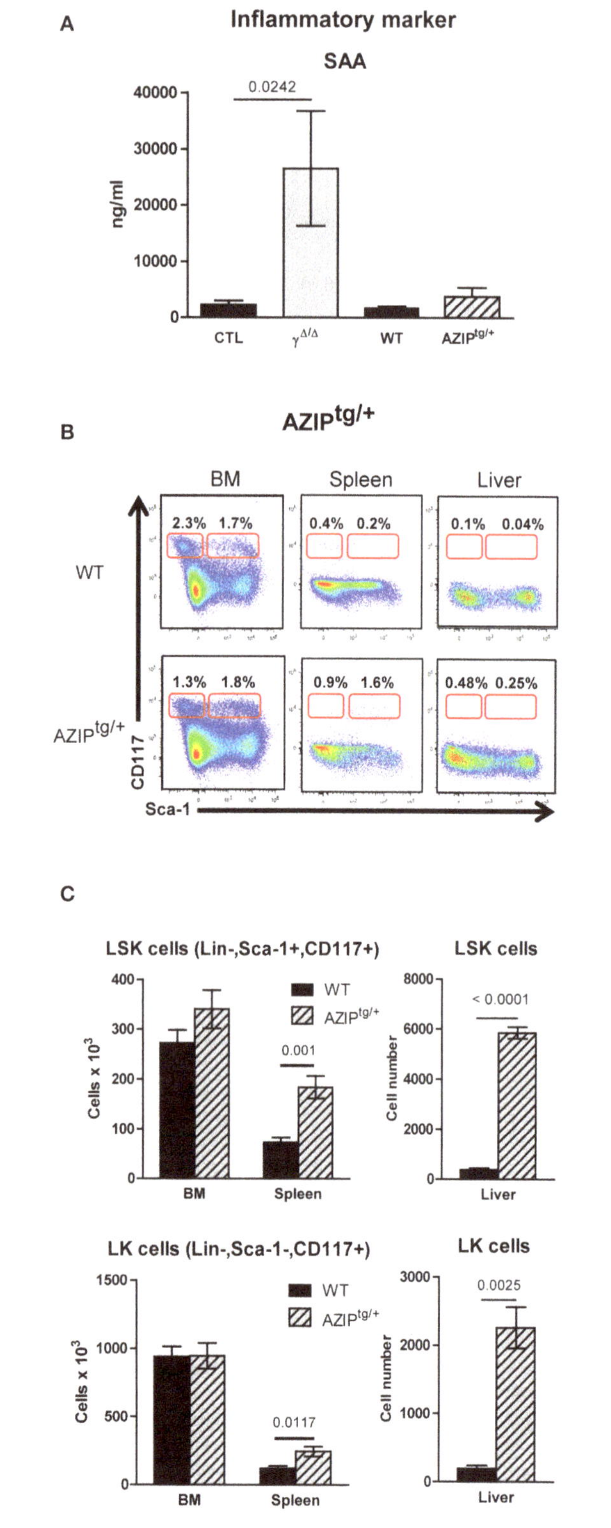

FIGURE 4 | Investigation of extramedullary hematopoiesis in AZIP$^{tg/+}$ mice. **(A)** Serum levels of the inflammatory marker Serum Amyloid A in *Pparg*$^{\Delta/\Delta}$ and in *AZIP*$^{tg/+}$, evaluated by ELISA. Mean ± SEM for 3 to 8 mice per genotype. **(B)** Representative FACS plots showing Sca-1 vs. CD117 staining on lineage-negative bone marrow (BM; left panels) and spleen (middle panels) and liver (right panels) cells from AZIP$^{tg/+}$ (lower row) mice and their wild-type (WT) littermates (upper row). The red frames on the left and right of each plot *(Continued)*

FIGURE 4 | indicate the gating and percentage of LK (Lineage-negative, Sca-1$^-$CD117$^+$) and LSK (Lineage-negative, Sca-1$^+$CD117$^+$) cells, respectively, expressed as a percentage of lineage-negative cells from each organ. **(C)** Histograms showing total numbers of LSK (left panel) and LK (right panel) cells in the BM, spleen and liver of WT control (dark bars) and AZIP$^{tg/+}$ (light hatched bars) mice. Mean ± SEM, $n = 3$–6 mice per genotype. All significant *p*-values are indicated above the corresponding bars.

in the reverse chimeras in the BM (**Figures 6A,B**), when wild-type cells were used to reconstitute the BM of irradiated *Pparg*$^{\Delta/\Delta}$ mice. However, in AZIP$^{tg/+}$ mice, which harbor no inflammation, increase of the LK cell population was observed in all progenitor subsets without alteration of the MEP to GMP ratio (**Figure 5C**). Consistent with this observation, mRNA expression levels of the myeloid-promoting transcription factor SFPI1/PU.1 were not increased in the bones of AZIP$^{tg/+}$ mice (**Figure 5D**). Altogether, these data suggest that the increased ratio of GMPs over MEPs is in part linked to the systemic inflammation, whereas the EMH is linked to the lipodystrophy context.

Another distinct feature between the phenotypes of *Pparg*$^{\Delta/\Delta}$ and AZIP$^{tg/+}$ mice is that no decrease is observed in the numbers of B lymphocytes in the BM of AZIP$^{tg/+}$ mice (**Supplementary Figures S6A,B**). Further analyses in *Pparg*$^{\Delta/\Delta}$ mice demonstrated more specifically that while the early immature B cell subsets (PreProB, ProPreB, PreBI and large and small PreBII) were similar in control and *Pparg*$^{\Delta/\Delta}$ mice, the numbers of later-stage B cells (IgM$^+$ immature and mature cells) were significantly decreased in the absence of PPARγ (data not shown). These observations, not seen in AZIP$^{tg/+}$ mice, are therefore unlikely to be directly due to the lack of adipocytes in the BM.

Altered HSC Retention in Lipodystrophic Mice BM Contributes to EMH in Peripheral Organs

The next question was therefore which common mechanism in these two models of lipodystrophy would promote EMH. One important systemic perturbation observed in these two models, which is directly due to the lack of adipose tissue, is a severe type 2 diabetes phenotype with hyperglycemia and hyperinsulinemia. To evaluate the possible impact of these metabolic disorders in the induction of EMH, we analyzed the occurrence of EMH in a well-characterized model of type 2 diabetes, the leptin-deficient *ob/ob* mice. In contrast to the *Pparg*$^{\Delta/\Delta}$ and AZIP$^{tg/+}$ mice, no increase in spleen size was observed in *ob/ob* mice (data not shown). Moreover, normal numbers of LSK and LK cells were observed in the spleen of *ob/ob* mice (**Supplementary Figures S6C,D**), thus ruling out metabolic perturbation as a possible cause of EMH.

As the EMH observed in *Pparg*$^{\Delta/\Delta}$ mice was not due to a cell autonomous defect in hematopoietic cells, and was reproduced in another model of lipodystrophy, we hypothesized that the lack of adipocytes or factors produced by adipocytes could be responsible for this phenomenon. Indeed, one mechanism by which peripheral organs such as the liver and the spleen harbor

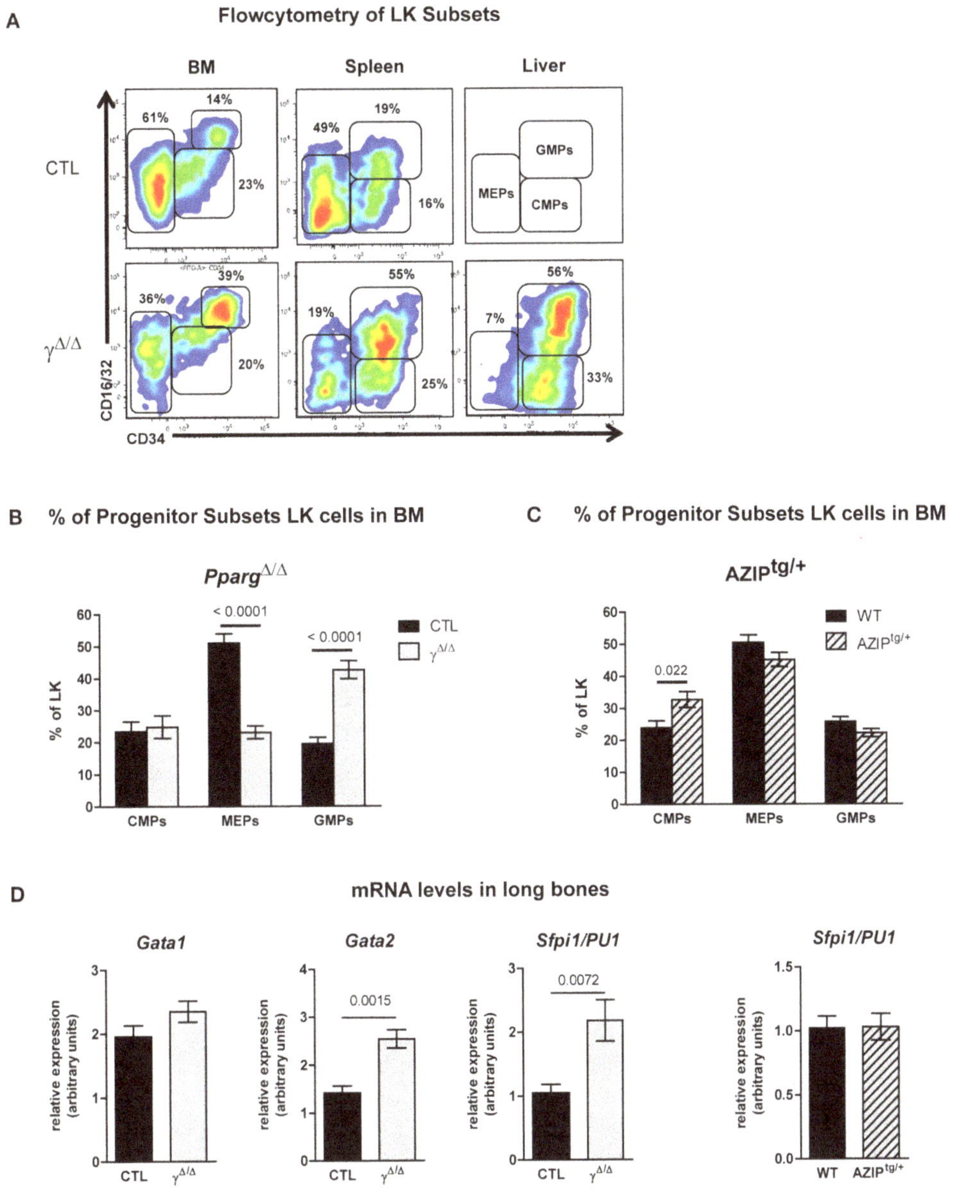

FIGURE 5 | FACS analyses of progenitor cell subsets in the LK population of the bone marrow (BM), spleen, and liver of Pparg$^{\Delta/\Delta}$ and AZIP$^{tg/+}$ mice. **(A)** Representative FACS plots of CD34 vs. CD16/32 expression in the LK subset of the BM (left panels), spleen (middle panels) and liver (right panels) of control (CTL, upper row) and *Pparg*$^{\Delta/\Delta}$ (lower row) mice. As there were insufficient liver cells to make a FACS plot for the CTL mice, the gating strategy for the progenitor subsets is indicated instead. The respective percentages of MEPs (CD34^{-}CD16/32^{-}), CMPs (CD34^{low}CD16/32^{-}), and GMPs (CD34^{+}CD16/32^{+}) are indicated in each plot. LK (Lineage-negative, Sca-1^{-},cKit-r /CD117^{+}); MEP (Megakaryocyte Erythroid Progenitor); CMP (Common Myeloid Progenitor); GMP (Granulocyte Monocyte Progenitor). **(B)** Histograms showing the proportion (%) of CMPs, MEPs and GMPs in the BM LK subset of control (dark bars) and *Pparg*$^{\Delta/\Delta}$ (light bars) mice. Mean ± SEM, $n = 7$–8 mice per genotype. **(C)** Histograms showing the proportion (%) of CMPs, MEPs, and GMPs in the BM LK subset of wild-type (dark bars) and AZIP$^{tg/+}$ (light hatched bars) mice. Mean ± SEM, $n = 7$ mice per genotype. **(D)** mRNA expression levels of the transcription factors *Gata1*, *Gata2*, *Sfpi1/PU1* evaluated by qRT-PCR in total cellular extracts from the long bones of control (dark bars) vs. *Pparg*$^{\Delta/\Delta}$ mice (light bars) or wild-type (dark bars) and AZIP$^{tg/+}$ (light hatched bars) mice. Mean ± SEM, $n = 5$–7 mice per genotype. All significant *p*-values are indicated above the corresponding bars.

HSC/progenitor cells is through egression of cells from the BM. This also occurs under normal homeostatic conditions, since small numbers of HSC/progenitor cells can be found, albeit at barely detectable levels, in the peripheral organs of normal mice (see for example **Figures 2A–C**).

The lack of adipocytes in the BM of *Pparg*$^{\Delta/\Delta}$ and AZIP$^{tg/+}$ mice may disrupt the local microenvironment. We thus explored whether the EMH observed in the absence of adipocytes resulted from an increase in cellular egress from the BM. As the CXCL12/CXCR4 axis is the main source of retention signals that maintain hematopoietic stem and progenitor cells (HSPCs) in the BM (26), we evaluated the expression levels of this cytokine (*Cxcl12*) and its receptor (*Cxcr4*) in mRNA isolated from the long bones. These extracts included both stromal and hematopoietic cell niche components. In the two models we studied, the levels of *Cxcl12* remained unaffected, whereas a significant reduction of *Cxcr4* was observed. Albeit it remains speculative, these results suggest that the retention of HSPCs in the BM might be impaired, contributing to the EMH in $Pparg^{\Delta/\Delta}$ and in $AZIP^{tg/+}$ mice. In contrast, *Cxcl12* is decreased in the spleen, whereas *Cxcr4* expression is not affected, indicating that these signals do not contribute to retaining HSCs in the spleen (**Figure 7**). The Sphingosine kinase/sphingosine 1-phosphate (S1P)/S1P receptor axis as well as the Parathyroid hormone (PTH) and its receptor PTHRP, two signals that play a role in this context (27, 28) are not different between the two genotypes (**Figure 7**), excluding their contribution to the phenotype.

Altogether, these results highlight that the occurrence of EMH in lipodystrophic mouse models results from a lack of adipocytes and is aggravated when systemic inflammation occurs.

DISCUSSION

In this study, we explored the role of adipocytes in BM homeostasis and regulation of hematopoiesis and showed that the total lipodystrophy in $Pparg^{\Delta/\Delta}$ mice is accompanied by a severe EMH that impacts upon all hematopoietic lineages. After a thorough analysis of the cell lineages found in the spleen and liver, we first demonstrated that the EMH observed in $Pparg^{\Delta/\Delta}$ mice is not a direct consequence of the lack of PPARγ in hematopoietic cells that normally express PPARγ (29, 30). Indeed, the EMH was reproduced when WT cells were used to reconstitute lethally irradiated $Pparg^{\Delta/\Delta}$ mice. We then observed EMH in an independent model of lipodystrophy ($AZIP^{tg/+}$). Albeit, we cannot exclude a contribution of inflammation in $Pparg^{\Delta/\Delta}$ mice, data from both models indicate that the most likely causes of EMH are linked to the lipodystrophy with possible local alterations of the BM microenvironment. Thus, the combination of the two experimental models of lipodystrophy used, $Pparg^{\Delta/\Delta}$ and $AZIP^{tg/+}$, allowed us to reveal an important contribution of adiposity in setting the appropriate BM microenvironment required for normal hematopoiesis.

There are three main known causes of EMH in the clinics and in experimental settings. The first one is associated with myelofibrosis disorders, which trigger a compensation in hematopoietic organs such as the spleen and liver to maintain functional hematopoiesis (31). Primary myelofibrosis begins as a myeloproliferative disorder and leads to an altered marrow with cellular abnormalities. Along this line, EMH has also been observed in mice carrying hypomorphic *Pparg* alleles and was shown to result from structural changes in the bones and thus reduced numbers of BM cells (32). In contrast, we found here that the BM in $Pparg^{\Delta/\Delta}$ and $AZIP^{tg/+}$ mice exhibited close to normal cell numbers, with neither myeloproliferation nor dramatic changes in the HSC population, excluding myelofibrosis as the cause of EMH. The second main cause of EMH is hypoxia, in which the increased need of red blood cell production is the trigger. The stress response to hypoxia in the context of hemoglobinopathy (33) stimulates erythropoiesis and increases hematocrit. Again, neither increases in erythropoiesis nor increased hematocrit were observed in the absence of PPARγ or in $AZIP^{tg/+}$ mice, making this hypothesis also unlikely.

The third main cause of EMH is the presence of severe systemic inflammation, particularly in rodents, where it is associated with a marked increase in granulopoiesis (17). Local skin inflammation is indeed observed in $Pparg^{\Delta/\Delta}$ mice and was associated with PPARγ-dependent scarring alopecia (18). However, this feature is specific to $Pparg^{\Delta/\Delta}$ mice and not found in $AZIP^{tg/+}$ mice. In addition, the blood levels of the inflammatory markers are significantly increased in $Pparg^{\Delta/\Delta}$ mice but not in $AZIP^{tg/+}$ mice. Thus, although we cannot rule out a contribution of inflammation, particularly in the case of the $Pparg^{\Delta/\Delta}$ mice, it does not explain the presence of EMH in $AZIP^{tg/+}$ mice. These distinct features in terms of inflammation also provide an explanation for the biased development of CMPs toward the myeloid lineage at the expense of the erythroid and megakaryocyte lineages seen only in $Pparg^{\Delta/\Delta}$ and not in $AZIP^{tg/+}$ mice. The inflammation seen in the former and not in the latter likely contributes to this shift in CMP commitment. The resulting relative decrease in the number of erythroblasts in the BM of $Pparg^{\Delta/\Delta}$ mice might thus be compensated for by active EMH.

Finally, although the three mouse models described in this study ($Pparg^{\Delta/\Delta}$, $AZIP^{tg/+}$, and *ob/ob*) are all affected by type 2 diabetes, the fact that *ob/ob* mice did not exhibit EMH excludes this systemic metabolic disorder as a common causative factor. Thus in this context, the most likely hypothesis is that adipocytes function to contribute to hematopoietic homeostasis in the BM.

The BM transfer experiment that we performed clearly indicates that the bone cavity micro-environment was involved in the EMH observed in our experimental models. The BM stem cell niche concept was first defined as a local microenvironment that maintains and regulates the function of stem and progenitor cells (1), and many cell types have been shown to be involved in these processes [reviewed in (2–4)]. BM adipocytes may or may not be considered as part of the niche *per se*, but they are present in large numbers and could contribute to the microenvironment in several ways. First, they play a role in bone homeostasis, which may indirectly affect the BM stem cell niche. This is due to the fact that adipocytes and osteoblasts are linked *via* their common mesenchymal progenitors, resulting in a balance between adipogenesis and osteoblastogenesis. PPARγ is central in this balance since this nuclear factor is a crucial regulator of MSC orientation toward adipocytes, as it's *ex vivo* or *in vitro* activation using synthetic agonists results in an adipogenic MSC phenotype, whereas it's pharmacological blockade or genetic deletion result in the opposite phenotype i.e., an osteoblastic phenotype (34, 35). Moreover, leptin and adiponectin, which are secreted by adipocytes, also exert a local and systemic role in bone homeostasis [reviewed in (36)]. Second, a direct function for adipocytes in supporting the proliferation of hematopoietic cells has been proposed, albeit the nature of this support function is not well described. It could combine energy sources and specific

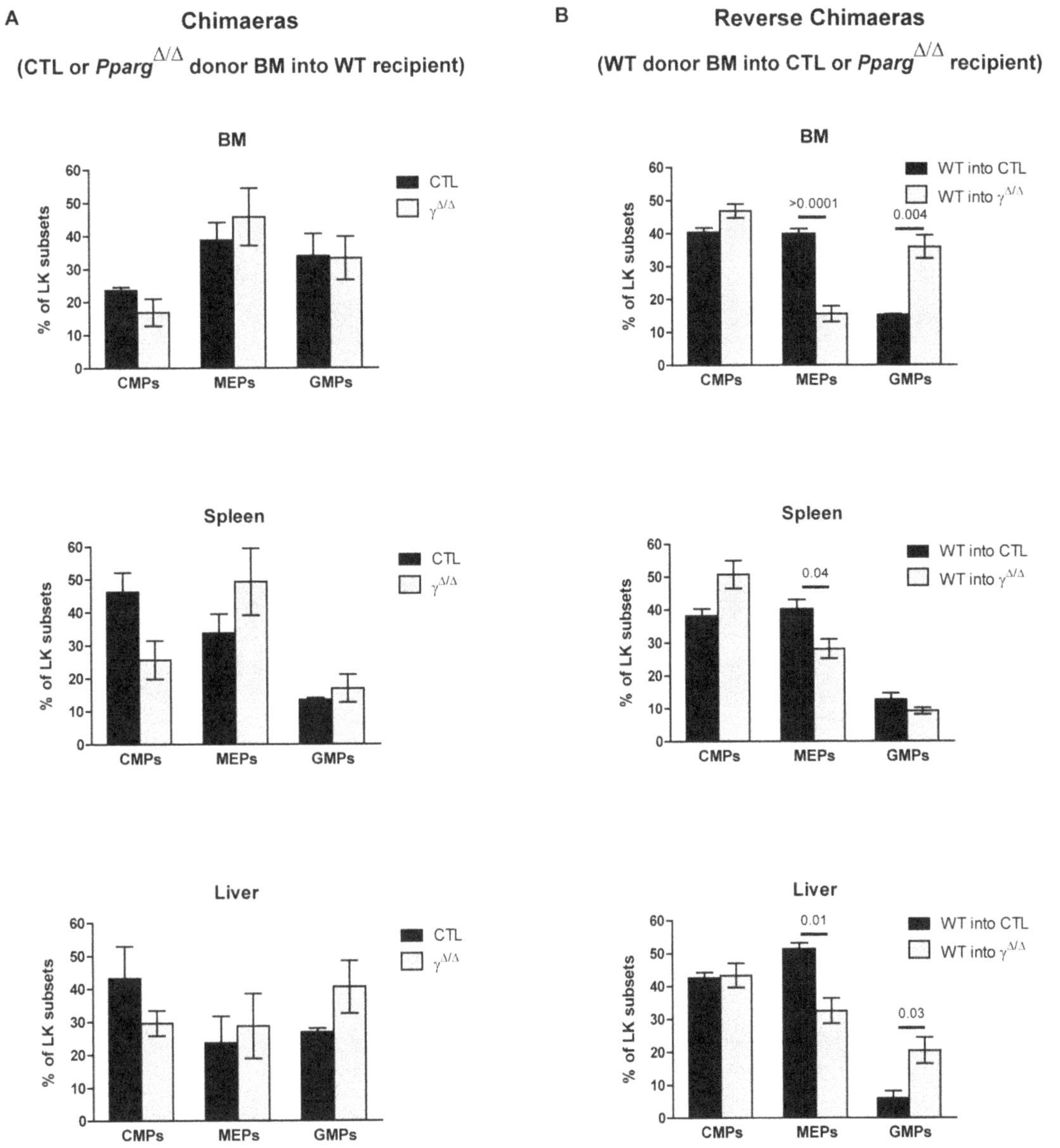

FIGURE 6 | FACS analyses of progenitor cell subsets in the LK population in chimeras and AZIP$^{tg/+}$ mice. **(A)** Chimeras using wild-type recipients and control or $Pparg^{\Delta/\Delta}$ donor BM. Hematopoietic reconstitution was evaluated by FACS analysis 3 months after the transfer (see also **Figure 3A**). The histograms show the proportion (%) of CMPs (CD34^{low}CD16/32^{-}), MEPs (CD34^{-}CD16/32^{-}), and GMPs (CD34^{+}CD16/32^{+}) in the LK cell subset, in the BM, the spleen and the liver of WT mice reconstituted with control (dark bars) or $Pparg^{\Delta/\Delta}$ (light bars) BM. Mean ± SEM, $n = 3$ mice per genotype. No significant p-value. **(B)** Reverse chimeras using wild-type (WT) control donor BM transferred into $Pparg^{\Delta/\Delta}$ or their littermate control (CTL) recipient. The histograms show the proportion (%) of CMPs, MEPs and GMPs in the LK cell subset in the BM, the spleen and the liver of control (dark bars) or $Pparg^{\Delta/\Delta}$ (light bars) mice reconstituted with wild-type donor BM. Mean ± SEM, $n = 3$ mice per genotype. All significant p-values are indicated above the corresponding bars.

adipokines, which have been proposed to mediate various aspects of HSC maintenance, quiescence and proliferation *in vitro* (9, 37, 38). In contrast, two reports have shown an anti-correlation between the number of adipocytes present in the bone cavity and the rapidity of recovery after BM irradiation (13, 39). One possible way to reconcile these conflicting observations is that the support provided by adipocytes may differ between *in vitro* and *in vivo* conditions as proposed by Spindler et al. (40). In agreement with our results, it is tempting to speculate on a specific role for BM adipocytes in this phenotype. However, our experiments do not exclude the possibility of a systemic cue directly related to the generalized lipoatrophy.

A possible consequence of an altered BM microenvironment is a modification of the balance between active retention and mobilization of HSCs. We showed that in the absence of PPARγ, all hematopoietic lineages are increased. Thus, the most likely explanation for the observed EMH is reduced BM colonization at birth or an increase in egress of HSCs and early progenitors

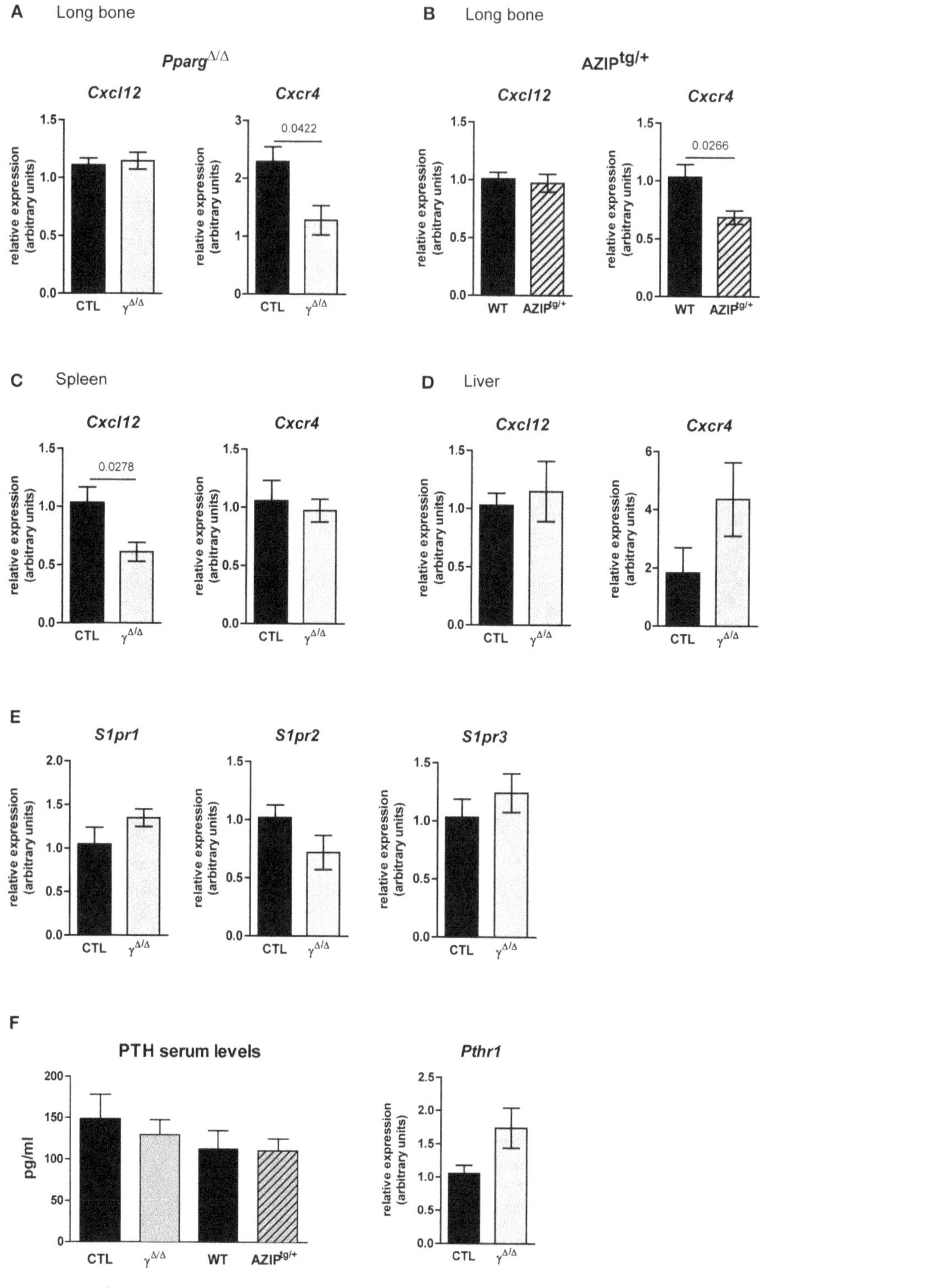

FIGURE 7 | Gene expression of key factors of cell egress from the BM in Pparg$^{\Delta/\Delta}$ and AZIP$^{tg/+}$ mice. **(A,B)** *Cxcl12* and *Cxcr4* mRNA expression in the long bones of *Pparg*$^{\Delta/\Delta}$ **(A)** and AZIP$^{tg/+}$ **(B)** mice and their controls, CTL and WT, respectively, as indicated. Mean ± SEM for 3 to 6 mice per genotype. **(C,D)** *Cxcl12* and *Cxcr4* mRNA expression in the spleen (**C**; Mean ± SEM for 5 mice per genotype) and the liver (**D**; Mean ± SEM for 6 to 7 mice per genotype) of *Pparg*$^{\Delta/\Delta}$ mice and their control. **(E)** Expression levels of Sphingosine Sphingosine kinase/sphingosine 1-phosphate receptors genes, *S1pr1, S1pr2, S1pr3*, in the long bone of *Pparg*$^{\Delta/\Delta}$ mice and their control. **(F)** Parathyroid hormone (PTH) serum levels and gene expression of its receptor PTHR1 in long bones of *Pparg*$^{\Delta/\Delta}$ mice and their control Mean ± SEM for 3 to 4 mice per genotype. All significant *p*-values are indicated above the corresponding bars.

from the BM. This is consistent with the fact that HSCs within the BM are very mobile cells, and that a small number of HSCs are constantly released into the circulation (41). Nevertheless, the best characterized mechanism of HSC and progenitor cell egress from the BM is the one provoked by pharmacological doses of G-CSF administered to patients for stem cell mobilization prior to autologous transplantation. This involves down-regulation of CXCL12, which is expressed by perivascular MSCs and CAR cells, as well as by osteoblast lineage cells. This decreased expression prevents interaction of CXCL12 with its receptor CXCR4 expressed by HSCs and progenitors, and the retention and survival of HSCs and progenitor cells in the BM (42, 43). In the models presented herein, *Cxcl12* expression levels in the BM were not altered, but gene expression of its receptor CXCR4 was significantly impaired. Pharmacological antagonists of CXCR4 are among the main recent innovations improving HSC mobilization in patients (44). Altogether, our observations are consistent with an alteration of the BM microenvironment due to the total lack of adipocytes, with loss of retention and/or increased egress of HSCs and progenitor cells from the BM to the peripheral organs, albeit this mechanistic hypothesis remains speculative. Nevertheless, we cannot completely exclude the contribution of an increased pool of splenic HSCs during development in both models of lipodystrophic mice. This could be due to reduced BM colonization at birth, when stem cell niches are being formed, or to an increased retention in spleen and liver, which are the primary sites of hematopoiesis before birth, although the decrease in CXCL12 expression in the spleen, does not favor this hypothesis.

The main limitation of the present study originates from the fact that mice, like most rodents, are more prone to develop EMH than humans. Nonetheless, our results strongly support the fact that lack or scarcity of adipocytes is deleterious for BM hematopoiesis. A deeper analysis of the adipocytes in the BM stem cell niche itself, more particularly with respect to their paracrine activity and cell-cell contacts may help to better define the role of adipocytes in cell retention/egress from the BM and highlight the importance of some key factors of interest for clinical situations of BM transfer. Alternately, and not exclusively, the search for a systemic cue linked to the generalized lipodystrophy might provide new avenues of research in hematopoiesis.

AUTHOR CONTRIBUTIONS

AW conceived the study, designed the experimental plan, performed all flow cytometry experiments, analyzed the data, wrote the manuscript, and acquired financial support for the project. HF designed the experimental plan, performed the experiments, analyzed the data, and contribute to the original draft preparation.

MS, CW, and MK performed experiments, analyzed the data, and prepared the vizualisation. FG, NB, and J-YJ contributed to the conceptualization, analyzed the data, and reviewed/edited the manuscript. FR and SL performed histology experiments, analyzed the data, and prepared the figure for the spleen characterization. DM performed experiments, analyzed the data, contribute to the conceptualization, and reviewed/edited the manuscript. BD conceived the study, designed the experimental plan, supervised the study, analyzed the data, wrote the manuscript, and acquired financial support for the project. All authors read and edited the manuscript. AW and BD are the guarantors of this work and, as such, had full access to all the data in the study and take responsibility for the integrity of the data and the accuracy of the data analyses.

ACKNOWLEDGMENTS

We are indebted to Charles Vinson for providing the AZIP mouse line. The authors would like to thank Danny Labes of the University of Lausanne Flow Cytometry Facility. We warmly thank Professors Andreas Trump, Olaia Naveiras, Ping-Chih Ho, Serge Ferrari, Marie-Thérèse Rubio, and Doctor Cécile Pochon for helpful discussions. This work was supported by the Etat de Vaud (BD and AW) the FNRS (BD), the Région Grand Est (J-YJ), the Fondation Arthritis (DM) and by the french PIA project Lorraine Université d'Excellence, reference ANR-15-IDEX-04-LUE (J-YJ and DM).

REFERENCES

1. Schofield R. The relationship between the spleen colony-forming cell and the haemopoietic stem cell. *Blood Cells* (1978) 4:7–25.
2. Kfoury Y, Scadden DT. Mesenchymal cell contributions to the stem cell niche. *Cell Stem Cell* (2015) 16:239–53. doi: 10.1016/j.stem.2015.02.019
3. Morrison SJ, Scadden DT. The bone marrow niche for haematopoietic stem cells. *Nature* (2014) 505:327–34. doi: 10.1038/nature12984
4. Nakamura-Ishizu A, Suda T. Hematopoietic stem cell niche: an interplay among a repertoire of multiple functional niches. *Biochim Biophys Acta* (2013) 1830:2404–9. doi: 10.1016/j.bbagen.2012.08.023
5. Rosen ED, Spiegelman BM. What we talk about when we talk about fat. *Cell* (2014) 156:20–44. doi: 10.1016/j.cell.2013.12.012
6. Luo L, Liu M. Adipose tissue in control of metabolism. *J Endocrinol.* (2016) 231:R77–99. doi: 10.1530/JOE-16-0211
7. Capeau J, Magre J, Caron-Debarle M, Lagathu C, Antoine B, Bereziat V, et al. Human lipodystrophies: genetic and acquired diseases of adipose tissue. *Endocr Dev.* (2010) 19:1–20. doi: 10.1159/000316893
8. Veldhuis-Vlug AG, Rosen CJ. Mechanisms of marrow adiposity and its implications for skeletal health. *Metabolism* (2017) 67:106–14. doi: 10.1016/j.metabol.2016.11.013
9. Claycombe K, King LE, Fraker PJ. A role for leptin in sustaining lymphopoiesis and myelopoiesis. *Proc Natl Acad Sci USA.* (2008) 105:2017–21. doi: 10.1073/pnas.0712053105
10. DiMascio L, Voermans C, Uqoezwa M, Duncan A, Lu D, Wu J, et al. Identification of adiponectin as a novel hemopoietic stem cell growth factor. *J Immunol.* (2007) 178:3511–20. doi: 10.4049/jimmunol.178.6.3511

11. Masamoto Y, Arai S, Sato T, Kubota N, Takamoto I, Kadowaki T, et al. Adiponectin enhances quiescence exit of murine hematopoietic stem cells and hematopoietic recovery through mTORC1 potentiation. *Stem Cells* (2017) 35:1835–48. doi: 10.1002/stem.2640
12. Zhou BO, Yu H, Yue R, Zhao Z, Rios JJ, Naveiras O, et al. Bone marrow adipocytes promote the regeneration of stem cells and haematopoiesis by secreting SCF. *Nat Cell Biol.* (2017) 19:891–903. doi: 10.1038/ncb3570
13. Naveiras O, Nardi V, Wenzel PL, Hauschka PV, Fahey F, Daley GQ. Bone-marrow adipocytes as negative regulators of the haematopoietic microenvironment. *Nature* (2009) 460:259–63. doi: 10.1038/nature08099
14. Sertorio M, Du W, Amarachintha S, Wilson A, Pang Q. *In vivo* RNAi screen unveils PPARgamma as a regulator of hematopoietic stem cell homeostasis. *Stem Cell Rep.* (2017) 8:1242–55. doi: 10.1016/j.stemcr.2017.03.008
15. Barak Y, Nelson MC, Ong ES, Jones YZ, Ruiz-Lozano P, Chien KR, et al. PPAR gamma is required for placental, cardiac, and adipose tissue development. *Mol Cell* (1999) 4:585–95. doi: 10.1016/S1097-2765(00)80209-9
16. Nadra K, Quignodon L, Sardella C, Joye E, Mucciolo A, Chrast R, et al. PPARgamma in placental angiogenesis. *Endocrinology* (2010) 151:4969–81. doi: 10.1210/en.2010-0131
17. Johns JL, Christopher MM. Extramedullary hematopoiesis: a new look at the underlying stem cell niche, theories of development, and occurrence in animals. *Vet Pathol.* (2012) 49:508–23. doi: 10.1177/0300985811432344
18. Sardella C, Winkler C, Quignodon L, Hardman JA, Toffoli B, Giordano Attianese GMP, et al. Delayed hair follicle morphogenesis and hair follicle dystrophy in a lipoatrophy mouse model of pparg total deletion. *J Invest Dermatol.* (2018) 138:500–10. doi: 10.1016/j.jid.2017.09.024
19. Moitra J, Mason MM, Olive M, Krylov D, Gavrilova O, Marcus-Samuels B, et al. Life without white fat: a transgenic mouse. *Genes Dev.* (1998) 12:3168–81. doi: 10.1101/gad.12.20.3168
20. Wilson A, Laurenti E, Oser G, van der Wath RC, Blanco-Bose W, Jaworski M, et al. Hematopoietic stem cells reversibly switch from dormancy to self-renewal during homeostasis and repair. *Cell* (2008) 135:1118–29. doi: 10.1016/j.cell.2008.10.048
21. Radtke F, Wilson A, Stark G, Bauer M, van Meerwijk J, MacDonald HR, et al. Deficient T cell fate specification in mice with an induced inactivation of Notch1. *Immunity* (1999) 10:547–58. doi: 10.1016/S1074-7613(00)80054-0
22. Link A, Vogt TK, Favre S, Britschgi MR, Acha-Orbea H, Hinz B, et al. Fibroblastic reticular cells in lymph nodes regulate the homeostasis of naive T cells. *Nat Immunol.* (2007) 8:1255–65. doi: 10.1038/ni1513
23. Toffoli B, Gilardi F, Winkler C, Soderberg M, Kowalczuk L, Arsenijevic Y, et al. Nephropathy in Pparg-null mice highlights PPARgamma systemic activities in metabolism and in the immune system. *PLoS ONE* (2017) 12:e0171474. doi: 10.1371/journal.pone.0171474
24. Wilson A, Trumpp A. Bone-marrow haematopoietic-stem-cell niches. *Nat Rev Immunol.* (2006) 6:93–106. doi: 10.1038/nri1779
25. Serwold T, Ehrlich LI, Weissman IL. Reductive isolation from bone marrow and blood implicates common lymphoid progenitors as the major source of thymopoiesis. *Blood* (2009) 113:807–15. doi: 10.1182/blood-2008-08-17ss3682
26. Karpova D, Bonig H. Concise review: CXCR4/CXCL12 signaling in immature hematopoiesis–lessons from pharmacological and genetic models. *Stem Cells* (2015) 33:2391–9. doi: 10.1002/stem.2054
27. Cyster JG, Schwab SR. Sphingosine-1-phosphate and lymphocyte egress from lymphoid organs. *Annu Rev Immunol.* (2012) 30:69–94. doi: 10.1146/annurev-immunol-020711-075011
28. Calvi LM, Adams GB, Weibrecht KW, Weber JM, Olson DP, Knight MC, et al. Osteoblastic cells regulate the haematopoietic stem cell niche. *Nature* (2003) 425:841–6. doi: 10.1038/nature02040
29. Choi JM, Bothwell AL. The nuclear receptor PPARs as important regulators of T-cell functions and autoimmune diseases. *Mol Cells.* (2012) 33:217–22. doi: 10.1007/s10059-012-2297-y
30. Ramon S, Bancos S, Thatcher TH, Murant TI, Moshkani S, Sahler JM, et al. Peroxisome proliferator-activated receptor gamma B cell-specific-deficient mice have an impaired antibody response. *J Immunol.* (2012) 189:4740–7. doi: 10.4049/jimmunol.1200956
31. Wolf BC, Neiman RS. Myelofibrosis with myeloid metaplasia: pathophysiologic implications of the correlation between bone marrow changes and progression of splenomegaly. *Blood* (1985) 65:803–9.
32. Cock TA, Back J, Elefteriou F, Karsenty G, Kastner P, Chan S, et al. Enhanced bone formation in lipodystrophic PPARgamma(hyp/hyp) mice relocates haematopoiesis to the spleen. *EMBO Rep.* (2004) 5:1007–12. doi: 10.1038/sj.embor.7400254
33. Tan TC, Tsao J, Cheung FC. Extramedullary haemopoiesis in thalassemia intermedia presenting as paraplegia. *J Clin Neurosci.* (2002) 9:721–5. doi: 10.1054/jocn.2001.1038
34. Rzonca SO, Suva LJ, Gaddy D, Montague DC, Lecka-Czernik B. Bone is a target for the antidiabetic compound rosiglitazone. *Endocrinology* (2004) 145:401–6. doi: 10.1210/en.2003-0746
35. Akune T, Ohba S, Kamekura S, Yamaguchi M, Chung UI, Kubota N, et al. PPARgamma insufficiency enhances osteogenesis through osteoblast formation from bone marrow progenitors. *J Clin Invest.* (2004) 113:846–55. doi: 10.1172/JCI200419900
36. Lecka-Czernik B, Stechschulte LA. Bone and fat: a relationship of different shades. *Arch Biochem Biophys.* (2014) 561:124–9. doi: 10.1016/j.abb.2014.06.010
37. Gimble JM, Robinson CE, Wu X, Kelly KA. The function of adipocytes in the bone marrow stroma: an update. *Bone* (1996) 19:421–8. doi: 10.1016/S8756-3282(96)00258-X
38. Glettig DL, Kaplan DL. Extending human hematopoietic stem cell survival *in vitro* with adipocytes. *Biores Open Access.* (2013) 2:179–85. doi: 10.1089/biores.2013.0006
39. Zhu RJ, Wu MQ, Li ZJ, Zhang Y, Liu KY. Hematopoietic recovery following chemotherapy is improved by BADGE-induced inhibition of adipogenesis. *Int J Hematol.* (2013) 97:58–72. doi: 10.1007/s12185-012-1233-4
40. Spindler TJ, Tseng AW, Zhou X, Adams GB. Adipocytic cells augment the support of primitive hematopoietic cells in vitro but have no effect in the bone marrow niche under homeostatic conditions. *Stem Cells Dev.* (2014) 23:434–41. doi: 10.1089/scd.2013.0227
41. Wright DE, Wagers AJ, Gulati AP, Johnson FL, Weissman IL. Physiological migration of hematopoietic stem and progenitor cells. *Science* (2001) 294:1933–6. doi: 10.1126/science.1064081
42. Foudi A, Jarrier P, Zhang Y, Wittner M, Geay JF, Lecluse Y, et al. Reduced retention of radioprotective hematopoietic cells within the bone marrow microenvironment in CXCR4-/- chimeric mice. *Blood* (2006) 107:2243–51. doi: 10.1182/blood-2005-02-0581
43. Sugiyama T, Kohara H, Noda M, Nagasawa T. Maintenance of the hematopoietic stem cell pool by CXCL12-CXCR4 chemokine signaling in bone marrow stromal cell niches. *Immunity* (2006) 25:977–88. doi: 10.1016/j.immuni.2006.10.016
44. Bonig H, Papayannopoulou T. Hematopoietic stem cell mobilization: updated conceptual renditions. *Leukemia* (2013) 27:24–31. doi: 10.1038/leu.2012.254

5

Interleukin-6 Interweaves the Bone Marrow Microenvironment, Bone Loss and Multiple Myeloma

***Danielle Harmer*[1,2], *Carolyne Falank*[1] *and Michaela R. Reagan*[1,2,3*]**

[1] Reagan Laboratory, Maine Medical Center Research Institute, Scarborough, ME, United States, [2] Graduate School of Biomedical Sciences and Engineering, University of Maine, Orono, ME, United States, [3] School of Medicine, Tufts University, Boston, MA, United States

Correspondence:
Michaela R. Reagan
mreagan@mmc.org

The immune system is strongly linked to the maintenance of healthy bone. Inflammatory cytokines, specifically, are crucial to skeletal homeostasis and any dysregulation can result in detrimental health complications. Interleukins, such as interleukin 6 (IL-6), act as osteoclast differentiation modulators and as such, must be carefully monitored and regulated. IL-6 encourages osteoclastogenesis when bound to progenitors and can cause excessive osteoclastic activity and osteolysis when overly abundant. Numerous bone diseases are tied to IL-6 overexpression, including rheumatoid arthritis, osteoporosis, and bone-metastatic cancers. In the latter, IL-6 can be released with growth factors into the bone marrow microenvironment (BMM) during osteolysis from bone matrix or from cancer cells and osteoblasts in an inflammatory response to cancer cells. Thus, IL-6 helps create an ideal microenvironment for oncogenesis and metastasis. Multiple myeloma (MM) is a blood cancer that homes to the BMM and is strongly tied to overexpression of IL-6 and bone loss. The roles of IL-6 in the progression of MM are discussed in this review, including roles in bone homing, cancer-associated bone loss, disease progression and drug resistance. MM disease progression often includes the development of drug-resistant clones, and patients commonly struggle with reoccurrence. As such, therapeutics that specifically target the microenvironment, rather than the cancer itself, are ideal and IL-6, and its myriad of downstream signaling partners, are model targets. Lastly, current and potential therapeutic interventions involving IL-6 and connected signaling molecules are discussed in this review.

Keywords: multiple myeloma, IL-6, interleukin 6, bone marrow, MSCs

INTRODUCTION

For many years, the skeletal system was regarded purely as a means for structural support and movement; however, abundant data have since been collected that reveal a complex bi-directional interaction between bone cells and surrounding bone marrow (BM) cells. BM is composed of a heterogeneous cell population including adipocytes, chondrocytes, endothelial cells, immune cells, fibroblasts, and two multipotent stem cell populations: mesenchymal stem cells (MSCs) and haematopoietic stem cells (HSCs). MSCs can differentiate into chondrocytes, bone marrow adipocytes (BMAs), and osteoblasts (bone-forming cells), while HSCs give rise to both the myeloid and lymphoid immune cell populations. The myeloid cell precursors are of particular interest as they can give rise to both innate monocyte/macrophage immune cells, but can also fuse and differentiate to form osteoclasts, the cells responsible for bone resorption.

BM cells are involved in activating and intensifying numerous signaling pathways that contribute to diseased states. The instigation of these signaling pathways can be coupled to the secretion of soluble factors by bone and stromal cells, alike. Such soluble factors include interleukin 6 (IL-6), insulin-like growth factor-1 (IGF-1), stromal cell-derived factor-1 (SDF-1), tumor necrosis factor alpha (TNF-α), interleukin-8 (IL-8), interleukin-17 (IL-17) and vascular endothelial growth factor (VEGF), which play roles in inflammation, immunosuppression, tumorigenesis, and osteolysis and thus contribute to many disease states. A number of these molecules activate NF-κB signaling, which is key in the BMM, as it binds to and activates important transcription factors and signaling cascades.

The NF-κB molecule associates with STAT3, which then induces the expression of wound healing and cancer gene products (1), such as anti-apoptotic proteins. Furthermore, STAT3 signaling results in the release of inflammatory molecules, such as IL-6 (2), SDF-1 (3), TNF-α (4), interleukin-1 (IL-1) and (IL-6) (5), which are all known to stimulate NF-κB signaling, thus creating a positive feedback loop and increased downstream inflammatory cytokine production (2). This vicious circle of NF-κB signaling can be detrimental to bone due to chronic inflammation and damage, yet it remains key in the maintenance of healthy bone, as it facilitates osteoclast differentiation and survival (6) and thus bone homeostasis.

Receptor activator of nuclear factor kappa-B ligand (RANKL) is a molecule expressed on osteoblasts which can facilitate the fusion of myeloid progenitors into osteoclasts (7). When RANKL binds to progenitor cells, it promotes NF-κB signaling, blockade of TNF receptor associated factor-3 (TRAF-3), promotion of NF-κB inducing kinase (NIK), and a consequential translocation of RelB and p52 (NF-κB2) into cell nuclei (8), which promotes signaling for osteoclastogenesis (8). MAPK pathways, particularly those involving p38, feed into this system, as they are both activated by NF-κB, but furthermore, are known to result in the production of RANKL. IL-1, for example, can stimulate RANKL via p38 in stromal cells thus promoting osteoclastogenesis (9). The extent of osteoclastogenesis is regulated by an equilibrium between RANKL and its inhibitor, osteoprotegerin (OPG).

The regulation of these bone signaling pathways is key in the limitation of bone disease. Inflammatory cytokines can disrupt ratios of RANKL:OPG and can result in excessive osteoclastogenesis. IL-6, is tied to excessive promotion of RANKL and inhibition of OPG and thus has been linked to bone osteolysis (10), osteoporosis (11), rheumatoid arthritis (11) and other bone-related pathologies. Osteolysis has further implications as it allows for the release of growth factors which promote the homing and survival of bone-metastatic cancers (12), such as prostate (13), breast (14) neuroblastoma (15), acute myeloid leukemia (AML) (16) and MM (17, 18).

MM is a blood cancer which epitomizes the crosstalk between the immune and bone systems. It is a commonly refractory, and thus recurrent, pathology characterized by uncontrollable clonal expansion of plasma cells. Myeloma cells grow in the BMM where they disrupt the delicate balance between bone growth and resorption through the secretion of factors that directly and indirectly promote osteoclasts and inhibit osteoblasts. This interaction between myeloma cells and the BMM, and the potential to activate dormant immune cells to kill myeloma cells in the BM, demonstrate exciting areas of osteoimmunology under scrutiny. It is the hope that a better understanding of the signals in the BM may allow for the identification of better targets and development of better combination therapies for MM and other bone disease. This review focuses on just one signaling pathway, IL-6, and its ability to promote both diseased and healthy states within the BMM. Since MM is strongly tied to IL-6, it will be used frequently as a disease example to emphasize the role of IL-6 in bone osteolysis, bone-metastatic cancer and general bone disease.

IL-6 AND BONE REMODELING

Healthy bone is maintained by continuous bone resorption and regrowth, which is held at equilibrium through numerous signaling cascades (19, 20). Osteoclasts secrete acidic collagenases that break down matrices and form resorption pits. Osteoblasts line the border of mineralized bone and produce and deposit collagen, osteocalcin, and osteopontin to form an osteoid matrix. Osteoblasts then calcify osteoid through deposition of calcium phosphate, calcium carbonate and hydroxyapatite. Osteocytes, or other systemic signals, control the balance of bone resorption and formation. Osteocytes, the most abundant cell type in bone, are mechanosensing cells that produce signaling molecules in response to changes in pressure, sheer stress, or BMM chemical signals. Sclerostin is a signaling molecule that is synthesized and secreted by osteocytes, and acts as a WNT inhibitor causing inhibited osteoblast differentiation and supporting adipogenesis (21). Osteocytes also secrete Dentin-Matrix-acidic-Phosphoprotein-1(DMP-1), Matrix-Extracellular-Phospho-glycoprotein (MEPE), RANKL, Fibroblast-Growth-Factor-23 (FGF-23) and Phosphate-regulating-neutral-Endopeptidase-X-linked (PHEX), all of which play roles in regulating bone mineralisation, cell fate or phosphate homeostasis (21, 22).

Inflammatory cytokines, such as IL-6 and IL-11, can modulate skeletal homeostasis and osteoclast differentiation. When IL-6 binds receptors on pre-osteoclasts, they promote osteoclastogenesis (23), resulting in increased levels of bone resorption (**Figure 1**). Along with its direct roles on osteoclastogenesis, IL-6 also alters bone remodeling; when activated by IL-6, osteoblasts induce JAK/STAT3 pathways and ultimately secrete pro-osteoclast mediators, including RANKL, IL-1, parathyroid hormone related protein (PTHrP), and prostaglandin E2 (PGE2) (12, 24–27). PGE2 and PTHrP are particularly interesting factors as both, along with parathyroid hormone (PTH) and active vitamin D [1,25(OH)2D3], have been shown to stimulate IL-6 and RANKL production in osteoblasts within the BMM (28, 29). Thus, PGE2 and PTHrP reside both upstream and downstream of IL-6 signaling, facilitating

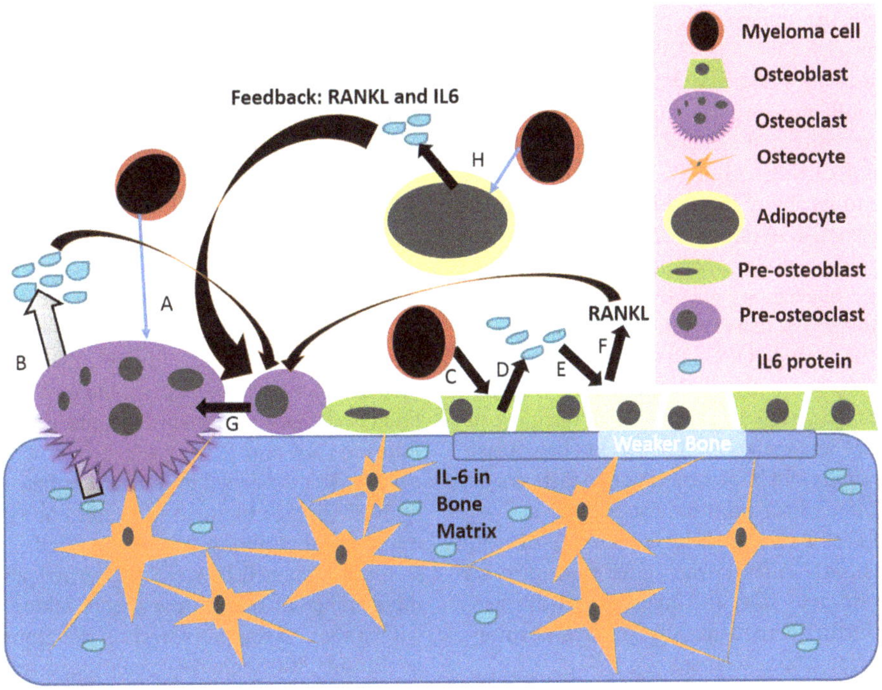

FIGURE 1 | Actions of IL-6 in the diseased bone marrow microenvironment. (A) Myeloma cells or other inflammatory triggers can induce osteoclast differentiation and osteolytic activity, which releases growth factors and IL-6 stored in the bone matrix (B). (C) Myeloma cells, or other inflammatory mediators, activate the release of IL-6 from osteoblasts (D); IL-6 then inhibits the activity of osteoblasts and induces their production of RANKL (E). (F,G) IL-6 from many sources, as well as RANKL from osteoblasts, induce pre-osteoclasts to differentiate into mature osteoclasts, which then resorb bone to induce greater release of stored growth factors, creating a vicious cycle. (H) Myeloma cells also alter bone marrow adipocytes to make a more supportive niche for tumor cells and to increase osteoclastic activity through IL-6 and other molecules.

a positive feedback loop that can exacerbate the detrimental pro-osteoclastic mechanisms seen in many diseased states. IL-6 can promote PTHrP secretion via TNF-α, which itself enhances osteoclastogenesis, bone loss and hypercalcaemia (30). The pathways that use osteoblastic mediation require the soluble IL-6 receptor (sIL-6R), as osteoblasts ordinarily express only low levels of the endogenous receptor (12). Soluble IL-6R forms as a result of cleavage or alternate splicing of IL-6R and is found in circulation in low numbers due to secretion from cells (31), commonly CD4 T cells (32). Therefore, it is necessary for IL-6 to meet and bind to sIL-6R within circulation, and then once bound, fuse with the osteoblastic membrane to trigger IL-6-inducible signaling pathways. Consequently, high levels of both IL-6 and sIL-6R are markers for osteolytic disorders, such as rheumatoid arthritis (10).

IL-6 also exacerbates osteolysis through inhibition of osteoblast differentiation, further disrupting the balance of healthy bone turnover. Both IL-6 and sIL-6R can cause a decrease in osteoblastic differentiation by reducing expression of genes involved in osteoblastic differentiation including alkaline phosphatase (ALP), Runx2 and osteocalcin (33). IL-6/sIL-6R signaling can also reduce the ability of osteoblasts to mineralise bone (**Figure 1**). This was determined to be a result of MEK/ERK and PI3K/AKT2 pathways; inhibiting these pathways increased expression of Runx2 and other mature osteoblastic phenotypes (33). Similarly, c-Src (a proto-oncogenic tyrosine kinase) has been shown to activate STAT3 and stimulate IL-6 within immature osteoblasts (34). This stimulation can induce expression of insulin-like growth factor 5 (IGFP5)—a molecule thought to act in a paracrine fashion to inhibit osteoclastogenesis (34). Overall, IL-6 has been shown to have anti-osteogenic and pro-osteoclastic effects leading to a net inhibition of bone.

IL-6 AND NON-CANCEROUS BONE DISEASE

Regulation of IL-6 plays a crucial role in bone maintenance and remodeling. Commonly, when chronic injury and/or inflammation occurs, it instigates overexpression of IL-6 within the BMM resulting in pro-osteoclastic pathways, osteopenia, osteoporosis, and an increased fracture risk (12). In fact, diseases characterized by excessive bone loss commonly coincide with IL-6 and RANKL overproduction (10). Numerous signaling molecules interact with IL-6 to accelerate bone disease including PGE2/COX2, PTH, 1,25(OH)2D3, estrogen, and VEGF, as described below.

PGE2 results from metabolism of the fatty acid arachidonic acid via cyclooxygenase-2 (COX-2). Overexpression of COX-2 is driven by IL-6 signaling and results in increased production PGE2 (35). PGE2 interacts with G-coupled receptors EP1, EP2, and EP4, which activate tissue-specific downstream signaling pathways (36). Inflammatory conditions such as rheumatoid arthritis and osteoarthritis appear are tied PGE2-induced inflammation (37). Mast cells (38), Th17 cells (39) and dendrites (40) can all be stimulated by PGE2 via EP2 and EP4, resulting in the release of pro-inflammatory cytokines, e.g., IL-6 (41). PGE2 is also linked to osteoclastogenesis and breakdown of juxta-articular-bone and cartilage (42). PGE2 further disrupts bone homeostasis due to its ability to inhibit OPG secretion by osteoblasts (27). Use of anti-IL-6 antibodies in osteoblastic and monocyte/macrophage-like cell lines demonstrated increased OPG secretion through alleviation of PGE2-driven inhibition (27), thus concluding that PGE2 increases IL-6 signaling, driving osteoclastogenesis in part through OPG inhibition.

Similar to PGE2, PTH acts both upstream and downstream of IL-6 signaling. This hormone is expressed in response to hypocalcaemia and, once in circulation, it acts upon osteoblasts to both increase their activity and induce secretion of factors such as RANKL and IL-6 (43), which promote osteoclastic activity. PTH-induced bone loss can be inhibited by blocking IL-6R with neutralizing antibodies (44). Patients who suffer from primary parathyroidism show elevated IL-6 and markers of increased bone resorption (45), further demonstrating how this hormone is involved in IL-6-associated bone diseases.

It would be overly simple to say that IL-6 is solely detrimental to bone, as recent *in vivo* work has shown a key role for it in bone repair. Transgenic mice overexpressing IL-6 have demonstrated enhanced bone loss, faulty osteoid ossification, and reduced osteoblast activity (46), but, other studies have also shown that IL-6 knock-out (KO) mice display abnormalities in bone architecture and delayed fracture healing (47). These IL-6 KO mice demonstrated delayed mineralization and remodeling of bone, with enhanced levels of collagen and cartilage at early stages of healing and reduced osteoclast number (47). This demonstrates a necessity for IL-6-induced bone loss in the correct repair of fractures. This is further evidenced in a diabetes-associated fracture model where reduced osteoclastic activity resulted in delayed repair (48).

IL-6 and Rheumatoid Arthritis (RA)

RA is a chronic, inflammatory condition prevalent in middle-aged people and is the leading cause of work-associated disability in the United States (49). Characterized by inflammation of the synovium of multiple joints of the body, sufferers exhibit pain and stiffness in hands, knees, wrists and feet. Progression of the disease results in detrimental damage to the joint and erosion of both the cartilage and bone. RA patients commonly express high levels of IL-6 intracellularly, which has been shown to have negative correlations clinically with bone mass density (BMD) (50). Increased vascular permeability and extravasation of fluid into synovial regions are key characteristics of RA and induce joint pain. Excess vascularization, a direct effect of IL-6-induced VEGF overexpression, enhances fluid build-up in joints (51). Antibodies against IL-6R can reduce VEGF expression in RA clinically (51).

In IL-6 KO mouse models, mice are protected against arthritis and have decreased osteoclast activity and bone loss (52). In addition, IL-6 neutralizing antibodies have been administered to mice in collagen-induced *in vivo* arthritis models, where they protected the mice from bone lesions and disease progression (53). Similarly, IL-6R antagonists have been shown to reduce osteoclastogenesis and reduce bone resorption in arthritic mouse models (54). The sIL-6R has also been shown to be of importance *in vivo,* as co-administration of mice with IL-6 and sIL-6R resulted in restoration of arthritic diseased states in IL-6 KO models (55). Having said this, some studies using male IL-6 KO mice demonstrated phenotypes of advanced osteoarthritis upon aging, complicating the story (56). Overall, most findings suggest that IL-6 induces RA initiation and progression (57).

Currently, targeting IL-6 therapeutically for RA has been successful in the clinic, although the negative side effects from this therapeutic approach should not be minimized. The U.S. Food and Drug Administration declined to approve Johnson & Johnson's RA anti-IL-6 drug called sirukumab, saying additional clinical data is needed to further evaluate its safety in September of 2017 (58). Sirukumab is a chimeric (murine-human) IgG1κ monoclonal antibody (mAb) that binds and neutralizes human IL-6. FDA panelists were concerned about an imbalance in the number of deaths in patients taking sirukumab compared with those taking a placebo, but Johnson & Johnson are continuing further development and testing of the drug (58). The most common causes of death were major heart problems, infection and cancers (58). However, Genentech's drug known as Actemra® (tocilizumab), the first humanized anti-IL-6 receptor agonist, has been FDA approved since 2010 for RA and was recently approved (November, 2018) as a prefilled autoinjector known as ACTPen™ for RA and patients with giant cell arthritis (GCA), active polyarticular juvenile idiopathic arthritis (PJIA) or active systemic juvenile idiopathic arthritis (SJIA) (59). Tocilizumab can cause serious side effects however (59), and hence safer options are still desired for patients with RA and other inflammatory diseases. Still, effects of tocilizumab on bone look promising, as different clinical trials have reported that patients experienced a decrease in osteogenic inhibitor DKK1, CTX-1 bone turnover markers, and in erosions of bone in the hands, and an increase in OPG with bone histology and P1NP bone formation markers in blood (60–65).

In May of 2017, Regeneron Pharmaceutical's Kevzara® (sarilumab), another IL-6 receptor antagonist, received FDA approval for treatment of adult patients with moderately to severely active RA (66). Similarly to the IL-6/IL-6R-targeting drugs, sarilumab also increases the risk of serious side effects that may lead to hospitalization or death, largely due to the suppression of the immune system (66). These therapies would be greatly improved if IL-6 could be targeted in the tissues or areas of interest rather than systemically. Moreover, better success may be achievable using bi-specific antibodies, such as one termed MT-6194 currently in preclinical studies targeting IL-17A and IL-6R (67). Research into these and other innovative ways to target IL-6 are crucial new directions for the next generation of anti-IL-6/IL-6R therapies, but as many of the current therapies already have FDA approval, despite toxicities, it is unlikely that pharmaceutical industries feel the financial incentive to move in this direction in their Research and Development departments. It may depend on academic scientists, doctors, patients, or companies that do not have a currently FDA approved anti-IL-6 therapeutic, to push for improvements and innovations in targeting IL-6.

IL-6 and Osteoporosis

Aging increases the production of inflammatory molecules, including IL-6, which explains some of the increased prevalence of inflammatory disorders (diabetes, lupus, and RA) in aging (68–70). Osteoporosis is also common in older and post-menopausal women due to a natural reduction in estrogen levels and high IL-6 levels, adding to increased osteoclastogenesis and pronounced osteopenia (71, 72). Ordinarily, the estrogen isomer 17-β-oestradiol (E2) reduces monocyte secretion of IL-6 and IL-8 (73), and thus after menopause, these pro-osteoclastic cytokines become more abundant (74). E2 interacts with the NFκB pathway, which is ordinarily held in an inactive state by coupling with an inhibitor known as IκBα (**Figure 2**). Certain signals result in IκBα becoming phosphorylated, uncoupling from NFκB and releasing it from its inactive state, allowing for signaling of downstream genes (75). Studies show that E2 promotes IκBα coupling to NFκB, keeping it in an inactivate state (76). This indicates how a loss in estrogen can result in increased IL-6 and NFκB signaling, and a consequential increase in bone loss and osteoporosis.

Bone loss induced by the E2-NFκB-IL-6 pathways can be reversed by administration of E2 (72) or anti-IL-6 neutralizing antibody (77–79). Clinically, post-menopausal women demonstrate an increased risk of osteoporosis, and patients with certain polymorphisms in the IL-6 promoter show further increases in bone resorption rates and reduction in BMD (80). This highlights how variation in IL-6 expression within patients can alter the risk of osteoporosis in estrogen-depleted environments. Currently, targeting IL-6 therapeutically for osteoporosis has not been explored, but this is an interesting clinical future direction that holds great potential if the side effects from these types of therapies can be minimized.

IL-6 AND BONE-METASTATIC CANCER

Paul Ehrlich first proposed the function of the immune system as the first line of defense against cancer in the early twentieth

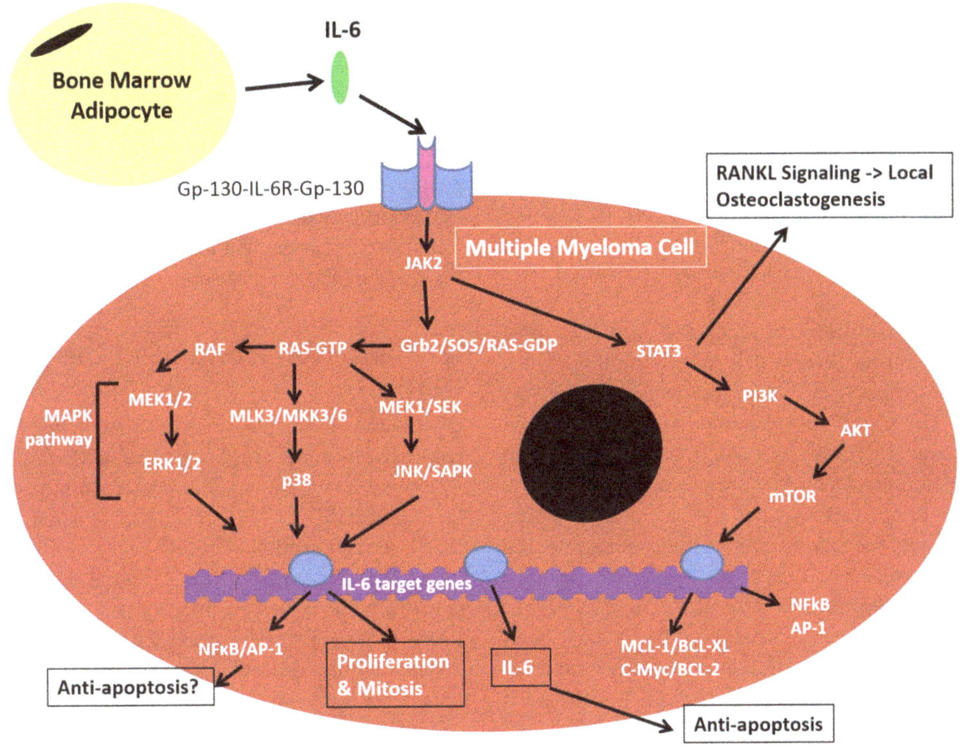

FIGURE 2 | IL-6 signaling in the tumor cell of the bone marrow niche. The bone marrow microenvironment augments MAPK and PI3K/Akt pathways resulting in anti-apoptotic and NF-κB signaling in multiple myeloma cells. Binding of IL-6 to IL-6R and Gp-130 co-receptors induces JAK-2 signaling. This signaling cascade diverges down STAT3/PI3K/Akt pathways and various MAPK pathways, including MEK/ERK. The former is associated with promoting anti-apoptotic proteins: MCL1, BCL-XL, BCL-2 and c-Myc, which contribute to drug resistance. STAT3/PI3K/Akt can also promote NF-κB signaling which results in release of angiogenic and inflammatory molecules, such as IL-6. This can feed into an autocrine positive feedback loop. IκBα can inhibit NFκB through coupling and this interaction can be maintained by certan signals, such as by estradiol. The IL-6 signaling pathway in MM cells is similar to that of bone marrow stromal cells and overall it promotes an inflammatory microenvironment in the bone which results in bone loss, increased tumor burden and disease progression. Bone marrow adipocytes (BMAs) are one cell within the bone microoenvironment thought to feed into this system through secretion of IL-6. This can promote anti-apoptosis and disease progrssion through NF-κB signaling. BMAs, thus, represent an ideal target for MM therapies in order to reduce drug resistance and relapse, instead of targeting the complicated, clonally expanding plasma cell.

century. Since then, the roles of immune and stromal cells, and their secretory repertoires, have been extensively studied in conjunction with cancer. Inflammation in particular has been shown to be key in promoting cancer proliferation and differentiation, with IL-6 being an integral player (81). Many cancer types have been shown to be associated with high serum IL-6 including colorectal (82), breast (83), and prostate cancer (84), as well as MM (85). These cancers induce phenotypic changes in the surrounding stromal cells, creating unique cell types, such as tumor-associated macrophage (TAMs) (86, 87) and cancer-associated fibroblasts (CAFs) (76, 77). These activated stromal cells, along with $CD4^+$ T cells and myeloid-derived suppressor cells (MDSCs), are the main sources of IL-6 in most tumor microenvironments, alongside the tumor cells themselves (88–92). Consequently, these BMM cells are associated with creating pro-oncogenic environments that promote proliferation and progression of cancer cells by favoring angiogenesis and metastasis, and inhibiting apoptosis (93–96). For example, knockdown of IL-6 by RNAi within CAFs can attenuate metastatic phenotypes *in vivo* (94). It is not surprising that level of IL-6 within the serum of various cancer patients is a key prognostic indicator for their response or disease progression (88). As a rule, high levels of IL-6 are associated with aggressive forms of cancers (97–100) and IL-6 levels can act as independent markers of prognosis in certain cancers (101). Furthermore, high expression of IL-6 has been more closely linked to recurrent tumors than primary tumors (102). IL-6 promotes proliferation (103), facilitates an epithelial-to-mesenchymal transition (94, 104) and enhances angiogenesis via VEGF stimulation (105, 106). Increased IL-6 in cancer cells results in subsequent release of IL-6 by stromal cells, thus feeding into the pro-tumoural feed-forward loop and exacerbating the diseased state (107–109).

Chemotherapeutics and ionizing radiation are the most common cancer therapies that work by disrupting DNA and protein synthesis pathways resulting in apoptosis. Yet both are known to stimulate oxidative stress, the NFκB pathway, and consequently IL-6 (110–114). IL-6 stimulation then counteracts the chemotherapy effect by promoting anti-apoptotic pathways to cause drug resistance (115). The anti-myeloma drug bortezomib targets the 26S subunit of the proteasome, the cellular machinery involved in degrading misfolded proteins, and causes an accumulation of unwanted/toxic proteins within cells (116). This accumulation of proteins is particularly seen in cells that already have dysfunctional or excessive protein-folding processes, such as myeloma cells (117). Misfolded protein accumulation results in increased ER stress, cell cycle arrest and programmed cell death (118). However, IL-6 has been shown to induce anti-apoptotic pathways in certain cancers, thus attenuating the efficacy of this drug (119–121). Gemcitabine is a nucleoside analog that causes termination of DNA synthesis (122). Gemcitabine targets fast-replicating cancer cells and resistance to this drug may also be tied to IL-6, as evidenced by a study where gemcitabine-resistance was observed in cancer cells treated with IL-6 and sIL-6R. This was thought to be due to a IL-6-prompted barricade of cells in G0/G1 cell cycle stages, preventing cells from entering the necessary cell-division stages necessary drug-induced replicative-associated destruction (26, 123–125).

As stated above, IL-6 also plays roles in apoptosis, which occurs due to cellular mishaps as a means to reduce malignancy. Interestingly, IL-6 has been shown to play both pro- and anti-apoptotic roles depending on tumor type. In some p53-wild-type breast and colon cancers, when tumors were treated with kinase inhibitors and general chemotherapies, IL-6 was shown to induce apoptosis via p53 and STAT5, with downstream signaling occurring through BAX [the reciprocal protein to anti-apoptotic BCL-2 (126)]. On the other hand, certain cancers, including many bone-metastases, have an opposing phenotype and demonstrate a sustained and even enhanced proliferation due to IL-6 and similar cytokines (113–115).

Bone metastatic cancer cells can become dormant within the BMM, thus protecting them from elimination by the immune system (127). It is common for these tumors to eventually become proliferative and induce osteoclastogenesis through secretion of soluble factors (128, 129). Melanoma cell lines have been shown to home to the bone and induce bone destruction through a TGF-β-IL-11 axis via osteoblasts (130), whilst other cancers facilitate similar pathways, such as TGF-β-RANKL-mediated destruction (131). IL-6 and its bone destructive roles can be tied to certain cancers, including MM and neuroblastoma, both of which induce IL-6 secretion from the surrounding stroma resulting in bone loss through the NFκB pathway (132, 133). MM cells derive from the immune plasma cell, home to the BM, cause bone destruction, and eventually become drug resistant. IL-6 plays a role in all these steps, so this review will focus on the effects of IL-6 in MM, as a disease model, from here on.

IL-6 and MM Homing to the Bone Marrow Niche

Chemokine gradients, such as that created by SDF-1, play a large role homing of cells to the BMM. The CXCR4-SDF1 axis is known to promote IL-6 expression in numerous cancers, including MM (3, 134), and other studies have also indicated that IL-6 may promote CXCR7-SDF1 or CXCR4-SDF1 signaling (135), and as such promote bone-homing (136). SDF1 is constitutively expressed by stromal cells and osteoblasts in the BMM (127, 128), and attracts $CXCR4^+$/$CXCR7^+$ haemopoietic or tumor cells to the BMM (137). B-cells, MM cells, and other bone metastatic cancer cells, including breast and melanoma cells, express CXCR4, which functions in the proliferation and migration of these cells to the SDF1-rich BMM (138–141). The CXCR4-SDF1 axis can also promote the expression of molecules that enable adhesion of cells to the endothelial lining of the BM sinus, such as VCAM1 (142). Additionally, α4β1 integrins can overexpressed due to CXCR4-SDF1 signaling, which can further enhance homing to the BM (142, 143). In contrast, TGF-β1 supresses expression of SDF-1 and has been shown to reduce BM stromal cell (BMSC) migration and adhesion, which could translate to a reduced ability to traffic to the BM (144). It is unsurprising that a CXCR4 inhibitor has been shown to disrupt

MM cell interaction with the BMM and thus increase sensitivity to treatment (145).

Myeloma cells also commonly express cell surface receptors CCR1 and CCR2 (146, 147), which bind MIP-1α and MCP1-3, respectively. Similar to SDF1, these ligands are expressed highly by BMSCs and promote myeloma cell migration and homing to the BMM (148, 149). All three receptor axes (CCR1, CCR2, CXCR4) are interesting from a clinical point of view as patients with low expression of these receptors have shown poor disease prognosis, associated with high serum β2 microglobulin and C-reactive protein (146). The former is a molecule secreted by B cells and acts as a marker of disease progression and poor prognosis in MM. The latter is a marker of systemic inflammation and again marks poor clinical prognosis in MM. It is possible that the downregulation of the receptors results in a reduced ability to home to and reside within the BMM and an increase in circulating myeloma cells, which may cause more systemic spreading of the disease. However, this contradicts our typical understanding that tumor cells are more protected in the BM, and thus cause worse outcomes when lodged in the bone rather than when in circulation. Interestingly, IL-6 KO mice are known to express lower levels of IL-2 (150), a cytokine known to promote CCR1 and CCR2 (151). Taken together, these data indicate that IL-6 may increase MM bone homing through promoting not only CXCR4 and possibly CCR2/3 signaling.

IL-6–Driven Bone Destruction in MM

MM also increases osteoclast number and activity, which leads to hypercalcaemia, renal-insufficiency, anemia, osteopenia and lesions in the bone. The breakdown of bone promotes chronic pain, increases fracture risk, and results in the release of bone-derived growth factors, which feed the tumor cells and promote disease progression (17, 18). This vicious cycle leads to a poor quality of life and ultimately results in prolific dissemination of these plasma cells throughout the body, a fatal condition known as plasma cell leukemia.

A number of factors feed into MM-bone loss including osteocyte-derived sclerostin. In MM patients, elevated circulating sclerostin levels are commonly seen, particularly in advanced stages (152). Sclerostin has anti-osteoblastic properties and anti-sclerostin therapeutics are currently being investigated for use in MM-associated bone loss pre-clinically (153, 154). Anti-sclerostin antibodies also reduce BM adiposity, and hence more research into their effects on bone or cancer though modulating BM adiposity is warranted (155, 156). DKK1 is another Wnt inhibitor involved in MM-mediated bone loss and disease progression that has been investigated as a target in MM bone loss (157). DKK1, like sclerostin, inhibits osteoblastogenesis by blocking differentiation of pre-osteoblasts by impeding the WNT signaling cascade (158). Recently, a bispecific antibody targeting sclerostin and DKK-1 has been shown to promote bone mass accrual and fracture repair in rodents and non-human primates (159). In addition to simply reducing numbers of mature osteoblasts, DKK1 also increases the number of undifferentiated BMSCs, and these undifferentiated BMSCs secrete higher IL-6 amounts than their differentiated counterparts (160), thus feeding into the IL-6-bone-destruction pathway described previously. Inhibition of IL-6 from MSC-conditioned media slowed the proliferation of DKK-1 secreting myeloma cells treated with this media, suggesting that in the myeloma environment, IL-6 increases bone resorption through promoting proliferation of DKK-1-secreting myeloma cells (160). However, in other contexts, a negative correlation between IL-6 and DKK1 was observed, implying that more research into the role of IL-6 in bone destruction would be useful (161).

IL-6 mediated bone loss also occurs due to direct expression and release of IL-6 by MM cells and consequential osteoclast activation. The mechanism of IL-6-mediated osteoclastogenesis is thought to be due primarily to activation of the JAK2/STAT3 axis, resulting in upregulation of RANKL molecules (24) (see **Figure 2**). This overthrows the fine balance between osteoclastic RANKL molecules and their inhibitor, OPG, pushing the equilibrium in favor of bone loss (162). In addition, IL-6 may also make preosteoclasts more sensitive to RANKL stimulation, presumably due to an IL-6-mediated upregulation of RANK receptors, which was previously shown in Paget's disease (163). *In vivo* studies have confirmed IL-6 mediated bone loss in both trabecular and endochondral bone; this bone loss is enhanced in the presence of MM cells and is associated with increased osteoclast differentiation (164). This finding is being investigated in phase II clinical trials, which are currently examining the efficacy of anti-IL-6 treatment on MM bone-loss (NCT01484275).

IL-6 and MM Disease Progression

MM begins as a condition known as monoclonal gammopathy of undetermined significance (MGUS), an asymptomatic stage where levels of immunoglobulin in the blood and risk of fracture are elevated. Blood serum IL-6 levels correspond to prognosis and progression of MM (85); prognosis is worse when levels exceed 7 pg/ml, with an average survival of 2.7 months compared to 53.7 months in those with lower levels (85). IL-6/STAT3 pathways are known to promote angiogenesis via enhancement of VEGF in MM (165). Osteoclasts are also known to secrete pro-angiogenic molecules, and thus in MM when both osteoclast number and activity is enhanced, there is also an increase in the development of vasculature (166). IL-6/STAT3 signaling not only promotes the creation of these new endothelial cells, but also stimulates Ras, Akt and MAPK pathways which promotes the survival of said MM cells (167).

IL-6–Mediated Drug Resistance and Survival in MM

Apoptosis involves the activation of caspase enzymes in a cascade ending in the activation and release of apoptosis-inducing factors from mitochondria. Apoptosis-inducing agents cause DNA fragmentation and chromatin condensation, which ultimately induces cell death (168). IL-6 promotes JAK/STAT3 and consequently PI3K/Akt and MEK/MAPK (169), (**Figure 2**); these pathways are known to upregulate anti-apoptosis proteins Mcl-1, Bcl-XL and c-Myc in primary MM cells, resulting in cell survival and chemotherapy resistance (170, 171). A number of antibodies have been investigated to neutralize IL-6, but little success has occurred clinically (172, 173). However, evidence indicates that indirect targeting of downstream anti-apoptosis mediators can help reverse the effects of IL-6. *In vitro,* anti-sense targeting strategies against MCL-1 sensitized MM cells to drugs by inhibiting these anti-apoptotic pathways (174). In addition, IL-6-mediated resistance was reversed by targeting CDC34 (175). This molecule is an ubiquitin-conjugating enzyme involved in proteasomal degradation. It has been tied to ubiquitination and degradation of IκBα, the NFκB inhibitor, and thus promotes drug resistance via NFκB signaling. Targeting other molecules within the JAK/STAT3 cascade also appears to aid in resistance reversal, as the Akt inhibitor, MK2206, has also been found to help overcome bortezomib resistance in MM cells induced by co-culturing with IL-6 or MSCs (176). [For more on IL-6 and proteasome inhibitor resistance in MM, we refer the reader to our recent review may (121)].

IL-6 may also cause drug resistance through epigenetic modulation proteins. IL-6 signals via STAT3 and enhances DNA methyltransferase 1, which promotes the methylation and thus deactivation of P53, facilitating cells to avoid cell cycle checkpoint destruction (177). This could clearly have unfavorable effects in MM, promoting drug resistance and/or disease progression. Initial studies into use of general histone deacetylase (HDAC) inhibitors were unfavorable (178), however, subsequent use of selective HDAC inhibitors, such as chidamide, have shown anti-MM and bone protective effect, showing synergistic effects with other therapies such as dexamethasone, carfilzomib and pomalidomide (179).

Bone Marrow Adipocyte (BMA)-Derived IL-6 Contribution to MM Progression

Obesity is an increasingly common condition which increases one's risk of cardiovascular disease, diabetes, certain cancers, and many other diseases. One link to cancer is due to the increased inflammatory state which occurs due to obesity (180). The excess storage of lipids within adipose tissues causes the release of inflammatory molecules, TNF-α and IL-6, and suppression of anti-inflammatory adiponectin (181). This creates a microenvironment of high oxidative stress and inflammation and results in damage to tissues, increasing one's risk of oncogenic mutations and tumorigenesis (180). Increased fat intake, which typically causes obesity over time, is linked to higher levels of BM adiposity in rodents (182); recently, BM adipocytes (BMAs) have been shown to play significant roles in MM drug resistance and disease progression (183), possibly through the secretion of soluble factors, such as IL-6 (184). BMAs have such a profound effect on MM that, clinically, obese and older populations, both of whom suffer from enhanced systemic inflammation and increased BMA levels, demonstrate higher risk of developing MM than other groups of people (185).

BMAs may contribute to disease progression in numerous ways. *In vitro* work has demonstrated an ability of BMAs extracted from MM patient femurs to support MM cell growth and protect them from chemotherapy-induced apoptosis (186). In addition, MM is known to increase expression of PGC-1α within BMAs, resulting in VEGF and GLUT-4 expression (187), which increases proliferation, angiogenesis and metastasis, as described above. BMAs have also been shown to increase expression of autophagic proteins within MM cells, which can promote drug resistance (186). Finally, BMA-derived IL-6 has been hypothesized to contribute to chemotherapy resistance due to an upregulation of anti-apoptotic proteins and inhibition of cell checkpoint proteins (**Figure 2**). The latter pathway remains unverified, yet studies are currently underway to investigate this further. If true, IL-6 and its downstream signaling molecules represent good targets for possible re-sensitization of MM cells in refractory disease. Investigation into the blockade of anti-apoptotic pathways downstream of IL-6 and other IL-6 mediated pathways is warranted. In addition, efforts should be made to find therapeutics that target BMAs specifically, and to investigate the secretory repertoires of all BMM cells to better understand and manipulate the microenvironment into one of anti-tumorigenicity.

Clinically Targeting IL-6 in Cancer

Despite extensive pre-clinical *in vitro* and *in vivo* support for the role of IL-6 in MM and other osteolytic bone cancers, clinical translation results have been dismal. Clinical trial results with siltuximab, formerly CNTO 328, in MM have been disheartening and no clinical trials in other bone cancers have been initiated as of yet. As presented in an abstract for the American Society of Hematology (ASH), 2017 annual meeting, IL-6 blockade did not add benefit to chemotherapy in a phase 2, randomized, double-blind, placebo-controlled multicenter study in patients with high-risk smoldering MM (188). A clinical trial examining if siltuximab can decrease symptom burden after autologous stem cell transplantation for patients with MM or AL amyloidosis is currently underway (ClinicalTrials.gov Identifier: NCT03315026). No data on MM and siltuximab was presented at the ASH 2018 conference. A study of CNTO 328 in Japan from 2011 to 2014 in relapsed or refractory MM patients was halted due to safety concerns (ClinicalTrials.gov Identifier: NCT01309412). An open-label, phase I trial of CTNO with lenalidomide, bortezomib and dexamethasone (RVD) was performed (ClinicalTrials.gov Identifier: NCT01531998), however the efficacy data were limited by the small number of patients since the trial was halted and did not proceed to phase II. The abandonment of the phase II trial was due to the negative outcomes from another phase II study of bortezomib-melphalan-prednisone (VMP) vs. VMP+siltuximab, which demonstrated no significant improvement in progression-free survival. After this finding, further development of siltuximab in symptomatic myeloma was halted by the sponsor (189). Trials have also been initiated examining the safety and efficacy of siltuximab in metastatic, hormone-refractory prostate cancer, renal and other solid tumors (ovarian, pancreatic, colorectal, and others), and the field is currently waiting to see the results of these trials (190).

Tocilizumab, a humanized anti-IL-6R mAb, is currently the subject of investigation in many clinical cancer trials. Current clinical trials are ongoing for metastatic HER2-positive breast cancer resistant to trastuzumab, lymphoblastic leukemia, pancreatic cancer, myeloid leukemia, B-cell chronic lymphocytic leukemia, non-Hodgkin's lymphoma, B-cell lymphoma, and diffuse large B-cell lymphoma (ClinicalTrials.gov). Trials in myeloma were terminated due to low accrual rate (ClinicalTrials.gov Identifier: NCT02057770). In Europe, there is currently a clinical trial to explore the use of tocilizumab in fibrous dysplasia of bone (FD), a rare, painful bone disease affecting one or several bones (191). If promising data result, more clinical trials may arise studying the drug for bone pain relief applications.

Unfortunately, overall, large randomized trials show no efficacy of IL-6 inhibitors in various cancers, particularly myeloma. These results are despite a full inhibition of C-reactive protein (CRP) production in treated patients, the numerous preclinical studies showing an involvement of IL-6 in these diseases, and initial short-term treatments demonstrating a dramatic inhibition of cancer cell proliferation *in vivo* (192). Similarly, a meta-review of 48 clinical studies concluded that inhibition of IL-6 has unknown and unproven effects on decreasing GI (gastric, pancreatic, colorectal, bile duct and gall bladder) cancer syndromes or improving quality of life (191). A likely explanation for this lack of efficacy is the plasticity of cancer cells and their ability to clonally evolve and develop subclones that are less dependent on IL-6. Moreover, many therapies targeting tumor cells already decrease IL-6 or pathways downstream of IL-6, so that no additive or synergistic effect is derived from the anti-IL-6 therapy. Still, anti-IL-6 therapeutics are able to neutralize IL-6 production *in vivo* and are safe and useful in inflammatory diseases and Castleman disease. Their application may hold promise in treatment of bone-resident cancers if more developed (e.g., bi-specific mAbs against tumor cells and IL-6, or against RANKL and IL-6) therapies can be developed to increase their efficacy. Moreover, getting the treatment more specifically to the cancer may allow for higher doses and less off-target effects, and thus better outcomes, and more research into tumor-homing drug delivery or targeted nanomedicine technology may accelerate this process. As we understand more about the role of the immune system in cancer and the ability for tumor cells to block the immune response, researchers and clinicians may be able to design anti-IL-6 clinical trials using patient populations that are identified to have a positive response to these therapies. Similarly, a better understanding of the full activity of anti-IL-6 therapy will mean that different combination regimens or dosing strategies may be designed to be optimal for different patient subgroups.

CONCLUSIONS

IL-6 is a pro-inflammatory cytokine that promotes NF-κB, MAPK and PI3K/Akt signaling. Together these pathways promote anti-apoptosis signaling and drug resistance in cancer cells, in addition to further inflammatory signaling. The latter contributes to bone destruction and osteopenia, which promotes homing of metastatic cancers to the bone marrow niche. Bone marrow adipocytes, as well as mesenchymal stromal cells, may be a source of IL-6 or other factors, that contribute to chemotherapy resistance in the bone microenvironment. Targeting of these adipocytes, or their secreted factors, may help alleviate refractory disease.

Because MM demonstrates such genetic heterogeneity and high levels of refractory disease, targeting the BMM, along with the tumor cell directly, is an ideal plan of attack. The IL-6 signaling pathway in MM cells promotes an inflammatory bone microenvironment that results in osteopenia, increased tumor burden and disease progression. Bone marrow adipocytes are one cell type within the bone microoenvironment thought to feed into this system through secretion of IL-6 and other adipokines. Thus, bone marrow adipocytes represent an ideal target for MM therapies in order to reduce drug resistance and relapse, instead of targeting the complicated, clonally expanding plasma cells. The more we learn, the better we can target such pathways and not only improve quality of life for patients, but hopefully extend that lifetime as well. As this dream has not become realized in the clinic yet, more efforts on understanding and maximizing the targeting of IL-6 and its downstream pathways may be necessary. Moreover, building mouse cancer models, or tissue-engineered 3D models, that more accurately model the effects of targeting IL-6 in the human should lead to better clinical results in the future and avoid the pitfalls of wasted time and money on unsuccessful clinical trials.

AUTHOR CONTRIBUTIONS

DH wrote the manuscript. CF and MR edited the manuscript. All authors approved the manuscript. MR takes responsibility for the manuscript.

ACKNOWLEDGMENTS

This review utilized services from core facilities at Maine Medical Center Research Institute, which are supported by NIH/NIGMS P20GM121301 (L. Liaw, PI), U54GM115516 (C. Rosen, PI), and P30GM106391 (R. Friesel, PI). The authors' work is also supported by start-up funds from the MMCRI, and a pilot grant from the American Cancer Society (Research Grant #IRG-16-191-33; Reagan, PI). The content is solely the responsibility of the authors and does not necessarily represent the official views of the NIH.

REFERENCES

1. Dauer DJ, Ferraro B, Song L, Yu B, Mora L, Buettner R, et al. Stat3 regulates genes common to both wound healing and cancer. *Oncogene* (2005) 24:3397. doi: 10.1038/sj.onc.1208469
2. Baeuerle PA, Henkel T. Function and activation of NF-kappaB in the immune system. *Annu Rev Immunol.* (1994) 12:141–79. doi: 10.1146/annurev.iy.12.040194.001041
3. Hideshima T, Chauhan D, Hayashi T, Podar K, Akiyama M, Gupta D, et al. The biological sequelae of stromal cell-derived factor-1α in multiple myeloma. *Mol Cancer Ther.* (2002) 1:539–44.
4. Hideshima T, Chauhan D, Schlossman R, Richardson P, Anderson KC. The role of tumor necrosis factor α in the pathophysiology of human multiple myeloma: therapeutic applications. *Oncogene* (2001) 20:4519. doi: 10.1038/sj.onc.1204623

5. Betts JC, Cheshire JK, Akirav S, Kishimotov T, Woo P. The Role of NF-KB and NF-IL6 transactivating factors in the synergistic activation of human serum amyloid A gene expression by interleukin- 1 and interleukin-6. *J Biol Chem.* (1993) 268:25624–31.
6. Xing L, Bushnell TP, Carlson L, Tai Z, Tondravi M, Siebenlist U, et al. NF-κB p50 and p52 expression is not required for RANK-expressing osteoclast progenitor formation but is essential for RANK- and cytokine-mediated osteoclastogenesis. *J Bone Miner Res.* (2009) 17:1200–10. doi: 10.1359/jbmr.2002.17.7.1200
7. Arai F, Miyamoto T, Ohneda O, Inada T, Sudo T, Brasel K, et al. Commitment and differentiation of osteoclast precursor cells by the sequential expression of C-Fms and receptor activator of nuclear factor κb (Rank) receptors. *J Exp Med.* (1999) 190:1741–54. doi: 10.1084/jem.190.12.1741
8. Franzoso G, Carlson L, Xing L, Poljak L, Shores EW, Brown KD, et al. Requirement for NF-κB in osteoclast and B-cell development. *Genes Dev.* (1997) 11:3482–96.
9. Wei S, Kitaura H, Zhou P, Ross FP, Teitelbaum SL. IL-1 mediates TNF-induced osteoclastogenesis. *J Clin Invest.* (2005) 115:282–90. doi: 10.1172/JCI200523394
10. Steeve KT, Marc P, Sandrine T, Dominique H, Yannick F. IL-6, RANKL, TNF-alpha/IL-1: interrelations in bone resorption pathophysiology. *Cytokine Growth Factor Rev.* (2004) 15:49–60. doi: 10.1016/j.cytogfr.2003.10.005
11. Hashizume M, Mihara M. The roles of interleukin-6 in the pathogenesis of rheumatoid arthritis. *Arthritis* (2011) 2011:765624. doi: 10.1155/2011/765624
12. Tawara K, Oxford JT, Jorcyk CL. Clinical significance of interleukin (IL)-6 in cancer metastasis to bone: potential of anti-IL-6 therapies. *Cancer Manag Res.* (2011) 3:177–189. doi: 10.2147/CMR.S18101
13. George DJ, Halabi S, Shepard TF, Sanford B, Vogelzang NJ, Small EJ, et al. The prognostic significance of plasma interleukin-6 levels in patients with metastatic hormone-refractory prostate cancer: results from cancer and leukemia group B 9480. *Clin Cancer Res.* (2005) 11:1815–20. doi: 10.1158/1078-0432.CCR-04-1560
14. Coleman RE, Rubens RD. The clinical course of bone metastases from breast cancer. *Br J Cancer* (1987) 55:61–6. doi: 10.1038/bjc.1987.13
15. Ara T, Song L, Shimada H, Keshelava N, Russell HV, Metelitsa LS, et al. Interleukin-6 in the bone marrow microenvironment promotes the growth and survival of neuroblastoma cells. *Cancer Res.* (2009) 69:329–37. doi: 10.1158/0008-5472.CAN-08-0613
16. Stevens AM, Miller JM, Munoz JO, Gaikwad AS, Redell MS. Interleukin-6 levels predict event-free survival in pediatric AML and suggest a mechanism of chemotherapy resistance. *Blood Adv.* (2017) 1:1387–97. doi: 10.1182/bloodadvances.2017007856
17. Hallek M, Bergsagel PL, Anderson KC. Multiple myeloma: increasing evidence for a multistep transformation process. *Blood* (1998) 91:3–21.
18. Kawano M, Hirano T, Matsuda T, Taga T, Horii Y, Iwato K, et al. Autocrine generation and requirement of BSF-2/IL-6 for human multiple myelomas. *Nature* (1988) 332:83–5. doi: 10.1038/332083a0
19. Hayrapetyan A, Jansen JA, van den Beucken JJJP. Signaling pathways involved in osteogenesis and their application for bone regenerative medicine. *Tissue Eng Part B Rev.* (2014) 21:75–87. doi: 10.1089/ten.teb.2014.0119
20. Thompson WR, Rubin CT, Rubin J. Mechanical regulation of signaling pathways in bone. *Gene* (2012) 503:179–193. doi: 10.1016/j.gene.2012.04.076
21. McDonald MM, Fairfield H, Falank C, Reagan MR. Adipose, bone, and myeloma: contributions from the microenvironment. *Calcif Tissue Int.* (2017) 100:433–48. doi: 10.1007/s00223-016-0162-2
22. Dallas SL, Prideaux M, Bonewald LF. The osteocyte: an endocrine cell … and more. *Endocr Rev.* (2013) 34:658–90. doi: 10.1210/er.2012-1026
23. Udagawa N, Takahashi N, Katagiri T, Tamura T, Wada S, Findlay D, et al. Interleukin (IL)-6 induction of osteoclast differentiation depends on IL-6 receptors expressed on osteoblastic cells but not on osteoclast progenitors. *J Exp Med.* (1995) 182:1461–8. doi: 10.1084/jem.182.5.1461
24. Hashizume M, Hayakawa N, Mihara M. IL-6 trans-signalling directly induces RANKL on fibroblast-like synovial cells and is involved in RANKL induction by TNF-α and IL-17. *Rheumatology* (2008) 47:1635–40. doi: 10.1093/rheumatology/ken363
25. O'Brien CA, Gubrij I, Lin SC, Saylors RL, Manolagas SC. STAT3 activation in stromal/osteoblastic cells is required for induction of the receptor activator of NF-κB ligand and stimulation of osteoclastogenesis by gp130-utilizing cytokines or interleukin-1 but not 1,25-dihydroxyvitamin D3 or parathyroid hormone. *J Biol Chem.* (1999) 274:19301–8.
26. Blanchard F, Duplomb L, Baud'huin M, Brounais B. The dual role of IL-6-type cytokines on bone remodeling and bone tumors. *Cytokine Growth Factor Rev.* (2009) 20:19–28. doi: 10.1016/j.cytogfr.2008.11.004
27. Liu X-H, Kirschenbaum A, Yao S, Levine AC. Cross-Talk between the interleukin-6 and prostaglandin E2 signaling systems results in enhancement of osteoclastogenesis through effects on the osteoprotegerin/Receptor Activator of Nuclear Factor-κB (RANK) ligand/RANK system. *Endocrinology* (2005) 146:1991–8. doi: 10.1210/en.2004-1167
28. Kozawa O, Suzuki A, Tokuda H, Kaida T, Uematsu T. Interleukin-6 synthesis induced by prostaglandin E2: cross-talk regulation by protein kinase C. *Bone* (1998) 22:355–60. doi: 10.1016/S8756-3282(97)00293-7
29. Gruber R, Nothegger G, Ho G-M, Willheim M, Peterlik M. Differential stimulation by PGE2 and calcemic hormones of IL-6 in stromal/osteoblastic cells. *Biochem Biophys Res Commun.* (2000) 270:1080–5. doi: 10.1006/bbrc.2000.2573
30. Devlin RD, Reddy SV, Savino R, Ciliberto G, Roodman GD. IL-6 mediates the effects of IL-1 or TNF, but Not PTHrP or 1,25(OH)2D3, on osteoclast-like cell formation in normal human bone marrow cultures. *J Bone Miner Res.* (1998) 13:393–9.
31. Csilla Holub M, Szalai C, Polgár A, Tóth S, Falus A. Generation of 'truncated' interleukin-6 receptor (IL-6R) mRNA by alternative splicing; a possible source of soluble IL-6R. *Immunol Lett.* (1999) 68:121–4.
32. Briso EM, Dienz O, Rincon M. Soluble IL-6R is produced by IL-6R ectodomain shedding in activated CD4 T cells. *J Immunol.* (2008) 180:7102–6. doi: 10.4049/jimmunol.180.11.7102
33. Kaneshiro S, Ebina K, Shi K, Higuchi C, Hirao M, Okamoto M, et al. IL-6 negatively regulates osteoblast differentiation through the SHP2/MEK2 and SHP2/Akt2 pathways in vitro. *J Bone Miner Metab.* (2014) 32:378–92. doi: 10.1007/s00774-013-0514-1
34. Peruzzi B, Cappariello A, Del Fattore A, Rucci N, De Benedetti F, Teti A. c-Src and IL-6 inhibit osteoblast differentiation and integrate IGFBP5 signalling. *Nat Commun.* (2012) 3:630. doi: 10.1038/ncomms1651
35. Liu X, Kirschenbaum A, Yao S, Levine ACBT-V& H. The role of the interleukin-6/gp130 signaling pathway in bone metabolism. In: Litwack G, editor. *Vitamins and Hormones.* London: Academic Press (2006). p. 341–55.
36. Breyer RM, Bagdassarian CK, Myers SA, Breyer MD. Prostanoid receptors: subtypes and signaling. *Annu Rev Pharmacol Toxicol.* (2001) 41:661–90. doi: 10.1146/annurev.pharmtox.41.1.661
37. Park JY, Pillinger MH, Abramson SB. Prostaglandin E2 synthesis and secretion: the role of PGE2 synthases. *Clin Immunol.* (2006) 119:229–40. doi: 10.1016/j.clim.2006.01.016
38. Morimoto K, Shirata N, Taketomi Y, Tsuchiya S, Segi-Nishida E, Inazumi T, et al. Prostaglandin E2–EP3 signaling induces inflammatory swelling by mast cell activation. *J Immunol.* (2014) 192:1130–7. doi: 10.4049/jimmunol.1300290
39. Yao C, Sakata D, Esaki Y, Li Y, Matsuoka T, Kuroiwa K, et al. Prostaglandin E2–EP4 signaling promotes immune inflammation through TH1 cell differentiation and TH17 cell expansion. *Nat Med.* (2009) 15:633. doi: 10.1038/nm.1968
40. Jia X-Y, Chang Y, Sun X-J, Dai X, Wei W. The role of prostaglandin E2 receptor signaling of dendritic cells in rheumatoid arthritis. *Int Immunopharmacol.* (2014) 23:163–9. doi: 10.1016/j.intimp.2014.08.024
41. Honda T, Segi-Nishida E, Miyachi Y, Narumiya S. Prostacyclin-IP signaling and prostaglandin E_2-P2/EP4 signaling both mediate joint inflammation in mouse collagen-induced arthritis. *J Exp Med.* (2006) 203:325–35. doi: 10.1084/jem.20051310
42. Fattahi MJ, Mirshafiey A. Prostaglandins and rheumatoid arthritis. *Arthritis* (2012) 2012:239310. doi: 10.1155/2012/239310
43. Löwik CWGM, van der Pluijm G, Bloys H, Hoekman K, Bijvoet OLM, Aarden LA, et al. Parathyroid hormone (PTH) and PTH-like protein (PLP) stimulate interleukin-6 production by osteogenic cells: a possible role of interleukin-6 in osteoclastogenesis. *Biochem Biophys Res Commun.* (1989) 162:1546–1552.

44. Greenfield EM, Shaw SM, Gornik SA, Banks MA. Adenyl cyclase and interleukin 6 are downstream effectors of parathyroid hormone resulting in stimulation of bone resorption. *J Clin Invest.* (1995) 96:1238–44. doi: 10.1172/JCI118157
45. Grey A, Mitnick M-A, Masiukiewicz U, Sun B-H, Rudikoff S, Jilka RL, et al. A role for interleukin-6 in parathyroid hormone-induced bone resorption *in Vivo* 1. *Endocrinology* (1999) 140:4683–90. doi: 10.1210/endo.140.10.7036
46. Fabrizio DB, Nadia R, Andrea DF, Barbara P, Rita P, Maurizio L, et al. Impaired skeletal development in interleukin-6–transgenic mice: a model for the impact of chronic inflammation on the growing skeletal system. *Arthritis Rheum.* (2006) 54:3551–63. doi: 10.1002/art.22175
47. Yang X, Ricciardi BF, Hernandez-Soria A, Shi Y, Camacho NP, Bostrom MPG. Callus mineralization and maturation are delayed during fracture healing in interleukin-6 knockout mice. *Bone* (2007) 41:928–36. doi: 10.1016/j.bone.2007.07.022
48. Kasahara T, Imai S, Kojima H, Katagi M, Kimura H, Chan L, et al. Malfunction of bone marrow derived osteoclasts and the delay of bone fracture healing in diabetic mice. *Bone* (2010) 47:617–25. doi: 10.1016/j.bone.2010.06.014
49. Theis KA, Roblin DW, Helmick CG, Luo R. Prevalence and causes of work disability among working-age U.S. adults, 2011–2013, NHIS. *Disabil Health J.* (2018) 11:108–15. doi: 10.1016/j.dhjo.2017.04.010
50. Verbruggen A, De Clerck LS, Bridts CH, Van Offel JF, Stevens WJ. Flow cytometrical determination of interleukin 1β, interleukin 6 and tumour necrosis factor α in monocytes of rheumatoid arthritis patients; relation with parameters of osteoporosis. *Cytokine* (1999) 11:869–74. doi: 10.1006/cyto.1998.0500
51. Hideko N, Jian S, Masamichi S, Keisuke H, Tadamitsu K, Kazuyuki Y, et al. Anti–interleukin-6 receptor antibody therapy reduces vascular endothelial growth factor production in rheumatoid arthritis. *Arthritis Rheum.* (2003) 48:1521–9. doi: 10.1002/art.11143
52. Wong PK, Quinn JM, Sims NA, van Nieuwenhuijze A, Campbell IK, Wicks IP. Interleukin-6 modulates production of T lymphocyte–derived cytokines in antigen-induced arthritis and drives inflammation-induced osteoclastogenesis. *Arthritis Rheum.* (2005) 54:158–68. doi: 10.1002/art.21537
53. Liang B, Song Z, Wu B, Gardner D, Shealy D, Song X-Y, et al. Evaluation of anti-IL-6 monoclonal antibody therapy using murine type II collagen-induced arthritis. *J Inflamm (Lond)* (2009) 6:10. doi: 10.1186/1476-9255-6-10
54. Tanaka K, Hashizume M, Mihara M, Yoshida H, Suzuki M, Matsumoto Y. Anti-interleukin-6 receptor antibody prevents systemic bone mass loss via reducing the number of osteoclast precursors in bone marrow in a collagen-induced arthritis model. *Clin Exp Immunol.* (2014) 175:172–80. doi: 10.1111/cei.12201
55. Nowell MA, Richards PJ, Horiuchi S, Yamamoto N, Rose-John S, Topley N, et al. Soluble IL-6 receptor governs IL-6 activity in experimental arthritis: blockade of arthritis severity by soluble glycoprotein 130. *J Immunol.* (2003) 171:3202–9. doi: 10.4049/jimmunol.171.6.3202
56. de Hooge ASK, van de Loo FAJ, Bennink MB, Arntz OJ, de Hooge P, van den Berg WB. Male IL-6 gene knock out mice developed more advanced osteoarthritis upon aging. *Osteoarthr Cartilage* (2005) 13:66–73. doi: 10.1016/j.joca.2004.09.011
57. Madhok R, Crilly A, Watson J, Capell HA. Serum interleukin 6 levels in rheumatoid arthritis: correlations with clinical and laboratory indices of disease activity. *Ann Rheum Dis.* (1993) 52:232–4. doi: 10.1136/ard.52.3.232
58. Clarke T. FDA declines to approve J&J arthritis drug sirukumab. *Reuters.* Washington, DC (2017).
59. *FDA Approves the ACTPen for Genentech's Actemra, a Single-Dose, Prefilled Autoinjector for the Treatment of Rheumatoid Arthritis, Giant Cell Arteritis and Two Forms of Juvenile Arthritis | Business Wire. BusinessWire (2018)* Available online at: https://www.businesswire.com/news/home/20181126005067/en/ (Accessed November 30, 2018)
60. Garnero P, Thompson E, Woodworth T, Smolen JS. Rapid and sustained improvement in bone and cartilage turnover markers with the antiâ€"interleukin-6 receptor inhibitor tocilizumab plus methotrexate in rheumatoid arthritis patients with an inadequate response to methotrexate: results from a substudy of the multicenter double-blind, placebo-controlled trial of tocilizumab in inadequate responders to methotrexate alone. *Arthritis Rheum.* (2010) 62:33–43. doi: 10.1002/art.25053
61. Hashimoto J, Garnero P, van der Heijde D, Miyasaka N, Yamamoto K, Kawai S, et al. Humanized anti-interleukin-6-receptor antibody (tocilizumab) monotherapy is more effective in slowing radiographic progression in patients with rheumatoid arthritis at high baseline risk for structural damage evaluated with levels of biomarkers, radiography, and BMI: data from the SAMURAI study. *Mod Rheumatol.* (2011) 21:10–5. doi: 10.3109/s10165-010-0325-3
62. Karsdal MA, Schett G, Emery P, Harari O, Byrjalsen I, Kenwright A, et al. IL-6 receptor inhibition positively modulates bone balance in rheumatoid arthritis patients with an inadequate response to anti-tumor necrosis factor therapy: biochemical marker analysis of bone metabolism in the tocilizumab RADIATE study (NCT00106522). *Semin Arthritis Rheum.* (2012) 42:131–9. doi: 10.1016/j.semarthrit.2012.01.004
63. Kanbe K, Nakamura A, Inoue Y, Hobo K. Osteoprotegerin expression in bone marrow by treatment with tocilizumab in rheumatoid arthritis. *Rheumatol Int.* (2012) 32:2669–74. doi: 10.1007/s00296-011-2021-9
64. Finzel S, Rech J, Schmidt S, Engelke K, Englbrecht M, Schett G. Interleukin-6 receptor blockade induces limited repair of bone erosions in rheumatoid arthritis: a micro CT study. *Ann Rheum Dis.* (2013) 72:396–400. doi: 10.1136/annrheumdis-2011-201075
65. Yeo L, Toellner K-M, Salmon M, Filer A, Buckley CD, Raza K, et al. Cytokine mRNA profiling identifies B cells as a major source of RANKL in rheumatoid arthritis. *Ann Rheum Dis.* (2011) 70:2022–8. doi: 10.1136/ard.2011.153312
66. Gillilan RE, Ayers SD, Noy N. Structural basis for activation of fatty acid-binding protein 4. *J Mol Biol.* (2007) 372:1246–60. doi: 10.1016/j.jmb.2007.07.040
67. Lyman M, Lieuw V, Richardson R, Timmer A, Stewart C, Granger S, et al. A bispecific antibody that targets IL-6 receptor and IL-17A for the potential therapy of patients with autoimmune and inflammatory diseases. *J Biol Chem.* (2018) 293:9326–34. doi: 10.1074/jbc.M117.818559
68. Maggio M, Guralnik JM, Longo DL, Ferrucci L. Interleukin-6 in aging and chronic disease: a magnificent pathway. *J Gerontol A Biol Sci Med Sci.* (2006) 61:575–84. doi: 10.1093/gerona/61.6.575
69. Ershler WB, Keller ET. Age-associated increased interleukin-6 gene expression, late-life diseases, and frailty. *Annu Rev Med.* (2000) 51:245–70. doi: 10.1146/annurev.med.51.1.245
70. Daynes RA, Araneo BA, Ershler WB, Maloney C, Li GZ, Ryu SY. Altered regulation of IL-6 production with normal aging. Possible linkage to the age-associated decline in dehydroepiandrosterone and its sulfated derivative. *J Immunol.* (1993) 150:5219–30.
71. Chisato M, Kenichiro K, Toshihide M, Osamu C, Yoshiko O, Maki A, et al. Endogenous bone-resorbing factors in estrogen deficiency: cooperative effects of IL-1 and IL-6. *J Bone Miner Res.* (2009) 10:1365–73. doi: 10.1002/jbmr.5650100914
72. Jilka RL, Hangoc G, Girasole G, Passeri G, Williams DC, Abrams JS, et al. Increased osteoclast development after estrogen loss: mediation by interleukin-6. *Science* (1992) 257:88–91.
73. Kramer PR, Kramer SF, Guan G. 17β-estradiol regulates cytokine release through modulation of CD16 expression in monocytes and monocyte-derived macrophages. *Arthritis Rheum.* (2004) 50:1967–75. doi: 10.1002/art.20309
74. Yasui T, Maegawa M, Tomita J, Miyatani Y, Yamada M, Uemura H, et al. Changes in serum cytokine concentrations during the menopausal transition. *Maturitas* (2007) 56:396–403. doi: 10.1016/j.maturitas.2006.11.002
75. Karin M. How NF-κB is activated: the role of the IκB kinase (IKK) complex. *Oncogene* (1999) 18:6867. doi: 10.1038/sj.onc.1203219
76. Sun WH, Keller ET, Stebler BS, Ershler WB. Estrogen inhibits phorbol ester-induced IκBα transcription and protein degradation. *Biochem Biophys Res Commun.* (1998) 244:691–5. doi: 10.1006/bbrc.1998.8324
77. Poli V, Balena R, Fattori E, Markatos A, Yamamoto M, Tanaka H, et al. Interleukin-6 deficient mice are protected from bone loss caused by estrogen depletion. *EMBO J.* (1994) 13:1189–96. doi: 10.1002/j.1460-2075.1994.tb06368.x

78. Li X, Zhou Z, Zhang Y, Yang H. IL-6 contributes to the defective osteogenesis of bone marrow stromal cells from the vertebral body of the glucocorticoid-induced osteoporotic mouse. *PLoS ONE* (2016) 11:e0154677. doi: 10.1371/journal.pone.0154677
79. Roland A, Christina B, Gerhard K, Jochen Z, Josef S, Georg S. Inhibition of interleukin-6 receptor directly blocks osteoclast formation *in vitro* and *in vivo*. *Arthritis Rheum.* (2009) 60:2747–56. doi: 10.1002/art.24781
80. Ferrari SL, Garnero P, Emond S, Montgomery H, Humphries SE, Greenspan SL. A functional polymorphic variant in the interleukin-6 gene promoter associated with low bone resorption in postmenopausal women. *Arthritis Rheum* (2001) 44:196–201. doi: 10.1002/1529-0131(200101)44:1<196::AID-ANR26>3.0.CO;2-5
81. Bromberg J, Wang TC. Inflammation and cancer: IL-6 and STAT3 complete the link. *Cancer Cell* (2009) 15:79–80. doi: 10.1016/j.ccr.2009.01.009
82. Hara M, Nagasaki T, Shiga K, Takahashi H, Takeyama H. High serum levels of interleukin-6 in patients with advanced or metastatic colorectal cancer: the effect on the outcome and the response to chemotherapy plus bevacizumab. *Surg Today* (2017) 47:483–9. doi: 10.1007/s00595-016-1404-7
83. Ma Y, Ren Y, Dai Z, Wu C, Ji Y, Xu J. IL-6, IL-8 and TNF-α levels correlate with disease stage in breast cancer patients. *Adv Clin Exp Med.* (2017) 26:421–6. doi: 10.17219/acem/62120.
84. Nakashima J, Tachibana M, Horiguchi Y, Oya M, Ohigashi T, Asakura H, et al. Serum Interleukin 6 as a prognostic factor in patients with prostate cancer. *Clin Cancer Res.* (2000) 6:2702–6.
85. Ludwig H, Nachbaur D, Fritz E, Krainer M, Huber H. Interleukin-6 is a prognostic factor in multiple myeloma. *Blood* (1991) 77:2794–5.
86. Franklin RA, Liao W, Sarkar A, Kim M V, Bivona MR, Liu K, et al. The cellular and molecular origin of tumor-associated macrophages. *Science* (2014) 344:921–5. doi: 10.1126/science.1252510
87. Van Overmeire E, Laoui D, Keirsse J, Bonelli S, Lahmar Q, Van Ginderachter JA. STAT of the union: dynamics of distinct tumor-associated macrophage subsets governed by STAT1. *Eur J Immunol.* (2014) 44:2238–42. doi: 10.1002/eji.201444870
88. Kumari N, Dwarakanath BS, Das A, Bhatt AN. Role of interleukin-6 in cancer progression and therapeutic resistance. *Tumor Biol.* (2016) 37:11553–72. doi: 10.1007/s13277-016-5098-7
89. Erreni M, Mantovani A, Allavena P. Tumor-associated Macrophages (TAM) and inflammation in colorectal cancer. *Cancer Microenviron.* (2011) 4:141–54. doi: 10.1007/s12307-010-0052-5
90. Wan S, Zhao E, Kryczek I, Vatan L, Sadovskaya A, Ludema G, et al. Tumor-associated macrophages produce interleukin 6 and signal via STAT3 to promote expansion of human hepatocellular carcinoma stem cells. *Gastroenterology* (2014) 147:1393–1404. doi: 10.1053/j.gastro.2014.08.039
91. Erez N, Truitt M, Olson P, Hanahan D. Cancer-associated fibroblasts are activated in incipient neoplasia to orchestrate tumor-promoting inflammation in an NF-κB-dependent manner. *Cancer Cell* (2010) 17:135–47. doi: 10.1016/j.ccr.2009.12.041
92. Karin M, Greten FR. NF-κB: linking inflammation and immunity to cancer development and progression. *Nat Rev Immunol.* (2005) 5:749. doi: 10.1038/nri1703
93. Zhang Y, Tang H, Cai J, Zhang T, Guo J, Feng D, et al. Ovarian cancer-associated fibroblasts contribute to epithelial ovarian carcinoma metastasis by promoting angiogenesis, lymphangiogenesis and tumor cell invasion. *Cancer Lett.* (2011) 303:47–55. doi: 10.1016/j.canlet.2011.01.011
94. Wu X, Tao P, Zhou Q, Li J, Yu Z, Wang X, et al. IL-6 secreted by cancer-associated fibroblasts promotes epithelial-mesenchymal transition and metastasis of gastric cancer via JAK2/STAT3 signaling pathway. *Oncotarget* (2017) 8:20741–50. doi: 10.18632/oncotarget.15119
95. Nagasaki T, Hara M, Nakanishi H, Takahashi H, Sato M, Takeyama H. Interleukin-6 released by colon cancer-associated fibroblasts is critical for tumour angiogenesis: anti-interleukin-6 receptor antibody suppressed angiogenesis and inhibited tumour–stroma interaction. *Br J Cancer* (2014) 110:469–78. doi: 10.1038/bjc.2013.748
96. Tang D, Gao J, Wang S, Ye N, Chong Y, Huang Y, et al. Cancer-associated fibroblasts promote angiogenesis in gastric cancer through galectin-1 expression. *Tumor Biol.* (2016) 37:1889–99. doi: 10.1007/s13277-015-3942-9
97. Silva EM, Mariano VS, Pastrez PRA, Pinto MC, Castro AG, Syrjanen KJ, et al. High systemic IL-6 is associated with worse prognosis in patients with non-small cell lung cancer. *PLoS ONE* (2017) 12:e0181125. doi: 10.1371/journal.pone.0181125
98. Chen M-F, Chen P-T, Lu MS, Lin PY, Chen W-C, Lee K-D. IL-6 expression predicts treatment response and outcome in squamous cell carcinoma of the esophagus. *Mol Cancer* (2013) 12:26. doi: 10.1186/1476-4598-12-26
99. Wu C-T, Chen M-F, Chen W-C, Hsieh C-C. The role of IL-6 in the radiation response of prostate cancer. *Radiat Oncol.* (2013) 8:159. doi: 10.1186/1748-717X-8-159
100. Heikkila K, Ebrahim S, Lawlor DA. Systematic review of the association between circulating interleukin-6 (IL-6) and cancer. *Eur J Cancer* (2008) 44:937–45. doi: 10.1016/j.ejca.2008.02.047
101. Shintani Y, Fujiwara A, Kimura T, Kawamura T, Funaki S, Minami M, et al. IL-6 secreted from cancer-associated fibroblasts mediates chemoresistance in NSCLC by increasing epithelial-mesenchymal transition signaling. *J Thorac Oncol.* (2016) 11:1482–92. doi: 10.1016/j.jtho.2016.05.025
102. Guo Y, Xu F, Lu T, Duan Z, Zhang Z. Interleukin-6 signaling pathway in targeted therapy for cancer. *Cancer Treat Rev.* (2012) 38:904–10. doi: 10.1016/j.ctrv.2012.04.007
103. Di G-H, Liu Y, Lu Y, Liu J, Wu C, Duan H-F. IL-6 secreted from senescent mesenchymal stem cells promotes proliferation and migration of breast cancer cells. *PLoS ONE* (2014) 9:e113572. doi: 10.1371/journal.pone.0113572
104. Sullivan NJ, Sasser AK, Axel AE, Vesuna F, Raman V, Ramirez N, et al. Interleukin-6 induces an epithelial–mesenchymal transition phenotype in human breast cancer cells. *Oncogene* (2009) 28:2940–7. doi: 10.1038/onc.2009.180
105. Wei L-H, Kuo M-L, Chen C-A, Chou C-H, Lai K-B, Lee C-N, et al. Interleukin-6 promotes cervical tumor growth by VEGF-dependent angiogenesis via a STAT3 pathway. *Oncogene* (2003) 22:1517. doi: 10.1038/sj.onc.1206226
106. Adachi Y, Aoki C, Yoshio-Hoshino N, Takayama K, Curiel DT, Nishimoto N.. Interleukin-6 induces both cell growth and VEGF production in malignant mesotheliomas. *Int J Cancer* (2006) 119:1303–11. doi: 10.1002/ijc.22006
107. Iliopoulos D, Hirsch HA, Struhl K. An epigenetic switch involving NF-κB, Lin28, let-7 microRNA, and IL6 links inflammation to cell transformation. *Cell* (2009) 139:693–706. doi: 10.1016/j.cell.2009.10.014
108. Iliopoulos D, Jaeger SA, Hirsch HA, Bulyk ML, Struhl K. STAT3 activation of miR-21 and miR-181b-1, via PTEN and CYLD, are part of the epigenetic switch linking inflammation to cancer. *Mol Cell* (2010) 39:493–506. doi: 10.1016/j.molcel.2010.07.023
109. Hendrayani S-F, Al-Harbi B, Al-Ansari MM, Silva G, Aboussekhra A. The inflammatory/cancer-related IL-6/STAT3/NF-κB positive feedback loop includes AUF1 and maintains the active state of breast myofibroblasts. *Oncotarget* (2016) 7:41974–85. doi: 10.18632/oncotarget.9633
110. Brach MA, Hass R, Sherman ML, Gunji H, Weichselbaum R, Kufe D. Ionizing radiation induces expression and binding activity of the nuclear factor kappa B. *J Clin Invest.* (1991) 88:691–5. doi: 10.1172/JCI115354
111. Veuger SJ, Hunter JE, Durkacz BW. Ionizing radiation-induced NF-κB activation requires PARP-1 function to confer radio-resistance. *Oncogene* (2009) 28:832–42. doi: 10.1038/onc.2008.439
112. Criswell T, Leskov K, Miyamoto S, Luo G, Boothman DA. Transcription factors activated in mammalian cells after clinically relevant doses of ionizing radiation. *Oncogene* (2003) 22:5813. doi: 10.1038/sj.onc.1206680
113. Zeligs KP, Neuman MK, Annunziata CM. Molecular pathways: the balance between cancer and the immune system challenges the therapeutic specificity of targeting nuclear factor-κB signaling for cancer treatment. *Clin Cancer Res.* (2016) 22:4302–8. doi: 10.1158/1078-0432.CCR-15-1374
114. Wu Z-H, Miyamoto S. Many faces of NF-κB signaling induced by genotoxic stress. *J Mol Med.* (2007) 85:1187–202. doi: 10.1007/s00109-007-0227-9
115. Kozakai N, Kikuchi E, Hasegawa M, Suzuki E, Ide H, Miyajima A, et al. Enhancement of radiosensitivity by a unique novel NF-κB inhibitor, DHMEQ, in prostate cancer. *Br J Cancer* (2012) 107:652–7. doi: 10.1038/bjc.2012.321
116. Selimovic D, Porzig BBOW, El-Khattouti A, Badura HE, Ahmad M, Ghanjati F, et al. Bortezomib/proteasome inhibitor triggers both apoptosis

and autophagy-dependent pathways in melanoma cells. *Cell Signal* (2013) 25:308–18. doi: 10.1016/j.cellsig.2012.10.004

117. Dou QP, Zonder JA. Overview of proteasome inhibitor-based anti-cancer therapies: perspective on bortezomib and second generation proteasome inhibitors versus future generation inhibitors of ubiquitin-proteasome system. *Curr Cancer Drug Targets* (2014) 14:517–36. doi: 10.2174/1568009614666140804154511
118. Periyasamy-Thandavan S, Jackson WH, Samaddar JS, Erickson B, Barrett JR, et al. Bortezomib blocks the catabolic process of autophagy via a cathepsin-dependent mechanism, affects endoplasmic reticulum stress, and induces caspase-dependent cell death in antiestrogen-sensitive and resistant ER+ breast cancer cells. *Autophagy* (2010) 6:19–35. doi: 10.4161/auto.6.1.10323
119. Yeong-Shiau P, Tzyh-Chyuan H, Shuang-En C, Ann-Lii C, Ming-Kuen L, Min-Liang K. Interleukin-6 is responsible for drug resistance and anti-apoptotic effects in prostatic cancer cells. *Prostate* (2004) 60:120–9. doi: 10.1002/pros.20057
120. Wei L-H, Kuo M-L, Chen C-A, Chou C-H, Cheng W-F, Chang M-C, et al. The anti-apoptotic role of interleukin-6 in human cervical cancer is mediated by up-regulation of Mcl-1 through a PI 3-K/Akt pathway. *Oncogene* (2001) 20:5799. doi: 10.1038/sj.onc.1204733
121. Farrell ML, Reagan MR. Soluble and cell–cell-mediated drivers of proteasome inhibitor resistance in multiple myeloma. *Front Endocrinol (Lausanne)* (2018) 9:218. doi: 10.3389/fendo.2018.00218
122. Gesto DS, Cerqueira NM, Fernandes PA, Ramos MJ. Gemcitabine: a critical nucleoside for cancer therapy. *Curr Med Chem.* (2012) 19:1076–87. doi: 10.2174/092986712799320682
123. Moran DM, Mattocks MA, Cahill PA, Koniaris LG, McKillop IH. Interleukin-6 (il-6) mediates g0/g1 growth arrest in hepatocellular carcinoma through a stat 3-dependent pathway. *J Surg Res.* (2008) 147:23–33. doi: 10.1016/j.jss.2007.04.022
124. Kortylewski M, Heinrich PC, Mackiewicz A, Schniertshauer U, Klingmüller U, Nakajima K, et al. Interleukin-6 and oncostatin M-induced growth inhibition of human A375 melanoma cells is STAT-dependent and involves upregulation of the cyclin-dependent kinase inhibitor p27/Kip1. *Oncogene* (1999) 18:3742.
125. Bellido T, O'Brien CA, Roberson PK, Manolagas SC. Transcriptional activation of the p21(WAF1,CIP1,SDI1) gene by interleukin-6 type cytokines. A prerequisite for their pro-differentiating and anti-apoptotic effects on human osteoblastic cells. *J Biol Chem.* (1998) 273:21137–44.
126. Chipoy C, Brounais B, Trichet V, Battaglia S, Berreur M, Oliver L, et al. Sensitization of osteosarcoma cells to apoptosis by oncostatin M depends on STAT5 and p53. *Oncogene* (2007) 26:6653. doi: 10.1038/sj.onc.1210492
127. Patel LR, Camacho DF, Shiozawa Y, Pienta KJ, Taichman RS. Mechanisms of cancer cell metastasis to the bone: a multistep process. *Future Oncol.* (2011) 7:1285–97. doi: 10.2217/fon.11.112
128. Tiedemann K, Hussein O, Sadvakassova G, Guo Y, Siegel PM, Komarova SV. Breast cancer-derived factors stimulate osteoclastogenesis through the Ca(2+)/protein kinase C and transforming growth factor-β/MAPK signaling pathways. *J Biol Chem.* (2009) 284:33662–70. doi: 10.1074/jbc.M109.010785
129. Tumber A, Hill PA. Breast cancer cells induce osteoclast formation by stimulating host IL-11 production and downregulating granulocyte/macrophage colony-stimulating factor. *Int J Cancer* (2004) 109:653–60. doi: 10.1002/ijc.20056
130. Yoshihiro M, Naoya F, Kazuo O, Takashi T. Stimulation of interleukin-11 production from osteoblast-like cells by transforming growth factor-β and tumor cell factors. *Int J Cancer* (1998) 71:422–8.
131. Goda Ta, Shimo S, Yoshihama Y, Mohammad N, Hassan M, Ibaragi S, et al. Bone destruction by invading oral squamous carcinoma cells mediated by the transforming growth factor-β signalling pathway. *Anticancer Res Int J Cancer Res Treat* (2010) 30:2615–23.
132. Sohara Y, Shimada H, DeClerck YA. Mechanisms of bone invasion and metastasis in human neuroblastoma. *Cancer Lett.* (2005) 228:203–9. doi: 10.1016/j.canlet.2005.01.059
133. Galson DL, Silbermann R, Roodman GD. Mechanisms of multiple myeloma bone disease. *Bonekey Rep.* (2012) 1:135. doi: 10.1038/bonekey.2012.135
134. Tang C-H, Chuang J-Y, Fong Y-C, Maa M-C, Way T-D, Hung C-H. Bone-derived SDF-1 stimulates IL-6 release via CXCR4, ERK and NF-κB pathways and promotes osteoclastogenesis in human oral cancer cells. *Carcinogenesis* (2008) 29:1483–92. doi: 10.1093/carcin/bgn045
135. Gazitt Y, Akay C. Mobilization of myeloma cells involves SDF-1/CXCR4 signaling and downregulation of VLA-4. *Stem Cells* (2008) 22:65–73. doi: 10.1634/stemcells.22-1-65
136. Aggarwal R, Ghobrial IM, Roodman GD. Chemokines in multiple myeloma. *Exp Hematol.* (2006) 34:1289–95. doi: 10.1016/j.exphem.2006.06.017
137. Aiuti A, Webb IJ, Bleul C, Springer T, Gutierrez-Ramos JC. The chemokine SDF-1 is a chemoattractant for human CD34(+) hematopoietic progenitor cells and provides a new mechanism to explain the mobilization of CD34(+) progenitors to peripheral blood. *J Exp Med.* (1997) 185:111–20. doi: 10.1084/jem.185.1.111
138. Nie Y, Waite J, Brewer F, Sunshine M-J, Littman DR, Zou Y-R. The role of CXCR4 in maintaining peripheral B cell compartments and humoral immunity. *J Exp Med.* (2004) 200:1145–56. doi: 10.1084/jem.20041185
139. Dürig J, Schmücker U, Dührsen U. Differential expression of chemokine receptors in B cell malignancies. *Leukemia* (2001) 15:752–6. doi: 10.1038/sj.leu.2402107
140. Moharita AL, Taborga M, Corcoran KE, Bryan M, Patel PS, Rameshwar P. SDF-1a regulation in breast cancer cells contacting bone marrow stroma is critical for normal hematopoiesis. *Blood* (2006) 108:3245–52. doi: 10.1182/blood-2006-01-017459
141. Bi J, Li P, Li C, He J, Wang Y, Zhang H, et al. The SDF-1/CXCR4 chemokine axis in uveal melanoma cell proliferation and migration. *Tumor Biol.* (2016) 37:4175–82. doi: 10.1007/s13277-015-4259-4
142. Sanz-Rodriguez F, Hidalgo A, Teixidó J. Chemokine stromal cell-derived factor-1α modulates VLA-4 integrin-mediated multiple myeloma cell adhesion to CS-1/fibronectin and VCAM-1. *Blood* (2001) 97:346–51. doi: 10.1182/blood.V97.2.346
143. Peled A, Kollet O, Ponomaryov T, Petit I, Franitza S, Grabovsky V, et al. The chemokine SDF-1 activates the integrins LFA-1, VLA-4, and VLA-5 on immature human CD34(+) cells: role in transendothelial/stromal migration and engraftment of NOD/SCID mice. *Blood* (2000) 95:3289–96.
144. Wright N, de Lera TL, García-Moruja C, Lillo R, García-Sánchez F, Caruz A, et al. Transforming growth factor-β1 down-regulates expression of chemokine stromal cell–derived factor-1: functional consequences in cell migration and adhesion. *Blood* (2003) 102:1978–84. doi: 10.1182/blood-2002-10-3190
145. Azab AK, Runnels JM, Pitsillides C, Moreau A-S, Azab F, Leleu X, et al. CXCR4 inhibitor AMD3100 disrupts the interaction of multiple myeloma cells with the bone marrow microenvironment and enhances their sensitivity to therapy. *Blood* (2009) 113:4341–51. doi: 10.1182/blood-2008-10-186668
146. Van de Broek I, Leleu X, Schots R, Facon T, Vanderkerken K, Van Camp B, et al. Clinical significance of chemokine receptor (CCR1, CCR2 and CXCR4) expression in human myeloma cells: the association with disease activity and survival. *Haematologica* (2006) 91:200–6.
147. Möller C, Strömberg T, Juremalm M, Nilsson K, Nilsson G. Expression and function of chemokine receptors in human multiple myeloma. *Leukemia* (2003) 17:203–10. doi: 10.1038/sj.leu.2402717
148. Broek I Vande, Asosingh K, Vanderkerken K, Straetmans N, Van Camp B, Van Riet I. Chemokine receptor CCR2 is expressed by human multiple myeloma cells and mediates migration to bone marrow stromal cell-produced monocyte chemotactic proteins MCP-1,-2 and-3. *Br J Cancer* (2003) 88:855–62. doi: 10.1038/sj.bjc.6600833
149. Nakayama T, Hieshima K, Izawa D, Tatsumi Y, Kanamaru A, Yoshie O. Cutting edge: profile of chemokine receptor expression on human plasma cells accounts for their efficient recruitment to target tissues. *J Immunol.* (2003) 170:1136–40. doi: 10.4049/jimmunol.170.3.1136
150. Ohshima S, Saeki Y, Mima T, Sasai M, Nishioka K, Nomura S, et al. Interleukin 6 plays a key role in the development of antigen-induced arthritis. *Proc Natl Acad Sci USA.* (1998) 95:8222–6. doi: 10.1073/pnas.95.14.8222
151. Loetscher P, Seitz M, Baggiolini M, Moser B. Interleukin-2 regulates CC chemokine receptor expression and chemotactic responsiveness in T lymphocytes. *J Exp Med.* (1996) 184:569–77. doi: 10.1084/jem.184.2.569
152. Terpos E, Christoulas D, Katodritou E, Bratengeier C, Gkotzamanidou M, Michalis E, et al. Elevated circulating sclerostin correlates with advanced

disease features and abnormal bone remodeling in symptomatic myeloma: reduction post-bortezomib monotherapy. *Int J cancer* (2012) 131:1466–71. doi: 10.1002/ijc.27342
153. McDonald MM, Reagan MR, Youlten SE, Mohanty ST, Seckinger A, Terry RL, et al. Inhibiting the osteocyte-specific protein sclerostin increases bone mass and fracture resistance in multiple myeloma. *Blood* (2017) 129:3452–64. doi: 10.1182/blood-2017-03-773341
154. Eda H, Santo L, Wein MN, Hu DZ, Cirstea DD, Nemani N, et al. Regulation of sclerostin expression in multiple myeloma by Dkk-1; a potential therapeutic strategy for myeloma bone disease. *J Bone Miner Res.* (2016) 31:1225–34. doi: 10.1002/jbmr.2789
155. Falank C, Fairfield H, Reagan MR. Reflections on cancer in the bone marrow: adverse roles of adipocytes. *Curr Mol Biol Rep.* (2017) 3:254–62. doi: 10.1007/s40610-017-0074-6
156. Fairfield H, Falank C, Harris E, Demambro V, McDonald M, Pettitt JAJ, et al. The skeletal cell-derived molecule sclerostin drives bone marrow adipogenesis. *J Cell Physiol.* (2017) 233:1156–67. doi: 10.1002/jcp.25976
157. Gavriatopoulou M, Dimopoulos M-A, Christoulas D, Migkou M, Iakovaki M, Gkotzamanidou M, et al. Dickkopf-1: a suitable target for the management of myeloma bone disease. *Expert Opin Ther Targets* (2009) 13:839–48. doi: 10.1517/14728220903025770
158. Tian E, Zhan F, Walker R, Rasmussen E, Ma Y, Barlogie B, et al. The role of the Wnt-signaling antagonist DKK1 in the development of osteolytic lesions in multiple myeloma. *N Engl J Med.* (2003) 349:2483–94. doi: 10.1056/NEJMoa030847
159. Florio M, Gunasekaran K, Stolina M, Li X, Liu L, Tipton B, et al. A bispecific antibody targeting sclerostin and DKK-1 promotes bone mass accrual and fracture repair. *Nat Commun.* (2016) 7:11505. doi: 10.1038/ncomms11505
160. Gunn WG, Conley A, Deininger L, Olson SD, Prockop DJ, Gregory CA. A crosstalk between myeloma cells and marrow stromal cells stimulates production of DKK1 and interleukin-6: a potential role in the development of lytic bone disease and tumor progression in multiple myeloma. *Stem Cells* (2006) 24:986–91. doi: 10.1634/stemcells.2005-0220
161. Yeremenko N, Zwerina K, Rigter G, Pots D, Fonseca JE, Zwerina J, et al. Brief report: tumor necrosis factor and interleukin-6 differentially regulate Dkk-1 in the inflamed arthritic joint. *Arthritis Rheumatol.* (2015) 67:2071–5. doi: 10.1002/art.39183
162. Wu Q, Zhou X, Huang D, JI Y, Kang F. IL-6 enhances osteocyte-mediated osteoclastogenesis by promoting JAK2 and RANKL activity *in vitro*. *Cell Physiol Biochem.* (2017) 41:1360–9. doi: 10.1159/000465455
163. Menaa C, Reddy SV, Kurihara N, Maeda H, Anderson D, Cundy T, et al. Enhanced RANK ligand expression and responsivity of bone marrow cells in Paget's disease of bone. *J Clin Invest.* (2000) 105:1833–8. doi: 10.1172/JCI9133
164. Rozen N, Ish-Shalom S, Rachmiel A, Stein H, Lewinson D. Interleukin-6 modulates trabecular and endochondral bone turnover in the nude mouse by stimulating osteoclast differentiation. *Bone* (2000) 26:469–74. doi: 10.1016/S8756-3282(00)00263-5
165. Dankbar B, Padró T, Leo R, Feldmann B, Kropff M, Mesters RM, et al. Vascular endothelial growth factor and interleukin-6 in paracrine tumor-stromal cell interactions in multiple myeloma. *Blood* (2000) 95:2630–6.
166. Tanaka Y, Abe M, Hiasa M, Oda A, Amou H, Nakano A, et al. Myeloma Cell-osteoclast interaction enhances angiogenesis together with bone resorption: a role for vascular endothelial cell growth factor and osteopontin. *Clin Cancer Res.* (2007) 13:816–23. doi: 10.1158/1078-0432.CCR-06-2258
167. Podar K, Anderson KC. The pathophysiologic role of VEGF in hematologic malignancies: therapeutic implications. *Blood* (2005) 105:1383–95. doi: 10.1182/blood-2004-07-2909
168. Candé C, Cohen I, Daugas E, Ravagnan L, Larochette N, Zamzami N, et al. Apoptosis-inducing factor (AIF): a novel caspase-independent death effector released from mitochondria. *Biochimie* (2002) 84:215–22. doi: 10.1016/S0300-9084(02)01374-3
169. Lu Z, Xu S. ERK1/2 MAP kinases in cell survival and apoptosis. *IUBMB Life* (2006) 58:621–31. doi: 10.1080/15216540600957438
170. Tu Y, Renner S, Xu F, Fleishman A, Taylor J, Weisz J, et al. BCL-X expression in multiple myeloma: possible indicator of chemoresistance. *Cancer Res.* (1998) 58:256–62.
171. Zhang B, Gojo I, Fenton RG. Myeloid cell factor−1 is a critical survival factor for multiple myeloma. *Blood* (2002) 99:1885–93. doi: 10.1182/blood.V99.6.1885
172. Voorhees PM, Manges RF, Sonneveld P, Jagannath S, Somlo G, Krishnan A, et al. A phase 2 multicentre study of siltuximab, an anti-interleukin-6 monoclonal antibody, in patients with relapsed or refractory multiple myeloma. *Br J Haematol.* (2013) 161:357–66. doi: 10.1111/bjh.12266
173. Orlowski RZ, Gercheva L, Williams C, Sutherland H, Robak T, Masszi T, et al. A phase ii, randomized, double-blind, placebo-controlled study of siltuximab (Anti-IL-6 mAb) and bortezomib versus bortezomib alone in patients with relapsed or refractory multiple myeloma. *Am J Hematol.* (2015) 90:42–9. doi: 10.1002/ajh.23868
174. Derenne S, Monia B, Dean NM, Taylor JK, Rapp M-J, Harousseau J-L, et al. Antisense strategy shows that Mcl-1 rather than Bcl-2 or Bcl-x(L) is an essential survival protein of human myeloma cells. *Blood* (2002) 100:194–9. doi: 10.1182/blood.V100.1.194
175. Chauhan D, Li G, Hideshima T, Podar K, Shringarpure R, Mitsiades C, et al. Blockade of ubiquitin-conjugating enzyme CDC34 enhances anti-myeloma activity of Bortezomib/Proteasome inhibitor PS-341. *Oncogene* (2004) 23:3597. doi: 10.1038/sj.onc.1207458
176. Xiang R-F, Wang Y, Zhang N, Xu W-B, Cao Y, Tong J, et al. MK2206 enhances the cytocidal effects of bufalin in multiple myeloma by inhibiting the AKT/mTOR pathway. *Cell Death Dis.* (2017) 8:e2776. doi: 10.1038/cddis.2017.188
177. Hodge DR, Peng B, Cherry JC, Hurt EM, Fox SD, Kelley JA, et al. Interleukin 6 supports the maintenance of p53 tumor suppressor gene promoter methylation. *Cancer Res.* (2005) 65:4673–82. doi: 10.1158/0008-5472.CAN-04-3589
178. Harada T, Hideshima T, Anderson KC. Histone deacetylase inhibitors in multiple myeloma: from bench to bedside. *Int J Hematol.* (2016) 104:300–9. doi: 10.1007/s12185-016-2008-0
179. He J, Chen Q, Yang Y, Li Y, Yang L, Huang H, et al. The novel subtype-selective histone deacetylase (HDAC) inhibitor, chidamide, exerts dual anti-myeloma and bone protective effect *in vitro* and *in vivo*. *Blood* (2017) 130:5392.
180. Okwan-Duodu D, Umpierrez GE, Brawley OW, Diaz R. Obesity-driven inflammation and cancer risk: role of myeloid derived suppressor cells and alternately activated macrophages. *Am J Cancer Res.* (2013) 3:21–33.
181. Ellulu MS, Patimah I, Khaza'ai H, Rahmat A, Abed Y. Obesity and inflammation: the linking mechanism and the complications. *Arch Med Sci.* (2017) 13:851–63. doi: 10.5114/aoms.2016.58928
182. Doucette CR, Horowitz MC, Berry R, MacDougald OA, Anunciado-Koza R, Koza RA, et al. A high fat diet increases bone Marrow Adipose Tissue (MAT) but does not alter trabecular or cortical bone mass in C57BL/6J mice. *J Cell Physiol.* (2015) 230:2032–7. doi: 10.1002/jcp.24954
183. Falank C, Fairfield H, Farrell M, Reagan MR. New bone cell type identified as driver of drug resistance in multiple myeloma: the bone marrow adipocyte. *Blood* (2017) 130 (Suppl. 1):122.
184. Fairfield H, Falank C, Avery L, Reagan MR. Multiple myeloma in the marrow: pathogenesis and treatments. *Ann N Y Acad Sci.* (2016) 1364:32–51. doi: 10.1111/nyas.13038
185. Friedman G, LJ H. Obesity and multiple myeloma. *Cancer Causes Control* (1994) 5: :479–83.
186. Liu Z, Xu J, He J, Liu H, Lin P, Wan X, et al. Mature adipocytes in bone marrow protect myeloma cells against chemotherapy through autophagy activation. *Oncotarget* (2015) 6:34329–41. doi: 10.18632/oncotarget.6020
187. Cao D, Zhou H, Zhao J, Jin L, Yu W, Yan H, et al. PGC-1α integrates glucose metabolism and angiogenesis in multiple myeloma cells by regulating VEGF and GLUT-4. *Oncol Rep.* (2014) 31:1205–10. doi: 10.3892/or.2014.2974

188. Brighton T, Harrison SJ, Ghez D, Weiss BM, Kirsch A, Magen H, et al. A phase 2, randomized, double-blind, placebo-controlled, multicenter study of siltuximab (Anti IL-6 monoclonal antibody) in patients with high-risk smoldering multiple myeloma. *Blood* (2017) 130:3155.
189. Shah JJ, Feng L, Thomas SK, Berkova Z, Weber DM, Wang M, et al. Siltuximab (CNTO 328) with lenalidomide, bortezomib and dexamethasone in newly-diagnosed, previously untreated multiple myeloma: an open-label phase I trial. *Blood Cancer J.* (2016) 6:e396. doi: 10.1038/bcj.2016.4
190. Rossi J-F, Négrier S, James ND, Kocak I, Hawkins R, Davis H, et al. A phase I/II study of siltuximab (CNTO 328), an anti-interleukin-6 monoclonal antibody, in metastatic renal cell cancer. *Br J Cancer* (2010) 103:1154–62. doi: 10.1038/sj.bjc.6605872
191. Chapurlat R. Fibrous dysplasia in the adult. *Bone Abstr.* (2016) 5:e396. doi: 10.1530/boneabs.5.CU2.2
192. Rossi J-F, Lu Z-Y, Jourdan M, Klein B. Interleukin-6 as a therapeutic target. *Clin Cancer Res.* (2015) 21:1248–57. doi: 10.1158/1078-0432.CCR-14-2291

6

Extracellular Matrices to Modulate the Innate Immune Response and Enhance Bone Healing

Andrés García-García and Ivan Martin**

Tissue Engineering, Department of Biomedicine, University Hospital Basel, University of Basel, Basel, Switzerland

***Correspondence:**
Andrés García-García
andres.garciagarcia@usb.ch
Ivan Martin
ivan.martin@usb.ch

Extracellular matrices (ECMs) have emerged as promising off-the-shelf products to induce bone regeneration, with the capacity not only to activate osteoprogenitors, but also to influence the immune response. ECMs generated starting from living cells such as mesenchymal stromal cells (MSCs) have the potential to combine advantages of native tissue-derived ECMs (e.g., physiological presentation of multiple regulatory factors) with those of synthetic ECMs (e.g., customization and reproducibility of composition). MSC-derived ECMs could be tailored by enrichment not only in osteogenic cytokines, but also in immunomodulatory factors, to skew the innate immune response toward regenerative processes. After reviewing the different immunoregulatory properties of ECM components, here we propose different approaches to engineer ECMs enriched in factors capable to regulate macrophage polarization, recruit host immune and mesenchymal cells, and stimulate the synthesis of other immunoinstructive cytokines. Finally, we offer a perspective on the possible evolution of the paradigm based on biological and chemico-physical design considerations, and the use of gene editing approaches.

Keywords: tissue engineering, extracelullar matrix, immunomodulation, bone repair, innate immune system, mesenchymal stromal cell, regenerative medicine

INTRODUCTION

Bone disorders have a worldwide prevalence since they can be derived from multiple causes, including orthopedic trauma, cancer or congenital diseases. Since it emerged in the early 90s, bone tissue engineering has aimed to develop innovative biological materials to improve bone repair and regeneration (1, 2). Among different biomaterials, extracellular matrices (ECMs) have been proposed as one of the best candidates to fabricate grafts for bone regeneration (3). Native tissue-derived ECMs represent a physiological solution providing not only structural support, but also multiple biomolecules capable to modulate the behavior of both resident and recruited cells in the context of bone healing (4–6). However, they exhibit limited reproducibility in their composition, can lead to pathogen transmission and lack the possibility of customization. Furthermore, native ECMs are rich in immunogenic molecules that can trigger an uncontrolled response and affect graft integration (7). Synthetic ECMs, typically in the form of hydrogels, have been developed as tunable alternatives, with promising results also in the context of bone repair (8). However, they still rely on the presentation of a limited set of signals, in ways which do not entirely recapitulate physiological processes. ECMs could be also generated from living cells, e.g., mesenchymal stromal cells (MSCs), using typical tissue engineering paradigms, and afterwards decellularized (9, 10). The resulting ECMs would in principle combine the advantages of a physiological system with the possibility of standardization (e.g., through the use of immortalized cell lines) and tunability (e.g., by genetic modification of the cells used) (11). Decellularization of the MSC-generated ECMs can also be designed to improve the immunogenic properties of the resulting material (12, 13).

Despite many advances, the need for quality improvement of engineered ECM (either synthetic or MSC-generated) for bone healing is still quite large (3). Along this line, ECMs might be enriched in morphogens or angiogenic factors to enhance bone regeneration. Importantly, multiple evidences have revealed that a proportionated and coordinated immune system response is essential to critically promote bone healing. Indeed, many studies in the past years have revealed a broad crosstalk between the skeletal and immune systems through many shared cytokines, molecular pathways and transcription factors. All these findings have contributed to define the so-called osteoimmunology field, in which engineering ECMs to modulate immune signals has become one of the spearhead (14). In this context, current strategies do not aim to suppress the immune response, but rather engineer ECM-derived materials to present osteoimmunomodulatory factors and instruct the inescapable immune response in favor of bone regeneration (15).

In this review, we describe firstly key aspects of the interplay between innate immunity and bone healing. Then, we highlight how some ECM components are able to modulate the innate immune response. Finally, we summarize different strategies proposed for ECMs enriched with innate immunoinstructive factors to improve bone regeneration.

INNATE IMMUNE SYSTEM IN BONE REPAIR

All bone substitute materials, as any other foreign structure, trigger a host immune reaction after implantation, which recapitulates the first steps of the classical immune response after bone injury (16, 17). In addition, implantation surgery is not more than a controlled injury. Therefore, understanding the immune cascade following bone injury is key to generate immunoinstructive scaffolds capable to enhance bone regeneration.

Immediately after any bone injury, vascular disruption generates a hematoma and triggers a quick and potent inflammatory reaction. Multiple blood and interstitial fluid proteins [e.g., Factor XII and tissue factor (TF)] adsorb the injury site and activate the blood coagulation cascade as well as the complement system (18). In this context, activated platelets play a critical role producing prothrombinases, which activate thrombin serin protease and allow the amplification of the coagulation process (19). All these proteins lead to a transient fibrin clot formation that constitutes the matrix for the recruitment of the first immune cells. In contrast with later stages, the onset of the acute inflammatory response is mostly governed by the innate immune system, whose main players are polymorphonuclear leukocytes (PMNs, neutrophils), monocytes and tissue-resident macrophages (20).

Circulating PMNs are quickly recruited by this chemoattractant protein matrix to the injury site. While they might contribute to fibrin clot formation (21), their main roles involve the release of proteolytic enzymes to promote tissue remodeling, and inflammatory cytokines (such as IL1β, TNFα, IL8, MCP1, or MIP1β) to recruit other myeloid cells and MSCs (15). Recruited monocytes release more cytokines and differentiate into macrophages. Both monocytes derived- and tissue resident macrophages have been revealed essential for successful bone formation (22). The relevance of this cell type resides in its capacity to exhibit different functional phenotypes in response to environmental cues (23). Initially, the inflammatory storm upon bone injury polarizes macrophages toward an activated M1 phenotype. M1 macrophages release more inflammatory cytokines to contribute to cell recruitment and dead cell clearing. At later stages, macrophages are alternatively polarized toward an anti-inflammatory M2 phenotype. These cells secrete tissue repair factors (IL10, IL1ra, TGFβ1, or VEGFα) to resolve the inflammation, recruit MSCs, promote angiogenesis and induce endochondral bone formation (24). Recruited MSCs undergo chondrogenic differentiation adjacent to the fracture site to form bone by endochondral ossification, while direct intramembranous ossification takes place under the periosteum (25). Interestingly, they also play a crucial paracrine role releasing immunosuppressive cytokines to resolve site inflammation. Human MSCs suppress innate immune cells migration, proliferation and differentiation through multiple pathways including Notch and PGE-2 signaling (26). Therefore, the coordinated crosstalk between MSCs/osteoprogenitor cells and macrophages is critically required for successful bone healing.

Following these principles, several studies have attempted to improve bone regeneration modulating either macrophage number or their polarization toward M1 or M2 phenotypes (27). On the one hand, it has been reported that the expression of some pro-inflammatory signals right after injury significantly improves bone healing. As examples, TNFα promotes postnatal intramembranous bone repair through the induction of osteoprogenitor cell recruitment or osteogenic cell activation (28), while IL1β administration could favor endochondral bone formation after injury (29, 30). Similarly, IL-6 family signaling was shown to stimulate bone formation during the inflammatory process (31). On the other hand, different studies have proposed that an anti-inflammatory M2 environment is more suitable for human MSC activity (32) and delivers osteoinductive signals (33). In this regard, IL4 administration could decrease bone degradation after joint replacement (34).

Accumulating evidences suggest that an appropriate transition from the inflammatory M1 to the anti-inflammatory M2 phenotype favors bone regeneration by endochondral ossification (24, 35). However, macrophage activation and polarization are very complex *in vivo*, since the exposition to multiple signaling leads to activation of macrophages with mixed functions. This is especially prominent in pathological conditions, where abnormal signaling might prime macrophages toward a profibrotic phenotype (36). Indeed, macrophage activation nomenclature has been recently revised to unify criteria for the diverse experimental scenarios (37).

In the context of ECM engineering, some researchers have used myeloid cells to improve ECM-derived grafts integration after implantation and/or promote bone healing after trauma or bone degeneration. Although the supplementation of ECM-derived grafts with peripheral blood monocytes did not seem to increase bone regeneration by itself (38), peripheral blood-derived macrophages were reported to be essential in the degradation and remodeling of ECM-based materials (39). Other studies have developed strategies to generate immunoinstructive ECMs by modulating macrophage polarization during bone healing and promote bone formation (40). However, the success of these approaches is often subjected to several variables like patient health, trauma size or ECM composition.

ECM COMPOSITION AND INNATE IMMUNITY

Many endogenous ECM components exhibit important immunomodulatory features that can decisively influence the innate immune response *in vivo* (41, 42). For example, the collagenous network is, together with the proteoglycans, the main component of bone tissue ECM that defines its mechano-physical features. However, collagen fibers exhibit motifs that can interact with some immune cell receptors. In particular, macrophages can specifically adhere to denatured forms of collagen type I fibers through their scavenger receptors (43). Furthermore, collagen fibers have been reported to affect metalloproteinase 9 (MMP9) secretion on the macrophage-like U937 cell line (44).

Hyaluronic acid is one of the most important glycosaminoglycan of native ECMs and it has been proposed to play a dual immunomodulatory role based on its molecular weight. Whereas, intact high molecular weight hyaluronic acid has a prominent anti-inflammatory effect inducing IL10 production by macrophages, damaged low molecular weight hyaluronic acid promotes a pro-inflammatory phenotype stimulating TNFα expression (45). Interestingly, this immune cells-hyaluronic acid crosstalk seems to be bidirectional, since monocyte activation can modulate its binding to hyaluronic acid too. More specifically, TNFα promotes monocytes-hyaluronic acid interactions through CD44 receptor, while IL4 administration is sufficient to abrogate this effect (46). Heparan sulfate, another important glycosaminoglycan that binds to ECM proteins to form proteoglycans, can also interact with the immune system to regulate cell adhesion, the availability of immune cytokines and leukocyte migration (47).

Importantly, not only components of native ECM have been reported to modulate the innate immunity. Fibrin is a molecule often used to build synthetic ECMs, which has been also shown to modulate macrophages behavior. This protein derives from fibrinogen after thrombin proteolytic activity and it is involved in the hemostatic clot formation after injury (48). Several studies have reported that fibrin could facilitate or block macrophages migration depending on its abundance in the matrix (49), and inhibit their pro-inflammatory properties (50). In contrast, fibrin degradation products induce leukocyte recruitment (51) and promote pro-inflammatory (IL1β, IL6) cytokines secretion by monocytes *in vitro* (52).

ECMs can also contain cryptic domains very similar to immune cytokines that are only exposed after proteolytic activity by metalloproteinases. In non-physiological conditions, the aberrant expression of these domains by exacerbated tissue remodeling can influence immune cell activation and survival (53, 54). Moreover, the decellularization step followed to generate non-immunogenic off-the-shelf grafts could also condition the immunomodulatory properties of ECM components. Pioneering work from Badylak using the bladder system showed that decellularized grafts preferentially induce an anti-inflammatory macrophage polarization, while cellular components trigger a pro-inflammatory polarization (55, 56).

Furthermore, different types of ECMs seem to induce a different innate immune response *in vivo*. For example, decellularized bone-derived ECM has a higher capacity to induce monocytes recruitment than cardiac ECMs, which might reflect the differential molecular composition of these matrices (57).

In summary, ECMs exhibit intrinsic immunomodulatory features which are mostly determined by their molecular composition. Therefore, a precise knowledge of the components of ECMs is essential to further develop their immunomodulatory properties with extrinsic factors.

EXOGENOUS DELIVERY OF SPECIFIC IMMUNOREGULATORS IN ENGINEERED ECMs TO MODULATE THE INNATE IMMUNE RESPONSE

In order to modulate the innate immune response upon implantation, pro-inflammatory or anti-inflammatory cytokines can be directly delivered into the grafts. To antagonize the pro-inflammatory effect of IL1β, inhibitors of IL1R1/MyD88 signaling were covalently cross-linked into fibrin matrix to improve MSC-based bone regeneration in mice (58).

Immune cytokines could be also delivered sequentially in order to facilitate the transition between the inflammatory and anti-inflammatory phases during bone healing. For instance, Spiller et al. physically adsorbed IFNγ onto the scaffolds and attached IL4 using biotin-streptavidin binding to drive the sequential polarization of macrophages from M1 to M2 phenotype. These scaffolds also exhibited increased vascularization upon *in vivo* implantation, which proved their functionality (59). Along the same line, another study confirmed that IL4 released from a nanometer-thickness coating is critical promoting the M1-to-M2 transition during bone tissue repair and improving implant integration (60). Recently, Schlundt et al. further demonstrated the importance of M2 macrophages to induce endochondral ossification in the context of bone healing. Indeed, they added IL4 and IL13 to the collagen scaffolds prior to insertion in an osteotomy model. In this way, they stimulated M2 macrophage polarization and improved bone regeneration (24).

In addition to interleukins, synthetic peptides represent an alternative way to modulate the immunomodulatory features of ECMs. The peptide Arg-Gly-Asp (RGD), contained in basement membranes components such as entactin or presented in photopolymerizable poly(ethylene glycol) (PEG)- based hydrogels, has been shown to enhance myeloid cells adhesion to the ECM (61, 62), while it induces macrophage polarization toward an anti-inflammatory profile via integrins interactions (63). As another example, a synthetic peptide binding to LAIR1, a receptor expressed in multiple immune cells, has been reported to reduce pro-inflammatory cytokines release by BM-derived macrophages. Interestingly, this effect was only observed when the peptide was linked to the scaffold surface (64). On the other side, TP508, a synthetic 23-aminoacid peptide representing a receptor-binding domain of human thrombin, promotes bone healing in a rat femoral fracture model by inducing inflammatory mediators release and angiogenesis (65). Adsorbed fibrinogen or scaffolds made of this material could also elicit a favorable immune response and improve the osteogenic capacity in a critical size bone defect in rats (66, 67). Among lipid compounds, specific prostaglandin agonists administration could enhance bone formation after injury avoiding systemic inflammation induction (68, 69). For example, prostaglandin E EP4 receptor agonist was shown to synergize with BMP2 and activate osteoprogenitor cells when delivered in a biodegradable copolymer composed by poly-D,L-lactic acid with random insertion of p-dioxanone and polyethylene glycol (70).

The anti-inflammatory properties of glucocorticoids are well-known. In particular, dexamethasone delivery in polydimethylsiloxane-based 3D scaffolds has been used to promote macrophage polarization toward an anti-inflammatory (M2) phenotype and suppress inflammatory pathways during the first week post-implantation (71). Dexamethasone delivery using poly (lactic-co-glycolic acid) microsphere/polyvinyl alcohol hydrogel composites has been shown to elicit an anti-angiogenic effect which could be overcame by co-administering VEGF (72).

Different approaches have been here discussed to deliver immunoregulatory factors into ECM in order to instruct the innate immune response *in vivo*. Nevertheless, the delivery of exogenous factors is subjected to several drawbacks including poor matrix penetration, diffusion, enzymatic degradation and thus uncontrolled doses. In addition, the delivery of few specific agents has been revealed inefficient in triggering a complete immune response *in vivo*. For this reason, different strategies have been developed to control the spatial and temporal delivery (73–75). Among them, 3D multilayer systems and intelligent hydrogels have been tested for the sequential release of several factors to ECM-based scaffolds (76, 77). Biomimetic biomaterials, like hydrogels, have been developed to achieve a molecular-level modulation. This includes strategies to immobilize incorporated factors by cross-linking and approaches based on protease-dependent degradation to release them (78). Other options to engineer immunoinstructive ECMs directly target MSCs or immune cells to modulate the natural production and release of immune factors by these cells.

ECM-DRIVEN ENDOGENOUS SYNTHESIS OF IMMUNOREGULATORS BY HOST CELLS TO MODULATE THE INNATE IMMUNE RESPONSE

Aiming to generate ECM grafts instructed to trigger a more physiological immune response, many researchers have tried to use several biological agents to stimulate host MSCs and/or immune cells to deliver key immune cytokines and enhance bone formation. Macrophage recruitment is critical for dead tissue clearance and modulate the inflammatory cascade in bone healing. Kim et al. used a sphingosine-1 phosphate agonist in combination with platelet-rich plasma to sequentially induce pro-inflammatory (TNFα) and anti-inflammatory (OPG, IL10, and TGFβ1) signals in order to promote macrophages recruitment and enhance bone healing (79). In contrast, adding high sulfated hyaluronan to collagen I-enriched ECMs impairs the secretion of IL1β, IL8, IL12, and TNFα, while it enhances the production of IL10 and CD163 expression in macrophages (80).

Interestingly, inorganic compounds like magnesium-doped calcium phosphate cement are also able to elicit a favorable innate immune reaction modulating macrophage activity to improve osteogenesis and angiogenesis. This compound represses TNFα and IL6 expression while it upregulates TGFβ1 in macrophages (81). Beyond macrophage activation, immunoregulators have been also used to modulate MSC behavior. For example, the combination of RGD peptide and 3D hyaluronic acid hydrogels can influence MSC integrin expression (82).

To sum up, these studies attempt to improve bone regeneration by targeting endogenous MSC/immune cells to produce themselves the cues critical for an orchestrated repair upon bone injury (83).

CONCLUSIONS AND PERSPECTIVES

In this work, we have reviewed some relevant aspects of the interplay between the innate immune system and osteogenesis in the context of bone healing. Then we have focused on the interactions between ECM components and innate immune cells to finally discuss some strategies followed to immune-instruct ECMs. However, many other critical aspects have not been discussed here.

As previously mentioned, the innate immunity plays an essential role during the initial phases after bone injury, promoting cell immunorecruitment and modulating the inflammatory environment (M1-to-M2 paradigm). Importantly, the adaptive immune response takes slowly part in this regulation to instruct the bone formation phase. Multiples studies have attempted to engineer ECM-based materials to modulate the adaptive immune response, specially targeting T cells (84). Indeed, many efforts are currently conducted to better coordinate the activity of both branches of the immune response after engineered graft implantation.

We have discussed how different ECM components, even in the absence of immunomodulatory factors, could modulate the innate immune response. The works studying these interactions reveal that ECM composition is an important factor to consider prior to any further immunoregulatory engineering. However, beyond its chemical properties, ECM physical features can also decisively modulate the immune response *in vivo* (85). Therefore, strategies to enrich ECMs in immunoinstructive factors should be coupled with the engineering of endogenous physical and chemical properties of the ECM used (86).

Different approaches have been proposed to improve the spatiotemporal delivery of growth factors to engineer "smart" ECMs. However, in most cases they only focus on osteogenic and angiogenic factors. Immunomodulatory ECM-like microspheres have been recently used to improve IL4 delivery and accelerate bone regeneration modulating macrophage polarization (87). Future studies should aim to a coordinated delivery of osteogenic, angiogenic and immune factors according to the natural stages of bone healing.

Genetic manipulation of MSCs has also emerged as an alternative to better control the dose and temporal delivery of osteogenic and angiogenic factors into engineered ECMs to improve bone regeneration process (88). Genetically modified MSCs could contribute directly to bone formation promoting osteoprogenitor cells differentiation, but also indirectly enhancing host cells recruitment. The most followed approaches involve the expression of the osteoinductive bone morphogenetic protein (BMP) family factors to stimulate bone repair. In particular, BMP2-overexpressing cells have been successfully used to speed up the repair of critical-size bone defects in rodent models (89, 90). Other overexpressed factors like Osterix aimed to induce osteogenic differentiation (91, 92). As a master regulator of angiogenesis, VEGF has been overexpressed in different cell types to favor tissue vascularization (93). A VEGF-overexpressing MSC line gives rise to ECMs with high VEGF content and superior vasculature in an ectopic implantation model (11). In addition to its angiogenic properties, VEGF could also modulate the immune response (94). Similarly, sphingosine 1-phosphate has been reported to enhance vascularization and bone formation (95), but at the same time it also plays multiple roles in the innate immunity (96). These works represent examples of how MSC can be genetically engineered to generate ECMs enhancing osteogenesis and vasculogenesis. An analogous approach could be pursued to overexpress specific osteoimmunomodulatory factors and thus generate immunoinstructive ECMs (**Figure 1**). In this context, MSCs overexpressing IL4 and IL10 have been proposed as promising tools to mitigate chronic inflammation diseases (such as arthritis) and promote tissue regeneration (97, 98). However, their capacity to generate immunoinstructive ECMs have not been yet explored. Moreover, the development of inducible cell lines might represent an interesting refinement to control the temporal expression of these key genes (98). Delivering candidate genes efficiently into the cells without viral vectors (which may carry safety concerns) remains an open challenge (99).

In summary, important advances have been achieved in the last years to improve the quality of immunoinstructive ECM-derived grafts and their immunogenicity after implantation.

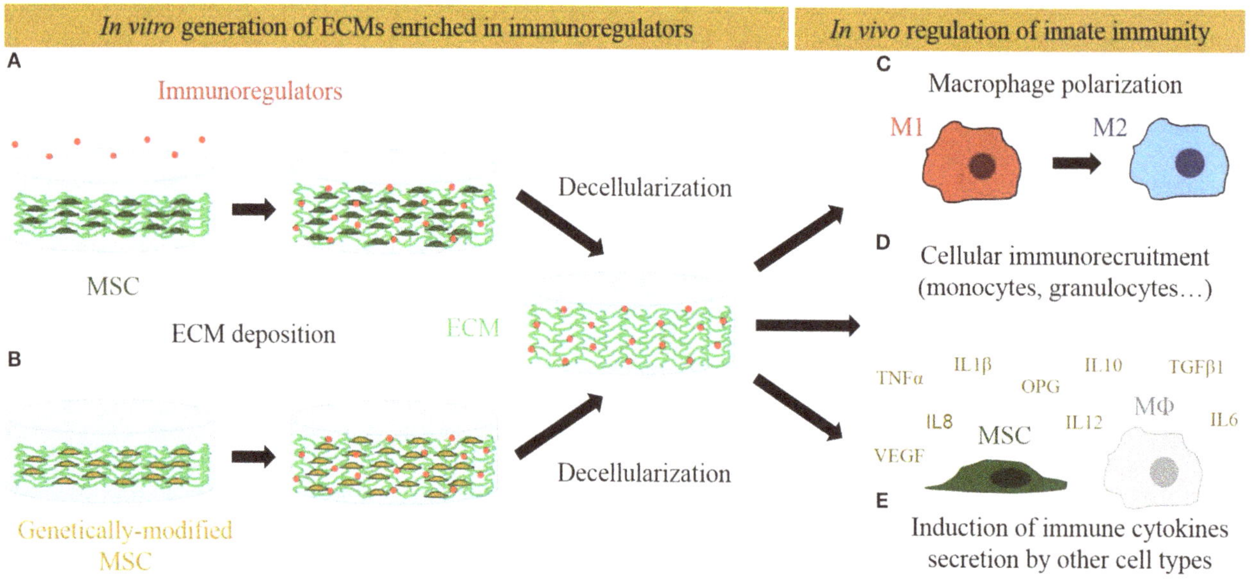

FIGURE 1 | Different *in vitro* approaches followed to deliver immunoregulators into ECM-derived scaffolds and their interactions with the innate immune system *in vivo*. **(A)** Immunoregulators can be directly supplemented and anchored into MSC-derived ECMs. **(B)** Alternatively, MSCs can be genetically edited to overexpress immunoregulators and seeded on scaffolds, where they will produce an ECM enriched in those factors. The tissues are later decellularized to generate cell-free ECMs. *In vivo*, these immunoinstructive ECMs can activate innate immunity at different levels: **(C)** induce macrophage polarization toward an anti-inflammatory M2 phenotype, **(D)** recruit immune cells, and **(E)** induce the secretion of immune cytokines by recruited mesenchymal stromal cells and macrophages (MΦ).

In the context of ECM engineering, immunoregulators can be exogenously delivered to enrich the biomaterial in specific cytokines and/or stimulate the endogenous synthesis of other factors by host cells. In this perspective, genetically modified MSCs represent a relevant alternative to control the spatiotemporal delivery of immunoregulators in order to engineer immunoinstructive ECMs promoting efficient bone repair.

AUTHOR CONTRIBUTIONS

AG-G and IM prepared the figures and wrote the manuscript.

FUNDING

Financial support was received from the Swiss National Science Foundation (Grant 310030-133110).

REFERENCES

1. Shrivats AR, McDermott MC, Hollinger JO. Bone tissue engineering: state of the union. *Drug Discov Today.* (2014) 19:781–6. doi: 10.1016/j.drudis.2014.04.010
2. Laurencin CT, Ambrosio AM, Borden MD, Cooper JA Jr. Tissue engineering: orthopedic applications. *Annu Rev Biomed Eng.* (1999) 1:19–46. doi: 10.1146/annurev.bioeng.1.1.19
3. Mansour A, Mezour MA, Badran Z, Tamimi F. (*) Extracellular matrices for bone regeneration: a literature review. *Tissue Eng Part A.* (2017) 23:1436–51. doi: 10.1089/ten.tea.2017.0026
4. Benders KE, van Weeren PR, Badylak SF, Saris DB, Dhert WJ, Malda J. Extracellular matrix scaffolds for cartilage and bone regeneration. *Trends Biotechnol.* (2013) 3:169–76. doi: 10.1016/j.tibtech.2012.12.004
5. Midwood KS, Williams LV, Schwarzbauer JE. Tissue repair and the dynamics of the extracellular matrix. *Int.J.Biochem.Cell Biol.* (2004) 36:1031–7. doi: 10.1016/j.biocel.2003.12.003
6. Vaday GG, Lider O. Extracellular matrix moieties, cytokines, and enzymes: dynamic effects on immune cell behavior and inflammation. *J.Leukoc.Biol.* (2000) 67:149–59. doi: 10.1002/jlb.67.2.149
7. Aamodt JM, Grainger DW. Extracellular matrix-based biomaterial scaffolds and the host response. *Biomaterials.* (2016) 86:68–82. doi: 10.1016/j.biomaterials.2016.02.003
8. Lutolf MP, Weber FE, Schmoekel HG, Schense JC, Kohler T, Muller R, et al. Repair of bone defects using synthetic mimetics of collagenous extracellular matrices. *Nat.Biotechnol.* (2003) 21:513–18. doi: 10.1038/nbt818
9. Sadr N, Pippenger BE, Scherberich A, Wendt D, Mantero S, Martin I, et al. Enhancing the biological performance of synthetic polymeric materials by decoration with engineered, decellularized extracellular matrix. *Biomaterials.* (2012) 33:5085–93. doi: 10.1016/j.biomaterials.2012.03.082
10. Clough BH, McCarley MR, Krause U, Zeitouni S, Froese JJ, McNeill EP, et al. Bone regeneration with osteogenically enhanced mesenchymal stem cells and their extracellular matrix proteins. *J.Bone Miner.Res.* (2015) 30:83–94. doi: 10.1002/jbmr.2320
11. Bourgine PE, Gaudiello E, Pippenger B, Jaquiery C, Klein T, Pigeot S, et al. Engineered extracellular matrices as biomaterials of tunable composition and function. *Adv Funct Mater.* (2017) 27:1605486. doi: 10.1002/adfm.201605486
12. Papadimitropoulos A, Scotti C, Bourgine P, Scherberich A, Martin I. Engineered decellularized matrices to instruct bone regeneration processes. *Bone.* (2015) 70:66–72. doi: 10.1016/j.bone.2014.09.007
13. Bourgine PE, Scotti C, Pigeot S, Tchang LA, Todorov A, Martin I. Osteoinductivity of engineered cartilaginous templates devitalized by inducible apoptosis. *Proc.Natl.Acad.Sci.USA.* (2014) 111:17426–31. doi: 10.1073/pnas.1411975111
14. Dziki JL, Huleihel L, Scarritt ME, Badylak SF. Extracellular matrix bioscaffolds as immunomodulatory biomaterials. *Tissue Eng Part A.* (2017) 23:1152–9. doi: 10.1089/ten.tea.2016.0538
15. Franz S, Rammelt S, Scharnweber D, Simon JC. Immune responses to implants - a review of the implications for the design of immunomodulatory biomaterials. *Biomaterials.* (2011) 32:6692–709. doi: 10.1016/j.biomaterials.2011.05.078
16. Londono R, Badylak SF. Biologic scaffolds for regenerative medicine: mechanisms of *in vivo* remodeling. *Ann.Biomed.Eng.* (2015) 43:577–92. doi: 10.1007/s10439-014-1103-8
17. Gerstenfeld LC, Cullinane DM, Barnes GL, Graves DT, Einhorn TA. Fracture healing as a post-natal developmental process: molecular, spatial, and temporal aspects of its regulation. *J.Cell Biochem.* (2003) 88:873–84. doi: 10.1002/jcb.10435
18. Gorbet MB, Sefton MV. Biomaterial-associated thrombosis: roles of coagulation factors, complement, platelets and leukocytes. *Biomaterials.* (2004) 25:5681–703. doi: 10.1016/j.biomaterials.2004.01.023
19. Johne J, Blume C, Benz PM, Pozgajova M, Ullrich M, Schuh K, et al. Platelets promote coagulation factor XII-mediated proteolytic cascade systems in plasma. *Biol.Chem.* (2006) 387:173–8. doi: 10.1515/BC.2006.023
20. Baht GS, Vi L, Alman BA. The role of the immune cells in fracture healing. *Curr Osteoporos Rep.* (2018) 16:138–45. doi: 10.1007/s11914-018-0423-2
21. Bastian OW, Koenderman L, Alblas J, Leenen LP, Blokhuis TJ. Neutrophils contribute to fracture healing by synthesizing fibronectin+ extracellular matrix rapidly after injury. *Clin Immunol.* (2016) 164:78–84. doi: 10.1016/j.clim.2016.02.001
22. Chang MK, Raggatt LJ, Alexander KA, Kuliwaba JS, Fazzalari NL, Schroder K, et al. Osteal tissue macrophages are intercalated throughout human and mouse bone lining tissues and regulate osteoblast function *in vitro* and *in vivo*. *J Immunol.* (2008) 181:1232–44. doi: 10.4049/jimmunol.181.2.1232
23. Mosser DM, Edwards JP. Exploring the full spectrum of macrophage activation. *Nat Rev Immunol.* (2008) 8:958–69. doi: 10.1038/nri2448
24. Schlundt C, El KT, Serra A, Dienelt A, Wendler S, Schell H, et al. Macrophages in bone fracture healing: their essential role in endochondral ossification. *Bone.* (2018) 106:78–89. doi: 10.1016/j.bone.2015.10.019
25. Einhorn TA. The cell and molecular biology of fracture healing. *Clin Orthop Relat Res.* (1998) 55:S7–21. doi: 10.1097/00003086-199810001-00003
26. Wang M, Yuan Q, Xie L. Mesenchymal stem cell-based immunomodulation: properties and clinical application. *Stem Cells Int.* (2018) 2018:3057624. doi: 10.1155/2018/3057624
27. Pajarinen J, Lin T, Gibon E, Kohno Y, Maruyama M, Nathan K, et al. Mesenchymal stem cell-macrophage crosstalk and bone healing, *Biomaterials.* (2019) 196:80–9. doi: 10.1016/j.biomaterials.2017.12.025
28. Gerstenfeld LC, Cho TJ, Kon T, Aizawa T, Cruceta J, Graves BD, et al. Impaired intramembranous bone formation during bone repair in the absence of tumor necrosis factor-alpha signaling. *Cells Tissues Organs.* (2001) 169:285–94. doi: 10.1159/000047893
29. Mumme M, Scotti C, Papadimitropoulos A, Todorov A, Hoffmann W, Bocelli-Tyndall C, et al. Interleukin-1beta modulates endochondral ossification by human adult bone marrow stromal cells. *Eur Cell Mater.* (2012) 24:224–36. doi: 10.22203/eCM.v024a16
30. Lange J, Sapozhnikova A, Lu C, Hu D, Li X, Miclau T III, et al. Action of IL-1beta during fracture healing. *J Orthop Res.* (2010) 28:778–84. doi: 10.1002/jor.21061
31. Guihard P, Danger Y, Brounais B, David E, Brion R, Delecrin J, et al. Induction of osteogenesis in mesenchymal stem cells by activated monocytes/macrophages depends on oncostatin M signaling, *Stem Cells.* (2012) 30:762–72. doi: 10.1002/stem.1040
32. Freytes DO, Kang JW, Marcos-Campos I, Vunjak-Novakovic G. Macrophages modulate the viability and growth of human mesenchymal stem cells. *J Cell Biochem.* (2013) 114:220–9. doi: 10.1002/jcb.24357
33. Champagne CM, Takebe J, Offenbacher S, Cooper LF. Macrophage cell lines produce osteoinductive signals that include bone morphogenetic protein-2. *Bone.* (2002) 30:26–31. doi: 10.1016/S8756-3282(01)00638-X

34. Rao AJ, Nich C, Dhulipala LS, Gibon E, Valladares R, Zwingenberger S, et al. Local effect of IL-4 delivery on polyethylene particle induced osteolysis in the murine calvarium. *J Biomed Mater Res A.* (2013) 101:1926–34. doi: 10.1002/jbm.a.34486
35. Sicari BM, Dziki JL, Siu BF, Medberry CJ, Dearth CL, Badylak SF. The promotion of a constructive macrophage phenotype by solubilized extracellular matrix. *Biomaterials.* (2014) 35:8605–12. doi: 10.1016/j.biomaterials.2014.06.060
36. Weidenbusch M, Anders HJ. Tissue microenvironments define and get reinforced by macrophage phenotypes in homeostasis or during inflammation, repair and fibrosis. *J Innate Immun.* (2012) 4:463–77. doi: 10.1159/000336717
37. Murray PJ, Allen JE, Biswas SK, Fisher EA, Gilroy DW, Goerdt S, et al. Macrophage activation and polarization: nomenclature and experimental guidelines. *Immunity.* (2014) 41:14–20. doi: 10.1016/j.immuni.2014.06.008
38. Todorov A, Scotti C, Barbero A, Scherberich A, Papadimitropoulos A, Martin I. Monocytes seeded on engineered hypertrophic cartilage do not enhance endochondral ossification capacity. *Tissue Eng Part A.* (2017) 23:708–15. doi: 10.1089/ten.tea.2016.0553
39. Valentin JE, Stewart-Akers AM, Gilbert TW, Badylak SF. Macrophage participation in the degradation and remodeling of extracellular matrix scaffolds. *Tissue Eng Part A.* (2009) 15:1687–94. doi: 10.1089/ten.tea.2008.0419
40. Alvarez MM, Liu JC, Trujillo-de SG, Cha BH, Vishwakarma A, Ghaemmaghami AM, et al. Delivery strategies to control inflammatory response: modulating M1-M2 polarization in tissue engineering applications. *J Control Release.* (2016) 240:349–63. doi: 10.1016/j.jconrel.2016.01.026
41. Rowley AT, Nagalla RR, Wang SW, Liu WF. Extracellular matrix-based strategies for immunomodulatory biomaterials engineering. *Adv Healthc Mater.* (2019) 8:e1801578. doi: 10.1002/adhm.201801578
42. Slivka PF, Dearth CL, Keane TJ, Meng FW, Medberry CJ, Riggio RT, et al. Fractionation of an ECM hydrogel into structural and soluble components reveals distinctive roles in regulating macrophage behavior. *Biomater Sci.* (2014) 2:1521–34. doi: 10.1039/C4BM00189C
43. Gowen BB, Borg TK, Ghaffar A, Mayer EP. Selective adhesion of macrophages to denatured forms of type I collagen is mediated by scavenger receptors. *Matrix Biol.* (2000) 19:61–71. doi: 10.1016/S0945-053X(99)00052-9
44. Veres SP, Brennan-Pierce EP, Lee JM. Macrophage-like U937 cells recognize collagen fibrils with strain-induced discrete plasticity damage. *J Biomed Mater Res A.* (2015) 103:397–408. doi: 10.1002/jbm.a.35156
45. Rayahin JE, Buhrman JS, Zhang Y, Koh TJ, Gemeinhart RA. High and low molecular weight hyaluronic acid differentially influence macrophage activation. *ACS Biomater Sci Eng.* (2015) 1:481–93. doi: 10.1021/acsbiomaterials.5b00181
46. Levesque MC, Haynes BF. TNFalpha and IL-4 regulation of hyaluronan binding to monocyte CD44 involves posttranslational modification of CD44. *Cell Immunol.* (1999) 193:209–18. doi: 10.1006/cimm.1999.1456
47. Collins LE, Troeberg L. Heparan sulfate as a regulator of inflammation and immunity. *J Leukoc Biol.* (2019) 105:81–92. doi: 10.1002/JLB.3RU0618-246R
48. Clark RA. Fibrin and wound healing. *Ann N Y Acad Sci.* (2001) 936:355–67. doi: 10.1111/j.1749-6632.2001.tb03522.x
49. Ciano PS, Colvin RB, Dvorak AM, McDonagh J, Dvorak HF. Macrophage migration in fibrin gel matrices. *Lab Invest.* (1986) 54:62–70.
50. Hsieh JY, Smith TD, Meli VS, Tran TN, Botvinick EL, Liu WF. Differential regulation of macrophage inflammatory activation by fibrin and fibrinogen. *Acta Biomater.* (2017) 47:14–24. doi: 10.1016/j.actbio.2016.09.024
51. Yakovlev S, Medved L. Effect of fibrinogen, fibrin, and fibrin degradation products on transendothelial migration of leukocytes. *Thromb Res.* (2018) 162:93–100. doi: 10.1016/j.thromres.2017.11.007
52. Robson SC, Shephard EG, Kirsch RE. Fibrin degradation product D-dimer induces the synthesis and release of biologically active IL-1 beta. IL-6 and plasminogen activator inhibitors from monocytes *in vitro*. *Br J Haematol.* (1994) 86:322–6. doi: 10.1111/j.1365-2141.1994.tb04733.x
53. Sorokin L. The impact of the extracellular matrix on inflammation. *Nat Rev Immunol.* (2010) 10:712–23. doi: 10.1038/nri2852
54. Reing JE, Zhang L, Myers-Irvin J, Cordero KE, Freytes DO, Heber-Katz E, et al. Degradation products of extracellular matrix affect cell migration and proliferation. *Tissue Eng Part A.* (2009) 15:605–14. doi: 10.1089/ten.tea.2007.0425
55. Brown BN, Valentin JE, Stewart-Akers AM, McCabe GP, Badylak SF. Macrophage phenotype and remodeling outcomes in response to biologic scaffolds with and without a cellular component. *Biomaterials.* (2009) 30:1482–91. doi: 10.1016/j.biomaterials.2008.11.040
56. Keane TJ, Londono R, Turner NJ, Badylak SF. Consequences of ineffective decellularization of biologic scaffolds on the host response. *Biomaterials.* (2012) 33:1771–81. doi: 10.1016/j.biomaterials.2011.10.054
57. Sadtler K, Allen BW, Estrellas K, Housseau F, Pardoll DM, Elisseeff JH. The scaffold immune microenvironment: biomaterial-mediated immune polarization in traumatic and nontraumatic applications. *Tissue Eng Part A.* (2017) 23:1044–53. doi: 10.1089/ten.tea.2016.0304
58. Martino MM, Maruyama K, Kuhn GA, Satoh T, Takeuchi O, Muller R, et al. Inhibition of IL-1R1/MyD88 signalling promotes mesenchymal stem cell-driven tissue regeneration. *Nat.Commun.* (2016) 7:11051. doi: 10.1038/ncomms11051
59. Spiller KL, Nassiri S, Witherel CE, Anfang RR, Ng J, Nakazawa KR, et al. Sequential delivery of immunomodulatory cytokines to facilitate the M1-to-M2 transition of macrophages and enhance vascularization of bone scaffolds. *Biomaterials.* (2015) 37:194–207. doi: 10.1016/j.biomaterials.2014.10.017
60. Hachim D, Lopresti ST, Yates CC, Brown BN. Shifts in macrophage phenotype at the biomaterial interface via IL-4 eluting coatings are associated with improved implant integration. *Biomaterials.* (2017) 112:95–107. doi: 10.1016/j.biomaterials.2016.10.019
61. Senior RM, Gresham HD, Griffin GL, Brown EJ, Chung AE. Entactin stimulates neutrophil adhesion and chemotaxis through interactions between its Arg-Gly-Asp (RGD) domain and the leukocyte response integrin. *J Clin Invest.* (1992) 90:2251–7. doi: 10.1172/JCI116111
62. Lynn AD, Kyriakides TR, Bryant SJ. Characterization of the *in vitro* macrophage response and *in vivo* host response to poly(ethylene glycol)-based hydrogels. *J Biomed Mater Res A.* (2010) 93:941–53. doi: 10.1002/jbm.a.32595
63. Zaveri TD, Lewis JS, Dolgova NV, Clare-Salzler MJ, Keselowsky BG. Integrin-directed modulation of macrophage responses to biomaterials. *Biomaterials.* (2014) 35:3504–15. doi: 10.1016/j.biomaterials.2014.01.007
64. Kim YK, Chu SH, Hsieh JY, Kamoku CM, Tenner AJ, Liu WF, et al. Incorporation of a ligand peptide for immune inhibitory receptor LAIR-1 on biomaterial surfaces inhibits macrophage inflammatory responses. *Adv Healthc Mater.* (2017) 6:1700707. doi: 10.1002/adhm.201700707
65. Wang H, Li X, Tomin E, Doty SB, Lane JM, Carney DH, et al. Thrombin peptide (TP508) promotes fracture repair by up-regulating inflammatory mediators, early growth factors, and increasing angiogenesis. *J Orthop Res.* (2005) 23:671–9. doi: 10.1016/j.orthres.2004.10.002
66. Santos SG, Lamghari M, Almeida CR, Oliveira MI, Neves N, Ribeiro AC, et al. Adsorbed fibrinogen leads to improved bone regeneration and correlates with differences in the systemic immune response. *Acta Biomater.* (2013) 9:7209–17. doi: 10.1016/j.actbio.2013.04.008
67. Vasconcelos DM, Goncalves RM, Almeida CR, Pereira IO, Oliveira MI, Neves N, et al. Fibrinogen scaffolds with immunomodulatory properties promote *in vivo* bone regeneration. *Biomaterials.* (2016) 111:163–78. doi: 10.1016/j.biomaterials.2016.10.004
68. Paralkar VM, Borovecki F, Ke HZ, Cameron KO, Lefker B, Grasser WA, et al. An EP2 receptor-selective prostaglandin E2 agonist induces bone healing. *Proc Natl Acad Sci USA.* (2003) 100:6736–40. doi: 10.1073/pnas.1037343100
69. Tanaka M, Sakai A, Uchida S, Tanaka S, Nagashima M, Katayama T, et al. Prostaglandin E2 receptor (EP4) selective agonist (ONO-4819.CD) accelerates bone repair of femoral cortex after drill-hole injury associated with local upregulation of bone turnover in mature rats. *Bone.* (2004) 34:940–8. doi: 10.1016/j.bone.2004.01.002
70. Toyoda H, Terai H, Sasaoka R, Oda K, Takaoka K. Augmentation of bone morphogenetic protein-induced bone mass by local delivery of a prostaglandin E EP4 receptor agonist. *Bone.* (2005) 37:555–62. doi: 10.1016/j.bone.2005.04.042
71. Jiang K, Weaver JD, Li Y, Chen X, Liang J, Stabler CL. Local release of dexamethasone from macroporous scaffolds accelerates islet transplant engraftment by promotion of anti-inflammatory M2 macrophages. *Biomaterials.* (2017) 114:71–81. doi: 10.1016/j.biomaterials.2016.11.004
72. Patil SD, Papadmitrakopoulos F, Burgess DJ. Concurrent delivery of dexamethasone and VEGF for localized inflammation

control and angiogenesis. *J Control Release.* (2007) 117:68–79. doi: 10.1016/j.jconrel.2006.10.013

73. Santo VE, Gomes ME, Mano JF, Reis RL. Controlled release strategies for bone, cartilage, and osteochondral engineering–part I: recapitulation of native tissue healing and variables for the design of delivery systems. *Tissue Eng Part B Rev.* (2013) 19:308–26. doi: 10.1089/ten.teb.2012.0138
74. Santo VE, Gomes ME, Mano JF, Reis RL. Controlled release strategies for bone, cartilage, and osteochondral engineering–part II: challenges on the evolution from single to multiple bioactive factor delivery. *Tissue Eng Part B Rev.* (2013) 19:327–52. doi: 10.1089/ten.teb.2012.0727
75. Vo TN, Kasper FK, Mikos AG. Strategies for controlled delivery of growth factors and cells for bone regeneration. *Adv Drug Deliv Rev.* (2012) 64:1292–309. doi: 10.1016/j.addr.2012.01.016
76. Yang SS, Jin LH, Park SH, Kim MS, Kim YJ, Choi BH, et al. Extracellular Matrix (ECM) multilayer membrane as a sustained releasing growth factor delivery system for rhTGF-beta3 in articular cartilage repair. *PLoS.ONE.* (2016) 11:e0156292. doi: 10.1371/journal.pone.0156292
77. Lee SC, Kwon IK, Park K. Hydrogels for delivery of bioactive agents: a historical perspective. *Adv Drug Deliv Rev.* (2013) 65:17–20. doi: 10.1016/j.addr.2012.07.015
78. Lienemann PS, Lutolf MP, Ehrbar M. Biomimetic hydrogels for controlled biomolecule delivery to augment bone regeneration. *Adv Drug Deliv Rev.* (2012) 64:1078–89. doi: 10.1016/j.addr.2012.03.010
79. Kim YH, Furuya H, Tabata Y. Enhancement of bone regeneration by dual release of a macrophage recruitment agent and platelet-rich plasma from gelatin hydrogels. *Biomaterials.* (2014) 35:214–24. doi: 10.1016/j.biomaterials.2013.09.103
80. Kajahn J, Franz S, Rueckert E, Forstreuter I, Hintze V, Moeller S, et al. Artificial extracellular matrices composed of collagen I and high sulfated hyaluronan modulate monocyte to macrophage differentiation under conditions of sterile inflammation. *Biomatter.* (2012) 2:226–36. doi: 10.4161/biom.22855
81. Wang M, Yu Y, Dai K, Ma Z, Liu Y, Wang J, et al. Improved osteogenesis and angiogenesis of magnesium-doped calcium phosphate cement via macrophage immunomodulation. *Biomater Sci.* (2016) 4:1574–83. doi: 10.1039/C6BM00290K
82. Lam J, Segura T. The modulation of MSC integrin expression by RGD presentation. *Biomaterials.* (2013) 34:3938–47. doi: 10.1016/j.biomaterials.2013.01.091
83. Lo SC, Tasso R. Harnessing endogenous cellular mechanisms for bone repair. *Front Bioeng Biotechnol.* (2017) 5:52. doi: 10.3389/fbioe.2017.00052
84. Julier Z, Park AJ, Briquez PS, Martino MM. Promoting tissue regeneration by modulating the immune system. *Acta Biomater.* (2017) 53:13–28. doi: 10.1016/j.actbio.2017.01.056
85. Hallmann R, Zhang X, Di RJ, Li L, Song J, Hannocks MJ, et al. The regulation of immune cell trafficking by the extracellular matrix. *Curr Opin Cell Biol.* (2015) 36:54–61. doi: 10.1016/j.ceb.2015.06.006
86. Andorko JI, Jewell CM. Designing biomaterials with immunomodulatory properties for tissue engineering and regenerative medicine. *Bioeng Transl Med.* (2017) 2:139–55. doi: 10.1002/btm2.10063
87. Hu Z, Ma C, Rong X, Zou S, Liu X. Immunomodulatory ECM-like microspheres for accelerated bone regeneration in diabetes mellitus. *ACS Appl Mater Interfaces.* (2018) 10:2377–90. doi: 10.1021/acsami.7b18458
88. Huang YC, Kaigler D, Rice KG, Krebsbach PH, Mooney DJ. Combined angiogenic and osteogenic factor delivery enhances bone marrow stromal cell-driven bone regeneration. *J Bone Miner Res.* (2005) 20:848–57. doi: 10.1359/JBMR.041226
89. Lieberman JR, Le LQ, Wu L, Finerman GA, Berk A, Witte ON, et al. Regional gene therapy with a BMP-2-producing murine stromal cell line induces heterotopic and orthotopic bone formation in rodents. *J Orthop Res.* (1998) 16:330–9. doi: 10.1002/jor.1100160309
90. Blum JS, Barry MA, Mikos AG, Jansen JA. *In vivo* evaluation of gene therapy vectors in *ex vivo*-derived marrow stromal cells for bone regeneration in a rat critical-size calvarial defect model. *Hum Gene Ther.* (2003) 14:1689–701. doi: 10.1089/104303403322611719
91. Tu Q, Valverde P, Chen J. Osterix enhances proliferation and osteogenic potential of bone marrow stromal cells. *Biochem Biophys Res Commun.* (2006) 341:1257–65. doi: 10.1016/j.bbrc.2006.01.092
92. Wu L, Wu Y, Lin Y, Jing W, Nie X, Qiao J, et al. Osteogenic differentiation of adipose derived stem cells promoted by overexpression of osterix. *Mol Cell Biochem.* (2007) 301:83–92. doi: 10.1007/s11010-006-9399-9
93. Jabbarzadeh E, Starnes T, Khan YM, Jiang T, Wirtel AJ, Deng M, et al. Induction of angiogenesis in tissue-engineered scaffolds designed for bone repair: a combined gene therapy-cell transplantation approach. *Proc Natl Acad Sci USA.* (2008) 105:11099–104. doi: 10.1073/pnas.0800069105
94. Vitale G, Dicitore A, Gentilini D, Cavagnini F. Immunomodulatory effects of VEGF: clinical implications of VEGF-targeted therapy in human cancer. *Cancer Biol Ther.* (2010) 9:694–8. doi: 10.4161/cbt.9.9.11691
95. Sefcik LS, Petrie Aronin CE, Wieghaus KA, Botchwey EA. Sustained release of sphingosine 1-phosphate for therapeutic arteriogenesis and bone tissue engineering. *Biomaterials.* (2008) 29:2869–77. doi: 10.1016/j.biomaterials.2008.03.017
96. Bryan AM, Del PM. Sphingosine-1-phosphate receptors and innate immunity. *Cell Microbiol.* (2018) 20:e12836. doi: 10.1111/cmi.12836
97. Choi JJ, Yoo SA, Park SJ, Kang YJ, Kim WU, Oh IH, et al. Mesenchymal stem cells overexpressing interleukin-10 attenuate collagen-induced arthritis in mice. *Clin Exp Immunol.* (2008) 153:269–76. doi: 10.1111/j.1365-2249.2008.03683.x
98. Lin T, Pajarinen J, Nabeshima A, Lu L, Nathan K, Yao Z, et al. Establishment of NF-kappaB sensing and interleukin-4 secreting mesenchymal stromal cells as an "on-demand" drug delivery system to modulate inflammation. *Cytotherapy.* (2017) 19:1025–34. doi: 10.1016/j.jcyt.2017.06.008
99. Ramamoorth M, Narvekar A. Non viral vectors in gene therapy- an overview. *J Clin Diagn Res.* (2015) 9:GE01–6. doi: 10.7860/JCDR/2015/10443.5394

7

Shear and Dynamic Compression Modulates the Inflammatory Phenotype of Human Monocytes *in vitro*

*Niamh Fahy, Ursula Menzel, Mauro Alini and Martin J. Stoddart**

AO Research Institute Davos, Davos, Switzerland

Correspondence:
Martin J. Stoddart
martin.stoddart@aofoundation.org

Monocytes and their derived macrophages are found at the site of remodeling tissue, such as fracture hematoma, that is exposed to mechanical forces and have been previously implicated in the reparative response. However, the mechanoresponsive of monocytes and macrophages to skeletal tissue-associated mechanical forces and their subsequent contribution to skeletal repair remains unclear. The aim of this study was to investigate the potential of skeletal tissue-associated loading conditions to modulate human monocyte activation and phenotype. Primary human monocytes or the human monocyte reporter cell line, THP1-Blue, were encapsulated in agarose and exposed to a combination of shear and compressive loading for 1 h a day for 3 consecutive days. Exposure of monocytes to mechanical loading conditions increased their pro-inflammatory gene and protein expression. Exposure of undifferentiated monocytes to mechanical loading conditions significantly upregulated gene expression levels of interleukin(IL)-6 and IL-8 compared to free swelling controls. Additionally, multiaxial loading of unstimulated monocytes resulted in increased protein secretion of TNF-α (17.1 $\pm$ 8.9 vs. 8 $\pm$ 7.4 pg/ml) and MIP-1α (636.8 $\pm$ 471.1 vs. 124.1 $\pm$ 40.1 pg/ml), as well as IL-13 (42.1 $\pm$ 19.8 vs. 21.7 $\pm$ 13.6) compared monocytes cultured under free-swelling conditions. This modulatory effect was observed irrespective of previous activation with the M1/pro-inflammatory differentiation stimuli lipopolysaccharide and interferon-γ or the M2/anti-inflammatory differentiation factor interleukin-4. Furthermore, mechanical shear and compression were found to differentially regulate nitric oxide synthase 2 (NOS2) and IL-12B gene expression as well as inflammatory protein production by THP1-Blue monocytes. The findings of this study indicate that human monocytes are responsive to mechanical stimuli, with a modulatory effect of shear and compressive loading observed toward pro-inflammatory mediator production. This may play a role in healing pathways that are mechanically regulated. An in depth understanding of the impact of skeletal tissue-associated mechanical loading on monocyte behavior may identify novel targets to maximize inflammation-mediated repair mechanisms.

Keywords: osteoimmunology, immune regulation, fracture repair, mechanoregulation, bone healing, macrophage

INTRODUCTION

The repair process following traumatic injury to the musculoskeletal system is known to be influenced by the mechanical environment. The natural course of bone healing can be intramembranous ossification resulting from stable fracture fixation and subsequent low interfragmentary motion, or endochondral ossification which is associated with moderate interfragmentary movement (1). In addition to driving fracture healing responses, mechanical forces of an appropriate magnitude are also key to maintaining cartilage homeostasis within the articulating joint (2).

A wound healing response is initiated during the process of bone fracture repair, as well as marrow stimulation techniques applied in cartilage repair strategies where the subchondral bone is penetrated. This involves inflammatory cell exudation or infiltration to the site of injury, followed by coagulation activation and fibrin clot formation, which is known to regulate monocyte chemotaxis and proliferation (3, 4). Monocytes and monocyte-derived macrophages are key immune effector cells playing a vital role in host defense, as well as contributing to tissue remodeling and repair (5). Macrophages are associated with a high degree of plasticity having the potential to change phenotype in response to environmental cues, and may be classified according to pro-inflammatory (M1) or anti-inflammatory (M2) subsets (5). Pro-inflammatory macrophages are associated with high production of pro-inflammatory cytokines and increased microbicidal activity, whereas anti-inflammatory macrophages are associated with wound healing and immunoregulatory functions (3, 6).

Infiltrating monocytes and macrophages may influence the success of musculoskeletal tissue repair processes. Macrophage depletion has been previously demonstrated to negatively impact endochondral ossification and subsequently delay bone fracture healing (7–9). Furthermore, monocyte and macrophage associated inflammatory cytokines such as IL-6 and TNF-α are known to promote bone repair, with inhibition of TNF-α signaling shown to delay both intramembranous and endochondral bone formation (10, 11). In contrast to bone healing, pro-inflammatory factors such as IL-1β and TNF-α produced by both activated monocytes and M1 polarized macrophages, induce destructive processes in cartilage tissue including catabolic enzyme expression and reduced extracellular matrix deposition (12–14). However, recruitment of anti-inflammatory macrophages to the site of subchondral drill holes within osteochondral defects using chitosan-glycerol phosphate composites was reported enhance subchondral bone repair and improve cartilage resurfacing, further highlighting the impact of macrophages on skeletal tissue repair (15). Monocytes and macrophages are found at the site of remodeling tissue that is exposed to mechanical forces and have been previously implicated in the reparative response (16–18). As the area of osteoimmunology gains in importance, the influence of mechanical stimulation on immune cell phenotype needs to be investigated in greater detail. However, the responsiveness of macrophages and monocytes, their lineage precursors, to mechanical forces that are native to skeletal tissues and the effect of such mechanical stimuli on macrophage phenotype requires further elucidation. Therefore, the aim of this study was to investigate the impact of mechanical shear and compressive loading on monocyte activation and phenotype. Unstimulated, M1 or M2-stimulated primary human monocytes as well as the human monocyte reporter cell line, THP1-Blue, were exposed to a combination of shear and compressive loading *in vitro*. Gene expression levels of inflammatory mediators and inflammatory protein secretion was assessed following 3 days of mechanical stimulation.

MATERIALS AND METHODS

Human Monocyte Isolation

Human monocytes were isolated from buffy coats left over from voluntary whole blood donations after informed consent of the donors according to the regulations of Swiss Red Cross Blood Service. Buffy coats were processed within 23 h after blood donation by centrifugation at 5,000 g for 15 min and subsequent separation on Compomat G5 (Fresenius, Oberdorf, Switzerland) using top-and-bottom 450 ml blood bag systems pre-filled with Citrate-Dextrose-Phosphate Solution (Fresenius). Buffy coats were anonymized prior to delivery from the Blood Service to AO Institute in line with the ethics code provided by the Swiss Drug Law (Heilmittelgesetz). For the isolation of peripheral blood mononuclear cells (PBMCs), each buffy coat was diluted at a 1:5 ratio with 0.1% bovine serum albumin (BSA) in phosphate buffered saline (PBS). Thirty milliliter of diluted buffy coat was layered on 15 ml of Ficoll and centrifuged at 1,000 g for 15 min without brake. Following centrifugation, the interphase layer containing PBMCs was removed and washed with 0.5% BSA/PBS containing 2 mM EDTA. Isolated PBMCs were labeled with 100 μl of anti-CD14 magnetic bead solution (Miltenyi Biotec Bergisch Gladbach, Germany) in the dark at 4°C for 20 min. Monocytes were isolated utilizing MACS LS Separation columns and a MidiMACS™ Separator (Miltenyi Biotec), according to manufacturer's instructions. Purity of isolated CD14+ cells was assessed by fluorescence activated cell sorting (FACS) analysis. 1×10^5 monocytes were incubated with APC-Cy7-conjugated anti-human CD14 antibody (BD pharmingen) for 20 min in the dark at 4°C. FACS analysis was performed using a BD Aria III machine, and data analyzed using BD FACS Diva 6.1.3 software (BD Biosciences). The average purity of CD14+ monocytes from all donors was found to be 95% (data not shown). Monocytes were isolated from two individual buffy coat donors and pooled per experiment.

THP1-Blue™ Cell Culture

The human monocyte reporter cell line THP1-Blue™ (InvivoGen, CA, USA) which expresses an NF-κB and AP-1-inducible secreted embryonic alkaline phosphatase (SEAP) reporter gene, was cultured in RPMI-1640 medium (2 mM L-glutamine; Gibco, Carlsbad, USA) supplemented with 1% penicillin/streptomycin (Gibco) and 10% heat inactivated fetal bovine serum (FBS; Pan Biotech, Aidenbach, Germany). Monocyte suspension cultures were maintained at a density of at 3–8 × 100,000 cells/ml.

Agarose Gel Seeding and Culture

To evaluate the effect of mechanical loading on monocyte phenotype, human primary monocytes and THP1-Blue cells were encapsulated in 2% low melting temperature agarose (Lonza) at a cell density of 3×10^6 monocytes per gel. In brief, a 4% agarose solution was prepared by dissolving low melting temperature agarose in sterile phosphate buffered saline and heated. The 4% agarose solution was cooled and mixed with an equal volume of cells suspended in pre-warmed culture media, composed of RPMI-1640 medium supplemented with 2 mM L-glutamine, 1% penicillin/streptomycin and 10% heat inactivated FBS. Two hundred and fifty microliters of cells/agarose suspension was added to a sterile cap of an Eppendorf tube and gels were allow to set at 37°C for 20 min. All agarose constructs were carefully removed from the Eppendorf cap, placed in a sterile PEEK sample holder and cultured with 2.5 ml of culture medium. To investigate the effect of mechanical loading on macrophage phenotype, CD14+ monocytes were stimulated with 10 ng/ml IFN-γ (PeproTech, Rocky Hill, NJ, USA) and 100 ng/ml lipopolysaccharide to induce differentiation toward a pro-inflammatory/M1 phenotype, 10 ng/ml IL-4 (PeproTech) for an anti-inflammatory/M2 phenotype or unstimulated for 72 h prior to loading. Agarose gels containing THP1-Blue monocytes were prepared 24 h prior to loading.

Mechanical Loading

CD14+ monocyte seeded agarose gels were mechanically loaded using a custom built multi-axial load bioreactor based on a 32 mm ceramic hip ball that can apply compression, shear or a combination of the two, to the sample as previously described (19, 20). Shear (±25° ball rotation at 1 Hz) and compression (10% compression superimposed on top of a 10% pre-strain at 1 Hz) loading was applied for 1 h a day for 3 consecutive days. This protocol was chosen as it has been shown to direct osteochondral differentiation of human MSCs and therefore we aimed to investigate similar loading patterns on the modulation of macrophage phenotype (21). Control gels were maintained in free-swelling conditions for the duration of the experiment. To investigate the effect of shear or compression alone on monocyte phenotype, THP1-Blue monocytes were stimulated with shear or compression alone as well as multiaxial loading for 1 h a day for 3 consecutive days. Control gels were maintained in free-swelling conditions for the duration of the experiment. Cell culture media was refreshed every 24 h prior to loading.

Reverse Transcription and PCR

Monocyte-seeded agarose gels were homogenized in 1 ml TRI reagent (Molecular Research Center Inc., Cincinnati, OH, USA). Homogenized samples were supplemented with 100 μl of 1-Bromo-3-chloropropane (Sigma-Aldrich) and processed according to manufacturer's instructions to achieve phase separation. Following phase separation the aqueous phase was removed, supplemented with an equal volume of 70% ethanol (Sigma-Aldrich) and transferred to a RNeasy spin column (Qiagen, Hilden, Germany). RNA was extracted using RNeasy mini spin columns according to manufacturer's instructions. The purity of isolated RNA was assessed using a NanoDrop spectrophotometer (Fisher Scientific, Delaware, USA) based on the absorbance ratios 260/280 nm and 260/230 nm. Reverse transcription was performed using random hexamer primers and TaqMan reverse transcription reagents (Applied Biosystems, Carlsbad, CA, USA). Quantitative real time PCR was performed in 10 μl reactions on cDNA using the Applied Biosystems QuantStudio 6 Flex Real Time PCR system (Applied Biosystems). Primers for cyclooxygenase(COX)-2 (*PTGS2*) were synthesized by Microsynth AG (Balgach, SG, Switzerland; **Table 1**). Gene expression assays for 18S ribosomal RNA (*18S*), interleukin(IL)-6 (*IL6*), IL-8 (*IL8*), IL-10 (*IL10*), tumor necrosis factor (TNF)-α (*TNF*), chemokine (C-C motif) ligand 18 (*CCL18*), mannose receptor CD206 (*MRC1*), nitric oxide synthase 2 (*NOS2*), and monocyte chemoattractant protein 1 (*CCL2*) were purchased from Applied Biosystems, Switzerland (**Table 1**). Gene expression levels were normalized to 18S rRNA, and relative expression calculated via a ΔΔCT comparison.

Cytokine Assays

Levels of IL-6, IL-8, and CCL18 in cell culture supernatant were quantified utilizing commercially available human IL-6 and CCL18 DuoSet ELISA kits according to manufacturer's instructions (R&D Systems, Minneapolis, Minnesota). Levels of IL-10, IL-13, IL-1β, C-X-C motif chemokine 10 (IP-10), macrophage-derived chemokine (MDC), monocyte chemoattractant protein-1 (MCP-1), macrophage inflammatory protein-1α (MIP-1α), and TNF-α were measured utilizing a Meso Scale Development multiplex assay according to manufacturer's instructions (Meso Scale Discovery, Maryland, USA).

Secreted Alkaline Phosphatase Assay

Secreted embryonic alkaline phosphatase (SEAP) levels were detected in cell culture supernatant using a QUANTI-Blue™ enzymatic assay (InvivoGen) according to manufacturer's instructions. SEAP levels were determined qualitatively following spectrophotometric measurement at 620 nm.

Statistical Analysis

IBM SPSS Statistics 21.0 (IBM, New York, USA) and GraphPad Prism software version 6 (GraphPad Software Inc., La Jolla, USA) were used for all statistical analysis. To take donor variability into account between primary monocyte donors, mixed models analysis was applied to test for statistical differences between loaded and free-swelling groups with monocyte donor considered a random factor. THP1-Blue monocyte data sets were analyzed using a Kruskal–Wallis test followed by Dunn's multiple comparisons test. For all analyses, differences were considered statistically significant at $P < 0.05$.

RESULTS

Pro-inflammatory Gene and Protein Expression by Differentially Activated Primary Human Monocytes Following Multiaxial Loading

Monocytes encapsulated in 2% agarose gel were unstimulated, LPS and IFN-γ or IL-4-stimulated for 3 days, prior to subjection

TABLE 1 | Gene expression assays utilized for quantitative real time PCR.

Gene name	Alias	Assay ID/Primer sequence
Human 18S rRNA (*18S*)	18S ribosomal RNA (18S rRNA)	Hs99999901_s1
Human interleukin-8 (*IL8*)	C-X-C motif chemokine ligand 8 (CXCL8)	Hs00174103_m1
Human interleukin-10 (*IL10*)	Cytokine Synthesis Inhibitory Factor (CSIF)	Hs00961622_m1
Human interleukin-6 (*IL6*)	B-Cell Stimulatory Factor (BSF)- 2	Hs00985639_m1
Human tumor necrosis factor (*TNF*)	Tumor Necrosis Factor (TNF)-α	Hs01113624_g1
Human chemokine (C-C motif) ligand 18 (*CCL18*)	Macrophage Inflammatory Protein (MIP)-4	Hs00268113_m1
Human mannose receptor, C type 1 (*MRC1*)	Macrophage Mannose Receptor (MMR, CD206)	Hs00267207_m1
Human C-C motif chemokine ligand 2 (*CCL2*)	Monocyte Chemoattractant Protein (MCP)-1	Hs00234140_m1
Human nitric oxide synthase 2 (*NOS2*)	Inducible Nitric Oxide Synthase (INOS)	Hs01075529_m1
Human interleukin 12B (*IL12B*)	Natural Killer Cell Stimulatory Factor	Hs01011518_m1
Human Prostaglandin-Endoperoxide Synthase 2 (*PTGS2*)	Cyclooxygenase (COX)-2	**Forward:** 5′-TTG TAC CCG GAC AGG ATT CTA TG-3′ **Reverse:** 5′-TGT TTG GAG TGG GTT TCA GAA ATA-3′ **Probe(5′FAM/3′ TAMRA):** 5′-GAA AAC TGC TCA ACA CCG GAA TTT TTG ACA A-3′

to multiaxial loading or free-swelling conditions and analysis of inflammatory gene and protein expression. Monocytes stimulated with LPS and IFN-γ had significantly higher gene expression levels of the pro-inflammatory genes *IL8* and *CCL2* under free-swelling conditions compared to IL-4 stimulated monocytes (10.3- and 28.3-fold increases, respectively), confirming their pro-inflammatory phenotype (**Figure 1A**). Additionally, IL-4 stimulated monocytes were associated with significantly higher *CCL18* expression compared to LPS and IFN-γ stimulated monocytes (41.5-fold increase), confirming their polarization toward an M2-like phenotype. Unstimulated primary human monocytes significantly upregulated gene expression levels of the pro-inflammatory genes *IL6* (5.9-fold change) and *IL8* (2.8-fold change) following 3 days of mechanical loading compared to monocytes cultured in free-swelling conditions (**Figure 1B**). Additionally, expression of the anti-inflammatory macrophage marker *IL10* was decreased in all four donors compared to free-swell controls, with gene expression levels undetectable in donors 1 and 3 following loading. No significant difference was observed in the expression levels of inflammatory mediators *CCL18*, *TNF*, and *CCL2*. Although a similar trend was observed toward inflammatory gene expression by LPS and IFN-γ activated monocytes following mechanical loading, larger variation was observed between donors and these findings were not statistically significant (**Figure 1C**). However, expression of *CCL2* was significantly decreased (1.9-fold decrease). Additionally, gene expression levels of *IL10* were also undetectable in LPS and IFN-γ stimulated monocytes from donors 1 and 3 following loading. In a similar manner to unstimulated monocytes, IL-4 activated cells were also associated with a significant increase in *IL6* (8.9-fold change) and decrease of *IL10* (3.1-fold) expression (**Figure 1D**).

Compared to free-swelling controls, mechanical loading of unstimulated monocytes significantly increased production of the pro-inflammatory mediators TNF-α (17.1 ± 8.9 vs. 8 ± 7.4 pg/ml) and MIP-1α (636.8 ± 471.1 vs. 124.1 ± 40.1 pg/ml), as well as IL-13 (42.1 ± 19.8 vs. 21.7 ± 13.6) (**Figure 2**). Protein levels of IL-10, CCL18, IP-10, MCP-1, MDC, and IL-1β produced by loaded unstimulated monocytes did not significantly differ from free-swelling controls. In a similar manner to gene expression levels, a trend toward an increase in IL-6 production was observed in response to loading of unstimulated monocytes. However, large donor variation was observed and this finding was not statically significant. Mechanical stimulation of LPS and IFN-γ stimulated monocytes significantly increased MDC levels in addition to TNF-α, MIP-1α, and IL-13 (**Figure 2**). In a similar manner to gene expression data, IL-4 activated monocytes were associated with significantly increased production of pro-inflammatory factors IL-6, IL-8, TNF-α, MIP-1α, IP-10, IL-13, IL-1β as well as IL-10 in response to mechanical loading, and decreased expression of CCL18 and MDC (**Figure 2**).

Inflammatory Gene and Protein Expression by THP1-Blue Monocytes Following Mechanical Shear or Compression

To evaluate the potential of mechanical shear or compression to differentially regulate inflammatory gene and protein expression by human monocytes, unstimulated THP1-Blue monocytes were subjected to multiaxial loading conditions, or mechanical shear or compression alone. THP1-Blue monocytes significantly upregulated gene expression levels of the pro-inflammatory markers *NOS2* and *IL12B* in response to compression alone compared to the combination of compression and shear, as well as shear alone following 3 days of loading (**Figure 3**). Gene expression levels of *IL6*, *IL-8*, *TNF-α*, *PTGS2*, *IL-10*, *CCL2*, and *CCL18* did not significantly differ between loading conditions, or compared to free-swelling controls at this time point. However, significantly increased levels of TNF-α, IL-10, IL-8, IL-13, and MDC were detected in the cell culture media

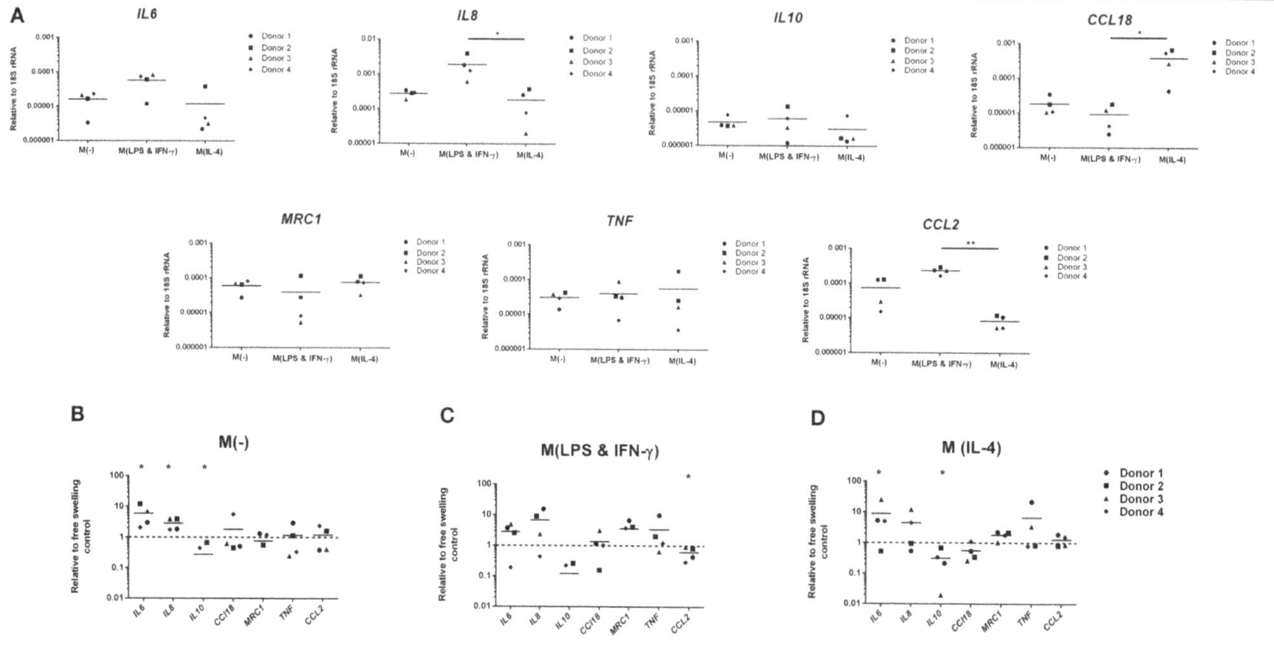

FIGURE 1 | Inflammatory gene expression by differentially activated primary human monocytes following multiaxial loading. **(A)** Gene expression by primary monocytes cultured for 6 days under free-swelling conditions as measured by real-time PCR. Gene expression levels were normalized to the housekeeper gene 18S rRNA. **(B)** Gene expression levels by unstimulated primary human monocytes, or LPS & IFN-γ **(C)** or IL-4 **(D)** stimulated monocytes following 3 days of multiaxial loading. Gene expression levels were normalized to the free swelling control, represented by the dashed line. Data is represented as dot plots including the median for 4 monocyte donors, each assessed in experimental triplicate. Missing points indicate undetectable gene expression. Statistical significance was determined utilizing a mixed model analysis, $^{*}P < 0.05$.

harvested from gels subjected to the combination of compression and shear, as well as compression and shear alone for 3 days compared to control (**Figure 4A**). Additionally, the application of compressive loading alone significantly upregulated IL-1β production by monocytes, whereas shear alone increased the release of MCP-1 compared to all other culture conditions. Levels of IL-6 and IP-10 did not significantly differ in response to any loading condition compared to free-swelling cultures. In addition to modulating inflammatory cytokine production, the application of both compression and shear or shear alone induced the release of secreted alkaline phosphatase by THP1-Blue monocytes, indicative of NF-κB and AP-1 transcription factor activation (**Figure 4B**).

DISCUSSION

Monocytes and their derived macrophages are considered key players in tissue remodeling and repair processes. Mechanical loading has been previously shown to influence the levels or pro and anti-inflammatory macrophages in a model of tendon healing (18). Additionally, cyclic strain has been reported to modulate macrophage polarization state toward a reparative phenotype which promoted extracellular matrix synthesis (22). Monocytes are found at the site of skeletal tissue injuries resulting from either traumatic bone fractures, or microdrilling of the subchondral bone to facilitate microfracture-mediated cartilage repair (23). However, the mechanoresponsive of monocytes and their derived macrophages to skeletal tissue-associated mechanical forces, and their subsequent contribution to skeletal repair remains unclear. The aim of this study was to investigate the potential of shear and compressive forces to modulate human monocyte activation and phenotype. In the present study, exposure of monocytes to mechanical loading conditions increased their production of pro-inflammatory mediators. Furthermore, mechanical loading modulated the production of inflammatory factors produced by monocytes irrespective of previous activation with the M1/pro-inflammatory differentiation stimuli LPS and IFN-γ or the M2/anti-inflammatory differentiation factor IL-4.

Bone fractures associated with less mechanical stability are known to heal via the process of endochondral ossification, involving inflammation, callus formation and tissue remodeling processes (1). Infiltration of macrophages into the fracture callus occurs at an early stage of fracture healing, and inhibition of macrophage recruitment impairs vascularization, decreases callus formation and delays repair (24). Macrophages are associated with a high degree of plasticity and can change phenotype according to environmental cues, encompassing both pro-inflammatory/M1 and anti-inflammatory/M2 phenotypes (5). In an experimental osteotomy model, M1-polarized macrophages were identified as the primary macrophage phenotype in the osteotomy area 24 h post-surgery (7). Interestingly, M1 polarized macrophages have also been reported to promote the osteogenic differentiation of bone

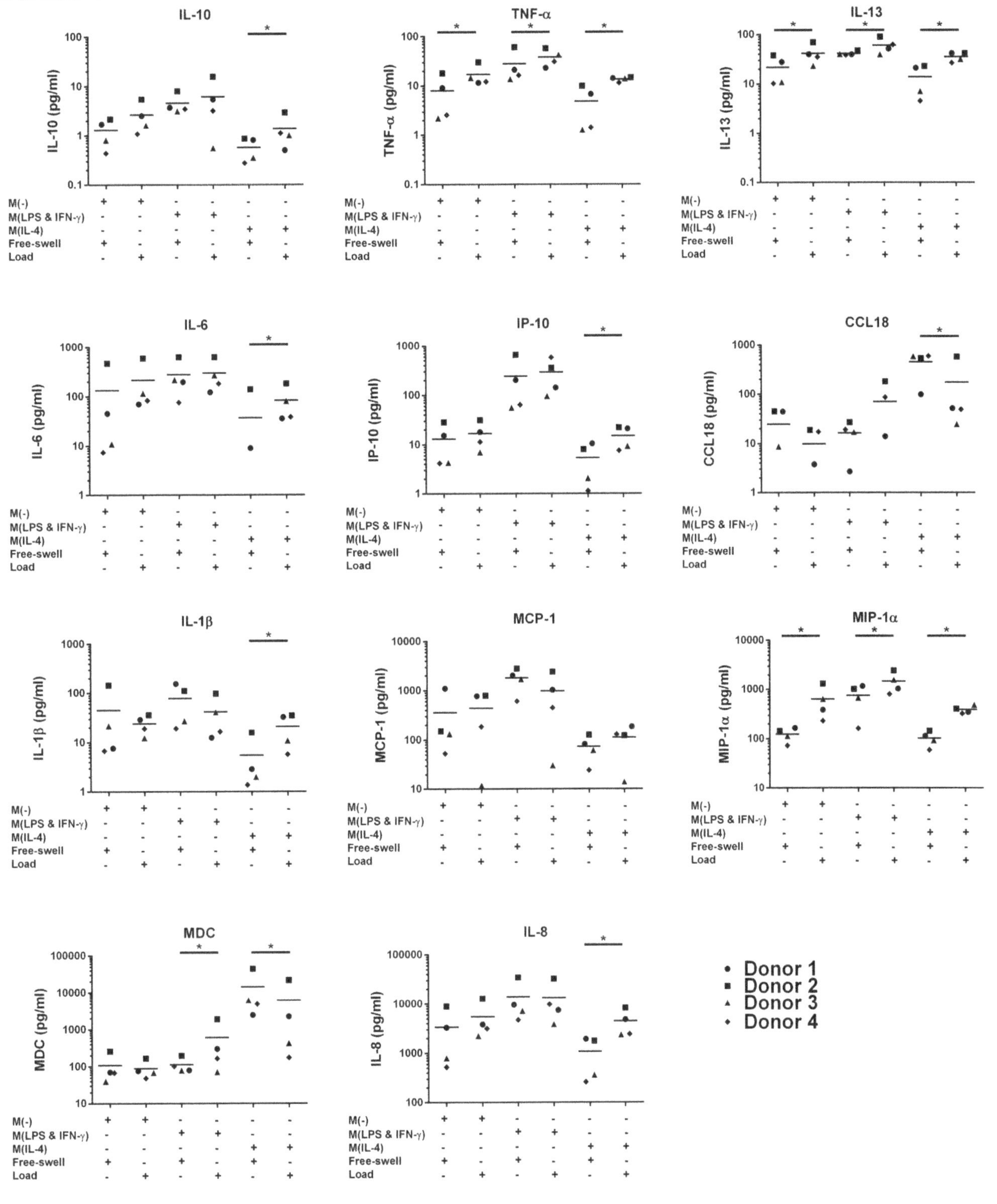

FIGURE 2 | Inflammatory mediator production by primary human monocytes following multiaxial loading. Levels of inflammatory mediators produced by primary monocytes following 3 days of multiaxial loading as quantified by ELISA and multiplex assay. Data is represented as dot plots including the median for 4 monocyte donors, each assessed in experimental triplicate. Missing points indicate undetectable protein levels. Statistical significance was determined utilizing a mixed model analysis, *$P < 0.05$. IL-6, Interleukin-6; IL-10, Interleukin-10; CCL18, chemokine (C-C motif) ligand 18; TNF-α, Tumor necrosis factor-α; MIP-1α, Macrophage inflammatory protein-1α; IP-10, C-X-C motif chemokine 10; MCP-1, Monocyte chemoattractant protein-1; IL-13, Interleukin-13; MDC, Macrophage-derived chemokine; IL-1β, Interleukin-1β; IL-8, Interleukin-8.

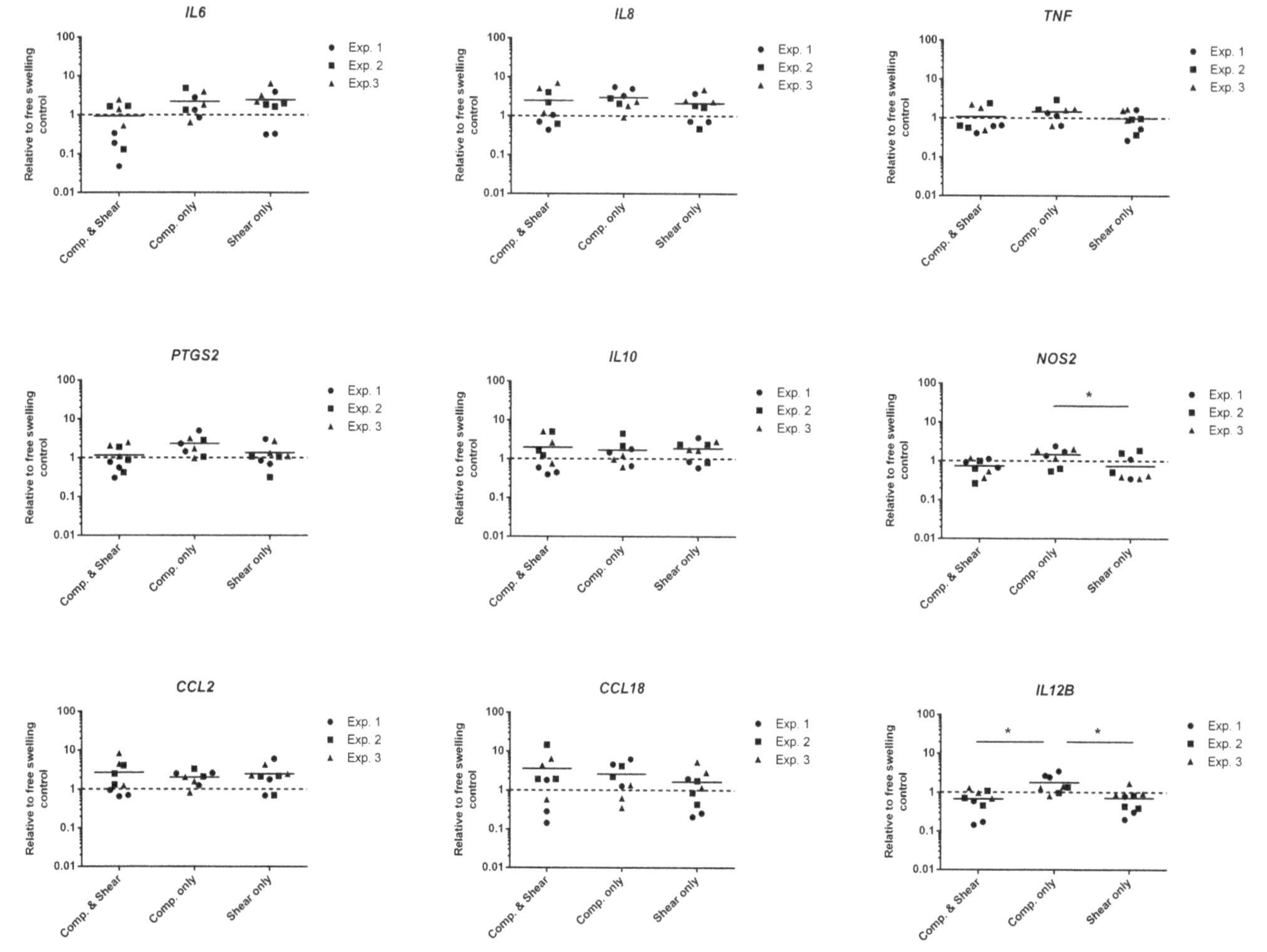

FIGURE 3 | Levels of inflammatory genes expressed by THP1-Blue monocytes in response to multiaxial loading, shear or compression alone. Gene expression by THP1-Blue monocytes following 3 days of multiaxial loading, shear, or compression alone as measured by real-time PCR. Gene expression levels were normalized to the free-swelling control, represented by the dashed line. Data is represented as dot plots including the median for three separate experiments, each assessed in experimental triplicate except for experiment 2 compression only group, which was assessed in duplicate. Statistical significance was determined by a Kruskal–Wallis test followed by Dunn's multiple comparisons test. $^*P < 0.05$. Comp, Compression.

marrow-derived mesenchymal stem cells (MSCs) (25). Furthermore, macrophage infiltration and prevalence of a M1-like phenotype has been observed in association with MSC-mediated bone repair *in vivo* (26, 27). In the present study, we have observed a skewing of monocyte activation toward a M1-like phenotype following 3 days of shear and compressive loading, highlighting the responsiveness of human monocytes to mechanical stimuli. These findings may shed some light on how the biomechanical environment may play a role in guiding monocyte/macrophage polarization, and potentially contribute to skeletal tissue repair.

In the present study, we have observed an increase in TNF-α, MIP-1α, and IL-13 protein production by unstimulated as well as LPS and IFN-γ and IL-4 activated monocytes following mechanical shear and compression. Two of four donors in the unstimulated group also substantially increased IL-6 production upon loading. Furthermore, levels of the pro-inflammatory cytokines IL-1β, IL-8, and IL-6 produced by IL-4 activated monocytes were increased following loading. Additionally, gene expression levels of IL-8 and IL-6 were increased by unstimulated primary human monocytes subjected to the combination of mechanical compression and shear. This could indicate that these factors would be induced within an unstable fracture. Previous reports have highlighted an influence of mechanical stimuli resulting from fracture fixation stability upon gene expression of matrix metalloproteinase (MMP)-9 and MMP-13 by fracture hematoma in rats (28). Both MMP-9 and MMP-13 are known to play a key role during the process of endochondral bone formation, facilitating extracellular matrix and cell migration (29). Additional studies have demonstrated an upregulation in the expression of genes involved in cartilage and skeletal development by callus tissue following mechanical stimulation, in a rat osteotomy model (30). However, the impact of mechanical stimuli upon the induction of inflammatory

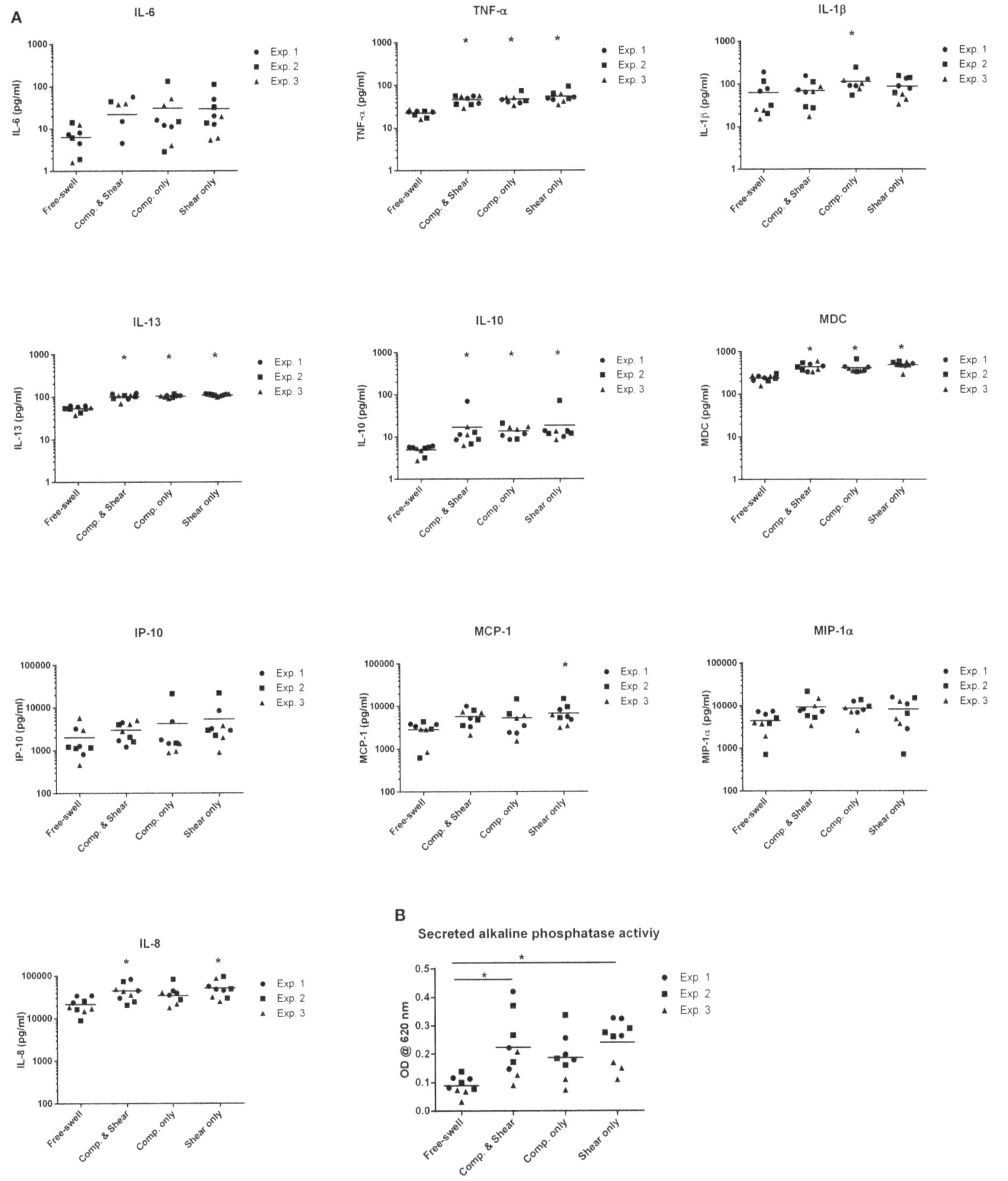

FIGURE 4 | Shear and compression differentially regulate inflammatory mediator expression by THP1-Blue monocytes. **(A)** Levels of inflammatory mediators produced by THP1-Blue monocytes following 3 days of multiaxial loading, shear or compression alone as measured by ELISA and multiplex assay. Protein levels were normalized to the free-swelling control, represented by the dashed line. Data is represented as dot plots including the median for 3 separate experiments, each assessed in experimental triplicate except for experiment 2 compression only group, which was assessed in duplicate. **(B)** SEAP levels detected in cell culture supernatant following 3 days of loading, as measured by spectrophotometric measurement. Statistical significance was determined by a Kruskal–Wallis test followed by Dunn's multiple comparisons test. *$P < 0.05$. IL-6, Interleukin-6; IL-10, Interleukin-10; CCL18, chemokine (C-C motif) ligand 18; TNF-α, Tumor necrosis factor-α; MIP-1α, Macrophage inflammatory protein-1α; IP-10, C-X-C motif chemokine 10; MCP-1, Monocyte chemoattractant protein-1; IL-13, Interleukin-13; MDC, Macrophage-derived chemokine; IL-1β, Interleukin-1β; IL-8, Interleukin-8; Comp, Compression.

gene expression by fracture hematoma *in vivo* requires further investigation. Production of IL-6 and TNF-α is characteristic of activated monocytes and pro-inflammatory M1 macrophages (5, 31). Both IL-6 and TNF-α signaling are known to play a key role in bone fracture healing (32, 33). Additionally, TNF-α is involved in osteoclastic bone resorption (34). Interestingly, in addition to acting as a chemotactic cytokine for monocytes and neutrophils, IL-8 has been reported by Ringe et al. to induce migration of human MSCs (35, 36). Furthermore, IL-8 is known to promote angiogenesis (37, 38). Mechanical stimulation of early human fracture hematoma has also been previously reported to result in increased production of the pro-angiogenic protein vascular endothelial growth factor (VEGF) (39). MIP-1α, also known as CCL3, has been previously implicated in the recruitment of macrophages to the site of injury during bone repair (40). In contrast to the observed upregulation of pro-inflammatory mediators by monocytes in response to mechanical loading, we also detected increased levels of IL-13 protein irrespective of cell activation with LPS and IFN-γ or IL-4. The pleiotropic cytokine IL-13 is known to polarize macrophages toward an M2 phenotype, encompassing anti-inflammatory and tissue repair subsets (41). Additionally, IL-13 is a key mediator of tissue fibrosis, reported to stimulate transforming growth factor (TGF)-β1 production by monocytes and macrophages, as well as increasing TGF-β1 activation (42, 43). TGF-β signaling may promote extracellular matrix deposition and tissue remodeling (44, 45). In addition to mediating tissue fibrosis and macrophage polarization, a role for IL-13 in osteoclast differentiation and bone resorption has been previously highlighted (46). Macrophages have been previously reported to change their phenotype throughout the course of bone healing, with a more predominant role of the M2 subset identified at later stages of repair (7). Given that in the current study loading of monocytes also resulted in production of the M2-polarization factor IL-13, whether a longer duration of loading may switch the balance from M1/M2 requires further investigation.

Having identified an influence of mechanical loading upon the phenotype of M1 or M2-differentiated as well as undifferentiated primary human monocytes, we next sought to investigate whether shear forces or compression alone may be responsible for this effect. In addition to compressive loading, cartilage in the articulating joint and fractures that have not been rigidly fixated, are also subjected to shear. Therefore, we next sought to examine whether shear or compression alone may exert differential effects on undifferentiated monocytes, to gain further insight into whether loading associated with various skeletal tissues may differentially modulate monocyte activation. The human monocyte cell line THP1-Blue™ was utilized to assess the effect of shear, compression or the combination of both on inflammatory mediator expression by monocytes. THP1-Blue™ cells are a reporter cell line, which express secreted embryonic alkaline phosphatase (SEAP) following activation of the transcription factors NF-κB and AP-1. Both NF-κB and AP-1 are activated in monocytes following toll-like receptor 4 (TLR4) stimulation and are involved in the induction of inflammatory gene expression (47). In a similar manner to primary human monocytes, the application of both compression and shear increased expression of inflammatory mediators TNF-α, IL-13, macrophage-derived chemokine (MDC), and IL-10. Interestingly, IL-10 is an anti-inflammatory cytokine but is also produced by monocytes in response to pro-inflammatory stimulation a part of a regulatory feedback mechanism (48). Furthermore, IL-10 is a factor also known to induce the differentiation of macrophages toward an anti-inflammatory phenotype (5). MDC is chemotactic for monocytes and is also considered a marker of M2 macrophages (49, 50). Additionally, we observed differential effects of compression or shear alone on monocyte phenotype. Application of compression alone increased expression of the pro-inflammatory genes *IL12B* and *NOS2* compared to shear alone or the combination of both stimuli. Interestingly, inducible nitric oxide synthase, which is encoded by the gene *NOS2*, has been previously shown to be expressed the initial phase of bone fracture repair (51). Compression alone also significantly increased IL-1β production compared to control, whereas shear alone was found to increase MCP-1. Furthermore, stimulation with both compression and shear or shear alone significantly increased SEAP expression compared to free-swelling controls, suggestive of potential TLR4 activation by monocytes in response to shear force (47). TLR4 has been previously implicated in the pro-inflammatory response of chondrocytes to high fluid shear, and increasing evidence highlights a role of TLR4 activation in inflammatory and catabolic processes associated with osteoarthritis pathogenesis (52–54). Our present findings may provide further insight to the mechanism of the effect of mechanical loading on monocyte activation, however further investigation is required to evaluate the effect of such mechanical stimuli directly on monocyte TLR expression and activation. These mechanically induced changes suggest that the initial monocyte containing hematoma would respond to mechanical motion by upregulating pro-inflammatory cytokines. This could be a danger signal that recruits cells to the site of damage and regulates their response. Rigid fixation would reduce this inflammatory signal leading to a different response. However, further investigation is required to fully determine the impact of mechanical stimuli resulting from fracture fixation stability upon monocyte behavior *in vivo*, and the subsequent influence of mechanically-stimulated monocytes upon skeletal tissue repair.

The findings of the present study highlight the mechanical sensitivity of human monocytes to skeletal tissue-associated loading conditions. Monocyte-derived macrophages have been previously shown to respond to mechanical strain *in vitro*, with an observed upregulation of MMP-1 and MMP-3 expression as well as the transcription factors c-fos and c-jun (55). Furthermore, Yang et al. highlighted a potential role of mechanical strain in the induction of monocyte to macrophage differentiation, mediated by upregulation of the monocyte differentiation-associated transcription factor PU.1 (55). In line with our findings, shear stress has also been shown to promote macrophage differentiation toward a pro-inflammatory M1-like phenotype in a model of atherosclerosis (56). Interestingly, extracellular physical cues resulting from surface stiffness have been reported to modulate TLR signaling by macrophages (57). However, whether these signaling pathways play a role in the responsiveness of monocytes and monocyte-derived macrophages to shear and compressive forces native to skeletal tissue requires further elucidation. This study has several limitations. Primary peripheral blood monocytes treated with LPS and IFN-γ or IL-4 were used as a model *in vitro* culture system to evaluate the effect of loading on M1 or M2-polarized cells, respectively. Investigation of the effect of mechanical loading on M1 and M2 pre-differentiated macrophages and a longer duration of study may be required to specifically examine the modulatory effect of mechanical loading on macrophage polarization state. Additionally, 2% agarose was used in this study as a cell-carrier system in our *in vitro* model to investigate the short-term response of human monocytes to skeletal tissue-associated mechanical stimuli. However, previous studies have highlighted an impact of different scaffold materials toward the cellular mechanical response (58). Therefore, further investigation may be required to determine whether monocyte interactions with different scaffold materials such as fibrin gels, as a more specific model of the wound healing phase of tissue repair, may determine their response to such mechanical stimuli. Furthermore, additional examination utilizing *in vivo* models of fracture healing is required to relate this observed induction of inflammatory mediators by mechanical loaded monocytes to skeletal tissue repair.

In conclusion, the findings of the present study indicate that human monocytes are responsive to mechanical stimuli, with a modulatory effect of shear and compressive loading observed toward pro-inflammatory mediator production. An in depth understanding of the impact of skeletal tissue-associated mechanical loading on monocyte behavior and their subsequent influence on local cellular responses and tissue repair processes, may identify novel strategies to maximize inflammation-mediated repair mechanisms. Furthermore, the findings of this study may provide insights for the development of novel rehabilitation medicine strategies to improve therapeutic outcome for skeletal tissue repair.

AUTHOR CONTRIBUTIONS

NF performed the experiments, processed samples, analyzed, and interpreted the data. UM processed samples and analyzed the data. MA supported in data analysis and interpretation. MS conceived and designed the study, and interpreted the data. NF, UM, MA, and MS drafted and critically revised the manuscript for important intellectual content. All authors have approved the final submitted manuscript.

FUNDING

This work was supported by the AO Foundation and the Swiss National Science Foundation (Grant no. 31003a_146375/1).

ACKNOWLEDGMENTS

We acknowledge the technical support of Dr. Reinhard Henschler and the team of Swiss Red Cross Blood Service Graubünden, CH-7000 Chur with buffy coats from whole blood donations.

REFERENCES

1. Claes L, Recknagel S, Ignatius A. Fracture healing under healthy and inflammatory conditions. *Nat Rev Rheumatol.* (2012) 8:133–43. doi: 10.1038/nrrheum.2012.1
2. Sanchez-Adams J, Leddy HA, McNulty AL, O'Conor CJ, Guilak F. The mechanobiology of articular cartilage: bearing the burden of osteoarthritis. *Curr Rheumatol Rep.* (2014) 16:451. doi: 10.1007/s11926-014-0451-6
3. Johnson K, Aarden L, Choi Y, De Groot E, Creasey A. The proinflammatory cytokine response to coagulation and endotoxin in whole blood. *Blood.* (1996) 87:5051–60.
4. Altieri DC. Proteases and protease receptors in modulation of leukocyte effector functions. *J Leukocyte Biol.* (1995) 58:120–7. doi: 10.1002/jlb.58.2.120
5. Mosser DM, Edwards JP. Exploring the full spectrum of macrophage activation. *Nat Rev Immunol.* (2008) 8:958–69. doi: 10.1038/nri2448
6. Murray PJ, Allen JE, Biswas SK, Fisher EA, Gilroy DW, Goerdt S, et al. Macrophage activation and polarization: nomenclature and experimental guidelines. *Immunity.* (2014) 41:14–20. doi: 10.1016/j.immuni.2014.06.008
7. Schlundt C, El Khassawna T, Serra A, Dienelt A, Wendler S, Schell H, et al. Macrophages in bone fracture healing: their essential role in endochondral ossification. *Bone.* (2018) 106:78–89. doi: 10.1016/j.bone.2015.10.019
8. Raggatt LJ, Wullschleger ME, Alexander KA, Wu AC, Millard SM, Kaur S, et al. Fracture healing via periosteal callus formation requires macrophages for both initiation and progression of early endochondral ossification. *Am J Pathol.* (2014) 184:3192–204. doi: 10.1016/j.ajpath.2014.08.017
9. Vi L, Baht GS, Whetstone H, Ng A, Wei Q, Poon R, et al. Macrophages promote osteoblastic differentiation *in-vivo*: implications in fracture repair and bone homeostasis. *J Bone Miner Res.* (2015) 30:1090–102. doi: 10.1002/jbmr.2422
10. Gerstenfeld LC, Cullinane DM, Barnes GL, Graves DT, Einhorn TA. Fracture healing as a post-natal developmental process: molecular, spatial, and temporal aspects of its regulation. *J Cell Biochem.* (2003) 88:873–84. doi: 10.1002/jcb.10435
11. Gerstenfeld LC, Cho TJ, Kon T, Aizawa T, Cruceta J, Graves BD, et al. Impaired intramembranous bone formation during bone repair in the absence of tumor necrosis factor-alpha signaling. *Cells Tissues Organs.* (2001) 169:285–94. doi: 10.1159/000047893
12. Westacott CI, Barakat AF, Wood L, Perry MJ, Neison P, Bisbinas I, et al. Tumor necrosis factor alpha can contribute to focal loss of cartilage in osteoarthritis. *Osteoarthr Cartil.* (2000) 8:213–21. doi: 10.1053/joca.1999.0292
13. Shakibaei M, John T, Schulze-Tanzil G, Lehmann I, Mobasheri A. Suppression of NF-kappaB activation by curcumin leads to inhibition of expression of cyclo-oxygenase-2 and matrix metalloproteinase-9 in human articular chondrocytes: implications for the treatment of osteoarthritis. *Biochem Pharmacol.* (2007) 73:1434–45. doi: 10.1016/j.bcp.2007.01.005
14. Johnson K, Hashimoto S, Lotz M, Pritzker K, Terkeltaub R. Interleukin-1 induces pro-mineralizing activity of cartilage tissue transglutaminase and factor XIIIa. *Am J Pathol.* (2001) 159:149–63. doi: 10.1016/S0002-9440(10)61682-3
15. Hoemann CD, Chen G, Marchand C, Tran-Khanh N, Thibault M, Chevrier A, et al. Scaffold-guided subchondral bone repair: implication

of neutrophils and alternatively activated arginase-1+ macrophages. *Am J Sports Med.* (2010) 38:1845–56. doi: 10.1177/0363546510369547
16. Hibino N, Yi T, Duncan DR, Rathore A, Dean E, Naito Y, et al. A critical role for macrophages in neovessel formation and the development of stenosis in tissue-engineered vascular grafts. *FASEB J.* (2011) 25:4253–63. doi: 10.1096/fj.11-186585
17. Arras M, Ito WD, Scholz D, Winkler B, Schaper J, Schaper W. Monocyte activation in angiogenesis and collateral growth in the rabbit hindlimb. *J Clin Invest.* (1998) 101:40–50. doi: 10.1172/JCI119877
18. Blomgran P, Blomgran R, Ernerudh J, Aspenberg P. A possible link between loading, inflammation and healing: immune cell populations during tendon healing in the rat. *Sci Rep.* (2016) 6:29824. doi: 10.1038/srep29824
19. Wimmer MA, Grad S, Kaup T, Hanni M, Schneider E, Gogolewski S, et al. Tribology approach to the engineering and study of articular cartilage. *Tissue Eng.* (2004) 10:1436–45. doi: 10.1089/ten.2004.10.1436
20. Neumann AJ, Gardner OF, Williams R, Alini M, Archer CW, Stoddart MJ. Human articular cartilage progenitor cells are responsive to mechanical stimulation and adenoviral-mediated overexpression of bone-morphogenetic protein 2. *PLoS ONE.* (2015) 10:e0136229. doi: 10.1371/journal.pone.0136229
21. Li Z, Kupcsik L, Yao SJ, Alini M, Stoddart MJ. Mechanical load modulates chondrogenesis of human mesenchymal stem cells through the TGF-beta pathway. *J Cell Mol Med.* (2010) 14:1338–46. doi: 10.1111/j.1582-4934.2009.00780.x
22. Ballotta V, Driessen-Mol A, Bouten CV, Baaijens FP. Strain-dependent modulation of macrophage polarization within scaffolds. *Biomaterials.* (2014) 35:4919–28. doi: 10.1016/j.biomaterials.2014.03.002
23. Hoff P, Gaber T, Strehl C, Schmidt-Bleek K, Lang A, Huscher D, et al. Immunological characterization of the early human fracture hematoma. *Immunol Res.* (2016) 64:1195–206. doi: 10.1007/s12026-016-8868-9
24. Xing Z, Lu C, Hu D, Yu YY, Wang X, Colnot C, et al. Multiple roles for CCR2 during fracture healing. *Dis Models Mech.* (2010) 3:451–8. doi: 10.1242/dmm.003186
25. Guihard P, Danger Y, Brounais B, David E, Brion R, Delecrin J, et al. Induction of osteogenesis in mesenchymal stem cells by activated monocytes/macrophages depends on oncostatin M signaling. *Stem Cells.* (2012) 30:762–72. doi: 10.1002/stem.1040
26. Tour G, Wendel M, Tcacencu I. Bone marrow stromal cells enhance the osteogenic properties of hydroxyapatite scaffolds by modulating the foreign body reaction. *J Tissue Eng Regen Med.* (2014) 8:841–9. doi: 10.1002/term.1574
27. Gamblin AL, Brennan MA, Renaud A, Yagita H, Lezot F, Heymann D, et al. Bone tissue formation with human mesenchymal stem cells and biphasic calcium phosphate ceramics: the local implication of osteoclasts and macrophages. *Biomaterials.* (2014) 35:9660–7. doi: 10.1016/j.biomaterials.2014.08.018
28. Ode A, Duda GN, Geissler S, Pauly S, Ode JE, Perka C, et al. Interaction of age and mechanical stability on bone defect healing: an early transcriptional analysis of fracture hematoma in rat. *PLoS ONE.* (2014) 9:e106462. doi: 10.1371/journal.pone.0106462
29. Ortega N, Behonick D, Stickens D, Werb Z. How proteases regulate bone morphogenesis. *Ann N Y Acad Sci.* (2003) 995:109–16. doi: 10.1111/j.1749-6632.2003.tb03214.x
30. Salisbury Palomares KT, Gerstenfeld LC, Wigner NA, Lenburg ME, Einhorn TA, Morgan EF. Transcriptional profiling and biochemical analysis of mechanically induced cartilaginous tissues in a rat model. *Arthritis Rheum.* (2010) 62:1108–18. doi: 10.1002/art.27343
31. Agbanoma G, Li C, Ennis D, Palfreeman AC, Williams LM, Brennan FM. Production of TNF-alpha in macrophages activated by T cells, compared with lipopolysaccharide, uses distinct IL-10-dependent regulatory mechanism. *J Immunol.* (2012) 188:1307–17. doi: 10.4049/jimmunol.1100625
32. Gerstenfeld LC, Cho TJ, Kon T, Aizawa T, Tsay A, Fitch J, et al. Impaired fracture healing in the absence of TNF-alpha signaling: the role of TNF-alpha in endochondral cartilage resorption. *J Bone Miner Res.* (2003) 18:1584–92. doi: 10.1359/jbmr.2003.18.9.1584
33. Yang X, Ricciardi BF, Hernandez-Soria A, Shi Y, Pleshko Camacho N, Bostrom MP. Callus mineralization and maturation are delayed during fracture healing in interleukin-6 knockout mice. *Bone.* (2007) 41:928–36. doi: 10.1016/j.bone.2007.07.022
34. Bertolini DR, Nedwin GE, Bringman TS, Smith DD, Mundy GR. Stimulation of bone resorption and inhibition of bone formation *in vitro* by human tumour necrosis factors. *Nature.* (1986) 319:516–8. doi: 10.1038/319516a0
35. Mukaida N. Pathophysiological roles of interleukin-8/CXCL8 in pulmonary diseases. *Am J Physiol Lung Cell Mol Physiol.* (2003) 284:L566–77. doi: 10.1152/ajplung.00233.2002
36. Ringe J, Strassburg S, Neumann K, Endres M, Notter M, Burmester GR, et al. Towards *in situ* tissue repair: human mesenchymal stem cells express chemokine receptors CXCR1, CXCR2 and CCR2, and migrate upon stimulation with CXCL8 but not CCL2. *J Cell Biochem.* (2007) 101:135–46. doi: 10.1002/jcb.21172
37. Brat DJ, Bellail AC, Van Meir EG. The role of interleukin-8 and its receptors in gliomagenesis and tumoral angiogenesis. *Neuro Oncol.* (2005) 7:122–33. doi: 10.1215/S1152851704001061
38. Li A, Dubey S, Varney ML, Dave BJ, Singh RK. IL-8 directly enhanced endothelial cell survival, proliferation, and matrix metalloproteinases production and regulated angiogenesis. *J Immunol.* (2003) 170:3369–76. doi: 10.4049/jimmunol.170.6.3369
39. Groothuis A, Duda GN, Wilson CJ, Thompson MS, Hunter MR, Simon P, et al. Mechanical stimulation of the pro-angiogenic capacity of human fracture haematoma: involvement of VEGF mechano-regulation. *Bone.* (2010) 47:438–44. doi: 10.1016/j.bone.2010.05.026
40. Kawao N, Tamura Y, Horiuchi Y, Okumoto K, Yano M, Okada K, et al. The tissue fibrinolytic system contributes to the induction of macrophage function and CCL3 during bone repair in mice. *PLoS ONE.* (2015) 10:e0123982. doi: 10.1371/journal.pone.0123982
41. Van Dyken SJ, Locksley RM. Interleukin-4- and interleukin-13-mediated alternatively activated macrophages: roles in homeostasis and disease. *Ann Rev Immunol.* (2013) 31:317–43. doi: 10.1146/annurev-immunol-032712-095906
42. Fichtner-Feigl S, Strober W, Kawakami K, Puri RK, Kitani A. IL-13 signaling through the IL-13alpha2 receptor is involved in induction of TGF-beta1 production and fibrosis. *Nat Med.* (2006) 12:99–106. doi: 10.1038/nm1332
43. Lee CG, Homer RJ, Zhu Z, Lanone S, Wang X, Koteliansky V, et al. Interleukin-13 induces tissue fibrosis by selectively stimulating and activating transforming growth factor beta(1). *J Exp Med.* (2001) 194:809–21. doi: 10.1084/jem.194.6.809
44. Burns WC, Twigg SM, Forbes JM, Pete J, Tikellis C, Thallas-Bonke V, et al. Connective tissue growth factor plays an important role in advanced glycation end product-induced tubular epithelial-to-mesenchymal transition: implications for diabetic renal disease. *J Am Soc Nephrol.* (2006) 17:2484–94. doi: 10.1681/ASN.2006050525
45. Zhu Z, Homer RJ, Wang Z, Chen Q, Geba GP, Wang J, et al. Pulmonary expression of interleukin-13 causes inflammation, mucus hypersecretion, subepithelial fibrosis, physiologic abnormalities, and eotaxin production. *J Clin Invest.* (1999) 103:779–88. doi: 10.1172/JCI5909
46. Palmqvist P, Lundberg P, Persson E, Johansson A, Lundgren I, Lie A, et al. Inhibition of hormone and cytokine-stimulated osteoclastogenesis and bone resorption by interleukin-4 and interleukin-13 is associated with increased osteoprotegerin and decreased RANKL and RANK in a STAT6-dependent pathway. *J Biol Chem.* (2006) 281:2414–29. doi: 10.1074/jbc.M510160200
47. Guha M, Mackman N. LPS induction of gene expression in human monocytes. *Cell Signal.* (2001) 13:85–94. doi: 10.1016/S0898-6568(00)00149-2
48. Donnelly RP, Freeman SL, Hayes MP. Inhibition of IL-10 expression by IFN-gamma up-regulates transcription of TNF-alpha in human monocytes. *J Immunol.* (1995) 155:1420–7.
49. Godiska R, Chantry D, Raport CJ, Sozzani S, Allavena P, Leviten D, et al. Human macrophage-derived chemokine (MDC), a novel chemoattractant for monocytes, monocyte-derived dendritic cells, and natural killer cells. *J Exp Med.* (1997) 185:1595–604. doi: 10.1084/jem.185.9.1595
50. Jaguin M, Houlbert N, Fardel O, Lecureur V. Polarization profiles of human M-CSF-generated macrophages and comparison of M1-markers in classically activated macrophages from GM-CSF and M-CSF origin. *Cell Immunol.* (2013) 281:51–61. doi: 10.1016/j.cellimm.2013.01.010
51. Zhu W, Diwan AD, Lin JH, Murrell GA. Nitric oxide synthase isoforms during fracture healing. *J Bone Miner Res.* (2001) 16:535–40. doi: 10.1359/jbmr.2001.16.3.535

52. Wang P, Zhu F, Tong Z, Konstantopoulos K. Response of chondrocytes to shear stress: antagonistic effects of the binding partners Toll-like receptor 4 and caveolin-1. *FASEB J.* (2011) 25:3401–15. doi: 10.1096/fj.11-184861
53. Kim HA, Cho ML, Choi HY, Yoon CS, Jhun JY, Oh HJ, et al. The catabolic pathway mediated by Toll-like receptors in human osteoarthritic chondrocytes. *Arthritis Rheum.* (2006) 54:2152–63. doi: 10.1002/art.21951
54. Bobacz K, Sunk IG, Hofstaetter JG, Amoyo L, Toma CD, Akira S, et al. Toll-like receptors and chondrocytes: the lipopolysaccharide-induced decrease in cartilage matrix synthesis is dependent on the presence of toll-like receptor 4 and antagonized by bone morphogenetic protein 7. *Arthritis Rheum.* (2007) 56:1880–93. doi: 10.1002/art.22637
55. Yang JH, Sakamoto H, Xu EC, Lee RT. Biomechanical regulation of human monocyte/macrophage molecular function. *Am J Pathol.* (2000) 156:1797–804. doi: 10.1016/S0002-9440(10)65051-1
56. Seneviratne AN, Cole JE, Goddard ME, Park I, Mohri Z, Sansom S, et al. Low shear stress induces M1 macrophage polarization in murine thin-cap atherosclerotic plaques. *J Mol Cell Cardiol.* (2015) 89(Pt B):168–72. doi: 10.1016/j.yjmcc.2015.10.034
57. Gruber E, Heyward C, Cameron J, Leifer C. Toll-like receptor signaling in macrophages is regulated by extracellular substrate stiffness and Rho-associated coiled-coil kinase (ROCK1/2). *Int Immunol.* (2018) 30:267–78. doi: 10.1093/intimm/dxy027
58. Hunter CJ, Mouw JK, Levenston ME. Dynamic compression of chondrocyte-seeded fibrin gels: effects on matrix accumulation and mechanical stiffness. *Osteoarthr Cartil.* (2004) 12:117–30. doi: 10.1016/j.joca.2003.08.009

8

Immune Modulation to Enhance Bone Healing—A New Concept to Induce Bone Using Prostacyclin to Locally Modulate Immunity

Sebastian Wendler[1,2†], *Claudia Schlundt*[1,2†], *Christian H. Bucher*[1,2], *Jan Birkigt*[3], *Christian J. Schipp*[1‡], *Hans-Dieter Volk*[2,4], *Georg N. Duda*[1,2,5] and *Katharina Schmidt-Bleek*[1,2*]

[1] Julius Wolff Institute and Center for Musculoskeletal Surgery, Charité–Universitätsmedizin Berlin, Berlin, Germany, [2] Berlin-Brandenburg Center for Regenerative Therapies, Charité–Universitätsmedizin Berlin, Berlin, Germany, [3] Department of Isotope Biogeochemistry, Helmholtz Centre for Environmental Research–UFZ, Leipzig, Germany, [4] Institute of Medical Immunology, Charité–Universitätsmedizin Berlin, Berlin, Germany, [5] Berlin Institute of Health Center for Regenerative Therapies, Berlin, Germany

***Correspondence:**
Katharina Schmidt-Bleek
katharina.schmidt-bleek@charite.de

† These authors shared first authorship

‡ Present Address:
Christian J. Schipp,
Department of Isotope Biogeochemistry, Helmholtz Centre for Environmental Research–UFZ, Leipzig, Germany

Within an aging population, fracture incidences will rise and with the augmented risks of impaired healing the overall risk of delayed bone regeneration will substantially increase in elderly patients. Thus, new strategies to rescue fracture healing in the elderly are highly warranted. Modulating the initial inflammatory phase toward a reduced pro-inflammation launches new treatment options for delayed or impaired healing specifically in the elderly. Here, we evaluated the capacity of the prostacyclin analog Iloprost to modulate the inflammatory phase toward a pro-regenerative milieu using *in vitro* as well as *in vivo* model systems. *In vitro*, Iloprost administration led to a downregulation of potential unfavorable CD8+ cytotoxic T cells as well as their pro-inflammatory cytokine secretion profile. Furthermore, Iloprost increased the mineralization capacity of osteogenic induced mesenchymal stromal cells through both direct as well as indirect cues. In an *in vivo* approach, Iloprost, embedded in a biphasic fibrin scaffold, decreased the pro-inflammatory and simultaneously enhanced the anti-inflammatory phase thereby improving bone healing outcome. Overall, our presented data confirms a possible strategy to modulate the early inflammatory phase in aged individuals toward a physiological healing by a downregulation of an excessive pro-inflammation that otherwise would impair healing. Further confirmation in phase I/II trials, however, is needed to validate the concept in a broader clinical evaluation.

Keywords: bone healing, immune modulation, prostacyclin analog, T cell, macrophage, immune cell, Iloprost

INTRODUCTION

Bone is one of the few tissues in the human body capable of regenerative, scar-free healing. Thus, a bony injury can result in complete restoration of form and function, a restitutio ad integrum. However, the complex bone healing process consisting of sequential, partly overlapping phases is prone to failure (1–4). Even in today's medical routine 5–10% of fracture patients suffer from delayed healing or a resulting non-union (5–7). Therefore, impaired bone repair after injury is still a clinically relevant problem, which will even further increase in the overall aging population

(8). Thus, a better and deeper understanding of the underlying biological mechanisms under unimpaired healing conditions is necessary for the development of novel therapeutic treatment strategies to improve unsuccessful bone regeneration.

The tight interaction of the immune system and bone healing has been recognized in the emerging research field of osteoimmunology. Especially the early phase of healing, the inflammatory phase seems to be a promising target for immunomodulatory approaches to enhance bone healing (9, 10). The pro-inflammatory reaction following injury (11) is an essential trigger or initiator of the healing process. However, a pronounced or prolonged pro-inflammatory reaction (due to a lack or damped anti-inflammatory phase) will negatively impact the healing process (12–14). Recently, specific subsets of the immune system have been shown to negatively influence bone formation: Effector and effector memory CD8+ T cells are producers of TNFα (tumor necrosis factor alpha) and IFNγ (interferon gamma), highly pro-inflammatory cytokines which have been found to deter osteogenic differentiation (15). Therefore, downregulation of the negative influence of immune cell subsets could potentially enhance bone healing. Anti-inflammatory cytokines such as interleukin (IL) 4/IL-13 further the M2/Th2 response, thus promoting the immune response triggered by tissue injury under a regulatory phenotype rather than a M1/Th1 pro-inflammatory phenotype. A proof of concept study showed that applying IL-4/IL-13 during the initial bone healing phase could indeed enhance bone formation (16). However, a distinct initiation of an anti-inflammation has not been evaluated so far.

Within this study, a prostacyclin (PGI_2) analog was tested as a possible immune modulatory drug to enhance bone formation. PGI_2 is a small molecule derived from arachidonic acid by cyclooxygenase-2 (Cox-2) and prostacyclin synthase. Endogenous PGI_2 is already well-known playing an important role in cardiovascular diseases due its vasodilatory function (17, 18). In recent years, a potential role of PGI_2 as immune modulatory agent was detected by promoting an anti-inflammatory and immunosuppressive effect (19, 20). In particular, the PGI_2 receptor (IP) is present on platelets, medullary thymocytes, neutrophils, dendritic cells, eosinophils, T regulatory cells, and activated T cells (21, 22). Thus, PGI_2 has an impact on both, cells of the innate, and of the adaptive immunity. Due to the strong interconnectivity of the immune system and the skeletal system during bone regeneration, PGI2 could represent a potential and promising agent to further bone fracture healing. In the context of bone injuries, the PGI2 analog Iloprost was already successfully used to treat bone marrow edema and avascular necrosis (23, 24). However, the effect of PGI_2 on the process of bone formation/regeneration was not analyzed by any study so far. In the here presented study, we investigated the immune modulatory effect of PGI_2 in the context of bone regeneration. Since the half-life of endogenous PGI_2 is very short, the PGI_2 analog Iloprost was used. Iloprost is approved as treatment for pulmonary arterial hypertension (25) and peripheral arterial occlusive disease (26), respectively. Within the here presented study, we focused on the immune suppressive capacities of Iloprost, especially on CD8+ T cells and macrophages. Immune modulatory properties were confirmed and the postulated positive osteogenic effect was verified *in vitro*. In a final proof of concept *in vivo* trial, the positive impact of an application of Iloprost during the early bone healing phase was demonstrated in a mouse osteotomy model.

MATERIALS AND METHODS

Animal Model

Female C57BL/6N (Charles River Laboratories, Wilmington, MA, USA) were used for the analysis of the bone healing capacity *in vivo*. All mice were purchased at an age of 8 weeks and mice were housed in small groups in our animal facility. Animals were kept for at least 4 weeks in the non-SPF area of the animal facility (area in the animal facility without filtered air supply for the cages and without additional barrier) to allow a higher environmental pathogen exposure to challenge and to moderately activate the adaptive immune system of the animals. All mice experiments were carried out with the ethical permission according to the principles and policies established by the Animal Welfare Act, the National Institutes of Health Guide for Care and Use of Laboratory Animals, and the National Animal Welfare Guidelines. All animal experiments were approved by the local legal representative animal rights protection authorities (Landesamt for Gesundheit und Soziales Berlin: G0008/12; T0119/14; T0249/11). All results are reported according the ARRIVE guidelines.

Sample Harvesting for the *in vitro* Analysis With Immune Cells

For the immunomodulatory analysis *in vitro*, femora, and humeri were harvested from C57BL/6N mice. To isolate the bone marrow, the epiphyses were cut off from the bones and the bone marrow was flashed out into RPMI 1640 media (Biochrom, Berlin, Germany). The bone marrow was pushed through a 40 μm cell strainer to get a single cell suspension. Residing erythrocytes were lysed for 4 min at room temperature (RT) in ACK lysing buffer (Gibco Life Technologies GmbH, Darmstadt, Germany). After centrifugation, cells were resuspended in 10 ml RPMI 1640 media and counted.

Isolation of CD8+ T Cells

CD8+ T cells were isolated from bones harvested from C57BL/6N mice. The isolation was performed via the *CD8 S-pluriBeads anti-ms* kit (pluriSelect Life Sciences, Leipzig, Germany). The isolation was carried out following the manufacturer's instructions. Briefly, complete bone marrow cells were resuspended in a 1:2 mixture of the isolation and wash buffer and 40 μl S-pluriBeads were added per 1 x 10^6 target cells and the mixture was incubated for 30 min at RT while continuous slowly shaking (horizontal roller mixer). Cell mixture was washed trough a S-pluriStrainer and target cells remained on the S-pluriStrainer. To detach the CD8+ T cells from the S-pluriBeads, detachment activation buffer D was added to the cells. Detached isolated cells were collected in a new tube, washed, and counted.

The purity of the isolated CD8+ T cells was confirmed by flow cytometry. The following antibodies were used: Life/Dead, α-CD3 PerCP, α-CD4 AF700, and α-CD8 eF450. The incubation with the antibodies was done on ice for 20 min. After the staining, cells were washed, fixed, and analyzed with a flow cytometer LSR II (Becton Dickinson Bioscience, Heidelberg, Germany).

Study Design for the *in vitro* Analysis of the Osteogenic and Osteoimmunological Effect of Iloprost

The objective of this study was to investigate the potential of the prostacyclin analoque Iloprost to improve bone healing. For this analysis, the osteogenic and osteoimmunological effect of Iloprost was first evaluated *in vitro*. Subsequently, Iloprost was inserted into a fibrin clot in order to confirm the pro-osteogenic potential of Iloprost in an *in vivo* proof of concept approach in a mouse osteotomy model. For the *in vitro* analysis, Iloprost was directly added to the osteogenic differentiation culture of bone marrow mesenchymal stromal cells (BM MSCs) isolated from the femur of C57BL/6N mice (**Figure 1**, left). To investigate an indirect effect of Iloprost on the mineralization capacity of osteogenic induced BM MSCs, all bone marrow cells or isolated CD8+ T cells from the bone marrow were stimulated with α-CD3/α-CD28 and the obtained conditioned media were added to the osteogenic differentiation culture of BM MSCs (**Figure 1**, right). The osteogenic differentiation was quantified based on mineralization by Alizarin Red staining.

Cell Stimulation for the Production of Conditioned Media

Bone marrow and isolated CD8+ T cells were stimulated by an α-CD3/α-CD28 stimulation for 2 days in 96 well-plates. The stimulation was performed in RPMI 1640 media supplemented with 10% fetal bovine serum (FBS), 1% penicillin/streptomycin (P/S), 50 μM β-mercaptoethanol, and 10 ng/ml IL-2. In the respective experimental setup, either PBS or 300 nM or 3 μM Iloprost were added to the culture. 5 x 10^5 cells in 225 μl were plated per well of a 96 well-plate. After the two stimulations, the supernatant was harvested (conditioned media) and stored at −80C.

Isolation and Polarization of Macrophages

1 x 10^6 isolated bone marrow cells were plated per well into a 96 well-plate and incubated for 3 days in RPMI complete media: RPMI 1640 supplemented with 50 ng/ml macrophage colony-stimulating factor (M-CSF), 1% P/S, 10% FBS, and 50 μM β-mercaptoethanol. Subsequently, RPMI complete media was replaced by the respective polarization media and cells were polarized for additional 3 days. For MΦ: RPMI complete media with PBS; M1: RPMI complete media with 20 ng/ml IFNγ and M2: 20 ng/ml IL-4/IL-13. The produced conditioned media was harvested and stored at −80°C. Macrophage monolayers were washed twice with PBS and fixed with 4% PFA/PBS for 10 min. Storage was done in PBS at 4°C for subsequent confirmation of polarization via immunofluorescence.

Immunofluorescence Staining of Polarized Macrophage Subsets

The immunofluorescence staining of polarized macrophages were realized on fixed cellular macrophage monolayers. Cells were shortly washed with PBS, permeabilized in 100 μl PBS supplemented with 0.1% Tween for 30 min and subsequently blocked for 30 min with PBS supplemented with 5% FBS. The following antibodies were used for the staining: α-CD68 FITC, α-CD206 PE, and α-CD80 AF647. Antibodies were incubated for 1 h in the dark at RT. Cells were washed with PBS and cell nuclei were stained with DAPI for 10 min in the dark at RT. Cell monolayers were washed twice with PBS and wells were kept at 4○C in the dark until imaging. Imaging was performed with a standard fluorescence microscope (Axio Observer, Carl Zeiss).

Investigation of the Immunomodulatory Effect of Iloprost

To investigate the immunomodulatory effect of Iloprost on immune cells, ELISA were performed analyzing the secretion of IFNγ, TNFα, and IL-10 as indicated. Frozen conditioned media were thawed and analyzed with respective ELISA kits following the manufacturer's protocol. ELISA was performed with a Mouse IFNγ ELISA Ready-SET-Go!®, Mouse TNFα ELISA Ready-SET-Go!®, and Mouse IL-10 ELISA Ready-SET-Go!® from eBioscience (Affymetrix, Santa Clara, CA USA). The samples were incubated at 4°C overnight. Final staining reactions were stopped with 1 M H_3PO_4 and absorbance values were acquired at 450 nm with a reference wavelength of 570 nm with Tecan Infinite M200 PRO (Tecan, Männedorf, Switzerland) and analyzed with i-control 1.9 software (Tecan, Männedorf, Switzerland).

Isolation and Cultivation of Mesenchymal Stromal Cells

At least 3 x 10^7 isolated bone marrow cells were cultured in expansion media: low glucose DMEM media supplemented with 10% FBS, 1% P/S, and 1% glutamax. Media exchange was performed twice a week to remove non-adherent cells until cultures were confluent. To detach the MSC monolayers, cells were washed once with PBS. TrypLE was added to the monolayer, incubated for 5 min at 37°C. The cell suspension was washed, centrifuged and the passaged cells were plated with increasing surface area.

Osteogenic Differentiation of MSCs and Quantification by Alizarin Red Staining

1.5 x 10^4 MSCs were seeded per well into a 96 well-plate. Cells were cultured in expansion media for 2 days. Subsequently, osteoinductive media was applied to the cells: low glucose DMEM media supplemented with 10% FBS, 100 nM dexamethasone, 10 mM β-glycerol phosphate, 50 μM L-ascorbate-2-phosphate, 1% P/S, and 1% glutamax. Osteogenic differentiation was stopped after 14 days including a media exchange every 3–4 days. When conditioned media of stimulated bone marrow or CD8+ T cells was supplemented, double concentrated osteoinductive media was mixed 1:2 with the respective conditioned media.

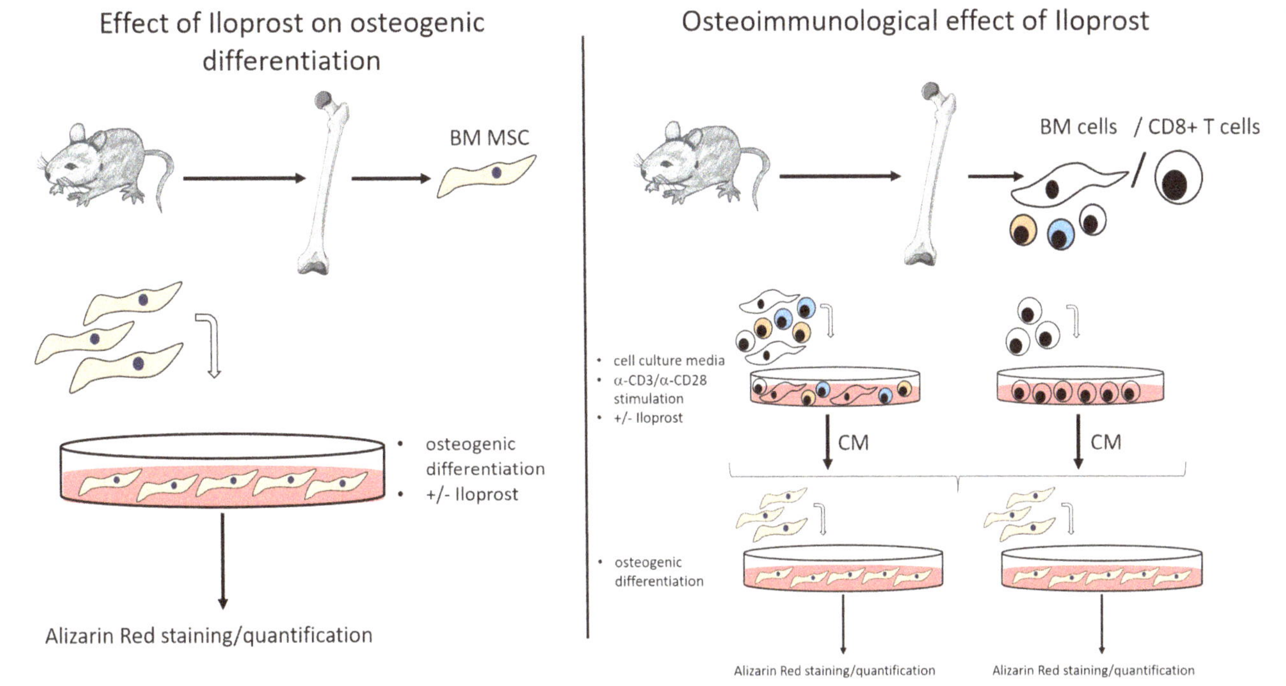

FIGURE 1 | Methodological scheme for the *in vitro* analysis of the osteogenic effect and osteoimmunological effect of Iloprost. BM MSC, bone marrow mesenchymal stromal cells; BM cells ,bone marrow cells; CM, conditioned media.

Alizarin Red staining was applied to quantify the osteogenic differentiation of the cultured MSCs. After a 14 days culture in osteoinductive media, well-plates were washed twice with PBS. Cell layers were fixed for 10 min at RT in 50 μl 4% paraformaldehyde/PBS (PFA/PBS). Cell nuclei were stained for DAPI for 10 min in the dark at RT. Cells were washed in ddH_2O and incubated with 0.5% Alizarin Red for 10 min at RT. Cells were washed five times with ddH_2O and cell layers were dried before imaging. For the quantification, Alizarin Red was detached with 10% cetylpyridinium chloride for 30 min at RT and optical density was measured and quantified with the plate reader Infinite M200 PRO (Tecan, Männedorf, Switzerland).

Chondrogenic Differentiation of MSCs and Quantification by Histomorphometry

3 x 10^5 MSCs were transferred into a 15 ml tube for the chondrogenic differentiation. Cells were centrifuged and chondrogenic induction media was carefully added to the cells without resuspension: high glucose DMEM media supplemented with 100 nM dexamethasone, 50 μg/ml L-ascorbate-2-phosphate, 350 μM L-proline, 2 mM sodium pyruvate, 6.25 μg/ml Insulin-transferrin-sodium selenite media supplement, 1.25 mg/ml bovine serum albumin, 5.35 μg/ml linoleic acid, 10 ng/ml TGF-β1, 10 ng/ml BMP-2, 1% P/S, and 1% glutamax. Pellets were cultured for 21 days under hypoxic conditions. Chondrogenic inductive media was changed twice a week.

For quantification, chondrogenic differentiated cell pellets were paraffin embedded, cut and stained with Alcian Blue (staining of the proteoglycans). Therefore, cell pellets were fixed for 2 h in 4% PFA/PBS, washed twice in PBS and dehydrated in an increasing alcohol series: 30 s in 70% EtOH, 20 min in 80% EtOH, 20 min 96% EtOH and twice 20 min in 100% EtOH. Cell pellets were incubated for 15 min in Xylol and subsequently paraffin embedded. Four micrometer thick sections were cut from three different areas of each pellet. Deparaffinized sections (incubation of the sections twice in Xylol for 10 min each and in a descending alcohol series) were washed in ddH_2O for 2 min, equilibrated in 3% acetic acid for 3 min, stained in 1% Alcian Blue for 45 min, washed in 3% acetic acid, washed in ddH_2O, and stained for cell nuclei in Nuclear Fast Red for 2 min. Pellets were shortly washed in ddH_2O and 70% EtOH. After an ascending alcohol series, pellets were incubated twice in Xylol, 10 min each, and embedded. Acquired images were quantified based on the blue values of bright field images.

Investigation of the Cellular Metabolic Activity by Prestoblue

Using the PrestoBlue Cell Viability Reagent (Thermo Fisher Scientific, Waltham, MA, USA), the metabolic activity of the stimulated cells was investigated after manufacturer's protocol. The reagent was diluted in RPMI complete media (for bone marrow cells) or low glucose DMEM (for MSCs), respectively, and applied to the cultured cells. After a 1 h incubation, the supernatant was collected and fluorescence top reading was performed at 560 nm excitation and 590 nm emission with the plate reader. For background correction, fluorescence values of no-cell control wells, which contained only reagent solution were averaged and subtracted from values of experimental wells.

Setting of an Osteotomy for the *in vivo* Analysis

The pro-regenerative potential of Iloprost was evaluated in a mouse osteotomy model. Therefore, mice were anesthetised by inhalation of Isoflurane. Before surgery, the animals received subcutaneous injection of the analgesic Buprenorphine (0.03 mg/kg s.c.) and of the antibiotic Clindamycin (0.02 ml s.c.). The operation area of the left femur was shaved and disinfected. The skin was opened by a longitudinal cut from the knee to the hip. The femur was bluntly exposed and stabilized by an external fixator (MouseExFix, RISystem AG, Davos, Switzerland). An osteotomy of 0.7 mm was introduced between the middle pins using a Gigli wire saw (RISystem AG, Davos, Switzerland). A biphasic fibrin clot (loaded with either 3 μM Iloprost or PBS) (Tissucol-kit Immuno, Baxter) was inserted into the osteotomy gap. The skin was closed and sutured. Mice were brought back to the cage and observed until they were fully mobile again. As post-operative analgesia, Tramadol hydrochloride (0.1 mg/ml) was added to the drinking water for 3 days.

Micro-Computed Tomography of Osteotomized Mouse Bones

To evaluate the healing outcome after Iloprost administration, fractured femora were harvested 21 days post-osteotomy and analyzed by μCT. Therefore, mice were euthanized by administering ketamine and xylazine (i.p., ketamine: 120 mg/kg, xylazine: 16 mg/kg) and cervical dislocation in deep anesthesia. After preparation of the femora, they were directly fixed in 4% PFA/PBS for 4 h at 4°C. Subsequently, the bones were dehydrated in an ascending sugar series: 10, 20, and 30%, for 24 h for each at 4°C. The bones were scanned in a μCT Viva 40 (SCANCO Medical AG, Brüttisellen, Switzerland). For the scan, the following parameters were used: 10.5 μm voxel size, 55keVp, and 145 uA. A gray value threshold was defined before analysis in order to be able to distinguish between mineralized and non-mineralized bone tissue (27). The global threshold for defining mineralized bone was set to 242, which corresponds to a mineralization of 369.9 mg hydroxyapatite (HA)/cm^2. The scanned volume of interest (VOI) included 190 slices around the middle of the fracture gap to the distal and proximal part of the femur, respectively. For the quantification of the μCT data, cortical bone was excluded from newly formed mineralized bone.

Histological and Immunohistological Analysis

For histological and immunohistological analysis, fractured bones were cryo embedded. Seven micrometer thick sections were cut and stained either for Movat's Pentachrome (overview staining) or the following cell types (immunofluorescence staining): CD4+ and CD8+ T cells, IFNγ-producing CD8+ T cells, osteoblasts, osteoclasts and differentially polarized macrophages.

The Movat pentachrome staining was done as follows: cryo-sections were thawed for 1 h at RT and fixed for 10 min in 4% PFA/PBS. Sections were washed twice in PBS/Tween-20 for 5 min. Subsequently, sections were incubated for 3 min in 3% acetic acid, for 30 min in 1% Alcian Blue/3% acetic acid, and differentiated for 5 min in 3% acetic acid. After washing in ddH_2O, sections were incubated for 1 h in ethyl alcohol, washed twice in tap water, shortly in ddH_2O and stained in iron hematoxylin (after Weigert) for 10 min. After washing with tap water, sections were incubated for 15 min in brilliant crocein-acid fuchsine. Tissue slides was shortly placed in 0.5% acidic acid, followed by a 20 min incubation in 5% phosphotungstic acid. After 1 min in 0.5% acetic acid, slides were incubated 3x à 5 min in 96% EtOH and stained with Saffron-du-Gatinais for 1 h. Subsequently, they were washed again 3x in 96% EtOH for 2 min each, 2x in Xylol for 10 min each and embedded.

Analysis of the immune cell subsets and osteoblasts, osteoclasts was done by immunofluorescence staining. All steps were performed at RT in a humidified chamber. Thawed cryo-sections were fixed for 20 min in 4% PFA/PBS/Tween-20 and washed twice with PBS/Tween-20. Sections were blocked in 1x TBS supplemented with 7% FBS and 0.05% Tween-20 for 1 h. Blocking buffer was decanted and the primary antibodies were applied to the respective section in the following combinations: (1) CD4+ and CD8+ T cells and osteoblasts: CD4 AF594, CD8 PE, osteocalcin; (2) IFNγ-producing CD8+ T cells: CD8 PE and IFNγ; and (3) differentially polarized macrophages: CD68 FITC, CD206 PE, and CD80 AF647. Tissue sections were washed in 1x TBS and, if necessary, incubated for 2 h with a secondary antibody: anti-rabbit AF647 for osteocalcin or anti-rat AF594 for IFNγ and for CD4. For the staining of osteoclasts, antigen retrieval was performed with ProteinaseK for 15 min on thawed cryo-sections. Sections were washed PBS/Tween-20 and fixed as described above. After washing and blocking, sections were stained for cathepsinK in 3.5% FBS, 0.025% Tween in tris-buffered saline (TBS) for 2 h. Sections were washed and stained for CD68 (FITC) and the secondary antibody for cathepsinK anti-rabbit AF647 in 3.5% FBS, 0.025% Tween in TBS for 2 h. Sections were washed, stained for cell nuclei with DAPI for 10 min and subsequently embedded. Sections were analyzed with a laser scanning microscope LSM 710 (Carl Zeiss AG, Oberkochen, Germany).

Statistics

The statistical evaluation of the presented data was done with the programs Graph Pad Prism and SPSS. Data were presented as dot plot graphs. Statistics were done by using the Mann-Whitney U test and data were statistically significant if $p \leq 0.05$. For comparison of more than two study groups the Bonferroni's *post-hoc* test was used.

RESULTS

Immunomodulatory Effects of Iloprost on Immune Cells

We first tested the immunomodulatory properties of Iloprost on murine immune and mesenchymal stromal cells (MSCs) *in vitro*.

Both, immune cells and MSCs are known to be essential for the early healing phase in bone regeneration.

In a first attempt, two different concentrations of Iloprost were tested on the whole bone marrow cellular composition: 300 nM and 3 μM. As readout, the secretion of the pro-inflammatory cytokines IFNγ and TNFα was analyzed. Both cytokines play an important role as signaling molecules in bone repair, especially in the early fracture healing phase. However, too high amounts of them negatively affect bone repair by diminishing the formation of mineralized matrix by MSCs (15). After a 2-day stimulation of the cells by the different concentrations of Iloprost, the concentration of secreted IFNγ and TNFα was significantly decreased in comparison to the control (PBS supplementation) (IFNγ: ~130 to ~55 ng/ml; TNFα: ~65 to ~40 pg/ml) (**Figures 2A,B**). Comparing the two different concentrations of Iloprost, the supplementation of the higher one (3 μM) led to an even more pronounced decrease of the secreted cytokines. As expected, non-activated cells showed almost no secretion of IFNγ and TNFα. The metabolic activity of the stimulated bone marrow cells was also downregulated by the supplementation of Iloprost in comparison to the control (**Figure 2C**).

In patients, we already showed that a too high amount of CD8+ T cells, one special subset of the adaptive immunity, negatively regulates successful bone repair (15). CD8+ T cells are one of the main producer of pro-inflammatory cytokines in the early bone repair phase. Therefore, as a next step, we evaluated the immunomodulatory effect of Iloprost on murine CD8+ T cells. CD8+ T cells were isolated via PluriBeads (pluriSelect) from bone marrow and spleen. The purity of the isolated cells was confirmed by flow cytometry after separation as well as after the duration of the *in vitro* stimulation and stayed above 80% (**Figure 3A**). Similar to the stimulation of the whole bone marrow cellular fraction, isolated CD8+ T cells showed a decreased secretion of IFNγ and TNFα under the presence of 3 μM Iloprost in comparison to the control (IFNγ: ~410 to ~250 ng/ml; TNFα: ~275 to ~180 pg/ml) (**Figures 3B,C**). The metabolic activity was again slightly downregulated by the Iloprost supplementation (**Figure S1**).

Besides cells of the adaptive immunity, also cellular compartments of the innate immune system play a key role in the early fracture healing phase. Macrophages are one of the first cells infiltrating the fracture area and are necessary for (a) the clearance of the cell debris as well as for (b) the recruitment of further cells important for the progression of the healing cascade due to their secreted cytokine profile (16, 28). We already demonstrated the importance of macrophages in bone regeneration using an *in vivo* mouse osteotomy model. After a chemically induced reduction of the macrophage cell population, a disturbed bone healing outcome was observed in comparison to the control group while an induction of the regulatory M2 macrophage phenotype (addition of IL-4/IL-13) lead to a significantly enhanced healing outcome (16). In the here presented study, we further tested whether the supplementation of Iloprost promotes simultaneously the downregulation of pro-inflammatory and the upregulation of anti-inflammatory cytokines by MΦ, M1, or M2 polarized macrophages, respectively (**Figure 4**). Regarding the secretion of TNFα, the supplementation of Iloprost led to a decreased secretion by MΦ as well as by pro-inflammatory M1 (~50 to ~20 pg/ml) (**Figure 4A**). Whereas, the secretion of the anti-inflammatory cytokine IL-10 was significantly upregulated in the M2 type, but unaffected in the MΦ and M1 macrophages (~290 to ~410 pg/ml) (**Figure 4B**). The polarization culture was confirmed by immune fluorescence staining of the stimulated and polarized cells (**Figure 4C**). MΦ macrophages were identified by the marker expression CD68 (green fluorescence signal). M1 were double positive for CD68 and CD80 (CD80: white fluorescence signal) and M2 double positive for CD68 and CD206 (CD206: red fluorescence signal). Cell nuclei were identified by DAPI (blue fluorescence signal).

Effects of Iloprost on the Osteogenic and Chondrogenic Differentiation Capacity of Mesenchymal Stromal Cells

MSCs are the precursor cells for cartilage producing chondrocytes and bone forming osteoblasts. During secondary bone healing, a cartilage template is first build. These chondrocytes further get hypertrophic, mineralize and are subsequently replaced by newly formed woven bone produced by osteoblasts. Thus, a cartilage template is indispensable for successful bone regeneration. Therefore, the osteogenic and chondrogenic differentiation capacity of MSCs was investigated under the influence of Iloprost. We tested again two different concentrations of Iloprost: 300 nM and 3 μM, respectively.

For the osteogenic differentiation, monolayers of MSCs cultured for 14 days in osteoinductive media were stained with Alizarin Red to reveal the calcification of the cells (**Figure 5**). The quantification of the Alizarin Red staining demonstrated that Iloprost had no negative effect on the osteogenic capacity of MSCs (**Figures 5A,B**). The metabolic activity as well as the cell number of the cultured MSCs were also unaffected by the presence of Iloprost in the osteoinductive media (**Figures 5C,D**).

After the demonstration that Iloprost is not affecting the mineralization capacity of MSCs, we evaluated the impact of Iloprost on their capacity to differentiate into the chondrogenic cell lineage. Representative images of Alcian Blue stained paraffin sections of cartilage pellets are presented in **Figure 6A**. The quantification of the Alcian Blue staining revealed no negative effect on the proteoglycan production of chondrogenically induced MSC pellets under the supplementation of Iloprost in comparison to the PBS control (**Figure 6B**).

Osteoimmunological Effect of Iloprost

In the first part of the study, we demonstrated that the supplementation of Iloprost promotes the functionality of immune cells toward both, a reduction of pro-inflammatory signals and an induction of anti-inflammatory ones. We further showed that Iloprost had no negative effect on the osteogenic as well as chondrogenic differentiation capacity of MSCs. Next, we wondered, whether the immune modulatory effect of Iloprost on immune cells is also influencing the osteogenic capacity of MSCs.

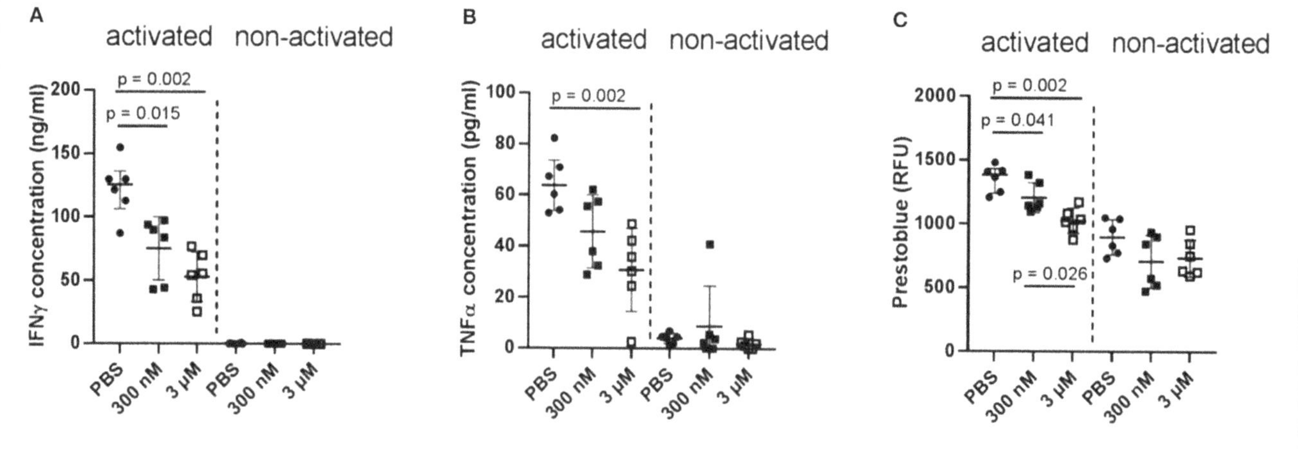

FIGURE 2 | Immunomodulatory effects of Iloprost on bone marrow cells. Bone marrow cells were stimulated for 2 days by α-CD3/α-CD28 in addition to either PBS or two different concentrations of Iloprost (300 nM or 3 µM, respectively). The following secreted cytokine concentrations were evaluated: IFNγ **(A)** and TNFα **(B)**. The metabolic activity of the stimulated bone marrow cells was measured via Prestoblue **(C)**. $n = 6$.

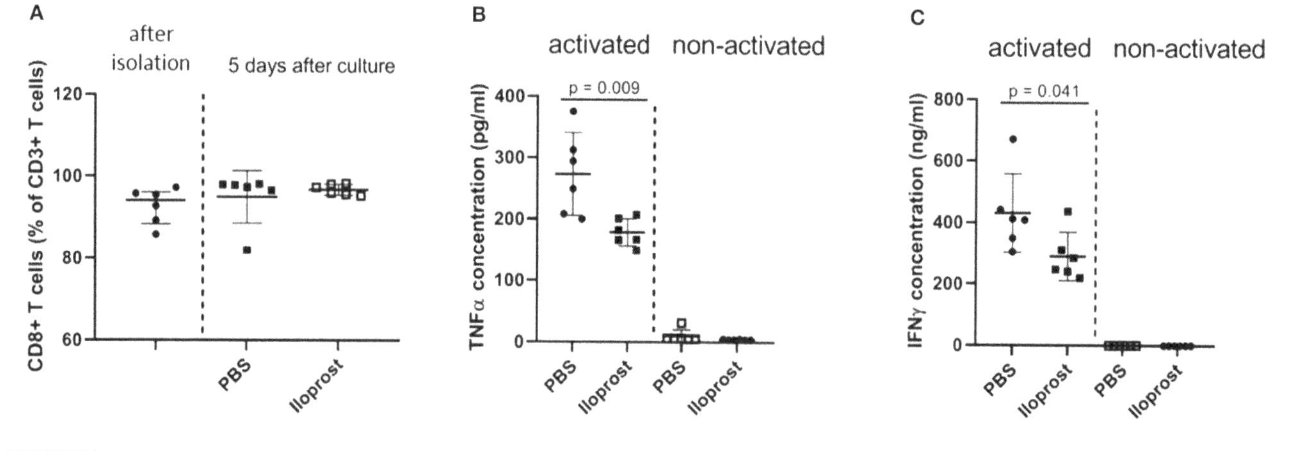

FIGURE 3 | Immunomodulatory effects of Iloprost on isolated CD8+ T cells. The purity of the isolated CD8+ T cells after bead-based separation as well as after *in vitro* stimulation was confirmed by flow cytometry **(A)**. CD8+ T cells were stimulated by α-CD3/α-CD28 in addition to either PBS or 3 µM Iloprost. The following secreted cytokine concentrations were evaluated: TNFα **(B)** and IFNγ **(C)**; $n = 6$.

Therefore, conditioned media (CM) of α-CD3/α-CD28 stimulated and Iloprost treated bone marrow cells and isolated CD8+ T cells, respectively, were added to the osteoinductive culture of MSCs. The CM of activated bone marrow cells significantly decreased the mineralization capacity of MSCs in comparison to the control (cultivated MSCs in osteoinductive media, OM) (**Figures 7A,B**). The supplementation of Iloprost during the α-CD3/α-CD28 stimulation of bone marrow cells was able to compensate partially the negative impact on mineralization induced by the activation (Iloprost, activated). CM of non-activated bone marrow cells had no effect on the mineralization capacity of MSCs (PBS, non-activated).

Repeating the analysis of the osteoimmunological effect of Iloprost on MSCs with isolated CD8+ T cells, similar results were obtained. CM of activated CD8+ T cells led to a significant decrease of mineralized matrix synthesis of cultured MSCs compared to the control (MSCs cultured in OM) (**Figures 8A,B**). Again, the supplementation of Iloprost to the stimulation of CD8+ T cells significantly improved the osteogenic matrix production by MSCs (**Figures 8A,B**; Iloprost, activated). However, this was still significantly lower in comparison to the OM control. CM of non-activated CD8+ T cells had no effect on the mineralization of MSCs (PBS, non-activated).

Summarizing the data from our *in vitro* study, we confirmed the immune modulatory effect of Iloprost on the secreted cytokine profile of immune cells. We also showed that Iloprost had no effect on the cartilage and bone forming capacity of MSCs. Thus, Iloprost is not negatively affecting the pro-regenerative functionality of MSCs. In a next step, we tested the capacity of Iloprost as a bone healing promoting agent in our mouse osteotomy model in a proof of concept *in vivo* approach.

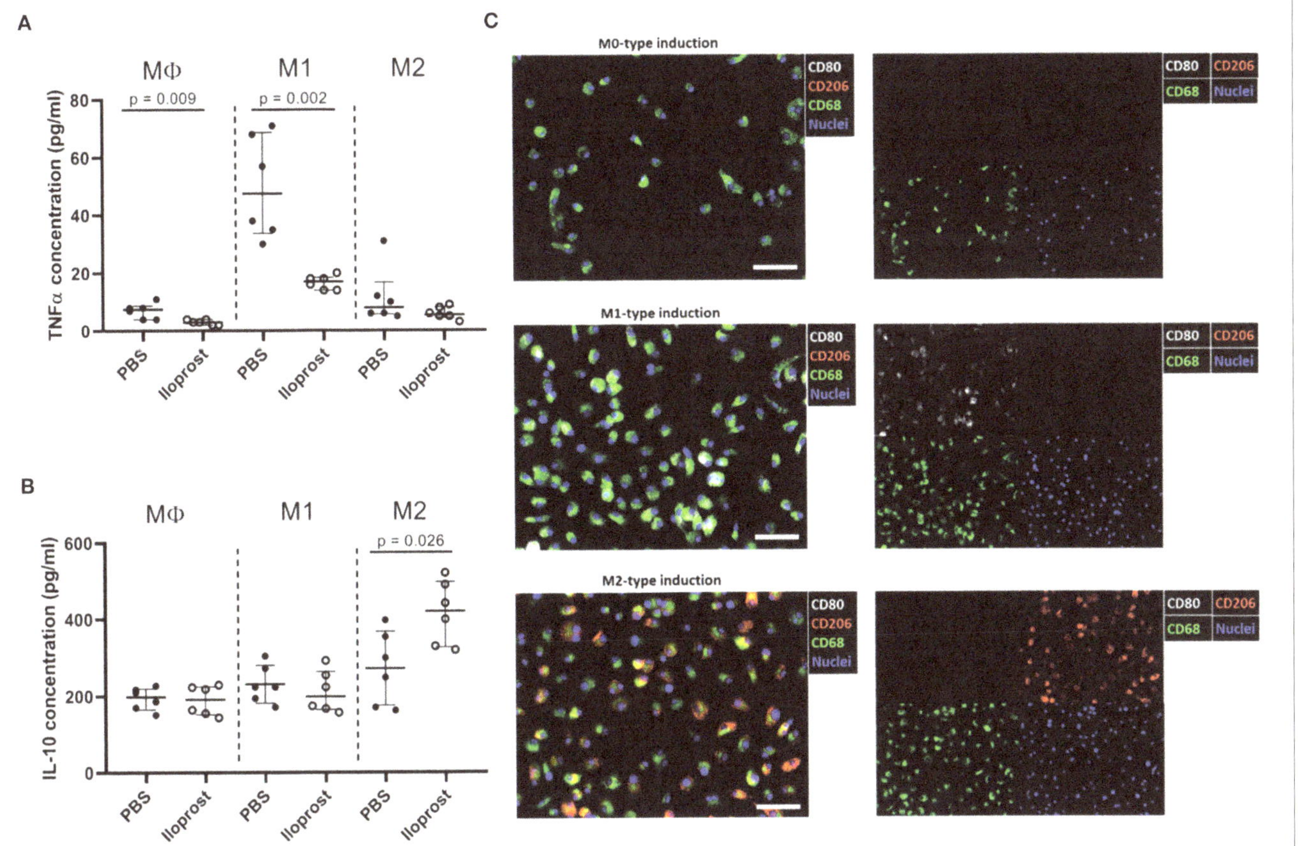

FIGURE 4 | Immunomodulatory effects of Iloprost on polarized bone marrow macrophages. Macrophages were polarized for 3 days toward the M1 or M2 type, supplemented with either PBS or 3 μM Iloprost. **(A,B)** The following secreted cytokine concentrations were evaluated: TNFα **(A)** and IL-10 **(B)** of M1-type induced and M2-type induced polarized macrophages, respectively. **(C)** Representative immune fluorescence images of unpolarised CD68+ MΦ macrophages (on top), CD68+CD80+ M1 macrophages (middle), and CD68+CD206+ M2 macrophages (bottom). Color code of the immune fluorescence images: CD68 = green, CD80 = white, CD206 = red, and cell nuclei = blue (DAPI). Scale bars: 100 μm; *n* = 6.

Iloprost–A Potent Agent to Promote Bone Fracture Healing *in vivo*?

In bone regeneration, a first pro-inflammatory phase is indispensable for the initiation of the healing cascade. Due to the anti-inflammatory effect of Iloprost via its effect on immune cell function shown *in vitro*, we chose an application strategy, where the applied Iloprost will be successively released from a biphasic fibrin scaffold, thus allowing the pro-inflammatory phase to proceed. Fibrous tissue is a component of the classical healing cascade in bone regeneration and thus represents an endogenous material, which is already present in the fracture gap. Furthermore, fibrin is biocompatible and biodegradable. Iloprost embedded in a fibrin clot was inserted during surgery in the osteotomy gap. Due to the biphasic structure of the fibrin scaffold, the included Iloprost would not be directly released in the fracture zone at the onset of the surgery but with a delay. This delay allows the initial pro-inflammatory phase to proceed and to initiate the healing cascade.

The healing outcome was evaluated 21 days post-surgery. The model was chosen to enable detection of healing enhancement–with a gap size of 0.7 mm the healing is not concluded after 21 days (control) (**Figure 9**, PBS). Regarding the Iloprost treated group, μCT analysis 21 days post-surgery showed an improved healing outcome of the mice receiving Iloprost in comparison to the control group (mice with fibrin scaffold, PBS supplementation) (**Figure 9**; Iloprost: mice with Iloprost supplementation; PBS: control group). The quantification of the μCT data confirmed the already visually seen improved healing by a significant increase of bone volume, total callus volume and the ratio of bone volume/total callus volume in the Iloprost treated animals with regard to the control (**Figures 9B–D**).

Next to the μCT evaluation, histological and immunohistological analyses were performed on cryosections of the fractured femora 3 days and 21 days post-osteotomy (**Figures 10, 11**). Movat Pentachrome staining was performed to evaluate the relative amount of mineralized bone, cartilage, connective tissue and bone marrow (**Figure 10**). In **Figure 10A**, representative Movat Pentachrome pictures are presented to illustrate the tissue formation in and around the osteotomy gap at the respective time point. Three days post-surgery, the fibrin scaffold was still visible within the osteotomy gap in both groups, the control (PBS) and Iloprost treated animals

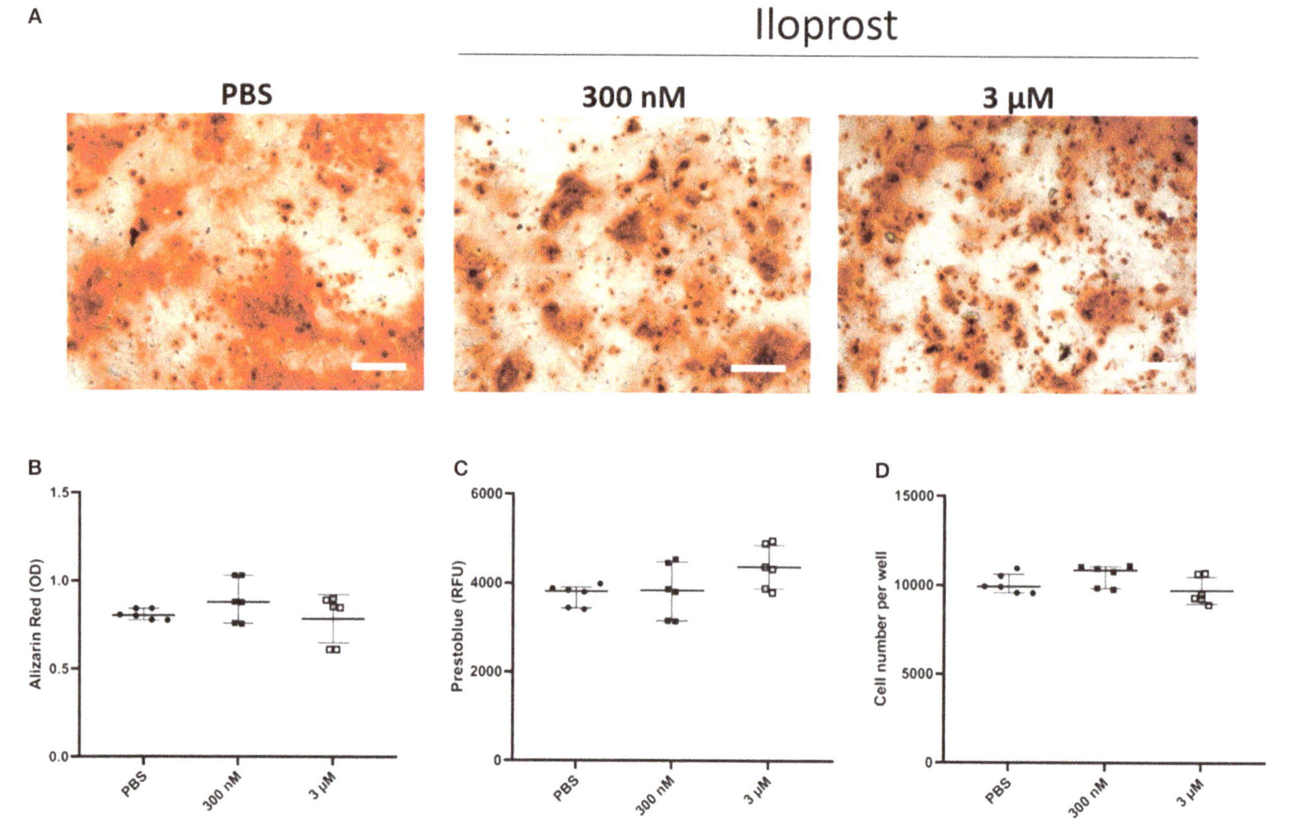

FIGURE 5 | Effect of Iloprost on mineralization capacity of osteogenically induced MSCs. Monolayers of MSCs were stained with Alizarin Red to visualize the formation of mineralized matrix. **(A,B)** Representative images of the Alizarin Red staining of cultured MSCs with osteoinductive media after 14 days of cultivation. Different concentrations of Iloprost were supplemented to the osteoinductive media (300 nM and 3 µM, respectively) **(A)**. Quantification of the Alizarin Red staining **(B)**. The metabolic activity of the cultured MSCs was measured by Prestoblue **(C)**. Determination of the cell number of the cultured MSCs under the different stimuli **(D)**. Scale bars: 200 µm; $n = 6$.

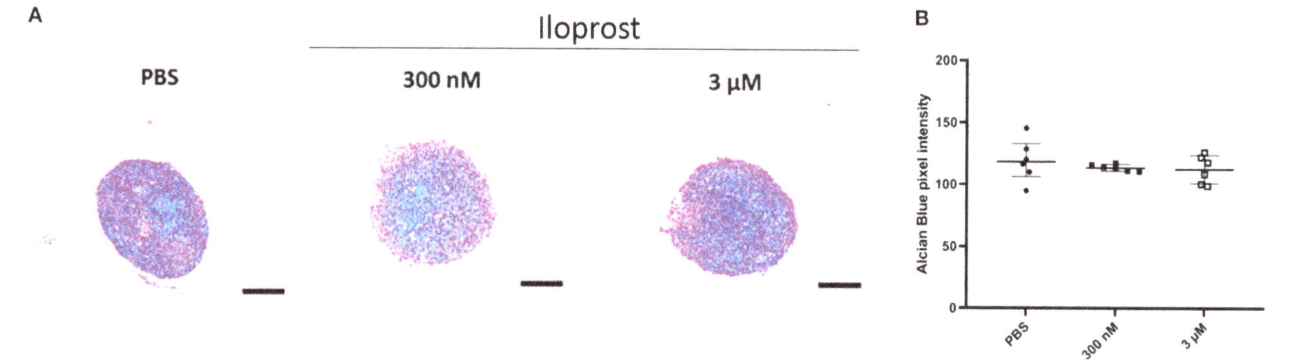

FIGURE 6 | Effect of Iloprost on cartilage formation capacity of chondrogenically induced MSCs. **(A)** Alcian Blue stained paraffin sections of cartilage pellets after 21 days of incubation in chondroinductive media, supplemented with different concentration of Iloprost (300 nM and 3 µM, respectively) or PBS as control. **(B)** Quantification of the Alcian Blue staining. Scale bars: 200 µm; $n = 6$.

(Iloprost), indicated by a red color after Movat's Pentachrome staining (**Figure 10A**, left). After 21 days, no fibrin scaffold was detected anymore in or around the osteotomy area (**Figure 10A**, right). Histomorphometrical analysis of the tissue distribution revealed a significantly higher amount of mineralized bone and cartilage tissue 21 days post-surgery in the Iloprost treated group in comparison to the control animals (**Figure 10B**). Three days post-osteotomy, both groups showed almost no proportion of mineralized bone or cartilage tissue. Both groups showed just slightly differences in the amount of connective tissue at both investigated time points (**Figure 10D**, connective tissue). Regarding the area of bone marrow, the

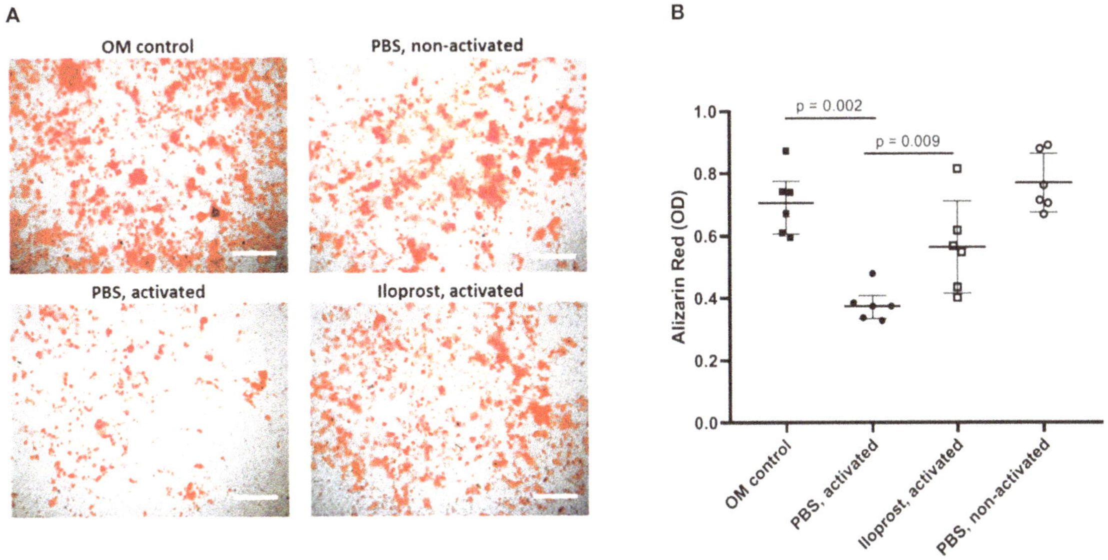

FIGURE 7 | Osteoimmunological effect of Iloprost treated bone marrow cells. α-CD3/α-CD28 activated bone marrow cells were cultured either with Iloprost or PBS as control. Obtained conditioned media was added to an osteogenic differentiation culture of MSCs and the secretion of mineralized matrix was measured by Alizarin Red staining. **(A)** Representative images of the Alizarin Red staining of the different culture conditions. **(B)** Quantification of the Alizarin Red signal. OM, osteoinductive media. Scale bars: 200 μm; *n* = 6.

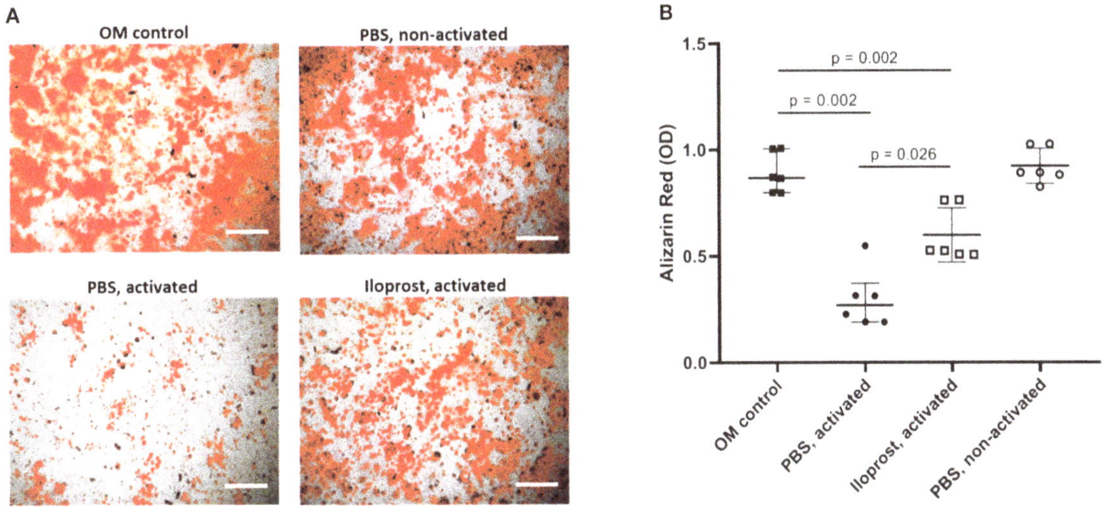

FIGURE 8 | Osteoimmunological effect of Iloprost treated isolated CD8+ T cells. Isolated α-CD3/α-CD28 activate CD8+ T cells were cultured either with Iloprost or PBS as control. Obtained conditioned media was added to an osteogenic differentiation culture of MSCs and the secretion of mineralized matrix was measured by Alizarin Red staining. **(A)** Representative images of the Alizarin Red staining of the different culture conditions. **(B)** Quantification of the Alizarin Red signal. OM, osteoinductive media. Scale bars: 200 μm; *n* = 6.

Iloprost treated mice displayed a slightly higher amount 21 days after surgery.

To better understand the impact and direct influence of Iloprost during the early phase of bone healing, immunohistochemical (IHC) analyses were performed on bone sections of mice sacrificed 3 days post-osteotomy. At this time point, Iloprost conducted its immune modulatory effect as shown below (**Figure 9**). In addition, around 3 days post-osteotomy, the starting shift of the pro-inflammatory into the anti-inflammatory phase is observed in our chosen mouse osteotomy model system.

First, the distribution of CD4+ and CD8+ T cells (identified by CD4 and CD8, respectively), as well as osteoblasts (identified by osteocalcin, OCN) was investigated in a defined region of interest (ROI) in and around the fracture zone (**Figures 11A,B**). Quantification of the analyzed bone sections revealed a

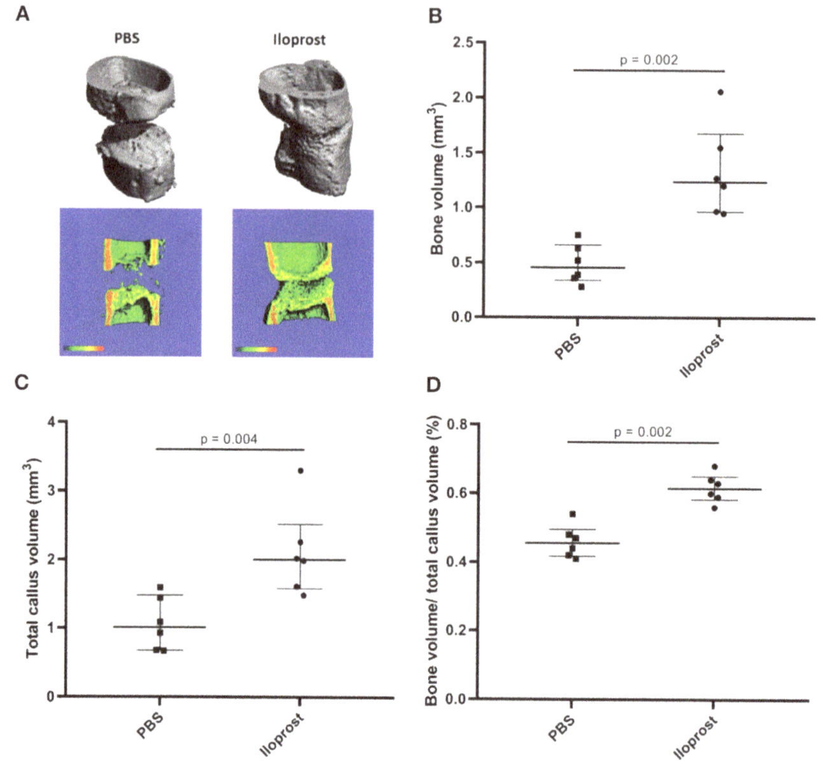

FIGURE 9 | Proof of concept approach of Iloprost to improve bone fracture healing *in vivo*. μCT analysis of the healing outcome 21 days post-osteotomy in a mouse osteotomy model. **(A)** Representative μCT images of the Iloprost treated (right) and control (left, PBS) group. The upper row shows the 3D reconstruction of the μCT measurement. In the lower row, 3D reconstruction was cut in the middle to evaluate the healing progression. The color code indicates the mineralization state, increasing from blue to red. **(B–D)** Quantification of the μCT results; $n = 6$.

significantly reduction of the relative amount of CD4+ and CD8+ T cells in the Iloprost treated mice in comparison to the control. The relative number of osteoblasts was not affected by Iloprost treatment. Next, we were interested in the IFNγ producing CD8+ T cells, which were already shown to be detrimental for successful bone repair. Iloprost treatment led to a clear decrease of IFNγ producing CD8+ T cells with regard to the control group (**Figure 11C**, highlighted by arrows). Next to the T cells, the distribution of MΦ, M1, and M2 type macrophages was also evaluated 3 days post-osteotomy. Corresponding to the chosen marker set for the *in vitro* analysis, CD68 was used as pan-macrophage marker, CD68 and CD80 for M1 and CD68 and CD206 for M2 (**Figure 11D**). Due to the Iloprost administration in the fracture zone, a simultaneous significant decrease of pro-inflammatory M1 and significant increase of anti-inflammatory and pro-regenerative M2 macrophages was detectable. In order to evaluate if Iloprost administration has an impact on bone resorption, osteoclasts were also investigated by IHC. Osteoclasts were identified by the myeloid-lineage marker CD68, the collagen digesting enzyme cathepsinK (CTSK) and presence of multiple nuclei (**Figure 11E**). No significant differences were observed in both groups 3 days post-osteotomy.

Summarizing the data from the proof of concept study in our *in vivo* mouse osteotomy model system, the pro-regenerative effect of Iloprost in bone healing was confirmed. We further revealed underlying changes in the immune cell composition in and around the fracture zone in the early inflammatory phase toward a reduced pro-inflammatory and increased anti-inflammatory cell phenotype caused by the application of Iloprost. Thus, Iloprost is a promising agent to improve bone regeneration by the downregulation of partial unfavorable pro-inflammatory and a simultaneous support of anti-inflammatory and pro-regenerative mediators.

DISCUSSION

Healing is impaired if a prolonged (pro-) inflammatory phase persists and an early anti-inflammatory stimulus is required. Thus, developing strategies that would ensure or even enhance anti-inflammatory stimuli appears mandatory. Iloprost is a well-known drug to treat diseases of the vascular system like pulmonary arterial hypertension and scleroderma (25, 29, 30). Its main function is conducted via vasodilatation (widening of blood vessels). Regarding the bone system, Iloprost is already successfully used to treat bone marrow oedema, partially also in the context of bone injuries (23, 24).

In the here presented study, the immune modulatory effect of the synthetic prostacyclin analog Iloprost was evaluated for

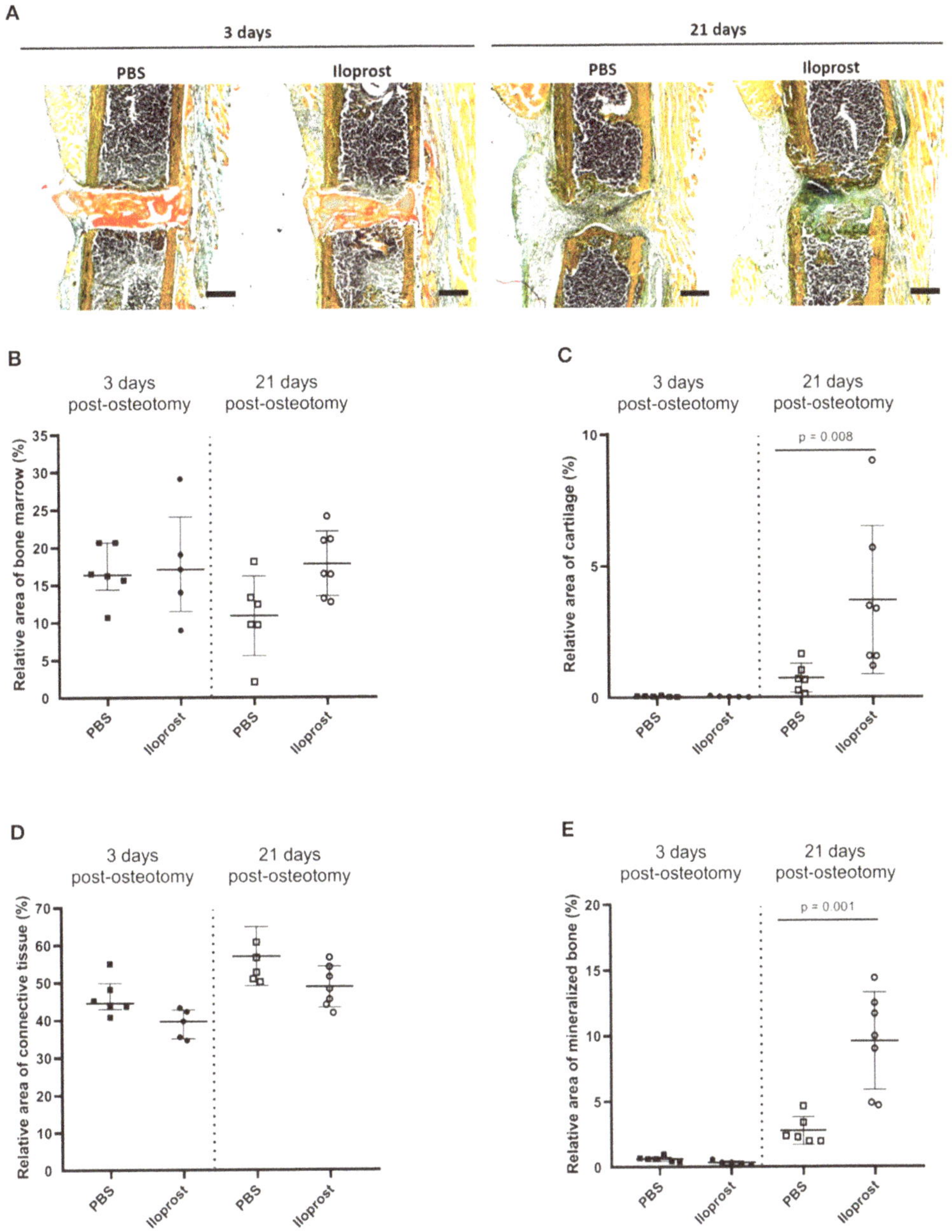

FIGURE 10 | Histological analysis of *in vivo* experiments in mouse osteotomies at days 3 and 21 post-osteotomy. **(A)** Representative Movat's pentachrome pictures are displayed for the respective time point and group. **(B–E)** Histomorphometrical analysis of the Movat Pentachrome stainings: **(B)** bone marrow, **(C)** cartilage tissue, **(D)** connective tissue, and **(E)** mineralized bone tissue. Color coding of the Movat Pentachrome staining: mineralized bone = yellow, cartilage = dark blue-green, connective tissue = light blue-green, muscle fibers = light orange, cell nuclei = purple, fibrin clot = red/orange. Scale bars equal 500 µm, $n = 6$.

bone fracture healing. The impact of Iloprost was investigated on immune cells and MSCs *in vitro* as well as in a well-established mouse osteotomy model *in vivo*. We demonstrated that the supplementation of Iloprost led to a decrease in the expression of pro-inflammatory cytokines by immune cells (T cells and macrophages) and thus promoted a shift in the function of these cells toward the anti-inflammatory path. The metabolic activity of the stimulated immune cells was also downregulated by Iloprost further supporting the observed decrease of the secreted pro-inflammatory cytokine profile. Iloprost had no negative effect on the osteogenic as well as chondrogenic function of MSCs. In an *in vivo* proof of concept approach, the pro-regenerative capacity of Iloprost as potential agent to further bone regeneration was confirmed, evaluated by an improved healing outcome after 21 days. Immunohistochemical analysis of the cellular

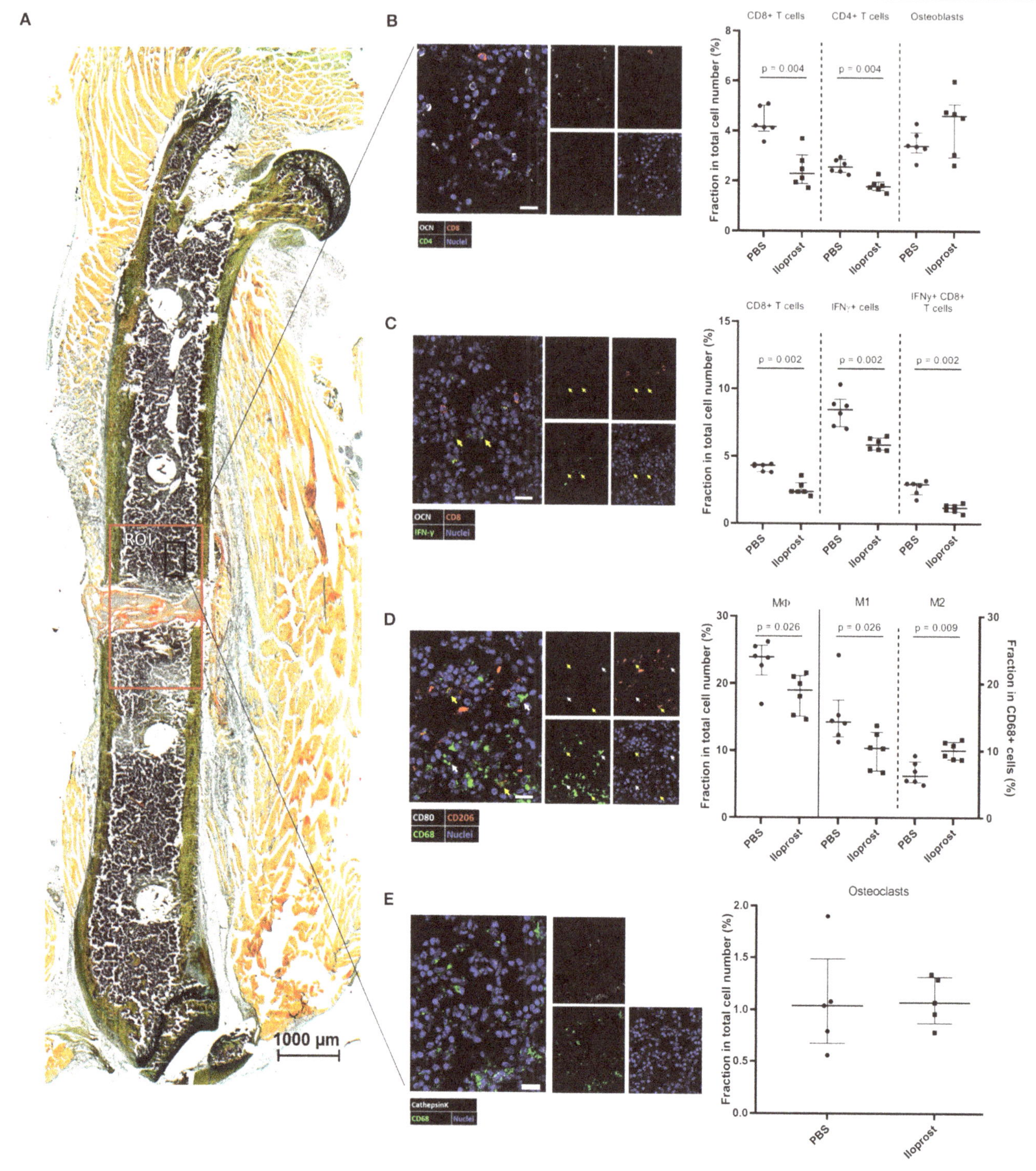

FIGURE 11 | Immunohistochemical (IHC) analysis of the distribution of immune cells in the fracture zone 3 days post-osteotomy. **(A)** A section of a fractured femur from the Iloprost treated group is displayed, Movat Pentachrome staining. The region of interest (ROI) for the quantitative analysis of IHC images is enlarged (red rectangle). The black rectangle represents the region from which the representative examples of the respective IHC staining for **(B)** CD4+ and CD8+ T cells and osteoblasts, **(C)** IFNγ producing CD8+ T cells; CD8+IFNγ+ cells = white indicator, **(D)** macrophages; M1-type macrophages = white indicator; M2-type macrophages = yellow indicator, and **(E)** osteoclasts were taken. The quantification of the cellular distributions are displayed in the corresponding dot plot graphs. Color code: Movat Pentachrome mineralized bone = yellow, cartilage = dark blue-green, connective tissue = light blue-green, muscle fibers = light orange, cell nuclei = purple, fibrin clot = red/orange; **(B)** osteoblasts = white, CD8+ T cells = red, CD4+ T cells = green and cell nuclei = blue; **(C)** osteoblasts = white, CD8+ T cells = red, IFNγ = green, cell nuclei = blue; **(D)** CD68 = green, CD80 = white, CD206 = red; **(E)** osteoclasts: double positive for cathepsinK = white and CD68 = green cell nuclei = blue. Scale bars: 20 µm (IHC) 1,000 µm (Movat Pentachrome); $n = 6$.

distribution in the fracture gap revealed a decrease of potential unfavorable IFNγ producing CD8+ cells as well as an increase of anti-inflammatory M2 macrophages in comparison to the control group due to Iloprost administration concurring with the *in vitro* results. Both are furthering the pro-regenerative pathway.

The signaling receptor for prostacyclin and thus also for Iloprost is found on a variety of different cell types, among others on cells of the innate as well as adaptive immunity. Iloprost signaling leads to an intracellular increase of cyclic adenosine monophosphate (cAMP) via the stimulation of the adenylyl cyclase. cAMP is an anti-inflammatory acting agent that suppresses the effector function of CD4+ and CD8+ T cells (31, 32). Here, we also observed a decrease of the secretion of the pro-inflammatory cytokines TNFα and IFNγ from whole bone marrow cells as well as (IFNγ producing) CD8+ T cells *in vitro* and *in vivo* under the presence of Iloprost. This observation demonstrates the immune modulatory effect of Iloprost on cellular components of the adaptive immunity toward a reduced pro-inflammatory and thus pro-regenerative phenotype. This finding was further confirmed by the increase of the pro-regenerative M2 type macrophages under the influence of Iloprost. The group of Alkhabit also showed an immune modulatory effect of Iloprost on macrophage polarization toward a pro-regenerative phenotype in an *in vivo* model system in rats, supporting our findings (33). Regarding bone fracture healing, possible negative effects of Iloprost on MSCs and bone forming osteoblasts as well as bone resorbing osteoclasts have to be considered. No possible negative effects by Iloprost on the osteogenic and chondrogenic capacities of MSCs were observed *in vitro*, further supporting the local application of Iloprost for bone healing scenarios *in vivo*. In a proof of concept approach, we evaluated the administration of Iloprost in a mouse osteotomy model system. Iloprost was inserted into a fibrin clot delivery system, from which the prostacyclin analog was successively released, which was shown by a downregulation of a pro-inflammatory cellular distribution around the fracture gap 3 days post osteotomy. The *in vivo* study confirmed the positive effect of Iloprost on bone regeneration. Animals treated with Iloprost showed a significantly improved bone healing outcome 21 days post-osteotomy compared to untreated control mice evaluated by μCT as well as histomorphometry after Movat's Pentachrome staining. The observed significantly enhanced bone formation in the Iloprost treated animals can be explained by an earlier starting of the regenerative process due to the down-regulated pro-inflammatory phase at the beginning of the healing cascade in comparison to the PBS treated control mice. Analysis of the cellular distribution of specific immune cells 3 days post-osteotomy in the fractured bones showed a clear tendency toward a reduced pro-inflammatory and increased anti-inflammatory cellular phenotype and cytokine secretion profile, as already observed in the preceding *in vitro* study. Furthermore, no effect on the relative amount of osteoblasts and osteoclasts in and around the fracture gap were detectable after Iloprost treatment 3 days post-osteotomy *in vivo*. *In vitro*, we also showed that the secreted cytokine milieu of activated and either Iloprost or untreated T cells has a significant impact on the osteogenic capacity of MSCs cultured in osteoinductive media. Our results showed a compensatory effect by the Iloprost treatment on the potential anti-regenerative cytokine milieu produced by activated T cells. Thus, the pro-regenerative effect of Iloprost is indirectly mediated on MSCs/osteoblasts by changes in the functionality of (pro-inflammatory) effector T cells participating in the bone regeneration cascade. Next to the effect of Iloprost on CD8+ T cells and macrophages, an influence on other immune cell could further impact bone healing *in vivo*. The early fracture healing phase is characterized by an infiltration of cells of the innate immunity like mast cells and neutrophils. For both, it was already shown, that the administration of prostacyclin analogs led to a reduced recruitment of these cells to the site of injury (34–36). Furthermore, an inhibitory function of Iloprost is reported for the secretion of effector cytokines of bone marrow dendritic cells as well as Th1 and Th2 CD4+ T cells *in vitro* (37). Thus, Iloprost is not only affecting the CD8+, but also the CD4+ T cell compartment in diminishing the (pro-inflammatory) effector cytokine secretion and thus function. One major key element of the potential of Iloprost to improve bone regeneration seems to be the time point of administration during the healing scenario. The group of Dogan reported an inhibitory effect of Iloprost on fracture repair in rats (38). There, Iloprost was administered by a daily injection for 5 days, starting at the time point of surgery. Due to the immune modulatory effect of Iloprost, a too early application of the drug could lead to an inhibition of the indispensable early pro-inflammatory phase initiating the healing cascade. This hypothesis is further supported by the reported effects of Iloprost on mast cells and neutrophils. Both cell types are indispensable for the early fracture healing phase to initiate the healing cascade. If Iloprost is administered directly at the time point of surgery/injury, it will inhibit the crucial recruitment of both cells types and will therefore disturbed the formation of the necessary cellular and cytokine milieu for a correct progression of the regeneration cascade (35, 36). Therefore, we used a fibrin clot for a (1) delayed and (2) successive release of Iloprost into the fracture gap thereby allowing the first pro-inflammatory phase to proceed. The positive impact of Iloprost in bone healing was already demonstrated in a small case study in the clinic for the treatment of subchondral stress fractures of the knee. Patients receiving Iloprost showed an improved healing of the stress fractures in comparison to the control group receiving the opioid analgesic Tramadol (39). Even though Iloprost is beneficial for bone healing applied systemically, this also bears considerable risks which would be circumvented by a local application as we proved in our proof of concept *in vivo* study. Thus, also in the treatment of patients, the possible pro-regenerative effect of Iloprost in bone healing was confirmed further supporting our *in vivo* and *in vitro* results.

CONCLUSION

In the here presented study, the anti-inflammatory impact of Iloprost was confirmed. Cellular components of the immune system play a key role in bone fracture healing. An overwhelming pro-inflammatory phase in the early fracture healing cascade is correlated with an impaired healing outcome (15). We demonstrated that Iloprost has the potential to compensate the partial unfavorable pro-inflammatory effect of effector T cells and is able to stimulate the formation of an anti-inflammatory and pro-regenerative cellular milieu improving fracture healing. In a consecutive step, this strategy has to be confirmed in clinical phase I/II trials.

AUTHOR CONTRIBUTIONS

SW, KS-B, GD, and H-DV: conceptual idea and design of the study. SW, CS, CB, CJS, and JB: data collection, analysis, and interpretation. SW, CS, CB, KS-B, GD, and H-DV: drafting of the manuscript. All authors revised the manuscript.

ACKNOWLEDGMENTS

We would like to thank Norma Schulz for her excellent technical assistance performing the described experiments. We acknowledge support from the German Research Foundation (DFG) and the Open Access Publication Fund of Charité–Universitätsmedizin Berlin. This work was supported by a grant from the German Research Foundation (FG 2195, DFG SCHM 2977, DU 298/21-1) and the Friede Springer Stiftung.

REFERENCES

1. Marsell R, Einhorn TA. The biology of fracture healing. *Injury*. (2011) 42:551–5. doi: 10.1016/j.injury.2011.03.031
2. Schmidt-Bleek K, Petersen A, Dienelt A, Schwarz C, Duda GN. Initiation and early control of tissue regeneration - bone healing as a model system for tissue regeneration. *Expert Opin Biol Ther*. (2014) 14:247–59. doi: 10.1517/14712598.2014.857653
3. Einhorn TA, Gerstenfeld LC. Fracture healing: mechanisms and interventions. *Nat Rev Rheumatol*. (2015) 11:45–54. doi: 10.1038/nrrheum.2014.164
4. Schmidt-Bleek K, Kwee BJ, Mooney DJ, Duda GN. Boon and bane of inflammation in bone tissue regeneration and its link with angiogenesis. *Tissue Eng Part B Rev*. (2015) 21:354–64. doi: 10.1089/ten.teb.2014.0677
5. Einhorn TA, Lane JM. Significant advances have been made in the way surgeons treat fractures. *Clin Orthop Relat Res*. (1998) 355:S2–3. doi: 10.1097/00003086-199810001-00001
6. Schlundt C, Bucher CH, Tsitsilonis S, Schell H, Duda GN, Schmidt-Bleek K. Clinical and research approaches to treat non-union fracture. *Curr Osteoporos Rep*. (2018) 16:155–68. doi: 10.1007/s11914-018-0432-1
7. Winkler TA, Duda GN, Schmidt-Bleek K. A review of biomaterials in bone defect healing, remaining shortcomings and future opportunities for bone tissue engineering. *Bone Joint Res*. (2018) 7:232–243. doi: 10.1302/2046-3758.73.BJR-2017-0270.R1
8. Gruber R, Koch H, Doll BA, Tegtmeier F, Einhorn TA, Hollinger JO. Fracture healing in the elderly patient. *Exp Gerontol*. (2006) 41:1080–93. doi: 10.1016/j.exger.2006.09.008
9. Bucher CH, Duda GN, Volk H-D, Schmidt-Bleek K. The role of immune reactivity in bone regeneration. In: Zorzi AR, de Miranda JB, editors. *Advanced Techniques in Bone Regeneration*. London: IntechOpen Limited (2016). p. 169–194. doi: 10.5772/62476
10. Schell H, Duda GN, Peters A, Tsitsilonis S, Johnson KA, Schmidt-Bleek K. The haematoma and its role in bone healing. *J Exp Orthop*. (2017) 4:5. doi: 10.1186/s40634-017-0079-3
11. Opal SM. Phylogenetic and functional relationships between coagulation and the innate immune response. *Crit Care Med*. (2000) 28:S77–80. doi: 10.1097/00003246-200009001-00017
12. Lienau J, Schmidt-Bleek K, Peters A, Haschke F, Duda GN, Perka C, et al. Differential regulation of blood vessel formation between standard and delayed bone healing. *J Orthop Res*. (2009) 27:1133–40. doi: 10.1002/jor.20870
13. Schmidt-Bleek K, Schell H, Kolar P, Pfaff M, Perka C, Buttgereit F, et al. Cellular composition of the initial fracture hematoma compared to a muscle hematoma: a study in sheep. *J Orthop Res*. (2009) 27:1147–51. doi: 10.1002/jor.20901
14. Lienau J, Schmidt-Bleek K, Peters A, Weber H, Bail HJ, Duda GN, et al. Insight into the molecular pathophysiology of delayed bone healing in a sheep model. *Tissue Eng Part A*. (2010) 16:191–9. doi: 10.1089/ten.tea.2009.0187
15. Reinke S, Geissler S, Taylor WR, Schmidt-Bleek K, Juelke K, Schwachmeyer V, et al. Terminally differentiated CD8(+) T cells negatively affect bone regeneration in humans. *Sci Transl Med*. (2013) 5:177ra136. doi: 10.1126/scitranslmed.3004754
16. Schlundt C, El Khassawna T, Serra A, Dienelt A, Wendler S, Schell H, et al. Macrophages in bone fracture healing: their essential role in endochondral ossification. *Bone*. (2018) 106:78–89. doi: 10.1016/j.bone.2015.10.019
17. Camacho M, Rodriguez C, Guadall A, Alcolea S, Orriols M, Escudero JR, et al. Hypoxia upregulates PGI-synthase and increases PGI(2) release in human vascular cells exposed to inflammatory stimuli. *J Lipid Res*. (2011) 52:720–31. doi: 10.1194/jlr.M011007
18. Mohite A, Chillar A, So SP, Cervantes V, Ruan KH. Novel mechanism of the vascular protector prostacyclin: regulating microRNA expression. *Biochemistry*. (2011) 50:1691–9. doi: 10.1021/bi101654w
19. Dorris SL, Peebles RS Jr. PGI2 as a regulator of inflammatory diseases. *Mediators Inflamm*. (2012) 2012:926968. doi: 10.1155/2012/926968
20. Muller T, Durk T, Blumenthal B, Herouy Y, Sorichter S, Grimm M, et al. Iloprost has potent anti-inflammatory properties on human monocyte-derived dendritic cells. *Clin Exp Allergy*. (2010) 40:1214–21. doi: 10.1111/j.1365-2222.2010.03558.x
21. Jaffar Z, Wan KS, Roberts K. A key role for prostaglandin I2 in limiting lung mucosal Th2, but not Th1, responses to inhaled allergen. *J Immunol*. (2002) 169:5997–6004. doi: 10.4049/jimmunol.169.10.5997
22. Lovgren AK, Jania LA, Hartney JM, Parsons KK, Audoly LP, Fitzgerald GA, et al. COX-2-derived prostacyclin protects against bleomycin-induced pulmonary fibrosis. *Am J Physiol Lung Cell Mol Physiol*. (2006) 291:L144–156. doi: 10.1152/ajplung.00492.2005
23. Disch AC, Matziolis G, Perka C. The management of necrosis-associated and idiopathic bone-marrow oedema of the proximal femur by intravenous iloprost. *J Bone Joint Surg Br*. (2005) 87:560–4. doi: 10.1302/0301-620X.87B4.15658
24. Jager M, Zilkens C, Bittersohl B, Matheney T, Kozina G, Blondin D, et al. Efficiency of iloprost treatment for osseous malperfusion. *Int Orthop*. (2011) 35:761–5. doi: 10.1007/s00264-010-0998-4
25. Roman A, Barbera JA, Escribano P, Sala ML, Febrer L, Oyaguez I, et al. Cost effectiveness of prostacyclins in pulmonary arterial hypertension. *Appl Health Econ Health Policy*. (2012) 10:175–88. doi: 10.2165/11630780-000000000-00000
26. Riemekasten G, Hoffmann U, Sunderkotter C, Weiss N, Kuhn A, Angiologisch-Dermatologisch-Rheumatologische DUE. [Management of digital ulcers in patients with systemic sclerosis]. *Dtsch Med Wochenschr*. (2012) 137:34–40. doi: 10.1055/s-0031-1298798
27. Bouxsein ML, Boyd SK, Christiansen BA, Guldberg RE, Jepsen KJ, Muller R. Guidelines for assessment of bone microstructure in rodents using micro-computed tomography. *J Bone Miner Res*. (2010) 25:1468–86. doi: 10.1002/jbmr.141

28. Abdelmagid SM, Barbe MF, Safadi FF. Role of inflammation in the aging bones. *Life Sci.* (2015) 123:25–34. doi: 10.1016/j.lfs.2014.11.011
29. Colaci M, Lumetti F, Giuggioli D, Guiducci S, Bellando-Randone S, Fiori G, et al. Long-term treatment of scleroderma-related digital ulcers with iloprost: a cohort study. *Clin Exp Rheumatol.* (2017) 35 (Suppl. 106):179–83.
30. Foti R, Visalli E, Amato G, Benenati A, Converso G, Farina A, et al. Long-term clinical stabilization of scleroderma patients treated with a chronic and intensive IV iloprost regimen. *Rheumatol Int.* (2017) 37:245–9. doi: 10.1007/s00296-016-3582-4
31. Zhou W, Hashimoto K, Goleniewska K, O'neal JF, Ji S, Blackwell TS, et al. Prostaglandin I2 analogs inhibit proinflammatory cytokine production and T cell stimulatory function of dendritic cells. *J Immunol.* (2007) 178:702–10. doi: 10.4049/jimmunol.178.2.702
32. D'amelio P, Cristofaro MA, D'amico L, Veneziano L, Roato I, Sassi F, et al. (2010). Iloprost modulates the immune response in systemic sclerosis. *BMC Immunol.* 11:62. doi: 10.1186/1471-2172-11-62
33. Alkhatib K, Poseno TM, Diaz Perez A, Durdik JM, Stenken JA. Iloprost affects macrophage activation and CCL2 concentrations in a microdialysis model in rats. *Pharm Res.* (2018) 35:20. doi: 10.1007/s11095-0 17-2277-1
34. Furuta GT, Schmidt-Choudhury A, Wang MY, Wang ZS, Lu L, Furlano RI, et al. Mast cell-dependent tumor necrosis factor alpha production participates in allergic gastric inflammation in mice. *Gastroenterology.* (1997) 113:1560–9. doi: 10.1053/gast.1997.v113.pm9352858
35. Kovtun A, Bergdolt S, Wiegner R, Radermacher P, Huber-Lang M, Ignatius A. The crucial role of neutrophil granulocytes in bone fracture healing. *Eur Cell Mater.* (2016) 32:152–62. doi: 10.22203/eCM.v032a10
36. Kroner J, Kovtun A, Kemmler J, Messmann JJ, Strauss G, Seitz S, et al. Mast cells are critical regulators of bone fracture-induced inflammation and osteoclast formation and activity. *J Bone Miner Res.* (2017) 32:2431–44. doi: 10.1002/jbmr.3234
37. Zhou W, Blackwell TS, Goleniewska K, O'neal JF, Fitzgerald GA, Lucitt M, et al. Prostaglandin I2 analogs inhibit Th1 and Th2 effector cytokine production by CD4 T cells. *J Leukoc Biol.* (2007) 81:809–17. doi: 10.1189/jlb.0606375
38. Dogan A, Duygun F, Kalender AM, Bayram I, Sungur I. Iloprost inhibits fracture repair in rats. *Chin Med J.* (2014) 127:2960–5. doi: 10.3760/cma.j.issn.0366-6999.20132862
39. Mayerhoefer ME, Kramer J, Breitenseher MJ, Norden C, Vakil-Adli A, Hofmann S, et al. MRI-demonstrated outcome of subchondral stress fractures of the knee after treatment with iloprost or tramadol: observations in 14 patients. *Clin J Sport Med.* (2008) 18:358–62. doi: 10.1097/JSM.0b013e31817f3e1c

9

The Uncovered Role of Immune Cells and NK Cells in the Regulation of Bone Metastasis

Ilaria Roato[1*] *and Massimo Vitale*[2]

[1] Center for Research and Medical Studies (CeRMS), A.O.U. Città della Salute e della Scienza di Torino, Turin, Italy, [2] UOC Immunologia, IRCCS Ospedale Policlinico San Martino Genova, Genoa, Italy

***Correspondence:**
Ilaria Roato
roato78@libero.it

Bone is one of the main metastatic sites of solid tumors like breast, lung, and prostate cancer. Disseminated tumor cells (DTCs) and cancer stem cells (CSCs) represent the main target to counteract bone metastatization. These cells often localize in bone marrow (BM) at level of pre-metastatic niche: they can remain dormant for years or directly grow and create bone lesion, according to the different stimulations received in BM. The immune system in bone marrow is dampened and represents an appealing site for DTCs/CSCs. NK cells have an important role in controlling tumor progression, but their involvement in bone metastasis formation is an interesting and not fully investigated issue. Indeed, whether NK cells can interfere with CSC formation, kill them at the site of primary tumor, during circulation or in the pre-metastic niche needs to be elucidated. This review focuses on different aspects that regulate DTC/CSC life in bone and how NK cells potentially control bone metastasis formation.

Keywords: bone metastases, NK cells, cancer stem cells, dormancy, immune response

INTRODUCTION

Although many cancer patients benefit from more efficient treatments of primary tumors and become long survivors, the overall probability to develop metastases is increasing, making this aspect of the disease a key target for researchers and clinicians (1). Bone is one of the main metastatic sites for different solid tumors including breast, lung, and prostate cancer (2). Bone metastasis formation and evolution is strongly influenced by a complex cross talk occurring among tumor, immune, and bone cells (3, 4). BM, besides cell precursors, contains different types of resident or recirculating mature immune cells, including Dendritic cells (DC), macrophages, granulocytes, myeloid derived suppressor cells (MDSCs), NK cells, and different T and B lymphocyte subsets. Although some of these cells (i.e., macrophages, granulocytes, lymphocytes, and NK cells) are endowed with effector functions and directly involved in pathogen elimination, virtually all BM immune cells can produce a variety of cytokines, chemokines, or other factors possibly influencing the local tissue homeostasis. Moreover, subtypes of bone cells, such as osteoclasts (OCs), originate from immune progenitors and use "immune" receptor/ligand pairs to rule their maturation and also to govern their bone degradation activity, a process significantly involved in metastasis formation (5).

Immune cells are poorly effective in the control of metastasis formation and growth, and this is true also for bone metastases, in spite of the consistency of the immune system in the bone niches. The definition of immunotherapeutic approaches in the metastatic disease is nevertheless attractive, especially considering NK cells, a subset of powerful effectors of the innate immunity endowed with anti-tumor activity. These cells have been shown to kill pro-metastatic tumor initiating cells and, recently, also to control metastases in animal models. On the other hand, NK cell heterogeneity and the complexity of their functional interactions with the local tumor microenvironment indicate that specific studies need to be addressed to define their role in bone metastases.

DTCS COLONIZE BONE MARROW AND ACTIVATE THE BONE METASTATIC VICIOUS CYCLE

In primary tumors, genetic, and epigenetic changes favor the switch of malignant cells to less differentiated forms through a process called epithelial-to-mesenchymal transition (EMT) (6). Cells rising from this switch can leave the primary tumor site becoming disseminated tumor cells (DTCs). DTCs can express cancer stem cell (CSC) profiles and properties such as resistance to chemotherapy and ability to home in BM for long time. Indeed, DTCs can migrate to distant organs and establish in BM at level of the premetastatic niches, which are induced by soluble factors or extra-cellular vescicles released in circulation by the primary tumor (7). The presence of DTCs in BM has clinical relevance, since it is associated to an increased risk to develop bone metastases (8–11).

In the BM, DTCs can also compete with hematopoietic stem cells (HSC) (12, 13) and establish in the niche by interacting with different elements including osteoblasts (OBs), endothelial cells, and Extracellular Matrix (ECM). OBs constitutively express CXCL12 and attract CXCR4-expressing tumor cells (14). Using mouse models, it has been shown that breast, lung, and prostate cancer cells overexpressing CXCR4 and CXCR7 increased their ability to extravasate and colonize bone (15, 16), and CXCR4 inhibition decreased bone and lung metastases (17, 18). Integrins and cadherins are other crucial factors for the interactions between DTCs and niches (16, 19). In breast cancer, the vascular-endothelial molecule-1 (VCAM-1) binds with high affinity $\alpha 4\beta 7$ and $\alpha 4\beta 1$ on OC precursors, leading to osteoclastogenesis, and $\alpha 4$ or VCAM-1 blocking antibodies effectively inhibit bone metastasis (20). Integrins can also interact with osteopontin (OPN), an ECM protein overexpressed in tumors and associated to tumor cell migration, metastases, and poor prognosis (21, 22).

Breast and prostate cancer DTCs can live in BM in a dormant state in pre-metastatic niche for years before starting to grow and to form metastases (5, 23). Indeed, the outgrowth of DTCs from dormant state, depends both on factors released by bone microenvironment, such as fibronectin, collagen I, and periostin (24), and by physical factors such as acid pH, hypoxia, high extracellular calcium concentration (25), which also cause disruption of the balanced physiological bone remodeling due to OC and OB activity (26). Remarkably, an increased OC activity generates the physical space for tumor expansion and induces the release from the bone matrix of molecules that further stimulate tumor cell proliferation, creating the vicious cycle (27, 28). Tumor cells in turn secrete PTHrP, activated vitamin D, tumor necrosis factor (TNF), matrix metalloproteinases (MMPs), interleukin-6 (IL-6), and other factors, which stimulate the expression of the receptor activator of nuclear factor NF-kB ligand (RANKL) on OBs, leading to the final stimulation of osteoclastogenesis from local OC precursors (3, 20).

INTERACTION BETWEEN IMMUNE SYSTEM AND BONE FAVOR TUMOR CELL SURVIVAL AND PROLIFERATION

A fundamental molecular link between immune system and bone is represented by the axis comprising RANKL, its receptor RANK, and the natural decoy receptor osteoprotegerin (OPG) (29, 30). RANK/RANKL interaction activates osteoclastogenesis, while OPG counteracts this effect by competing with RANK to bind RANKL (31). OBs and BM stromal cells are the main producers of both RANKL and OPG in physiological conditions (32), however, B or activated T cells can influence the RANKL/OPG ratio, end eventually osteoclastogenesis by producing OPG or RANKL, respectively (33). Literature data report that T cells could directly carry on a modulatory action on OCs through production of different factors such as IL-7, RANKL, TNFα (34–38). Circulating OC precursors from bone metastatic patients have been shown to differentiate into mature OCs in a T cell dependent way, in the absence of the classical OC inducers M-CSF, and RANKL (39). On the other hand, in mouse models, it has been shown that T cells exert a fundamental anti-tumor effect, regardless of OC status. Indeed, PLCγ2-KO mice, with dysfunctional OCs and impaired T-cell activation, showed increased bone tumor growth despite protection from bone loss, whereas Lyn-KO mice with numerous OCs and increased T-cell responses, showed impaired tumor growth in bone despite enhanced OC activity and osteolysis. The injection of antigen-specific wild-type cytotoxic CD8(+) T cells in both these mouse models normalized tumor growth in bone, suggesting their important role in the regulation of tumor bone metastases (40). T cells can limit tumor cell diffusion by releasing IFNγ, which also affects osteoclastogenesis, indeed lack of IFNγ has been related to the increase of bone metastases (41).

Tumor cells modify the surrounding microenvironment, indeed it has been shown that BM from breast cancer patients differed from that of healthy subjects in its cellular composition as well as the activation status of cells from the innate immune system (macrophages, NK cells) and from the adaptive immune system (T cell subsets) (42). Many immature and suppressor immune cell types are present in bone, such as T regulatory cells, which must maintain a balanced immune-reactivity (43), and MDSCs, which stimulate osteoclastogenesis (44). In breast cancer, infiltrating T regulatory cells produce RANKL, promoting OC differentiation, activity, and subsequent bone lesions (45).

MDSCs are increased in cancer patients from 2 up to 25% (46) suppressing innate and adaptive immune response, thus sustaining tumor growth and metastatization (47). In breast cancer, MDSCs, derived from bone metastatic microenvironment, can differentiate into mature and functional OCs *in vitro* (48).

NK CELLS ARE ENDOWED WITH POWERFUL ANTI-TUMOR FUNCTIONS

NK cells can kill a variety of tumor cells of different origin and types (49–52). This wide range of reactivity is ensured by the expression at the cell surface of several receptors capable of activating or inhibiting the main functions of NK cells, including the release of cytolytic granules (49, 53). Thus, thanks to their HLA-I-specific inhibitory receptors and a complex and heterogeneous group of activating receptors, NK cells can sense the HLA-I expression decrease that often characterizes tumor cells and recognize different ligands that can be variably induced on cells undergoing tumor transformation (**Table 1**). Different patterns of NK receptors are engaged during contact with pathological or non-pathological cells, regulating the activation, and the intensity of the cytolytic response (49, 50, 53, 54). Most NK cells express the FcγIII-receptor (CD16), which is a strong activator of cytotoxicity and enables NK cells to mediate the Antibody-Dependent Cellular Cytotoxicity (ADCC).

NK cells can attack tumor cells by releasing pro-apoptotic factors, including TNF-α and Tumor necrosis factor-related apoptosis-inducing ligand (TRAIL) (69, 70), or cytokines capable of inhibiting tumor cell proliferation and promoting the inflammatory response, such as IFN-γ. In addition, NK cells can release chemokines (CCL3, CCL4, CCL5, and XCL1) capable of attracting T cells, DC, and monocytes (71, 72) and give rise to specific cross-talks promoting and regulating the adaptive anti-tumor response (73–75). Finally, NK cells can also amplify their recruitment at the tumor site by releasing a chemotactic form of HMGB1 molecule upon interaction with tumor cells (76).

In order to appropriately evaluate the role of NK cells in the control of tumors it should be also considered that the NK cell population is rather heterogeneous as it includes different cell subsets, each characterized by peculiar functional capabilities (77). In humans, the CD56brightCD16dim/neg ($CD56^{bright}$) and the CD56dim/CD16bright ($CD56^{dim}$) cells represent the two most studied NK cell types. The $CD56^{bright}$ NK cells largely produce IFN-γ in response to monokines but are poorly cytotoxic. These cells constitute 5–10% of circulating NK cells, and, in line with their pattern of chemokine and homing receptors (i.e., CD62L, CCR7, CXCR3, and CXCR4), represent most LN-NK cells and an important fraction of tissue NK cells in different organs. The $CD56^{dim}$ cells release IFN-γ upon triggering of major activating receptors (NKp46, NKp30, NKp44, and CD16) and are highly cytotoxic. They represent 90–95% of PB NK cells and predominate in spleen, lungs, and kidney although in different percentages. Moreover, CD56dim NK cells express chemokine receptors (CXCR1, CX_3CR1, and CXCR4)

TABLE 1 | Overview of the major NK cell receptors and Ligands involved in tumor cell recognition.

	NK Receptor	Ligand(s)	Ligand expression on tumor cells	References
Inhibitory receptors	KIRs*	HLA-I (HLA-A,B,C)	Down-regulated in certain tumor cells	(50, 54)
	CD94:NKG2A	HLA-E (non-classical HLA-I)	Down-regulated in certain tumor cells	(50, 54, 55)
	LILRB1	HLA-I (HLA-A,B,C)	Down-regulated in certain tumor cells	(50, 54)
		HLA-G (non-classical HLA-I)	Up-regulated in certain tumors	(55–57)
Activating receptors	NKp46	HSPG	Up-regulated/modified in different tumor cells	(58, 59)
		Complement Factor P (properdin)	?	(60)
		Additional still unknown ligands**		(50, 61)
	NKp44	HSPG	Up-regulated/modified in different tumor cells	(58, 59)
		MLL5 isoform	Ectopically expressed at the cell surface of tumor cells of hematologic and solid tumors	(62)
		PDGF-DD	Soluble factor released by several tumors (induces NKp44-dependent cytokine release)	(63)
		Nidogen-1	Decoy extracellular ligand expressed by different tumor cell lines (inhibits NKp44-dependent cytokine release)	(64)
	NKp30	HSPG	Up-regulated/modified in different tumor cells	(58, 59)
		BAT3	Up-regulated in different tumor cells (released in exosomes)	(65)
		B7-H6	Highly expressed in different tumor cells	(66)
	NKG2D	MICA/B, ULBP1-6	Up-regulated in tumors of epithelial and non-epithelial origins	(67)
	DNAM-1	CD155, CD112	Up-regulated in many tumor cell types	(68)

**KIRs, Killer-cell immunoglobulin-like receptor; NKG2A, Natural Killer Group 2 A; LILRB1, Leukocyte Immunoglobulin Like Receptor B1; NKG2D, Natural Killer Group 2 D; DNAM-1, DNAX Accessory Molecule-1; HLA, Human Leukocyte Antigen; HSPG, Heparan Sulfate Proteoglycans; MLL5, mixed-lineage leukemia protein-5; PDGF-DD, platelet-derived growth factor—isoform dimer DD; BAT3, human leukocyte antigen (HLA)-B-associated transcript 3; MIC, MHC class I chain-related protein; ULBP, UL16 binding proteins.*

***Different tumor cell lines bind recombinant soluble NKp46 receptors and/or are killed by NK cells in a NKp46-dependent way but the putative ligand on these cells has not yet been identified.*

that allow their possible recruitment to inflamed peripheral tissues (77, 78). The assessment of NK cells in tissues and the definition of their anti-tumor potential are rather complicated. Indeed, tissues comprise both potentially cytotoxic NK cells that recirculate from PB, but also stably resident cells expressing specific markers of tissue retention (CD69, CD49a, and CD103) and chemokine receptors (CCR5, CXCR6) (79–82). These latter cells may display unique functions, possibly organ-specific, not necessarily oriented to tumor cell killing.

ROLE OF NK CELLS IN THE CONTROL OF SOLID TUMORS AND METASTATIC SPREAD

Several studies using different mice models have documented that NK cells can control tumor insurgence, growth, and metastasis dissemination (83–86). Remarkably, the role of NK cells in the control of tumors has also been suggested in different human studies. In a 11-year follow-up study on more than 8,000 healthy individuals, Imai et al. initially showed that insurgence of tumors of different types inversely correlated with the levels of natural cytotoxic activity of peripheral blood lymphocytes (87). More recently, different groups have found correlations between the quantity and the quality of tumor infiltrating or PB-NK cells and a more favorable prognosis or the lower number of metastases at diagnosis (88). In this last decade, it has also become evident that a plethora of mechanisms of tumor escape can strongly reduce the efficacy of NK cells. Within the tumor microenvironment, different immune suppressor cells (including Tregs and MDSCs), tumor-associated fibroblasts (TAF), and tumor cells can produce soluble factors (TGF-β, PGE2, IDO-derived kynurenine) which inhibit expression and function of the major activating receptors (89, 90). Similar effects on activating receptors are induced also by soluble decoy ligands shed by tumor cells or released as extracellular molecules (64, 89, 91, 92). Finally, exposure to hypoxia, which often characterizes tumor tissues, can also cause activating receptor down-regulation (93). Remarkably, some of these suppressive mechanisms, such as those induced by hypoxia and TAFs, appear to minimally affect the ADCC function (94). On the other hand, hypoxia and tumor cells can modulate the repertoire of chemokine receptors on NK cells and favor the preferential recruitment of CD56bright cells (poorly cytotoxic and unable to mediate ADCC) (95). The NK-cell recruitment into neoplastic tissues may also be influenced by the chemokine profile induced in the tumor microenvironment. Human lung and breast tumors have been shown to express higher CCL19 (a CD56bright cell attracting chemokine) and lower CXCL12 compared to their normal tissue counterpart (96), while in mice, BM with MM showed increased CXCL9 and CXCL10, decreased CXCL12, down-modulation of CXCR3 on NK cells, and selective reduction of KLRG1^{-} cytotoxic NK cells (97). Collectively, the above-described mechanisms can account for the observation that in different tumor tissues the NK cell infiltrate is often limited or constituted by CD56bright or altered (poorly functional) CD56^{dim} cells (50, 89).

Another important issue regards the so-called immune-checkpoints. Different pairs of receptor-ligands are available to the immune system to regulate or terminate excessive (dangerous) responses. Some of these receptors, such as PD-1, TIM-3, TIGIT, and SIGIRR, can be also expressed by NK cells, especially by those associated to tumors, and control different NK cell functions including cytotoxicity. Blocking or overcoming these checkpoints, by specific monoclonal antibodies or activating cytokines can improve the NK-mediated control of carcinogenesis or metastasis formation (98–101).

THE AMBIGUOUS ROLE OF THE NK:CSC CROSS-TALK IN THE CONTROL OF METASTASIS FORMATION

Whether NK cells can interfere with CSC formation, or kill CSC at the site of primary tumor, during circulation, or in the pre-metastatic niches represents an interesting and still incompletely investigated issue. Several reports have indicated that NK cells can kill tumor cells with features of CSC derived from different tumors (glioma, melanoma, colon, prostate, and breast) (102). Consistent with these findings, CSCs of different origins have been shown to express or even up-regulate the ligands for NKG2D, DNAM1, and NKp30 NK-activating receptors and cells undergoing EMT showed up-regulated NKG2D-Ls (88, 102). In addition, EMT induction in lung cancer cells could promote increased NK cell-mediated metastasis-specific immunosurveillance in RAG1$^{-/-}$ mice (103). On the other hand, it has also been shown that NK cells could induce melanoma cells to undergo EMT, upregulate the expression of stemness markers, reduce proliferative capability, thus acquiring characteristics reminiscent of the CSC phenotype. Moreover, EMT increased ability of melanoma cells to suppress NK cell cytotoxicity against tumor cells (104).

IS THERE ANY ROLE FOR NK CELLS IN BONE METASTASES?

Although the role of NK cells in contrasting bone metastases has been recently suggested in breast cancer preclinical models (105), an established knowledge on this issue is still lacking. BM is where NK cells mature and differentiate from CD34+ progenitors; therefore, it contains precursors at different stages. Once NK cells have matured, changes in the expression of the key receptors CXCR4 and S1P5 (down- and up-regulated, respectively) drive their egress from the CXCL12-containing BM and their recruitment to blood where the S1P5-ligand S1P is abundant (106). Besides the immature NK cell precursors, BM also contains a reservoir of mature NK cells, recirculating from the blood, which can be mobilized upon inflammatory stimuli (107). BM also includes a substantial population of resident CXCR6+CD69+ NK (BMrNK) cells, which may be poorly effective against tumor cells. Indeed, compared to classical NK cells, BMrNK cells display lower proliferative capacity, cytolytic granule content, DNAM1, and higher TIGIT expression (108).

The heterogeneity of the NK cells in the BM and their still poorly defined interaction with the metastatic niche, together with the possible cross-talk between PB-NK and CSC/EMT cells add a layer of complexity to the issue of how NK cells can influence bone metastasis formation and progression (**Figure 1**). In the bone, the RANK-RANK-L axis, whose deregulation is important in metastasis formation, also influences NK cells. The signaling of RANK-L in leukemia cells can induce the release of NK-suppressing factors (109), whereas, under inflammatory conditions (knee arthritis) NK cells can stimulate OCs through activation of RANKL pathway (110). NK cells can either favor or inhibit generation of OCs depending on the release of TNF-α or IFN-γ, respectively (111, 112). On the other hand, OCs have been shown to contribute to the induction of efficient NK cells, capable of inhibiting growth of poorly differentiated tumors in humanized BLT mice (113). This effect is in line with the ability of OCs to produce NK-stimulating cytokines such as IL-12, IL-15, and IL-18. Finally, OCs are targets of NK cells, as they express MHC class I molecules at low levels and are killed by IL-2 treated NK cells (114).

CONCLUDING REMARKS

Understanding the reason why and how in many patients' metastases can overcome the surveillance of NK cells is still poorly understood. Studies are rapidly progressing to define how to properly activate NK cells by cytokine combinations and unleash their potential by blocking their checkpoint receptors. The crucial mechanisms that govern entrance and egress of NK cells in the bone metastatic niche and modulate the NK cell killing capability within the bone lesions are lacking. Addressing these questions will significantly increase

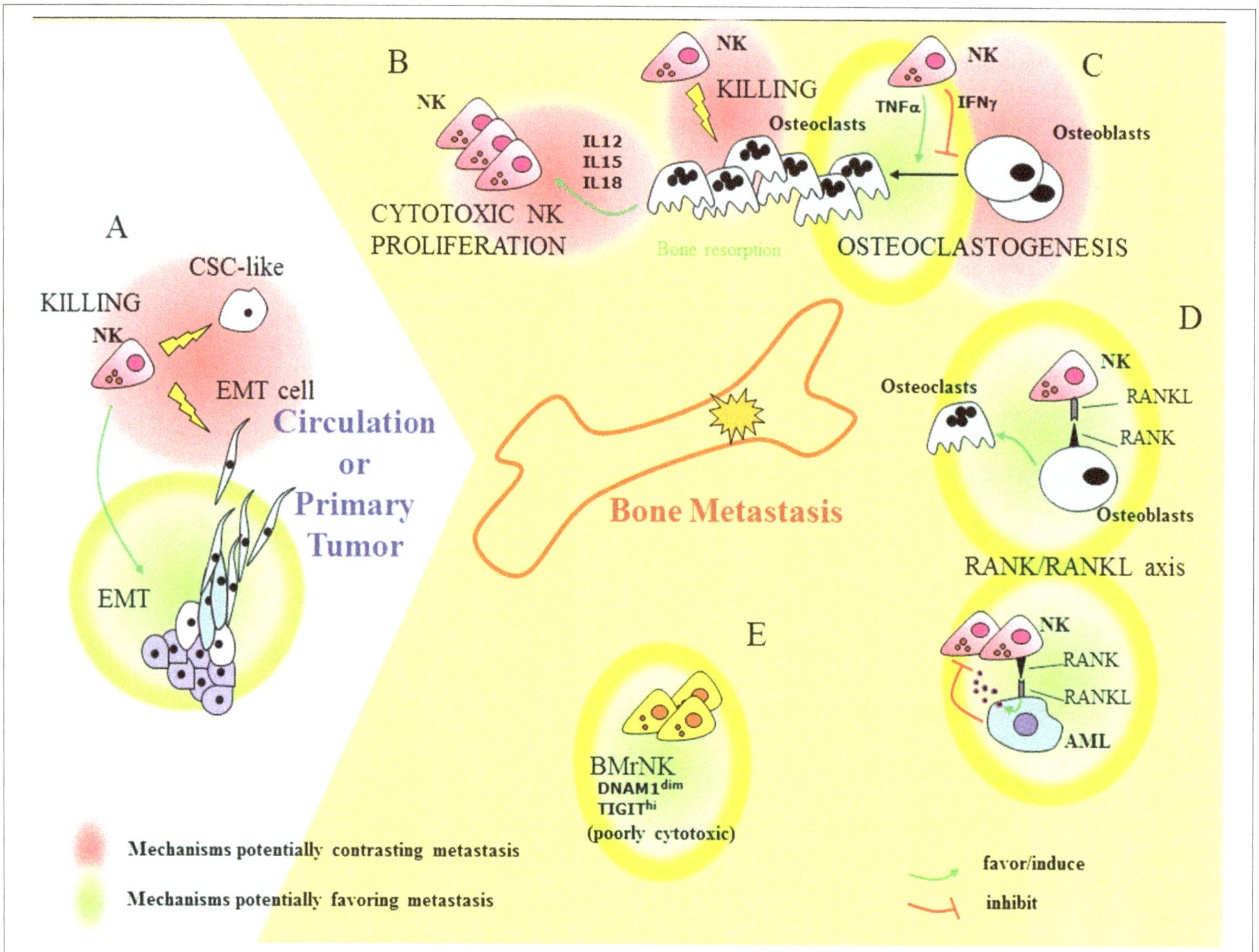

FIGURE 1 | Understanding how NK cells can influence bone metastasis. Outside and inside the bone (light blue and yellow fields, respectively), different functional interactions involving BM resident, recirculating, or PB NK cells can have contrasting effects on bone metastasis formation and tumor progression. **(A)** At the site of primary tumors NK cells may favor EMT. On the other hand, NK cells can kill pro-metastatic tumor cells, such as cells that have undergone EMT (EMT cells), and cells with features of CSC (CSC-like). **(B)** OCs can induce proliferation of highly cytotoxic NK cells via the release of IL12, IL15, and IL18. **(C)** The interaction of NK cells with OCs gives rise to contrasting effects: NK cells can either favor or inhibit generation of OCs depending on the release of TNF-α or IFN-γ, respectively and kill OCs. **(D)** The RANK/RANKL axis may play a role in the cross-talk between NK cells and bone microenvironment: the signaling of RANK-L in leukemia cells (AML) can induce the release of NK-suppressing factors; on the other hand, RANKL-expressing NK cells provide signals for OC generation. **(E)** Besides recirculating PB-NK cells, BM also contains resident poorly cytotoxic NK cells (BMrNK) which may hardly eliminate tumor cells.

the therapeutic options for NK cells in the treatment of bone metastatic disease.

AUTHOR CONTRIBUTIONS

IR revised the literature and wrote the paragraphs concerning bone metastasis. MV revised the literature and wrote the paragraphs concerning NK cells.

FUNDING

This work was supported by the CRT Foundations, Fondazione Ricerca Molinette ONLUS (IR) and Associazione Italiana Ricerca sul Cancro AIRC under grants: IG 2014 project n. 15428 (MV), 5 × 1000 Min Sal. 2013 (MV) and Roche Foundation: Bando per la Ricerca Roche 2017.

REFERENCES

1. Macedo F, Ladeira K, Pinho F, Saraiva N, Bonito N, Pinto L, et al. Bone metastases: an overview. *Oncol Rev.* (2017) 11:321. doi: 10.4081/oncol.2017.321
2. Coleman RE. Clinical features of metastatic bone disease and risk of skeletal morbidity. *Clin Cancer Res.* (2006) 12 (20 Pt 2):6243s–9s. doi: 10.1158/1078-0432.CCR-06-0931
3. Mundy GR. Metastasis to bone: causes, consequences and therapeutic opportunities. *Nat Rev Cancer.* (2002) 2:584–93. doi: 10.1038/nrc867
4. D'Amico L, Roato I. The impact of immune system in regulating bone metastasis formation by osteotropic tumors. *J Immunol Res.* (2015) 2015:143526. doi: 10.1155/2015/143526
5. Li L, Bhatia R. Stem cell quiescence. *Clin Cancer Res.* (2011) 17:4936–41. doi: 10.1158/1078-0432.CCR-10-1499
6. Tam WL, Weinberg RA. The epigenetics of epithelial-mesenchymal plasticity in cancer. *Nat Med.* (2013) 19:1438–49. doi: 10.1038/nm.3336
7. Peinado H, Zhang H, Matei IR, Costa-Silva B, Hoshino A, Rodrigues G, et al. Pre-metastatic niches: organ-specific homes for metastases. *Nat Rev Cancer.* (2017) 17:302–17. doi: 10.1038/nrc.2017.6
8. Braun S, Vogl FD, Naume B, Janni W, Osborne MP, Coombes RC, et al. A pooled analysis of bone marrow micrometastasis in breast cancer. *N Engl J Med.* (2005) 353:793–802. doi: 10.1056/NEJMoa050434
9. Pantel K, Brakenhoff RH, Brandt B. Detection, clinical relevance and specific biological properties of disseminating tumour cells. *Nat Rev Cancer.* (2008) 8:329–40. doi: 10.1038/nrc2375
10. Bartkowiak K, Kwiatkowski M, Buck F, Gorges TM, Nilse L, Assmann V, et al. Disseminated tumor cells persist in the bone marrow of breast cancer patients through sustained activation of the unfolded protein response. *Cancer Res.* (2015) 75:5367–77. doi: 10.1158/0008-5472.CAN-14-3728
11. Janni W, Vogl FD, Wiedswang G, Synnestvedt M, Fehm T, Juckstock J, et al. Persistence of disseminated tumor cells in the bone marrow of breast cancer patients predicts increased risk for relapse–a European pooled analysis. *Clin Cancer Res.* (2011) 17:2967–76. doi: 10.1158/1078-0432.CCR-10-2515
12. Calvi LM, Adams GB, Weibrecht KW, Weber JM, Olson DP, Knight MC, et al. Osteoblastic cells regulate the haematopoietic stem cell niche. *Nature.* (2003) 425:841–6. doi: 10.1038/nature02040
13. Zhang J, Niu C, Ye L, Huang H, He X, Tong WG, et al. Identification of the haematopoietic stem cell niche and control of the niche size. *Nature.* (2003) 425:836–41. doi: 10.1038/nature02041
14. Broxmeyer HE, Orschell CM, Clapp DW, Hangoc G, Cooper S, Plett PA, et al. Rapid mobilization of murine and human hematopoietic stem and progenitor cells with AMD3100, a CXCR4 antagonist. *J Exp Med.* (2005) 201:1307–18. doi: 10.1084/jem.20041385
15. Kang Y, Siegel PM, Shu W, Drobnjak M, Kakonen SM, Cordon-Cardo C, et al. A multigenic program mediating breast cancer metastasis to bone. *Cancer Cell.* (2003) 3:537–49. doi: 10.1016/S1535-6108(03)00132-6
16. Wang H, Yu C, Gao X, Welte T, Muscarella AM, Tian L, et al. The osteogenic niche promotes early-stage bone colonization of disseminated breast cancer cells. *Cancer Cell.* (2015) 27:193–210. doi: 10.1016/j.ccell.2014.11.017
17. Richert MM, Vaidya KS, Mills CN, Wong D, Korz W, Hurst DR, et al. Inhibition of CXCR4 by CTCE-9908 inhibits breast cancer metastasis to lung and bone. *Oncol Rep.* (2009) 21:761–7. doi: 10.3892/or_00000282
18. Bertolini G, D'Amico L, Moro M, Landoni E, Perego P, Miceli R, et al. Microenvironment-modulated metastatic CD133+/CXCR4+/EpCAM- lung cancer-initiating cells sustain tumor dissemination and correlate with poor prognosis. *Cancer Res.* (2015) 75:3636–49. doi: 10.1158/0008-5472.CAN-14-3781
19. Chu K, Cheng CJ, Ye X, Lee YC, Zurita AJ, Chen DT, et al. Cadherin-11 promotes the metastasis of prostate cancer cells to bone. *Mol Cancer Res.* (2008) 6:1259–67. doi: 10.1158/1541-7786.MCR-08-0077
20. Lu X, Mu E, Wei Y, Riethdorf S, Yang Q, Yuan M, et al. VCAM-1 promotes osteolytic expansion of indolent bone micrometastasis of breast cancer by engaging alpha4beta1-positive osteoclast progenitors. *Cancer Cell.* (2011) 20:701–14. doi: 10.1016/j.ccr.2011.11.002
21. Rudland PS, Platt-Higgins A, El-Tanani M, De Silva Rudland S, Barraclough R, Winstanley JH, et al. Prognostic significance of the metastasis-associated protein osteopontin in human breast cancer. *Cancer Res.* (2002) 62:3417–27.
22. Anborgh PH, Mutrie JC, Tuck AB, Chambers AF. Role of the metastasis-promoting protein osteopontin in the tumour microenvironment. *J Cell Mol Med.* (2010) 14:2037–44. doi: 10.1111/j.1582-4934.2010.01115.x
23. Shiozawa Y, Pedersen EA, Havens AM, Jung Y, Mishra A, Joseph J, et al. Human prostate cancer metastases target the hematopoietic stem cell niche to establish footholds in mouse bone marrow. *J Clin Invest.* (2011) 121:1298–312. doi: 10.1172/JCI43414
24. Oskarsson T, Batlle E, Massague J. Metastatic stem cells: sources, niches, and vital pathways. *Cell Stem Cell.* (2014) 14:306–21. doi: 10.1016/j.stem.2014.02.002
25. Lou Y, McDonald PC, Oloumi A, Chia S, Ostlund C, Ahmadi A, et al. Targeting tumor hypoxia: suppression of breast tumor growth and metastasis by novel carbonic anhydrase IX inhibitors. *Cancer Res.* (2011) 71:3364–76. doi: 10.1158/0008-5472.CAN-10-4261
26. Chiang AC, Massague J. Molecular basis of metastasis. *N Engl J Med.* (2008) 359:2814–23. doi: 10.1056/NEJMra0805239
27. Roodman GD. Mechanisms of bone metastasis. *N Engl J Med.* (2004) 350:1655–64. doi: 10.1056/NEJMra030831
28. Bussard KM, Gay CV, Mastro AM. The bone microenvironment in metastasis; what is special about bone? *Cancer Metastasis Rev.* (2008) 27:41–55. doi: 10.1007/s10555-007-9109-4
29. Hofbauer LC, Kuhne CA, Viereck V. The OPG/RANKL/RANK system in metabolic bone diseases. *J Musculoskelet Neuronal Interact.* (2004) 4:268–75.
30. Santini D, Perrone G, Roato I, Godio L, Pantano F, Grasso D, et al. Expression pattern of receptor activator of NFkappaB (RANK) in a series of primary solid tumors and related bone metastases. *J Cell Physiol.* (2011) 226:780–4. doi: 10.1002/jcp.22402
31. Kostenuik PJ, Shalhoub V. Osteoprotegerin: a physiological and pharmacological inhibitor of bone resorption. *Curr Pharm Des.* (2001) 7:613–35. doi: 10.2174/1381612013397807
32. Manolagas SC. Birth and death of bone cells: basic regulatory mechanisms and implications for the pathogenesis and treatment of osteoporosis. *Endocr Rev.* (2000) 21:115–37. doi: 10.1210/er.21.2.115
33. Li Y, Toraldo G, Li A, Yang X, Zhang H, Qian WP, et al. B cells and T cells are critical for the preservation of bone homeostasis and attainment of peak bone mass *in vivo*. *Blood.* (2007) 109:3839–48. doi: 10.1182/blood-2006-07-037994
34. Weitzmann MN, Roggia C, Toraldo G, Weitzmann L, Pacifici R. Increased production of IL-7 uncouples bone formation from bone resorption during estrogen deficiency. *J Clin Invest.* (2002) 110:1643–50. doi: 10.1172/JCI0215687
35. Lee SK, Kalinowski JF, Jastrzebski SL, Puddington L, Lorenzo JA. Interleukin-7 is a direct inhibitor of *in vitro* osteoclastogenesis. *Endocrinology.* (2003) 144:3524–31. doi: 10.1210/en.2002-221057

36. Colucci S, Brunetti G, Rizzi R, Zonno A, Mori G, Colaianni G, et al. T cells support osteoclastogenesis in an *in vitro* model derived from human multiple myeloma bone disease: the role of the OPG/TRAIL interaction. *Blood.* (2004) 104:3722–30. doi: 10.1182/blood-2004-02-0474
37. Roato I, Brunetti G, Gorassini E, Grano M, Colucci S, Bonello L, et al. IL-7 up-regulates TNF-alpha-dependent osteoclastogenesis in patients affected by solid tumor. *PLoS ONE.* (2006) 1:e124. doi: 10.1371/journal.pone.0000124
38. Giuliani N, Colla S, Sala R, Moroni M, Lazzaretti M, La Monica S, et al. Human myeloma cells stimulate the receptor activator of nuclear factor-kappa B ligand (RANKL) in T lymphocytes: a potential role in multiple myeloma bone disease. *Blood.* (2002) 100:4615–21. doi: 10.1182/blood-2002-04-1121
39. Roato I, Grano M, Brunetti G, Colucci S, Mussa A, Bertetto O, et al. Mechanisms of spontaneous osteoclastogenesis in cancer with bone involvement. *FASEB J.* (2005) 19:228–30. doi: 10.1096/fj.04-1823fje
40. Zhang K, Kim S, Cremasco V, Hirbe AC, Collins L, Piwnica-Worms D, et al. CD8+ T cells regulate bone tumor burden independent of osteoclast resorption. *Cancer Res.* (2011) 71:4799–808. doi: 10.1158/0008-5472.CAN-10-3922
41. Xu Z, Hurchla MA, Deng H, Uluckan O, Bu F, Berdy A, et al. Interferon-gamma targets cancer cells and osteoclasts to prevent tumor-associated bone loss and bone metastases. *J Biol Chem.* (2009) 284:4658–66. doi: 10.1074/jbc.M804812200
42. Feuerer M, Rocha M, Bai L, Umansky V, Solomayer EF, Bastert G, et al. Enrichment of memory T cells and other profound immunological changes in the bone marrow from untreated breast cancer patients. *Int J Cancer.* (2001) 92:96–105. doi: 10.1002/1097-0215(200102)9999:9999<::AID-IJC1152>3.0.CO;2-Q
43. Zou L, Barnett B, Safah H, Larussa VF, Evdemon-Hogan M, Mottram P, et al. Bone marrow is a reservoir for CD4+CD25+ regulatory T cells that traffic through CXCL12/CXCR4 signals. *Cancer Res.* (2004) 64:8451–5. doi: 10.1158/0008-5472.CAN-04-1987
44. Almand B, Clark JI, Nikitina E, van Beynen J, English NR, Knight SC, et al. Increased production of immature myeloid cells in cancer patients: a mechanism of immunosuppression in cancer. *J Immunol.* (2001) 166:678–89. doi: 10.4049/jimmunol.166.1.678
45. Tan W, Zhang W, Strasner A, Grivennikov S, Cheng JQ, Hoffman RM, et al. Tumour-infiltrating regulatory T cells stimulate mammary cancer metastasis through RANKL-RANK signalling. *Nature.* (2011) 470:548–53. doi: 10.1038/nature09707
46. Zea AH, Rodriguez PC, Atkins MB, Hernandez C, Signoretti S, Zabaleta J, et al. Arginase-producing myeloid suppressor cells in renal cell carcinoma patients: a mechanism of tumor evasion. *Cancer Res.* (2005) 65:3044–8. doi: 10.1158/0008-5472.CAN-04-4505
47. Kusmartsev S, Gabrilovich DI. Role of immature myeloid cells in mechanisms of immune evasion in cancer. *Cancer Immunol Immunother.* (2006) 55:237–45. doi: 10.1007/s00262-005-0048-z
48. Sawant A, Ponnazhagan S. Myeloid-derived suppressor cells as osteoclast progenitors: a novel target for controlling osteolytic bone metastasis. *Cancer Res.* (2013) 73:4606–10. doi: 10.1158/0008-5472.CAN-13-0305
49. Moretta L, Pietra G, Montaldo E, Vacca P, Pende D, Falco M, et al. Human NK cells: from surface receptors to the therapy of leukemias and solid tumors. *Front Immunol.* (2014) 5:87. doi: 10.3389/fimmu.2014.00087
50. Cantoni C, Grauwet K, Pietra G, Parodi M, Mingari MC, Maria AD, et al. Role of NK cells in immunotherapy and virotherapy of solid tumors. *Immunotherapy.* (2015) 7:861–82. doi: 10.2217/imt.15.53
51. Guillerey C, Huntington ND, Smyth MJ. Targeting natural killer cells in cancer immunotherapy. *Nat Immunol.* (2016) 17:1025–36. doi: 10.1038/ni.3518
52. Chiossone L, Dumas PY, Vienne M, Vivier E. Natural killer cells and other innate lymphoid cells in cancer. *Nat Rev Immunol.* (2018) 18:671–88. doi: 10.1038/s41577-018-0061-z
53. Vivier E, Raulet DH, Moretta A, Caligiuri MA, Zitvogel L, Lanier LL, et al. Innate or adaptive immunity? The example of natural killer cells. *Science.* (2011) 331:44–9. doi: 10.1126/science.1198687
54. Moretta L, Bottino C, Pende D, Vitale M, Mingari MC, Moretta A. Different checkpoints in human NK-cell activation. *Trends Immunol.* (2004) 25:670–6. doi: 10.1016/j.it.2004.09.008
55. Lopez-Botet M, Llano M, Navarro F, Bellon T. NK cell recognition of non-classical HLA class I molecules. *Semin Immunol.* (2000) 12:109–19. doi: 10.1006/smim.2000.0213
56. Carosella ED, Moreau P, Lemaoult J, Rouas-Freiss N. HLA-G: from biology to clinical benefits. *Trends Immunol.* (2008) 29:125–32. doi: 10.1016/j.it.2007.11.005
57. Rebmann V, Nuckel H, Duhrsen U, Grosse-Wilde H. HLA-G in B-chronic lymphocytic leukaemia: clinical relevance and functional implications. *Semin Cancer Biol.* (2007) 17:430–5. doi: 10.1016/j.semcancer.2007.06.011
58. Hecht ML, Rosental B, Horlacher T, Hershkovitz O, De Paz JL, Noti C, et al. Natural cytotoxicity receptors NKp30, NKp44 and NKp46 bind to different heparan sulfate/heparin sequences. *J Proteome Res.* (2009) 8:712–20. doi: 10.1021/pr800747c
59. Blackhall FH, Merry CL, Davies EJ, Jayson GC. Heparan sulfate proteoglycans and cancer. *Br J Cancer.* (2001) 85:1094–8. doi: 10.1054/bjoc.2001.2054
60. Narni-Mancinelli E, Campisi L, Bassand D, Cazareth J, Gounon P, Glaichenhaus N, et al. Memory CD8+ T cells mediate antibacterial immunity via CCL3 activation of TNF/ROI+ phagocytes. *J Exp Med.* (2007) 204:2075–87. doi: 10.1084/jem.20070204
61. Sivori S, Vitale M, Morelli L, Sanseverino L, Augugliaro R, Bottino C, et al. p46, a novel natural killer cell-specific surface molecule that mediates cell activation. *J Exp Med.* (1997) 186:1129–36. doi: 10.1084/jem.186.7.1129
62. Baychelier F, Sennepin A, Ermonval M, Dorgham K, Debre P, Vieillard V. Identification of a cellular ligand for the natural cytotoxicity receptor NKp44. *Blood.* (2013) 122:2935–42. doi: 10.1182/blood-2013-03-489054
63. Barrow AD, Edeling MA, Trifonov V, Luo J, Goyal P, Bohl B, et al. Natural killer cells control tumor growth by sensing a growth factor. *Cell.* (2018) 172:534–48.e19. doi: 10.1016/j.cell.2017.11.037
64. Gaggero S, Bruschi M, Petretto A, Parodi M, Zotto GD, Lavarello C, et al. Nidogen-1 is a novel extracellular ligand for the NKp44 activating receptor. *Oncoimmunology.* (2018) 7:e1470730. doi: 10.1080/2162402X.2018.1470730
65. Pogge von Strandmann E, Simhadri VR, von Tresckow B, Sasse S, Reiners KS, Hansen HP, et al. Human leukocyte antigen-B-associated transcript 3 is released from tumor cells and engages the NKp30 receptor on natural killer cells. *Immunity.* (2007) 27:965–74. doi: 10.1016/j.immuni.2007.10.010
66. Brandt CS, Baratin M, Yi EC, Kennedy J, Gao Z, Fox B, et al. The B7 family member B7-H6 is a tumor cell ligand for the activating natural killer cell receptor NKp30 in humans. *J Exp Med.* (2009) 206:1495–503. doi: 10.1084/jem.20090681
67. Raulet DH, Gasser S, Gowen BG, Deng W, Jung H. Regulation of ligands for the NKG2D activating receptor. *Annu Rev Immunol.* (2013) 31:413–41. doi: 10.1146/annurev-immunol-032712-095951
68. Bottino C, Castriconi R, Pende D, Rivera P, Nanni M, Carnemolla B, et al. Identification of PVR (CD155) and Nectin-2 (CD112) as cell surfaceligands for the human DNAM-1 (CD226) activating molecule. *J Exp Med.* (2003) 198:557–67. doi: 10.1084/jem.20030788
69. Takeda K, Hayakawa Y, Smyth MJ, Kayagaki N, Yamaguchi N, Kakuta S, et al. Involvement of tumor necrosis factor-related apoptosis-inducing ligand in surveillance of tumor metastasis by liver natural killer cells. *Nat Med.* (2001) 7:94–100. doi: 10.1038/83416
70. Plenker D, Bertrand M, de Langen AJ, Riedel R, Lorenz C, Scheel AH, et al. Structural alterations of MET trigger response to MET kinase inhibition in lung adenocarcinoma patients. *Clin Cancer Res.* (2018) 24:1337–43. doi: 10.1158/1078-0432.CCR-17-3001
71. Fauriat C, Long EO, Ljunggren HG, Bryceson YT. Regulation of human NK-cell cytokine and chemokine production by target cell recognition. *Blood.* (2010) 115:2167–76. doi: 10.1182/blood-2009-08-238469
72. Bottcher JP, Bonavita E, Chakravarty P, Blees H, Cabeza-Cabrerizo M, Sammicheli S, et al. NK cells stimulate recruitment of cDC1 into the tumor microenvironment promoting cancer immune control. *Cell.* (2018) 172:1022–37.e14. doi: 10.1016/j.cell.2018.01.004
73. Moretta L, Ferlazzo G, Bottino C, Vitale M, Pende D, Mingari MC, et al. Effector and regulatory events during natural killer-dendritic cell interactions. *Immunol Rev.* (2006) 214:219–28. doi: 10.1111/j.1600-065X.2006.00450.x

74. Bellora F, Castriconi R, Dondero A, Reggiardo G, Moretta L, Mantovani A, et al. The interaction of human natural killer cells with either unpolarized or polarized macrophages results in different functional outcomes. *Proc Natl Acad Sci USA*. (2010) 107:21659–64. doi: 10.1073/pnas.1007654108
75. Ardolino M, Zingoni A, Cerboni C, Cecere F, Soriani A, Iannitto ML, et al. DNAM-1 ligand expression on Ag-stimulated T lymphocytes is mediated by ROS-dependent activation of DNA-damage response: relevance for NK-T cell interaction. *Blood*. (2011) 117:4778–86. doi: 10.1182/blood-2010-08-300954
76. Parodi M, Pedrazzi M, Cantoni C, Averna M, Patrone M, Cavaletto M, et al. Natural Killer (NK)/melanoma cell interaction induces NK-mediated release of chemotactic High Mobility Group Box-1 (HMGB1) capable of amplifying NK cell recruitment. *Oncoimmunology*. (2015) 4:e1052353. doi: 10.1080/2162402X.2015.1052353
77. Freud AG, Mundy-Bosse BL, Yu J, Caligiuri MA. The broad spectrum of human natural killer cell diversity. *Immunity*. (2017) 47:820–33. doi: 10.1016/j.immuni.2017.10.008
78. Bjorkstrom NK, Ljunggren HG, Michaelsson J. Emerging insights into natural killer cells in human peripheral tissues. *Nat Rev Immunol*. (2016) 16:310–20. doi: 10.1038/nri.2016.34
79. Marquardt N, Beziat V, Nystrom S, Hengst J, Ivarsson MA, Kekalainen E, et al. Cutting edge: identification and characterization of human intrahepatic CD49a+ NK cells. *J Immunol*. (2015) 194:2467–71. doi: 10.4049/jimmunol.1402756
80. Cuff AO, Robertson FP, Stegmann KA, Pallett LJ, Maini MK, Davidson BR, et al. Eomeshi NK cells in human liver are long-lived and do not recirculate but can be replenished from the circulation. *J Immunol*. (2016) 197:4283–91. doi: 10.4049/jimmunol.1601424
81. Hudspeth K, Donadon M, Cimino M, Pontarini E, Tentorio P, Preti M, et al. Human liver-resident CD56(bright)/CD16(neg) NK cells are retained within hepatic sinusoids via the engagement of CCR5 and CXCR6 pathways. *J Autoimmun*. (2016) 66:40–50. doi: 10.1016/j.jaut.2015.08.011
82. Aw Yeang HX, Piersma SJ, Lin Y, Yang L, Malkova ON, Miner C, et al. Cutting Edge: human CD49e- NK cells are tissue resident in the liver. *J Immunol*. (2017) 198:1417–22. doi: 10.4049/jimmunol.1601818
83. Smyth MJ, Thia KY, Street SE, Cretney E, Trapani JA, Taniguchi M, et al. Differential tumor surveillance by natural killer (NK) and NKT cells. *J Exp Med*. (2000) 191:661–8. doi: 10.1084/jem.191.4.661
84. Guerra N, Tan YX, Joncker NT, Choy A, Gallardo F, Xiong N, et al. NKG2D-deficient mice are defective in tumor surveillance in models of spontaneous malignancy. *Immunity*. (2008) 28:571–80. doi: 10.1016/j.immuni.2008.02.016
85. Lakshmikanth T, Burke S, Ali TH, Kimpfler S, Ursini F, Ruggeri L, et al. NCRs and DNAM-1 mediate NK cell recognition and lysis of human and mouse melanoma cell lines *in vitro* and *in vivo*. *J Clin Invest*. (2009) 119:1251–63. doi: 10.1172/JCI36022
86. Iguchi-Manaka A, Kai H, Yamashita Y, Shibata K, Tahara-Hanaoka S, Honda S, et al. Accelerated tumor growth in mice deficient in DNAM-1 receptor. *J Exp Med*. (2008) 205:2959–64. doi: 10.1084/jem.20081611
87. Imai K, Matsuyama S, Miyake S, Suga K, Nakachi K. Natural cytotoxic activity of peripheral-blood lymphocytes and cancer incidence: an 11-year follow-up study of a general population. *Lancet*. (2000) 356:1795–9. doi: 10.1016/S0140-6736(00)03231-1
88. Lopez-Soto A, Gonzalez S, Smyth MJ, Galluzzi L. Control of metastasis by NK cells. *Cancer Cell*. (2017) 32:135–54. doi: 10.1016/j.ccell.2017.06.009
89. Vitale M, Cantoni C, Pietra G, Mingari MC, Moretta L. Effect of tumor cells and tumor microenvironment on NK-cell function. *Eur J Immunol*. (2014) 44:1582–92. doi: 10.1002/eji.201344272
90. Vacca P, Munari E, Tumino N, Moretta F, Pietra G, Vitale M, et al. Human natural killer cells and other innate lymphoid cells in cancer: friends or foes? *Immunol Lett*. (2018) 201:14–9. doi: 10.1016/j.imlet.2018.11.004
91. Reinart N, Nguyen PH, Boucas J, Rosen N, Kvasnicka HM, Heukamp L, et al. Delayed development of chronic lymphocytic leukemia in the absence of macrophage migration inhibitory factor. *Blood*. (2013) 121:812–21. doi: 10.1182/blood-2012-05-431452
92. Schlecker E, Fiegler N, Arnold A, Altevogt P, Rose-John S, Moldenhauer G, et al. Metalloprotease-mediated tumor cell shedding of B7-H6, the ligand of the natural killer cell-activating receptor NKp30. *Cancer Res*. (2014) 74:3429–40. doi: 10.1158/0008-5472.CAN-13-3017
93. Balsamo M, Manzini C, Pietra G, Raggi F, Blengio F, Mingari MC, et al. Hypoxia downregulates the expression of activating receptors involved in NK-cell-mediated target cell killing without affecting ADCC. *Eur J Immunol*. (2013) 43:2756–64. doi: 10.1002/eji.201343448
94. Costa D, Vene R, Benelli R, Romairone E, Scabini S, Catellani S, et al. Targeting the epidermal growth factor receptor can counteract the inhibition of natural killer cell function exerted by colorectal tumor-associated fibroblasts. *Front Immunol*. (2018) 9:1150. doi: 10.3389/fimmu.2018.01150
95. Parodi M, Raggi F, Cangelosi D, Manzini C, Balsamo M, Blengio F, et al. Hypoxia modifies the transcriptome of human NK cells, modulates their immunoregulatory profile, and influences NK cell subset migration. *Front Immunol*. (2018) 9:2358. doi: 10.3389/fimmu.2018.02358
96. Carrega P, Bonaccorsi I, Di Carlo E, Morandi B, Paul P, Rizzello V, et al. CD56(bright)perforin(low) noncytotoxic human NK cells are abundant in both healthy and neoplastic solid tissues and recirculate to secondary lymphoid organs via afferent lymph. *J Immunol*. (2014) 192:3805–15. doi: 10.4049/jimmunol.1301889
97. Ponzetta A, Benigni G, Antonangeli F, Sciume G, Sanseviero E, Zingoni A, et al. Multiple myeloma impairs bone marrow localization of effector natural killer cells by altering the chemokine microenvironment. *Cancer Res*. (2015) 75:4766–77. doi: 10.1158/0008-5472.CAN-15-1320
98. Molgora M, Bonavita E, Ponzetta A, Riva F, Barbagallo M, Jaillon S, et al. IL-1R8 is a checkpoint in NK cells regulating anti-tumour and anti-viral activity. *Nature*. (2017) 551:110–4. doi: 10.1038/nature24293
99. Pesce S, Greppi M, Tabellini G, Rampinelli F, Parolini S, Olive D, et al. Identification of a subset of human natural killer cells expressing high levels of programmed death 1: a phenotypic and functional characterization. *J Allergy Clin Immunol*. (2017) 139:335–46 e3. doi: 10.1016/j.jaci.2016.04.025
100. Seo H, Jeon I, Kim BS, Park M, Bae EA, Song B, et al. IL-21-mediated reversal of NK cell exhaustion facilitates anti-tumour immunity in MHC class I-deficient tumours. *Nat Commun*. (2017) 8:15776. doi: 10.1038/ncomms15776
101. Zhang Q, Bi J, Zheng X, Chen Y, Wang H, Wu W, et al. Blockade of the checkpoint receptor TIGIT prevents NK cell exhaustion and elicits potent anti-tumor immunity. *Nat Immunol*. (2018) 19:723–32. doi: 10.1038/s41590-018-0132-0
102. Voutsadakis IA. Expression and function of immune ligand-receptor pairs in NK cells and cancer stem cells: therapeutic implications. *Cell Oncol*. (2018) 41:107–21. doi: 10.1007/s13402-018-0373-9
103. Chockley PJ, Chen J, Chen G, Beer DG, Standiford TJ, Keshamouni VG. Epithelial-mesenchymal transition leads to NK cell-mediated metastasis-specific immunosurveillance in lung cancer. *J Clin Invest*. (2018) 128:1384–96. doi: 10.1172/JCI97611
104. Huergo-Zapico L, Parodi M, Cantoni C, Lavarello C, Fernandez-Martinez JL, Petretto A, et al. NK-cell editing mediates epithelial-to-mesenchymal transition via phenotypic and proteomic changes in melanoma cell lines. *Cancer Res*. (2018) 78:3913–25. doi: 10.1158/0008-5472.CAN-17-1891
105. Bottos A, Gotthardt D, Gill JW, Gattelli A, Frei A, Tzankov A, et al. Decreased NK-cell tumour immunosurveillance consequent to JAK inhibition enhances metastasis in breast cancer models. *Nat Commun*. (2016) 7:12258. doi: 10.1038/ncomms12258
106. Mayol K, Biajoux V, Marvel J, Balabanian K, Walzer T. Sequential desensitization of CXCR4 and S1P5 controls natural killer cell trafficking. *Blood*. (2011) 118:4863–71. doi: 10.1182/blood-2011-06-362574
107. Bernardini G, Sciume G, Santoni A. Differential chemotactic receptor requirements for NK cell subset trafficking into bone marrow. *Front Immunol*. (2013) 4:12. doi: 10.3389/fimmu.2013.00012
108. Melsen JE, Lugthart G, Vervat C, Kielbasa SM, van der Zeeuw SAJ, Buermans HPJ, et al. Human bone marrow-resident natural killer cells have a unique transcriptional profile and resemble resident memory CD8(+) T cells. *Front Immunol*. (2018) 9:1829. doi: 10.3389/fimmu.2018.01829
109. Schmiedel BJ, Werner A, Steinbacher J, Nuebling T, Buechele C, Grosse-Hovest L, et al. Generation and preclinical characterization of a Fc-optimized GITR-Ig fusion protein for induction of NK cell reactivity against leukemia. *Mol Ther*. (2013) 21:877–86. doi: 10.1038/mt.2013.11

110. Soderstrom K, Stein E, Colmenero P, Purath U, Muller-Ladner U, de Matos CT, et al. Natural killer cells trigger osteoclastogenesis and bone destruction in arthritis. *Proc Natl Acad Sci USA*. (2010) 107:13028–33. doi: 10.1073/pnas.1000546107
111. Lam J, Takeshita S, Barker JE, Kanagawa O, Ross FP, Teitelbaum SL. TNF-alpha induces osteoclastogenesis by direct stimulation of macrophages exposed to permissive levels of RANK ligand. *J Clin Invest*. (2000) 106:1481–8. doi: 10.1172/JCI11176
112. Takayanagi H, Ogasawara K, Hida S, Chiba T, Murata S, Sato K, et al. T-cell-mediated regulation of osteoclastogenesis by signalling cross-talk between RANKL and IFN-gamma. *Nature*. (2000) 408:600–5. doi: 10.1038/35046102
113. Kaur K, Topchyan P, Kozlowska AK, Ohanian N, Chiang J, Maung PO, et al. Super-charged NK cells inhibit growth and progression of stem-like/poorly differentiated oral tumors *in vivo* in humanized BLT mice; effect on tumor differentiation and response to chemotherapeutic drugs. *Oncoimmunology*. (2018) 7:e1426518. doi: 10.1080/2162402X.2018.1426518
114. Tseng HC, Kanayama K, Kaur K, Park SH, Park S, Kozlowska A, et al. Bisphosphonate-induced differential modulation of immune cell function in gingiva and bone marrow *in vivo*: role in osteoclast-mediated NK cell activation. *Oncotarget*. (2015) 6:20002–25. doi: 10.18632/oncotarget.4755

10

The RANKL-RANK Axis: A Bone to Thymus Round Trip

Cristina Sobacchi[1,2], *Ciro Menale*[1,2] *and Anna Villa*[1,3*]

[1] *Milan Unit, Institute for Genetic and Biomedical Research (CNR-IRGB), Milan, Italy,* [2] *Humanitas Clinical and Research Center IRCCS, Rozzano, Italy,* [3] *San Raffaele Telethon Institute for Gene Therapy (SR-Tiget), IRCCS San Raffaele Scientific Institute, Milan, Italy*

Correspondence:
Anna Villa
villa.anna@hsr.it

The identification of Receptor activator of nuclear factor kappa B ligand (RANKL) and its cognate receptor Receptor activator of nuclear factor kappa B (RANK) during a search for novel tumor necrosis factor receptor (TNFR) superfamily members has dramatically changed the scenario of bone biology by providing the functional and biochemical proof that RANKL signaling via RANK is the master factor for osteoclastogenesis. In parallel, two independent studies reported the identification of mouse RANKL on activated T cells and of a ligand for osteoprotegerin on a murine bone marrow-derived stromal cell line. After these seminal findings, accumulating data indicated RANKL and RANK not only as essential players for the development and activation of osteoclasts, but also for the correct differentiation of medullary thymic epithelial cells (mTECs) that act as mediators of the central tolerance process by which self-reactive T cells are eliminated while regulatory T cells are generated. In light of the RANKL-RANK multi-task function, an antibody targeting this pathway, denosumab, is now commonly used in the therapy of bone loss diseases including chronic inflammatory bone disorders and osteolytic bone metastases; furthermore, preclinical data support the therapeutic application of denosumab in the framework of a broader spectrum of tumors. Here, we discuss advances in cellular and molecular mechanisms elicited by RANKL-RANK pathway in the bone and thymus, and the extent to which its inhibition or augmentation can be translated in the clinical arena.

Keywords: osteoclasts, denosumab, thymus, central tolerance, rheumatoid arthritis, osteoporosis, tumor

INTRODUCTION

Receptor activator of nuclear factor kappa B (RANK) and its ligand (RANKL), encoded, respectively, by the *Tumor necrosis factor receptor superfamily member 11A* (*Tnfrsf11a*) and the *Tumor necrosis factor ligand superfamily member 11* (*Tnfsf11*) genes, constitute a receptor-ligand pair initiating a signaling pathway of paramount relevance in many pathophysiological contexts (1). They have been described in the context of T cell-dendritic cell interactions (2), in bone and in the immune system (3, 4), thus triggering the start of the osteoimmunology era. This axis has revealed an unexpected role in the thermoregulation by the central nervous system (5) and in mammary epithelium development during pregnancy and progesterone-driven breast cancer (3, 6). The RANKL-RANK axis has also been involved in diverse immune-mediated diseases affecting the bone (7–9) as well as other tissues (10), and in cancer settings (11). Overall, this pathway has emerged as a potential target of therapy in a wide range of conditions; which at the same time implies monitoring many different physiological functions when interfering with this axis.

As schematically depicted in **Figure 1**, here we focus on advances in cellular and molecular mechanisms elicited by RANKL-RANK signaling in two functionally related compartments: the bone and the thymus. Moreover, we review novel perspectives to translate inhibition or enhancement of this pathway in the clinic.

RANKL-RANK AXIS IN THE BONE

The identification of RANKL-RANK signaling in bone represents a milestone in bone biology (12, 13). Its indispensable role in osteoclast formation is clearly demonstrated by the complete absence of osteoclasts in the *Rankl*$^{-/-}$ and *Rank*$^{-/-}$ murine models (3, 4, 14, 15), as well as in their human counterpart, i.e., patients affected by RANKL-deficient and RANK-deficient osteoclast-poor Autosomal Recessive Osteopetrosis (16, 17). Nonetheless, the possibility of RANKL-independent osteoclastogenesis, particularly in pathologic conditions, has been a matter of a long-lasting debate (18–22) and a general consensus in the field has not been reached, yet.

RANKL is mainly produced by stromal cells in bone, in normal conditions, and primarily by osteocytes (23–25). RANKL is mostly membrane-bound and can be shed to form a soluble protein; the former is sufficient for most functions, while the latter contributes to physiological bone remodeling, as recently demonstrated in mice expressing a sheddase-resistant form of RANKL (26).

The membrane functional receptor RANK is mainly expressed by cells of hematopoietic origin, including also osteoclasts and their precursors, and has been recently detected also in Mesenchymal Stem Cells (MSCs) (27, 28), raising the intriguing hypothesis of an autocrine/paracrine loop in these cells (**Figure 1A**).

The RANKL-RANK signaling pathway in the osteoclast lineage comprises a plethora of molecules (29). Essentially, upon engagement by its ligand, RANK recruits a number of adaptors (most importantly, TNF Receptor-Associated Factor 6, TRAF6) (30), which converge on kinases activation, including Phosphoinositide-3-Kinase (PI3K) and Mitogen Activated Protein (MAP) kinases. This promotes nuclear translocation and activation of transcription factors, Nuclear Factor of Activated T cell 1 (NFATc1) (31), c-fos (32), and Nuclear Factor kappa B (NF-κB) (33), comprising the master regulator of the osteoclast-specific transcriptional program. The RANKL-RANK pathway interacts with costimulatory signals from immunoreceptor tyrosine based activation (ITAM)-motif containing proteins, further regulating NFATc1 activation (34, 35).

RANKL signaling during osteoclastogenesis results in the generation of reactive oxygen species (ROS), which further stimulate osteoclast formation and bone resorption (36). On the other hand, a variety of antioxidant mechanisms monitors ROS levels and the reciprocal control between these opposite functions (i.e., ROS production and scavenging) importantly impacts on bone homeostasis (37–39).

The RANKL-RANK axis is counterbalanced by the soluble decoy receptor osteoprotegerin (OPG) (40), which is itself controlled by many ligands, including the TNF-Related Apoptosis Inducing Ligand (TRAIL), von Willebrand factor (vWF), and glycosaminoglycans (GAGs) (41). Moreover, the Leucine-rich repeat-containing G protein-coupled receptor 4 (LGR4) is an additional membrane receptor for RANKL, competing with RANK for ligand binding and negatively regulating osteoclastogenesis through the inhibition of NFATc1 activation (42). LGR4 acts also as an R-spondin receptor in bone marrow MSCs and has been recently demonstrated as a key molecule in mesoderm-derived tissue development and MSC differentiation (43), whether RANKL might be involved in this specific context has to be investigated (**Figure 1A**).

The recognition of the crucial role of RANKL-RANK signaling in osteoclast biology led to the development of the anti-RANKL antibody denosumab, a fully human Immunoglobulin (Ig) G2 monoclonal antibody with high affinity and specificity for human soluble and membrane-bound RANKL (44). Specifically, denosumab binds to the DE loop region of the ligand, which is one of the surface loop structures interacting with the functional receptor on responding cells (44). Denosumab is used as an antiresorptive drug for diverse indications, such as osteoporosis (45), primary bone tumors (46), and osteolytic bone metastases (47). Its use is under evaluation also in other fields, such as solid tumors (11) and Rheumatoid Arthritis (48), and has been very recently proposed in the prevention of BRCA1-associated breast cancer (49). Finally, denosumab administration has been considered in the field of rare diseases too, for example for the treatment of persistent severe hypercalcemia after hematopoietic stem cell transplantation in patients affected by Autosomal Recessive Osteopetrosis (50), in patients affected by Fibrous Dysplasia (51), or by Osteogenesis Imperfecta, even though

---

Abbreviations: ACPA, Anti-Citrullinated Protein Antibodies; AIRE, Auto Immune Regulator; anti-CarP, anti-Carbamylated Protein; anti-CCP2, anti-Cyclic Citrullinated Peptide 2; Bcl-xl, B-cell lymphoma-extra-large; CCL20, C-C Motif Chemokine Ligand 20; CCR5, C-C chemokine receptor type 5; CCR6, C-C chemokine receptor type 6; cTEC, cortical Thymic Epithelial Cell; CXCR3, C-X-C Motif Chemokine Receptor 3; CXCR4, C-X-C Motif Chemokine Receptor 4; bDMARDs, biological Disease-Modifying Anti-Rheumatic Drugs; DETC, dendritic epidermal T cell; DP, Double Positive; FTOC, fetal thymic organ culture; GAGs, glycosaminoglycans; IL-1, Interleukin 1; IL-6, Interleukin 6; IL-17, Interleukin 17; IFNβ, Interferon beta; IFNAR, Interferon-α/β receptor; IRF7, Interferon Regulatory Factor 7; ITAM, Immunoreceptor Tyrosine-based Activation Motif; LGR4, Leucine Rich Repeat Containing G Protein-Coupled Receptor 4; LTα Lymphotoxin α; LTi, Lymphoid Tissue inducer cells; MAP kinase, Mitogen Activated Protein kinase; MHC, Major Histocompatibility Complex; MSCs, Mesenchymal Stem Cells; mTEC, medullary Thymic Epithelial Cell; NFATc1, Nuclear Factor Of Activated T Cells 1; NF-κB, Nuclear Factor kappa B; OPG, Osteoprotegerin; OVX, ovariectomized; PI3K, Phosphoinositide 3-kinase; RA, Rheumatoid Arthritis; RANK, Receptor Activator of Nuclear Factor kappa B; RANKL, Receptor Activator of Nuclear Factor kappa B Ligand; RF, Rheumatoid Factor; ROS, Reactive Oxygen Species; SP, Single Positive; STAT1, Signal Transducer and Activator of Transcription 1; TCR, T Cell Receptor; Th1, T helper 1 cells; Th17, T helper 17 cells; TNFα, Tumor Necrosis Factor α; TNFR, Tumor Necrosis Factor Receptor; TNFRSF11A, Tumor Necrosis Factor Receptor Superfamily Member 11A; TNFSF11, Tumor Necrosis Factor Ligand Superfamily Member 11; TRAF6, TNF Receptor-Associated Factor 6; TRAIL, TNF-Related Apoptosis Inducing Ligand; TRAs, Tissue Restricted Antigens; Treg, T regulatory cells; vWF, von Willebrand factor; XCL-1, X-C Motif Chemokine Ligand 1; ZAP-70, Zeta Chain Of T Cell Receptor Associated Protein Kinase 70.

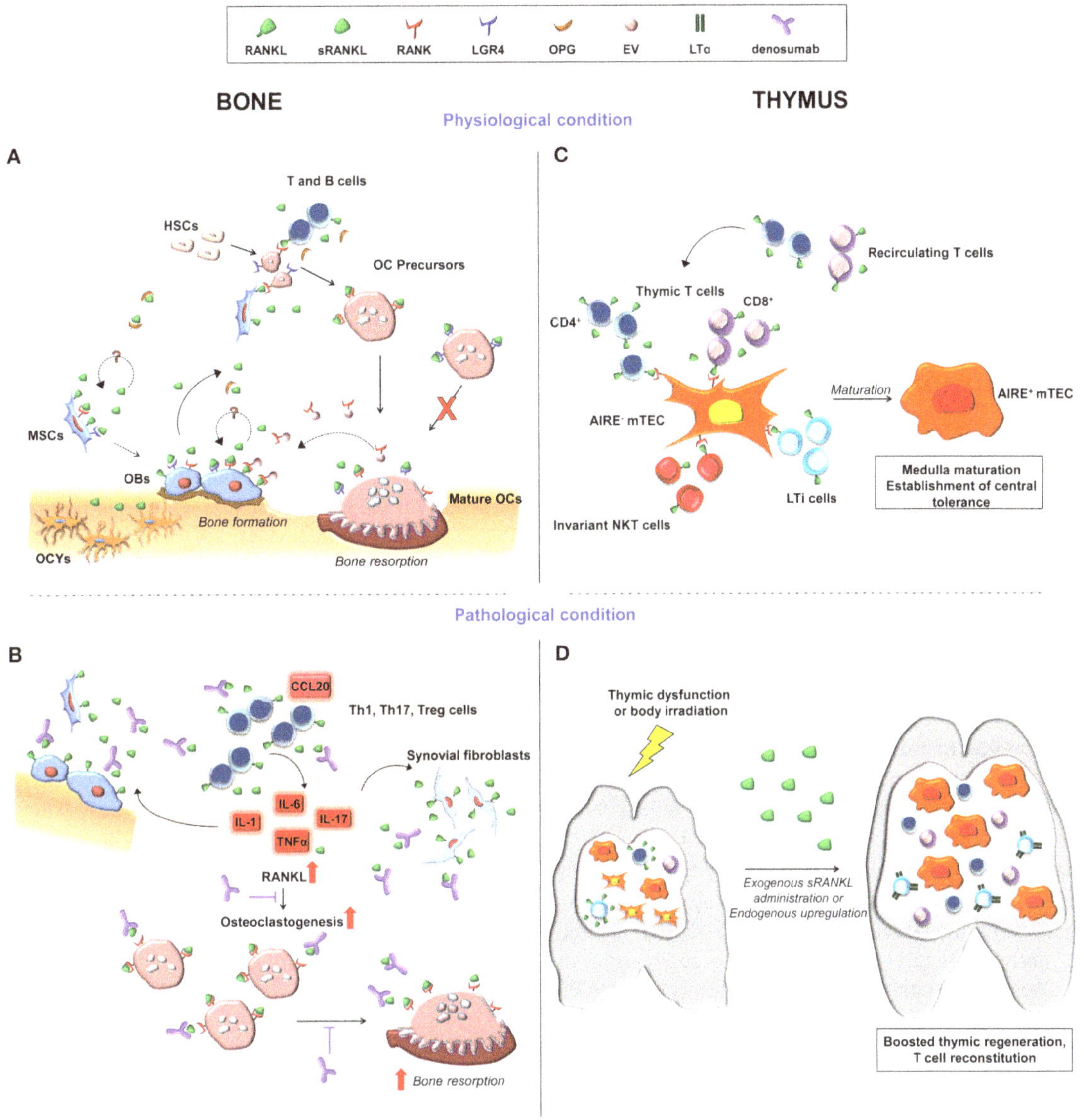

FIGURE 1 | Schematic representation of cellular and molecular players involved in RANKL-RANK signaling axis in the bone and thymus in physiological and in pathological conditions. **(A)** Membrane-bound and soluble RANKL produced by cells of the osteoblast lineage and by immune cells induce osteoclastogenesis upon its binding to RANK on osteoclast precursors. OPG is the soluble decoy receptor for RANKL. Moreover, RANKL binding to LGR4 on osteoclasts hinders their maturation. RANK expression by MSC and osteoblasts points to a potential RANKL autoregulatory mechanism affecting bone formation. In addition, osteoclast-derived RANK-expressing extracellular vesicles (EV) trigger a reverse signaling on osteoblast. **(B)** The inflammatory bone environment in pathological condition, such as osteoporosis and rheumatoid arthritis, results in increased production of RANKL by immune cells, osteoblastic cells and synovial fibroblasts. This exacerbates osteoclast generation and bone loss, which are target of denosumab treatment. **(C)** In the thymus, RANKL produced by resident and recirculating T cells, invariant NKT and LTi cells fosters mTEC AIRE expression and maturation via RANK receptor, allowing correct establishment of central tolerance. **(D)** In the presence of thymic dysfunction, pharmacological sRANKL administration boosts thymic regeneration, and T cell reconstitution. Similarly, in the early phases of thymic regeneration after body irradiation, $CD4^+$ and LTi cells upregulate RANKL. This results in increased expression of LTα in LTi cells. OBs, osteoblasts; OCs, osteoclasts; OCYs, osteocytes.

some variability in the clinical outcome has been reported (52) (**Figure 1B**).

Clinical case series and a recent analysis of the FREEDOM and FREEDOM Extension Trials about osteoporosis treatment with the anti-RANKL antibody have pointed to an increased risk of multiple vertebral fractures after denosumab discontinuation due to a rebound in bone resorption (53, 54), thus raising a note of caution. In an attempt to identify potential alternative antiresorptive therapies, scientific interest about natural compounds possibly interfering with the RANKL-RANK axis (e.g., flavonoids, alkaloid compounds, triterpenoids, polysaccharides as well as monomeric sugars) has been growing exponentially, as demonstrated by the number of publications evaluating this kind of approach (55–58).

In parallel, recent papers pointed to an unexpected osteogenic function of RANKL through (at least) two different, not mutually exclusive mechanisms: an autocrine-paracrine loop activated by RANKL binding to its receptor(s) on MSCs (27); and a reverse signaling elicited by osteoclast-derived RANK-expressing extracellular vesicles, which might induce membrane-RANKL clustering on osteoblasts (59, 60). This might represent an additional means for osteoblast-osteoclast crosstalk. As a perspective, it might be exploited by means of a new drug with two simultaneous activities: dampening of bone resorption by preventing RANKL binding to RANK receptors on the osteoclasts, and stimulating osteogenesis by triggering RANKL signaling in the osteoblasts (**Figure 1A**).

Actually, the biological relevance of these new findings in the framework of the overall bone homeostasis has to be clearly defined; for the sake of completeness, opposite results have been reported by others (28). Nevertheless, the possibility of an osteogenic function of RANKL is worth further investigations since it could pave the way to the development of new therapeutic strategies, thus fulfilling a medical need.

RANKL-RANK AXIS IN THE THYMUS

The thymus is a primary lymphoid organ responsible for the development of T lymphocytes expressing a T cell repertoire capable of responding to a diverse array of foreign antigens but tolerant to self-antigens (61, 62). Migrant lymphoid progenitors, arising in the liver during embryonic life and in the bone marrow in postnatal life, enter the thymus where they undergo different phases of differentiation throughout a complex journey from the cortical region to the medullary compartment (63). The early phases of thymocyte differentiation strictly depend on stromal derived signals mediated by the interaction of $CD4^+CD8^+$ double positive (DP) T cell precursors with cortical thymic epithelial cells (cTECs) and indirectly by the production of soluble factors (**Figure 1C**). cTECs foster lineage commitment during the early stages of T cell differentiation (double negative, DN, stage) through the expression of Notch ligand Delta-like 4 (64, 65) and mediate positive selection of DP T cells by presenting a broad array of self-peptides via major histocompatibility complex (MHC) class I and II molecules. This process results in the survival of thymocytes, which migrate into the thymic medulla where T cells are negatively selected to single positive (SP) $CD4^+CD8^-$ and $CD8^+CD4^-$ T cells (66). Mature medullary thymic epithelial cells (mTECs) mediate central tolerance process by expressing the transcriptional coactivator AutoImmune Regulator (AIRE), which drives the expression of self-antigens, including tissue restricted antigens (TRAs) leading to the clonal deletion of autoreactive T cells, while inducing the generation of regulatory T cells (67, 68), and the intra-thymic positioning of X-C Motif Chemokine Ligand 1 $(XCL1)^+$ dendritic cells (69).

Various factors modulate the development and maturation of the thymic epithelial compartment, including several signal transducers regulating NF-κB pathway and the NF-κB family member RelB (70–76). Signaling mediated by four receptors of the tumor necrosis factor family [RANK, OPG, CD40, and lymphotoxin (LT) β receptor] acts as important modulator of thymic microenvironment along with the cross talk between thymocytes and TECs (77–79). In addition, the Ets transcription factor family member Spi-B, which was found to be associated with autoimmune phenomena (80), mediates OPG expression via a negative feedback regulatory loop thus limiting the development of mature TECs (81). RANKL is mainly produced by $CD4^+$ cells, a small subset of $CD8^+$ cells, invariant (Natural Killer T) NKT cells and $CD4^+CD3^-$ lymphoid tissue inducer (LTi) cells (82, 83). Of note, during embryonic life at the initial stages of thymus development, invariant $V\gamma5^+$ dendritic epidermal T cells (DETCs) and $V\gamma5^+$ γδ T cells T cells contribute to central tolerance establishment by promoting $CD80^-Aire^-$ mTECs to become $CD80^+Aire^+$ mTECs (84–86) thus supporting a critical role for RANK signaling in the interaction between fetal γδ T cell progenitors and mTECs (87, 88). Of note, these immune cell subsets provide different physiological levels of RANKL and CD40 Ligand (CD40L) during ontogeny. During fetal life, mTEC development is controlled by the expression of RANKL by LTi and invariant $V\gamma5^+$ DETC progenitors, while after birth is controlled by RANKL and CD40L produced by αβ T Cell Receptor $(TCR)^{high}$ $CD4^+$ thymocytes (89).

Transgenic mice expressing Venus, a fluorescent protein to track RANK expression, showed that this receptor is mainly expressed by mTECs at different stages of differentiation (90). Moreover, activated T cells recirculating to the thymus further contribute to the production of RANKL (91). Thus, it is tempting to speculate that the increased production of RANKL may support the skewing toward mTEC lineage, with consequent maturation of T cells leading to the exhaustion of the progenitor pool. These observations might explain the age-related changes observed in thymic epithelium during aging or thymic dysmorphology found in some pathological conditions (92, 93).

Extensive *in vitro* and *in vivo* studies have further confirmed the relevant role of the RANKL-RANK axis in the establishment and maintenance of the central tolerance process. *In vitro* stimulation of fetal thymic organ culture (FTOC) with recombinant RANKL or agonistic anti-RANK antibody results in the upregulation of CD80 and Aire expression by mTECs (87, 94). In parallel, mice deficient in TCRα or murine models with a reduced number of $CD4^+$ T cells for instance lacking molecules of the MHC II complex have a dramatic reduction in $Aire^+$ cells and decreased mTEC compartment (95, 96). Other molecular players contribute to TEC differentiation and among them a peculiar role is played by the interferon regulatory factor 7/interferon β/ interferon-α/β receptor/signal transducer and activator of transcription 1 (IRF7/IFNβ/IFNAR/STAT1) pathway (97). During embryonic life, the absence of RANK or RANKL severely affects mTEC maturation resulting in the complete loss of $Aire^+$ mTECs (87, 94, 98). However, after birth other factors compensate the absence of RANK signaling allowing the maturation of few $Aire^+$ mTECs (94). Furthermore, OPG is expressed by mTECs and genetically deletion in mice causes enlargement of the medulla area (82, 90). Overall, these data indicate that the RANKL-RANK axis is essential for the correct differentiation and development of mTECs and for the formation of the thymic medulla and consequent establishment of self-tolerance (**Figure 1C**). Consistently with the role of

RANKL as a potent mTEC inducer and indirectly as a key player in the control of central tolerance, systemic administration of soluble RANKL (sRANKL) can be considered to treat primary or secondary thymic dysfunction (99). Transgenic mice constitutively overexpressing human sRANKL displayed thymic medulla enlargement (100) and increased number of Aire$^+$ mTECs (101). Interestingly, during *in vivo* administration of recombinant soluble RANKL (sRANKL) to cure the bone defect in *Rankl*$^{-/-}$ mice, we observed a dramatic effect of the cytokine on thymic architecture (102) further confirming data reported in literature. Pharmacological sRANKL treatment induced expansion of the medulla in *Rankl*$^{-/-}$ mice and increase of Aire$^+$ mTECs. Improvement of thymic epithelium resulted in higher frequency of CD4$^+$ and CD8$^+$ SP and reduction of double positive thymocytes (102). These data suggest that the exogenous administration of RANKL may be a new therapeutic strategy to boost thymic regeneration. In line with this, compelling evidence indicate that upon body irradiation CD4$^+$ cells and LTi cells up-regulate RANKL in the early phase of thymic regeneration. Upon tissue damage, RANKL mediates the increased expression of LTα by LTi cells and reduces the expression of pro-apoptotic genes while increases the expression of the B-cell lymphoma-extra large (Bcl-xl) anti-apoptotic gene (103). The administration of RANKL to wild-type animals confirmed its crucial role in thymic recovery by enhancing TECs, thymocyte numbers, and in parallel increasing vasculature. Improved T cell reconstitution is also mediated by the increased expression of adhesion molecules and chemokines, which foster thymus homing of lymphoid progenitors. Remarkably, since RANKL is the master gene of osteoclastogenesis, it is tempting to speculate that the increased osteoclast activity may also boost hematopoiesis and consequent migration of thymic progenitors. Overall, these *in vivo* findings confirm the therapeutic effect of RANKL suggesting its putative use to boost immune reconstitution in transplanted elderly patients or in patients affected by primary thymic epithelial defects (104–106) (**Figure 1D**). Conversely, transient inhibition of RANKL in murine models indicate its effect on thymic negative selection of self-reactive T cells specific for tumor antigens, and resulting in an improvement of antitumor immune response (107, 108). However, *in vivo* inhibition of RANKL during prenatal life in rats and mice or long-life inhibition after birth did not show gross effects on innate or humoral immune response (109), thus supporting a possible repurposing of denosumab as anti-tumoral agent in combinatorial treatments and extending its use in the clinical arena.

T CELLS AND RANKL-RANK SIGNALING IN BONE PATHOLOGY

The overall picture described highlighted the importance of the RANKL-RANK axis in the bone and thymus compartments: in the former, RANKL-RANK signaling influences the bone remodeling process regulating bone cells activities; in the latter, it is pivotal in thymic cell development and T cell maturation and functioning.

After maturation, T cells exert their function centrally and in all the other peripheral organs, going back also to the bone. Although T cell levels represent about 3–8% of total nucleated bone marrow cells in homeostatic conditions (110), in pathological settings T cell recruitment from the periphery may occur and induce molecular and metabolic changes in bone cells, contributing to the bone loss phenotype associated with various conditions such as post-menopausal osteoporosis and Rheumatoid Arthritis (RA) (**Figure 1B**).

In post-menopausal osteoporotic patients an increase in RANKL production by activated T cells (and B cells, too), alone or in combination with TNFα, has been reported (111, 112). A similar finding has been shown in surgically ovariectomized (OVX) pre-menopausal women (113), further confirming the causative link between estrogen deprivation, T cell activation and RANKL-mediated bone loss previously observed in the murine model (114). Accordingly, 17β-estradiol inhibits thymic expansion after OVX in mice and T cell development, and protects against bone loss, while selective estrogen receptor modulators exhibit agonistic activity on bone but do not affect T lymphopoiesis (115). Of note, a study in thymectomized pre-menopausal women showed a drop in T cell counts after surgery, as expected, with enhanced activation and production of osteoclastogenic factors by the remaining T cells (116). On the other hand, the authors of the study hypothesized that the establishment of not clarified compensatory mechanisms could be responsible for maintaining bone density at levels similar to euthymic age-matched controls.

Another example of bone-thymus interplay is RA, a chronic inflammatory autoimmune disease characterized by joint inflammation, involving mainly synovial membranes, and bone and cartilage destruction (117, 118). In this condition, the synovium and articular tissues are highly enriched in inflammatory leukocytes, likely due to cell recruitment in the inflamed tissue (119), sustained by resident stromal cells of mesenchymal origin (120). The inflammatory process in the joints is suggested to enhance bone loss in patients with RA, in particular when Anti-Citrullinated Protein Antibodies (ACPA), Rheumatoid Factor (RF) and anti-Carbamylated Protein Antibodies (anti-CarP) are present (121, 122). Most of the T cells recruited from the circulation are T helper 1 (Th1), Th17, and Treg cells (123), which express C-X-C Motif Chemokine Receptor 3 (CXCR3), CXCR4, C-C chemokine receptor type 5 (CCR5), and CCR6 (mainly on Th17 cells) receptors that permit their entry into the inflammatory site upon attraction by the high levels of chemokines (e.g., CCL20) found in arthritic joints (124–126). The relevant presence of these cells exacerbates bone erosion by osteoclasts located at the interface between the synovial membrane and bone (48). The pathological bone loss is not compensated by osteoblast-repairing activity since this process is inhibited by synovial inflammation (127). Pro-inflammatory cytokines, such as IL-1, IL-6, and more importantly TNFα and IL-17 are produced in the inflamed synovium and strongly induce RANKL production through the activation of NF-κB pathway in synovial cells and T cells, which in turn massively activate osteoclasts (22, 48, 128). In patients with early RA, RANKL plasma levels have been associated with bone destruction and with radiological progression of the disease after 24 months of follow-up (129). Moreover, the combined presence of increased RANKL levels and the positivity for anti-Cyclic Citrullinated Peptide 2 (anti-CCP2) antibodies correlated with a more destructive process. These data were confirmed in a case-control study conducted in RA pre-symptomatic patients, where RANKL plasma levels were higher in pre-symptomatic individuals as compared to control subjects, increased over time until the onset of RA symptoms and were associated with levels of inflammatory cytokines. However, the positivity for ACPA/RF/anti-CarP preceded the rise of RANKL plasma levels (129).

Based on this, preventing bone erosion by targeting RANKL-RANK axis could be an effective strategy for intervention (130). In fact, taking into account that RANKL-RANK axis is a pivotal immune modulator in DC development and function, in memory B cells, Th17, and Treg cells (131), RANKL blockade might modulate the immune response thus contributing to limit pathological bone erosion and joint damage occurring in RA.

In a phase II trial (Denosumab in patients with RheumatoId arthritis on methotrexate to Validate inhibitory effect on bone Erosion -DRIVE- study) on Japanese RA patients treated with methotrexate, denosumab significantly inhibited the progression of bone erosion at 12 months, and preserved the bone mineral density (132). In addition, in a retrospective cohort trial, the decrease of bone erosion in patients treated with denosumab in combination with biological disease-modifying anti-rheumatic drugs (bDMARDs), at 12 months was significantly higher as compared to denosumab alone, with no adverse effects. Therefore, blocking RANKL-RANK signaling in RA patients by the addition of denosumab to conventional treatment agents may represent a potential new therapeutic option for patients to limits RA pathological outcome (**Figure 1B**).

Importantly, RA is primarily an autoimmune disease, in which defects in central and peripheral T cell tolerance are involved. Altered intra-thymic selection for the removal of autoreactive T cells may have a great impact on the onset of T cell mediated autoimmune disease (133). In the SKG strain murine model of autoimmune arthritis, bearing a spontaneous point mutation in Zeta Chain of T Cell Receptor Associated Protein Kinase 70 (ZAP-70), alterations in αβ TCR signaling in the thymus have been linked to the escape of autoreactive T cells from negative selection, playing an essential role in immune response in the periphery (134). In turn, the onset of RA may be due to impaired peripheral tolerance mechanisms, mainly elicited by Treg cells, in controlling autoreactive T cells (135, 136). In addition, recirculation of peripheral T cells back to the thymus has been described, and the re-entering cells (mainly Treg cells) might alter central tolerance and induce the deletion of thymic antigen presenting cell populations. This could be considered a mechanism for silencing autoreactive T cells in an RA setting where impaired thymic functions are present (133). Whether alteration of this process may be linked to T cell mediated autoimmunity is still not clear and how T cell production in the thymus and their effector functions in the periphery regulate tolerance maintenance needs further investigation from a therapeutic point of view.

Overall, although targeting RANKL-RANK axis in RA with a RANKL antagonist can improve bone and joints pathological features, it remains to be defined whether an effect on central tolerance and autoimmune reactions is achieved too, because of RANKL requirement for the correct thymic development and production of functional T cells.

Finally, interest has recently grown in another field, i.e., regarding the possibility to exploit immune-related mechanisms based on RANKL-RANK signaling in cancer settings for therapeutic purposes (11). In malignancies with enhanced RANKL expression, such as Multiple Myeloma, denosumab alone is well-known to be effective in terms of overall survival and skeletal-related events (137). In different tumor types that usually have low expression of RANKL, denosumab treatment combined with immune check-point inhibitors might lead to a cross-modulation of antitumor immunity (138, 139). The mechanisms proposed are various: denosumab might act on RANKL-expressing tumor infiltrating lymphocytes and relieve their anticancer activity that is otherwise blocked by engagement of the ligand with RANK receptor on cells of the tumor microenvironment (138, 139). Moreover, RANKL antagonists might put a break on central tolerance by transiently inhibiting negative selection in the thymus, resulting in the release of self-specific T cells in the periphery (108). Finally, the activation of reverse-signaling pathways might be proposed (140, 141), in line with mechanisms described in bone (142). At present, all these possibilities require further investigations; their elucidation might shed light on novel therapeutic perspectives.

CONCLUSIONS

The RANKL-RANK axis exerts pleiotropic effects and consistently involves an ever-increasing number of molecular and cellular players. In the bone and thymus compartments, where the crucial role of RANKL signaling was recognized first, novel functions have recently been discovered. This extends our understanding of the basic biology of these tissues and has translational implications in terms of current therapies monitoring. In particular, opposite effects are expected in the case of blocking or activating the RANKL-RANK pathway on bone and immune tolerance: while used as an antiresorptive drug, the anti-RANKL antibody denosumab might have adverse effects on the establishment of central tolerance, which would deserve attention. On the other hand, recent advances might support efforts toward drug repurposing strategies and development of new medicines, based on limitations of those currently available.

AUTHOR CONTRIBUTIONS

All authors listed have made a substantial, direct and intellectual contribution to the work, and approved it for publication.

FUNDING

The original work was supported by the Italian Telethon Grant C5, the European Community's Seventh Framework

Program (FP7/2007-2013, SYBIL Project), PRIN Project (2015F3JHMB_004), and by Programma Nazionale per la Ricerca-Consiglio Nazionale delle Ricerche Aging Project to AV. CM is recipient of an ECTS Basic Research Fellowship.

ACKNOWLEDGMENTS

We acknowledge the many authors whose original contribution in the field has not been cited in this mini review for the sake of brevity.

REFERENCES

1. Rao S, Cronin SJF, Sigl V, Penninger JM. RANKL and RANK: from mammalian physiology to cancer treatment. *Trends Cell Biol.* (2018) 28:213–23. doi: 10.1016/j.tcb.2017.11.001
2. Anderson DM, Maraskovsky E, Billingsley WL, Dougall WC, Tometsko ME, Roux ER, et al. A homologue of the TNF receptor and its ligand enhance T-cell growth and dendritic-cell function. *Nature.* (1997) 390:175–9. doi: 10.1038/36593
3. Kong YY, Yoshida H, Sarosi I, Tan HL, Timms E, Capparelli C, et al. OPGL is a key regulator of osteoclastogenesis, lymphocyte development and lymph-node organogenesis. *Nature.* (1999) 397:315–23. doi: 10.1038/16852
4. Kim N, Odgren PR, Kim DK, Marks SC Jr, Choi Y. Diverse roles of the tumor necrosis factor family member TRANCE in skeletal physiology revealed by TRANCE deficiency and partial rescue by a lymphocyte-expressed TRANCE transgene. *Proc Natl Acad Sci USA.* (2000) 97:10905–10. doi: 10.1073/pnas.200294797
5. Hanada R, Leibbrandt A, Hanada T, Kitaoka S, Furuyashiki T, Fujihara H, et al. Central control of fever and female body temperature by RANKL/RANK. *Nature.* (2009) 462:505–9. doi: 10.1038/nature08596
6. Schramek D, Leibbrandt A, Sigl V, Kenner L, Pospisilik JA, Lee HJ, et al. Osteoclast differentiation factor RANKL controls development of progestin-driven mammary cancer. *Nature.* (2010) 468:98–102. doi: 10.1038/nature09387
7. Hofbauer LC, Schoppet M. Clinical implications of the osteoprotegerin/RANKL/RANK system for bone and vascular diseases. *JAMA.* (2004) 292:490–5. doi: 10.1001/jama.292.4.490
8. Han YK, Jin Y, Miao YB, Shi T, Lin XP. Improved RANKL production by memory B cells: a way for B cells promote alveolar bone destruction during periodontitis. *Int Immunopharmacol.* (2018) 64:232–7. doi: 10.1016/j.intimp.2018.08.033
9. Tanaka S, Tanaka Y, Ishiguro N, Yamanaka H, Takeuchi T. RANKL: a therapeutic target for bone destruction in rheumatoid arthritis. *Mod Rheumatol.* (2018) 28:9–16. doi: 10.1080/14397595.2017.1369491
10. Guerrini MM, Okamoto K, Komatsu N, Sawa S, Danks L, Penninger JM, et al. Inhibition of the TNF family cytokine RANKL prevents autoimmune inflammation in the central nervous system. *Immunity.* (2015) 43:1174–85. doi: 10.1016/j.immuni.2015.10.017
11. Ahern E, Smyth MJ, Dougall WC, Teng MWL. Roles of the RANKL-RANK axis in antitumour immunity - implications for therapy. *Nat Rev Clin Oncol.* (2018) 15:676–93. doi: 10.1038/s41571-018-0095-y
12. Nakagawa N, Kinosaki M, Yamaguchi K, Shima N, Yasuda H, Yano K, et al. RANK is the essential signaling receptor for osteoclast differentiation factor in osteoclastogenesis. *Biochem Biophys Res Commun.* (1998) 253:395–400. doi: 10.1006/bbrc.1998.9788
13. Yasuda H, Shima N, Nakagawa N, Yamaguchi K, Kinosaki M, Mochizuki S, et al. Osteoclast differentiation factor is a ligand for osteoprotegerin/osteoclastogenesis-inhibitory factor and is identical to TRANCE/RANKL. *Proc Natl Acad Sci USA.* (1998) 95:3597–602. doi: 10.1073/pnas.95.7.3597
14. Dougall WC, Glaccum M, Charrier K, Rohrbach K, Brasel K, De Smedt T, et al. RANK is essential for osteoclast and lymph node development. *Genes Dev.* (1999) 13:2412–24. doi: 10.1101/gad.13.18.2412
15. Li J, Sarosi I, Yan XQ, Morony S, Capparelli C, Tan HL, et al. RANK is the intrinsic hematopoietic cell surface receptor that controls osteoclastogenesis and regulation of bone mass and calcium metabolism. *Proc Natl Acad Sci USA.* (2000) 97:1566–71. doi: 10.1073/pnas.97.4.1566
16. Sobacchi C, Frattini A, Guerrini MM, Abinun M, Pangrazio A, Susani L, et al. Osteoclast-poor human osteopetrosis due to mutations in the gene encoding RANKL. *Nat Genet.* (2007) 39:960–2. doi: 10.1038/ng2076
17. Guerrini MM, Sobacchi C, Cassani B, Abinun M, Kilic SS, Pangrazio A, et al. Human osteoclast-poor osteopetrosis with hypogammaglobulinemia due to TNFRSF11A (RANK) mutations. *Am J Hum Genet.* (2008) 83:64–76. doi: 10.1016/j.ajhg.2008.06.015
18. Kobayashi K, Takahashi N, Jimi E, Udagawa N, Takami M, Kotake S, et al. Tumor necrosis factor alpha stimulates osteoclast differentiation by a mechanism independent of the ODF/RANKL-RANK interaction. *J Exp Med.* (2000) 191:275–86. doi: 10.1084/jem.191.2.275
19. Kim N, Kadono Y, Takami M, Lee J, Lee SH, Okada F, et al. Osteoclast differentiation independent of the TRANCE-RANK-TRAF6 axis. *J Exp Med.* (2005) 202:589–95. doi: 10.1084/jem.20050978
20. O'Brien W, Fissel BM, Maeda Y, Yan J, Ge X, Gravallese EM, et al. RANK-independent osteoclast formation and bone erosion in inflammatory arthritis. *Arthritis Rheumatol.* (2016) 68:2889–900. doi: 10.1002/art.39837
21. Tsukasaki M, Hamada K, Okamoto K, Nagashima K, Terashima A, Komatsu N, et al. LOX fails to substitute for RANKL in osteoclastogenesis. *J Bone Miner Res.* (2017) 32:434–9. doi: 10.1002/jbmr.2990
22. Mbalaviele G, Novack DV, Schett G, Teitelbaum SL. Inflammatory osteolysis: a conspiracy against bone. *J Clin Invest.* (2017) 127:2030–9. doi: 10.1172/JCI93356
23. Nakashima T, Hayashi M, Fukunaga T, Kurata K, Oh-Hora M, Feng JQ, et al. Evidence for osteocyte regulation of bone homeostasis through RANKL expression. *Nat Med.* (2011) 17:1231–4. doi: 10.1038/nm.2452
24. Xiong J, Onal M, Jilka RL, Weinstein RS, Manolagas SC, O'Brien CA. Matrix-embedded cells control osteoclast formation. *Nat Med.* (2011) 17:1235–41. doi: 10.1038/nm.2448
25. Fujiwara Y, Piemontese M, Liu Y, Thostenson JD, Xiong J, O'Brien CA. RANKL (receptor activator of NFkB ligand) produced by osteocytes is required for the increase in B cells and bone loss caused by estrogen deficiency in mice. *J Biol Chem.* (2016) 291:24838–50. doi: 10.1074/jbc.M116.742452
26. Xiong J, Cawley K, Piemontese M, Fujiwara Y, Zhao H, Goellner JJ, et al. Soluble RANKL contributes to osteoclast formation in adult mice but not ovariectomy-induced bone loss. *Nat Commun.* (2018) 9:2909. doi: 10.1038/s41467-018-05244-y
27. Schena F, Menale C, Caci E, Diomede L, Palagano E, Recordati C, et al. Murine Rankl(-/-) mesenchymal stromal cells display an osteogenic differentiation defect improved by a RANKL-expressing lentiviral vector. *Stem Cells.* (2017) 35:1365–77. doi: 10.1002/stem.2574
28. Chen X, Zhi X, Wang J, Su J. RANKL signaling in bone marrow mesenchymal stem cells negatively regulates osteoblastic bone formation. *Bone Res.* (2018) 6:34. doi: 10.1038/s41413-018-0035-6
29. Okamoto K, Nakashima T, Shinohara M, Negishi-KOGA T, Komatsu N, Terashima A, et al. Osteoimmunology: the conceptual framework unifying the immune and skeletal systems. *Physiol Rev.* (2017) 97:1295–349. doi: 10.1152/physrev.00036.2016
30. Kobayashi N, Kadono Y, Naito A, Matsumoto K, Yamamoto T, Tanaka S, et al. Segregation of TRAF6-mediated signaling pathways clarifies its role in osteoclastogenesis. *EMBO J.* (2001) 20:1271–80. doi: 10.1093/emboj/20.6.1271
31. Kim K, Lee SH, Ha Kim J, Choi Y, Kim N. NFATc1 induces osteoclast fusion via up-regulation of Atp6v0d2 and the dendritic cell-specific transmembrane protein (DC-STAMP). *Mol Endocrinol.* (2008) 22:176–85. doi: 10.1210/me.2007-0237
32. Matsuo K, Owens JM, Tonko M, Elliott C, Chambers TJ, Wagner EF. Fosl1 is a transcriptional target of c-Fos during osteoclast differentiation. *Nat Genet.* (2000) 24:184–7. doi: 10.1038/72855
33. Abu-Amer Y. NF-kappaB signaling and bone resorption. *Osteoporos Int.* (2013) 24:2377–86. doi: 10.1007/s00198-013-2313-x
34. Kim HS, Kim DK, Kim AR, Mun SH, Lee SK, Kim JH, et al. Fyn positively regulates the activation of DAP12 and FcRgamma-mediated costimulatory

signals by RANKL during osteoclastogenesis. *Cell Signal.* (2012) 24:1306–14. doi: 10.1016/j.cellsig.2012.02.014
35. Li S, Miller CH, Giannopoulou E, Hu X, Ivashkiv LB, Zhao B. RBP-J imposes a requirement for ITAM-mediated costimulation of osteoclastogenesis. *J Clin Invest.* (2014) 124:5057–73. doi: 10.1172/JCI71882
36. Lee NK, Choi YG, Baik JY, Han SY, Jeong DW, Bae YS, et al. A crucial role for reactive oxygen species in RANKL-induced osteoclast differentiation. *Blood.* (2005) 106:852–9. doi: 10.1182/blood-2004-09-3662
37. Gambari L, Lisignoli G, Cattini L, Manferdini C, Facchini A, Grassi F. Sodium hydrosulfide inhibits the differentiation of osteoclast progenitor cells via NRF2-dependent mechanism. *Pharmacol Res.* (2014) 87:99–112. doi: 10.1016/j.phrs.2014.06.014
38. Tan P, Guan H, Xie L, Mi B, Fang Z, Li J, et al. FOXO1 inhibits osteoclastogenesis partially by antagnozing MYC. *Sci Rep.* (2015) 5:16835. doi: 10.1038/srep16835
39. Kim HS, Nam ST, Mun SH, Lee SK, Kim HW, Park YH, et al. DJ-1 controls bone homeostasis through the regulation of osteoclast differentiation. *Nat Commun.* (2017) 8:1519. doi: 10.1038/s41467-017-01527-y
40. Simonet WS, Lacey DL, Dunstan CR, Kelley M, Chang MS, Luthy R, et al. Osteoprotegerin: a novel secreted protein involved in the regulation of bone density. *Cell.* (1997) 89:309–19. doi: 10.1016/S0092-8674(00)80209-3
41. Baud'huin M, Duplomb L, Teletchea S, Lamoureux F, Ruiz-Velasco C, Maillasson M, et al. Osteoprotegerin: multiple partners for multiple functions. *Cytokine Growth Factor Rev.* (2013) 24:401–9. doi: 10.1016/j.cytogfr.2013.06.001
42. Luo J, Yang Z, Ma Y, Yue Z, Lin H, Qu G, et al. LGR4 is a receptor for RANKL and negatively regulates osteoclast differentiation and bone resorption. *Nat Med.* (2016) 22:539–46. doi: 10.1038/nm.4076
43. Sun P, Jia K, Zheng C, Zhu X, Li J, He L, et al. Loss of Lgr4 inhibits differentiation, migration and apoptosis, and promotes proliferation in bone mesenchymal stem cells. *J Cell Physiol.* (2018). doi: 10.1002/jcp.27927. [Epub ahead of print].
44. Lacey DL, Boyle WJ, Simonet WS, Kostenuik PJ, Dougall WC, Sullivan JK, et al. Bench to bedside: elucidation of the OPG-RANK-RANKL pathway and the development of denosumab. *Nat Rev Drug Discov.* (2012) 11:401–19. doi: 10.1038/nrd3705
45. Lewiecki EM. New and emerging concepts in the use of denosumab for the treatment of osteoporosis. *Ther Adv Musculoskelet Dis.* (2018) 10:209–23. doi: 10.1177/1759720X18805759
46. Savvidou OD, Bolia IK, Chloros GD, Papanastasiou J, Koutsouradis P, Papagelopoulos PJ. Denosumab: current use in the treatment of primary bone tumors. *Orthopedics.* (2017) 40:204–10. doi: 10.3928/01477447-20170627-04
47. Zheng H, Li W, Kang Y. Tumor-stroma interactions in bone metastasis: molecular mechanisms and therapeutic implications. *Cold Spring Harb Symp Quant Biol.* (2016) 81:151–61. doi: 10.1101/sqb.2016.81.030775
48. Tanaka Y, Ohira T. Mechanisms and therapeutic targets for bone damage in rheumatoid arthritis, in particular the RANK-RANKL system. *Curr Opin Pharmacol.* (2018) 40:110–9. doi: 10.1016/j.coph.2018.03.006
49. Sigl V, Jones LP, Penninger JM. RANKL/RANK: from bone loss to the prevention of breast cancer. *Open Biol.* (2016) 6:160230. doi: 10.1098/rsob.160230
50. Shroff R, Beringer O, Rao K, Hofbauer LC, Schulz A. Denosumab for post-transplantation hypercalcemia in osteopetrosis. *N Engl J Med.* (2012) 367:1766–7. doi: 10.1056/NEJMc1206193
51. Rotman M, Hamdy NAT, Appelman-Dijkstra NM. Clinical and translational pharmacological aspects of the management of fibrous dysplasia of bone. *Br J Clin Pharmacol.* (2018). doi: 10.1111/bcp.13820. [Epub ahead of print].
52. Li G, Jin Y, Levine MAH, Hoyer-Kuhn H, Ward L, Adachi JD. Systematic review of the effect of denosumab on children with osteogenesis imperfecta showed inconsistent findings. *Acta Paediatr.* (2018) 107:534–7. doi: 10.1111/apa.14154
53. Tsourdi E, Langdahl B, Cohen-Solal M, Aubry-Rozier B, Eriksen EF, Guanabens N, et al. Discontinuation of Denosumab therapy for osteoporosis: a systematic review and position statement by ECTS. *Bone.* (2017) 105:11–7. doi: 10.1016/j.bone.2017.08.003
54. Roux S, Massicotte MH, Huot Daneault A, Brazeau-Lamontagne L, Dufresne J. Acute hypercalcemia and excessive bone resorption following anti-RANKL withdrawal: case report and brief literature review. *Bone.* (2019) 120:482–6. doi: 10.1016/j.bone.2018.12.012
55. An J, Hao D, Zhang Q, Chen B, Zhang R, Wang Y, et al. Natural products for treatment of bone erosive diseases: the effects and mechanisms on inhibiting osteoclastogenesis and bone resorption. *Int Immunopharmacol.* (2016) 36:118–31. doi: 10.1016/j.intimp.2016.04.024
56. Hong G, Zhou L, Shi X, He W, Wang H, Wei Q, et al. Bajijiasu abrogates osteoclast differentiation via the suppression of RANKL signaling pathways through NF-kappaB and NFAT. *Int J Mol Sci.* (2018) 18:E203. doi: 10.3390/ijms18010203
57. Wang Q, Yao L, Xu K, Jin H, Chen K, Wang Z, et al. Madecassoside inhibits estrogen deficiency-induced osteoporosis by suppressing RANKL-induced osteoclastogenesis. *J Cell Mol Med.* (2019) 23:380–94. doi: 10.1111/jcmm.13942
58. Xu Q, Chen G, Liu X, Dai M, Zhang B. Icariin inhibits RANKL-induced osteoclastogenesis via modulation of the NF-kappaB and MAPK signaling pathways. *Biochem Biophys Res Commun.* (2019) 508:902–6. doi: 10.1016/j.bbrc.2018.11.201
59. Ikebuchi Y, Aoki S, Honma M, Hayashi M, Sugamori Y, Khan M, et al. Coupling of bone resorption and formation by RANKL reverse signalling. *Nature.* (2018) 561:195–200. doi: 10.1038/s41586-018-0482-7
60. Sone E, Noshiro D, Ikebuchi Y, Nakagawa M, Khan M, Tamura Y, et al. The induction of RANKL molecule clustering could stimulate early osteoblast differentiation. *Biochem Biophys Res Commun.* (2018) 509:435–40. doi: 10.1016/j.bbrc.2018.12.093
61. Koch U, Radtke F. Mechanisms of T cell development and transformation. *Annu Rev Cell Dev Biol.* (2011) 27:539–62. doi: 10.1146/annurev-cellbio-092910-154008
62. Shah DK, Zuniga-Pflucker JC. An overview of the intrathymic intricacies of T cell development. *J Immunol.* (2014) 192:4017–23. doi: 10.4049/jimmunol.1302259
63. Petrie HT, Zuniga-Pflucker JC. Zoned out: functional mapping of stromal signaling microenvironments in the thymus. *Annu Rev Immunol.* (2007) 25:649–79. doi: 10.1146/annurev.immunol.23.021704.115715
64. Koch U, Fiorini E, Benedito R, Besseyrias V, Schuster-Gossler K, Pierres M, et al. Delta-like 4 is the essential, nonredundant ligand for Notch1 during thymic T cell lineage commitment. *J Exp Med.* (2008) 205:2515–23. doi: 10.1084/jem.20080829
65. Hirano K, Negishi N, Yazawa M, Yagita H, Habu S, Hozumi K. Delta-like 4-mediated Notch signaling is required for early T-cell development in a three-dimensional thymic structure. *Eur J Immunol.* (2015) 45:2252–62. doi: 10.1002/eji.201445123
66. Rodrigues PM, Peterson P, Alves NL. Setting up the perimeter of tolerance: insights into mTEC physiology. *Trends Immunol.* (2018) 39:2–5. doi: 10.1016/j.it.2017.11.001
67. Aschenbrenner K, D'Cruz LM, Vollmann EH, Hinterberger M, Emmerich J, Swee LK, et al. Selection of Foxp3+ regulatory T cells specific for self antigen expressed and presented by Aire+ medullary thymic epithelial cells. *Nat Immunol.* (2007) 8:351–8. doi: 10.1038/ni1444
68. Anderson G, Takahama Y. Thymic epithelial cells: working class heroes for T cell development and repertoire selection. *Trends Immunol.* (2012) 33:256–63. doi: 10.1016/j.it.2012.03.005
69. Lei Y, Ripen AM, Ishimaru N, Ohigashi I, Nagasawa T, Jeker LT, et al. Aire-dependent production of XCL1 mediates medullary accumulation of thymic dendritic cells and contributes to regulatory T cell development. *J Exp Med.* (2011) 208:383–94. doi: 10.1084/jem.20102327
70. Burkly L, Hession C, Ogata L, Reilly C, Marconi LA, Olson D, et al. Expression of relB is required for the development of thymic medulla and dendritic cells. *Nature.* (1995) 373:531–6. doi: 10.1038/373531a0
71. Weih F, Carrasco D, Durham SK, Barton DS, Rizzo CA, Ryseck RP, et al. Multiorgan inflammation and hematopoietic abnormalities in mice with a targeted disruption of RelB, a member of the NF-kappa B/Rel family. *Cell.* (1995) 80:331–40. doi: 10.1016/0092-8674(95)90416-6
72. Kajiura F, Sun S, Nomura T, Izumi K, Ueno T, Bando Y, et al. NF-kappa B-inducing kinase establishes self-tolerance in a thymic stroma-dependent manner. *J Immunol.* (2004) 172:2067–75. doi: 10.4049/jimmunol.172.4.2067
73. Akiyama T, Maeda S, Yamane S, Ogino K, Kasai M, Kajiura F, et al. Dependence of self-tolerance on TRAF6-directed development

of thymic stroma. *Science.* (2005) 308:248–51. doi: 10.1126/science.1105677

74. Nitta T, Ohigashi I, Nakagawa Y, Takahama Y. Cytokine crosstalk for thymic medulla formation. *Curr Opin Immunol.* (2011) 23:190–7. doi: 10.1016/j.coi.2010.12.002
75. Sun L, Luo H, Li H, Zhao Y. Thymic epithelial cell development and differentiation: cellular and molecular regulation. *Protein Cell.* (2013) 4:342–55. doi: 10.1007/s13238-013-3014-0
76. Bichele R, Kisand K, Peterson P, Laan M. TNF superfamily members play distinct roles in shaping the thymic stromal microenvironment. *Mol Immunol.* (2016) 72:92–102. doi: 10.1016/j.molimm.2016.02.015
77. Lkhagvasuren E, Sakata M, Ohigashi I, Takahama Y. Lymphotoxin beta receptor regulates the development of CCL21-expressing subset of postnatal medullary thymic epithelial cells. *J Immunol.* (2013) 190:5110–7. doi: 10.4049/jimmunol.1203203
78. Danzl NM, Jeong S, Choi Y, Alexandropoulos K. Identification of novel thymic epithelial cell subsets whose differentiation is regulated by RANKL and Traf6. *PLoS ONE.* (2014) 9:e86129. doi: 10.1371/journal.pone.0086129
79. Fujihara C, Williams JA, Watanabe M, Jeon H, Sharrow SO, Hodes RJ. T cell-B cell thymic cross-talk: maintenance and function of thymic B cells requires cognate CD40-CD40 ligand interaction. *J Immunol.* (2014) 193:5534–44. doi: 10.4049/jimmunol.1401655
80. Liu X, Invernizzi P, Lu Y, Kosoy R, Lu Y, Bianchi I, et al. Genome-wide meta-analyses identify three loci associated with primary biliary cirrhosis. *Nat Genet.* (2010) 42:658–60. doi: 10.1038/ng.627
81. Akiyama N, Shinzawa M, Miyauchi M, Yanai H, Tateishi R, Shimo Y, et al. Limitation of immune tolerance-inducing thymic epithelial cell development by Spi-B-mediated negative feedback regulation. *J Exp Med.* (2014) 211:2425–38. doi: 10.1084/jem.20141207
82. Hikosaka Y, Nitta T, Ohigashi I, Yano K, Ishimaru N, Hayashi Y, et al. The cytokine RANKL produced by positively selected thymocytes fosters medullary thymic epithelial cells that express autoimmune regulator. *Immunity.* (2008) 29:438–50. doi: 10.1016/j.immuni.2008.06.018
83. White AJ, Lucas B, Jenkinson WE, Anderson G. Invariant NKT cells and control of the thymus medulla. *J Immunol.* (2018) 200:3333–9. doi: 10.4049/jimmunol.1800120
84. Zuklys S, Balciunaite G, Agarwal A, Fasler-Kan E, Palmer E, Hollander GA. Normal thymic architecture and negative selection are associated with Aire expression, the gene defective in the autoimmune-polyendocrinopathy-candidiasis-ectodermal dystrophy (APECED). *J Immunol.* (2000) 165:1976–83. doi: 10.4049/jimmunol.165.4.1976
85. White AJ, Withers DR, Parnell SM, Scott HS, Finke D, Lane PJ, et al. Sequential phases in the development of Aire-expressing medullary thymic epithelial cells involve distinct cellular input. *Eur J Immunol.* (2008) 38:942–7. doi: 10.1002/eji.200738052
86. Montero-Herradon S, Garcia-Ceca J, Zapata AG. Altered maturation of medullary TEC in EphB-deficient Thymi is recovered by RANK signaling stimulation. *Front Immunol.* (2018) 9:1020. doi: 10.3389/fimmu.2018.01020
87. Rossi SW, Kim MY, Leibbrandt A, Parnell SM, Jenkinson WE, Glanville SH, et al. RANK signals from CD4(+)3(−) inducer cells regulate development of Aire-expressing epithelial cells in the thymic medulla. *J Exp Med.* (2007) 204:1267–72. doi: 10.1084/jem.20062497
88. Roberts NA, White AJ, Jenkinson WE, Turchinovich G, Nakamura K, Withers DR, et al. Rank signaling links the development of invariant gammadelta T cell progenitors and Aire(+) medullary epithelium. *Immunity.* (2012) 36:427–37. doi: 10.1016/j.immuni.2012.01.016
89. Desanti GE, Cowan JE, Baik S, Parnell SM, White AJ, Penninger JM, et al. Developmentally regulated availability of RANKL and CD40 ligand reveals distinct mechanisms of fetal and adult cross-talk in the thymus medulla. *J Immunol.* (2012) 189:5519–26. doi: 10.4049/jimmunol.1201815
90. Mccarthy NI, Cowan JE, Nakamura K, Bacon A, Baik S, White AJ, et al. Osteoprotegerin-mediated homeostasis of rank+ Thymic epithelial cells does not limit Foxp3+ regulatory T cell development. *J Immunol.* (2015) 195:2675–82. doi: 10.4049/jimmunol.1501226
91. Yin C, Pei XY, Shen H, Gao YN, Sun XY, Wang W, et al. Thymic homing of activated CD4(+) T cells induces degeneration of the thymic epithelium through excessive RANK signaling. *Sci Rep.* (2017) 7:2421. doi: 10.1038/s41598-017-02653-9
92. Shanley DP, Aw D, Manley NR, Palmer DB. An evolutionary perspective on the mechanisms of immunosenescence. *Trends Immunol.* (2009) 30:374–81. doi: 10.1016/j.it.2009.05.001
93. Sato K, Kato A, Sekai M, Hamazaki Y, Minato N. Physiologic thymic involution underlies age-dependent accumulation of senescence-associated CD4(+) T cells. *J Immunol.* (2017) 199:138–48. doi: 10.4049/jimmunol.1602005
94. Akiyama T, Shimo Y, Yanai H, Qin J, Ohshima D, Maruyama Y, et al. The tumor necrosis factor family receptors RANK and CD40 cooperatively establish the thymic medullary microenvironment and self-tolerance. *Immunity.* (2008) 29:423–37. doi: 10.1016/j.immuni.2008.06.015
95. Irla M, Hugues S, Gill J, Nitta T, Hikosaka Y, Williams IR, et al. Autoantigen-specific interactions with CD4+ thymocytes control mature medullary thymic epithelial cell cellularity. *Immunity.* (2008) 29:451–63. doi: 10.1016/j.immuni.2008.08.007
96. Irla M, Guerri L, Guenot J, Serge A, Lantz O, Liston A, et al. Antigen recognition by autoreactive CD4(+) thymocytes drives homeostasis of the thymic medulla. *PLoS ONE.* (2012) 7:e52591. doi: 10.1371/journal.pone.0052591
97. Otero DC, Baker DP, David M. IRF7-dependent IFN-beta production in response to RANKL promotes medullary thymic epithelial cell development. *J Immunol.* (2013) 190:3289–98. doi: 10.4049/jimmunol.1203086
98. Mouri Y, Yano M, Shinzawa M, Shimo Y, Hirota F, Nishikawa Y, et al. Lymphotoxin signal promotes thymic organogenesis by eliciting RANK expression in the embryonic thymic stroma. *J Immunol.* (2011) 186:5047–57. doi: 10.4049/jimmunol.1003533
99. Lin J, Yang L, Silva HM, Trzeciak A, Choi Y, Schwab SR, et al. Increased generation of Foxp3(+) regulatory T cells by manipulating antigen presentation in the thymus. *Nat Commun.* (2016) 7:10562. doi: 10.1038/ncomms10562
100. Mizuno A, Kanno T, Hoshi M, Shibata O, Yano K, Fujise N, et al. Transgenic mice overexpressing soluble osteoclast differentiation factor (sODF) exhibit severe osteoporosis. *J Bone Miner Metab.* (2002) 20:337–44. doi: 10.1007/s007740200049
101. Ohigashi I, Nitta T, Lkhagvasuren E, Yasuda H, Takahama Y. Effects of RANKL on the thymic medulla. *Eur J Immunol.* (2011) 41:1822–7. doi: 10.1002/eji.201141480
102. Lo Iacono N, Blair HC, Poliani PL, Marrella V, Ficara F, Cassani B, et al. Osteopetrosis rescue upon RANKL administration to Rankl(-/-) mice: a new therapy for human RANKL-dependent ARO. *J Bone Min Res.* (2012) 27:2501–10. doi: 10.1002/jbmr.1712
103. Lopes N, Vachon H, Marie J, Irla M. Administration of RANKL boosts thymic regeneration upon bone marrow transplantation. *Embo Mol Med.* (2017) 9:835–51. doi: 10.15252/emmm.201607176
104. Poliani PL, Vermi W, Facchetti F. Thymus microenvironment in human primary immunodeficiency diseases. *Curr Opin Allergy Clin Immunol.* (2009) 9:489–95. doi: 10.1097/ACI.0b013e3283327e5c
105. Toubert A, Glauzy S, Douay C, Clave E. Thymus and immune reconstitution after allogeneic hematopoietic stem cell transplantation in humans: never say never again. *Tissue Antigens.* (2012) 79:83–9. doi: 10.1111/j.1399-0039.2011.01820.x
106. Da Rocha LKA, De Barros SF, Bandeira F, Bollini A, Testa LHD, Simione AJ, et al. Thymopoiesis in pre- and post-hematopoietic stem cell transplantation. *Front Immunol.* (2018) 9:1889. doi: 10.3389/fimmu.2018.01889
107. Khan IS, Mouchess ML, Zhu ML, Conley B, Fasano KJ, Hou Y, et al. Enhancement of an anti-tumor immune response by transient blockade of central T cell tolerance. *J Exp Med.* (2014) 211:761–8. doi: 10.1084/jem.20131889
108. Bakhru P, Zhu ML, Wang HH, Hong LK, Khan I, Mouchess M, et al. Combination central tolerance and peripheral checkpoint blockade unleashes antimelanoma immunity. *JCI Insight.* (2017) 2:93265. doi: 10.1172/jci.insight.93265
109. Stolina M, Dwyer D, Ominsky MS, Corbin T, Van G, Bolon B, et al. Continuous RANKL inhibition in osteoprotegerin transgenic mice and rats suppresses bone resorption without impairing lymphorganogenesis or functional immune responses. *J Immunol.* (2007) 179:7497–505. doi: 10.4049/jimmunol.179.11.7497

110. Di Rosa F, Gebhardt T. Bone marrow T cells and the integrated functions of recirculating and tissue-resident memory T cells. *Front Immunol.* (2016) 7:51. doi: 10.3389/fimmu.2016.00051
111. Eghbali-Fatourechi G, Khosla S, Sanyal A, Boyle WJ, Lacey DL, Riggs BL. Role of RANK ligand in mediating increased bone resorption in early postmenopausal women. *J Clin Invest.* (2003) 111:1221–30. doi: 10.1172/JCI200317215
112. D'Amelio P, Grimaldi A, Di Bella S, Brianza SZM, Cristofaro MA, Tamone C, et al. Estrogen deficiency increases osteoclastogenesis up-regulating T cells activity: a key mechanism in osteoporosis. *Bone.* (2008) 43:92–100. doi: 10.1016/j.bone.2008.02.017
113. Adeel S, Singh K, Vydareny KH, Kumari M, Shah E, Weitzmann MN, et al. Bone loss in surgically ovariectomized premenopausal women is associated with T lymphocyte activation and thymic hypertrophy. *J Investig Med.* (2013) 61:1178–83. doi: 10.2310/JIM.0000000000000016
114. Toraldo G, Roggia C, Qian WP, Pacifici R, Weitzmann MN. IL-7 induces bone loss *in vivo* by induction of receptor activator of nuclear factor kappa B ligand and tumor necrosis factor alpha from T cells. *Proc Natl Acad Sci USA.* (2003) 100:125–30. doi: 10.1073/pnas.0136772100
115. Bernardi AI, Andersson A, Stubelius A, Grahnemo L, Carlsten H, Islander U. Selective estrogen receptor modulators in T cell development and T cell dependent inflammation. *Immunobiology.* (2015) 220:1122–8. doi: 10.1016/j.imbio.2015.05.009
116. D'Amelio P, Grimaldi A, Bernabei P, Pescarmona GP, Isaia G. Immune system and bone metabolism: does thymectomy influence postmenopausal bone loss in humans? *Bone.* (2006) 39:658–65. doi: 10.1016/j.bone.2006.03.009
117. Takayanagi H. New developments in osteoimmunology. *Nat Rev Rheumatol.* (2012) 8:684–9. doi: 10.1038/nrrheum.2012.167
118. Smolen JS, Aletaha D, Barton A, Burmester GR, Emery P, Firestein GS, et al. Rheumatoid arthritis. *Nat Rev Dis Primers.* (2018) 4:18001. doi: 10.1038/nrdp.2018.1
119. Mcinnes IB, Schett G. The pathogenesis of rheumatoid arthritis. *N Engl J Med.* (2011) 365:2205–19. doi: 10.1056/NEJMra1004965
120. Dakin SG, Coles M, Sherlock JP, Powrie F, Carr AJ, Buckley CD. Pathogenic stromal cells as therapeutic targets in joint inflammation. *Nat Rev Rheumatol.* (2018) 14:714–26. doi: 10.1038/s41584-018-0112-7
121. Harre U, Georgess D, Bang H, Bozec A, Axmann R, Ossipova E, et al. Induction of osteoclastogenesis and bone loss by human autoantibodies against citrullinated vimentin. *J Clin Invest.* (2012) 122:1791–802. doi: 10.1172/JCI60975
122. Bugatti S, Bogliolo L, Vitolo B, Manzo A, Montecucco C, Caporali R. Anti-citrullinated protein antibodies and high levels of rheumatoid factor are associated with systemic bone loss in patients with early untreated rheumatoid arthritis. *Arthritis Res Ther.* (2016) 18:226. doi: 10.1186/s13075-016-1116-9
123. Komatsu N, Takayanagi H. Immune-bone interplay in the structural damage in rheumatoid arthritis. *Clin Exp Immunol.* (2018) 194:1–8. doi: 10.1111/cei.13188
124. Hirota K, Yoshitomi H, Hashimoto M, Maeda S, Teradaira S, Sugimoto N, et al. Preferential recruitment of CCR6-expressing Th17 cells to inflamed joints via CCL20 in rheumatoid arthritis and its animal model. *J Exp Med.* (2007) 204:2803–12. doi: 10.1084/jem.20071397
125. Komatsu N, Okamoto K, Sawa S, Nakashima T, Oh-Hora M, Kodama T, et al. Pathogenic conversion of Foxp3+ T cells into TH17 cells in autoimmune arthritis. *Nat Med.* (2014) 20:62–8. doi: 10.1038/nm.3432
126. Nevius E, Gomes AC, Pereira JP. Inflammatory cell migration in rheumatoid arthritis: a comprehensive review. *Clin Rev Allergy Immunol.* (2016) 51:59–78. doi: 10.1007/s12016-015-8520-9
127. Baum R, Gravallese EM. Bone as a target organ in rheumatic disease: impact on osteoclasts and osteoblasts. *Clin Rev Allergy Immunol.* (2016) 51:1–15. doi: 10.1007/s12016-015-8515-6
128. Hayer S, Bauer G, Willburger M, Sinn K, Alasti F, Plasenzotti R, et al. Cartilage damage and bone erosion are more prominent determinants of functional impairment in longstanding experimental arthritis than synovial inflammation. *Dis Model Mech.* (2016) 9:1329–38. doi: 10.1242/dmm.025460
129. Boman A, Kokkonen H, Arlestig L, Berglin E, Rantapaa-Dahlqvist S. Receptor activator of nuclear factor kappa-B ligand (RANKL) but not sclerostin or gene polymorphisms is related to joint destruction in early rheumatoid arthritis. *Clin Rheumatol.* (2017) 36:1005–12. doi: 10.1007/s10067-017-3570-4
130. Chiu YG, Ritchlin CT. Denosumab: targeting the RANKL pathway to treat rheumatoid arthritis. *Expert Opin Biol Ther.* (2017) 17:119–28. doi: 10.1080/14712598.2017.1263614
131. Walsh MC, Choi Y. Biology of the RANKL-RANK-OPG System in Immunity, Bone, and Beyond. *Front Immunol.* (2014) 5:511. doi: 10.3389/fimmu.2014.00511
132. Takeuchi T, Tanaka Y, Ishiguro N, Yamanaka H, Yoneda T, Ohira T, et al. Effect of denosumab on Japanese patients with rheumatoid arthritis: a dose-response study of AMG 162 (Denosumab) in patients with RheumatoId arthritis on methotrexate to Validate inhibitory effect on bone Erosion (DRIVE)-a 12-month, multicentre, randomised, double-blind, placebo-controlled, phase II clinical trial. *Ann Rheum Dis.* (2016) 75:983–90. doi: 10.1136/annrheumdis-2015-208052
133. Cosway E, Anderson G, Garside P, Prendergast C. The thymus and rheumatology: should we care? *Curr Opin Rheumatol.* (2016) 28:189–95. doi: 10.1097/BOR.0000000000000251
134. Tanaka S, Maeda S, Hashimoto M, Fujimori C, Ito Y, Teradaira S, et al. Graded attenuation of TCR signaling elicits distinct autoimmune diseases by altering thymic T cell selection and regulatory T cell function. *J Immunol.* (2010) 185:2295–305. doi: 10.4049/jimmunol.1000848
135. Flores-Borja F, Jury EC, Mauri C, Ehrenstein MR. Defects in CTLA-4 are associated with abnormal regulatory T cell function in rheumatoid arthritis. *Proc Natl Acad Sci USA.* (2008) 105:19396–401. doi: 10.1073/pnas.0806855105
136. Cribbs AP, Kennedy A, Penn H, Read JE, Amjadi P, Green P, et al. Treg cell function in rheumatoid arthritis is compromised by ctla-4 promoter methylation resulting in a failure to activate the indoleamine 2,3-dioxygenase pathway. *Arthritis Rheumatol.* (2014) 66:2344–54. doi: 10.1002/art.38715
137. Raje N, Terpos E, Willenbacher W, Shimizu K, Garcia-Sanz R, Durie B, et al. Denosumab versus zoledronic acid in bone disease treatment of newly diagnosed multiple myeloma: an international, double-blind, double-dummy, randomised, controlled, phase 3 study. *Lancet Oncol.* (2018) 19:370–81. doi: 10.1016/S1470-2045(18)30072-X
138. Ahern E, Harjunpaa H, Barkauskas D, Allen S, Takeda K, Yagita H, et al. Co-administration of RANKL and CTLA4 antibodies enhances lymphocyte-mediated antitumor immunity in mice. *Clin Cancer Res.* (2017) 23:5789–801. doi: 10.1158/1078-0432.CCR-17-0606
139. Ahern E, Harjunpaa H, O'Donnell JS, Allen S, Dougall WC, Teng MWL, et al. RANKL blockade improves efficacy of PD1-PD-L1 blockade or dual PD1-PD-L1 and CTLA4 blockade in mouse models of cancer. *Oncoimmunology.* (2018) 7:e1431088. doi: 10.1080/2162402X.2018.1431088
140. Chen NJ, Huang MW, Hsieh SL. Enhanced secretion of IFN-gamma by activated Th1 cells occurs via reverse signaling through TNF-related activation-induced cytokine. *J Immunol.* (2001) 166:270–6. doi: 10.4049/jimmunol.166.1.270
141. Secchiero P, Corallini F, Barbarotto E, Melloni E, Di Iasio MG, Tiribelli M, et al. Role of the RANKL/RANK system in the induction of interleukin-8 (IL-8) in B chronic lymphocytic leukemia (B-CLL) cells. *J Cell Physiol.* (2006) 207:158–64. doi: 10.1002/jcp.20547
142. Zhang S, Wang X, Li G, Chong Y, Zhang J, Guo X, et al. Osteoclast regulation of osteoblasts via RANKRANKL reverse signal transduction *in vitro*. *Mol Med Rep.* (2017) 16:3994–4000. doi: 10.3892/mmr.2017.7039

11

Activation of Shc1 Allows Oncostatin M to Induce RANKL and Osteoclast Formation More Effectively than Leukemia Inhibitory Factor

Emma Persson[1†‡], Pedro P. C. Souza[2,3†], Thais Floriano-Marcelino[2], Howard Herschel Conaway[4], Petra Henning[5] and Ulf H. Lerner[1,5]*

[1] Department of Molecular Periodontology, Umeå University, Umeå, Sweden, [2] Bone Biology Research Group, Department of Physiology and Pathology, School of Dentistry, São Paulo State University (UNESP), Araraquara, Brazil, [3] School of Dentistry, Federal University of Goiás, Goiânia, Brazil, [4] Department of Physiology and Biophysics, University of Arkansas for Medical Sciences, Little Rock, AR, United States, [5] Department of Internal Medicine and Clinical Nutrition, Centre for Bone and Arthritis Research, Institute for Medicine, Sahlgrenska Academy, University of Gothenburg, Gothenburg, Sweden

***Correspondence:**
Ulf H. Lerner
ulf.lerner@gu.se

† These authors have contributed equally to this work

***‡ Present Address:**
Emma Persson,
Department of Radiation Sciences, Umeå University, Umeå, Sweden

Background and Purpose: The gp130 family of cytokines signals through receptors dimerizing with the gp130 subunit. Downstream signaling typically activates STAT3 but also SHP2/Ras/MAPK pathways. Oncostatin M (OSM) is a unique cytokine in this family since the receptor (OSMR) activates a non-redundant signaling pathway by recruitment of the adapter Shc1. We have studied the functional relevance of Shc1 for OSM-induced bone resorption.

Experimental Approach: Osteoblasts were stimulated with OSM and STAT3 and Shc1 activations were studied using real-time PCR and Western blots. The role of STAT3 and Shc1 for OSM-induced RANKL expression and osteoclast formation was studied by silencing their mRNA expressions. Effects of OSM were compared to those of the closely related cytokine leukemia inhibitory factor (LIF).

Key Results: OSM, but not LIF, induced the mRNA and protein expression of Shc1 and activated phosphorylation of Shc1 in the osteoblasts. Silencing of Shc1 decreased OSM-induced activation of STAT3 and RANKL expression. Silencing of STAT3 had no effect on activation of Shc1, but prevented the OSM-mediated increase of RANKL expression. Silencing of either Shc1 or STAT3 in osteoblasts decreased formation of osteoclasts in OSM-stimulated co-cultures of osteoblasts and macrophages. In agreement with these observations, OSM was a more potent and robust stimulator than LIF of RANKL formation and bone resorption in mouse calvariae and osteoclast formation in bone marrow cultures.

Conclusions and Implications: Activation of the Shc1-dependent STAT3 signaling is crucial for OSM-induced osteoclast formation. Inhibition of Shc1 is a potential mechanism to specifically inhibit OSM-induced bone resorption.

Keywords: OSM, LIF, RANKL, Shc1, osteoclast, bone resorption

INTRODUCTION

Oncostatin M (OSM) belongs to the gp130 family of cytokines. It was discovered as a cytokine released from macrophage differentiated U-937 histiocytic lymphoma cells that inhibited proliferation of melanoma cells (1). OSM has also been reported to be expressed in monocytes, dendritic cells, T-cells, neutrophils (2), intestinal stromal cells (3), osteoblasts (4, 5) and osteocytes (5). Several studies have shown that OSM is involved in a wide variety of functions (2, 6), including bone remodeling (7), embryologic development, liver regeneration, haematopoiesis (8), tumorigenic progression and metastasis formation (9, 10), as well as inflammatory processes such as pulmonary fibrosis (11, 12), asthma (13), inflammatory bowel disease (3), periodontal disease (14), rheumatoid arthritis (15) and neurogenic heterotopic ossifications (16).

Cytokines in the gp130 family bind to cell surface receptor (R) subunits, and the ligand-receptor complex interacts with the transmembrane protein gp130 for signal propagation. Activation of the OSMR triggers heterodimerization between the ligand-receptor complex and one gp130 subunit (2). Human OSM can induce signaling through both the OSMR and the receptor for leukemia inhibitory factor (LIF), a closely related cytokine in the gp130 family, whereas mouse OSM acts mainly through the OSMR:gp130 heterodimer (2, 6), although it has been shown that mouse OSM can stimulate bone formation by decreasing sclerostin expression after LIFR-induced activation of STAT3 (5).

OSM stimulates bone resorption in organ cultures (17) and enhances osteoclast formation in crude bone marrow cell cultures (18, 19), effects which are associated with increased expression of receptor activator of NF-κB ligand (RANKL) (17, 18). Interestingly, OSM is more potent and effective than LIF as a stimulator of osteoclast formation in co-cultures of mouse osteoblasts and bone marrow cells (20). The bone phenotype of mice in which the *Osm* gene has been deleted has not been reported, but mice globally deficient in the *Osmr* have increased bone mass and a decreased number of osteoclasts (5), findings which are in agreement with *in vitro* observations showing OSM increasing osteoclast numbers and stimulating bone resorption.

The OSMR has no intrinsic tyrosine kinase activity, but dimerization with gp130 activates the JAK-STAT (Janus kinase and signal transducer and activator of transcription) pathway. JAKs are constitutively connected to the membrane-proximal regions of gp130 and OSMR and, upon activation, JAKs trans-phosphorylate several Tyr residues in the intracellular domains of gp130 and OSMR. In the mouse OSMR, JAK2 is preferentially bound and its activation leads to phosphorylation of Tyr^{917} and Tyr^{945} in the OSMR and subsequent recruitment of the transcription factor STAT3 (21, 22). Recruitment of STAT3 to gp130 is mediated by JAK-dependent phosphorylation of $Tyr^{767}/Tyr^{814}/Tyr^{905}/Tyr^{915}$ (23). Once phosphorylated by JAKs, activated STAT3 dimers translocate to the nucleus and bind to specific DNA sequences in promoter regions of a variety of target genes. JAK-dependent phosphorylation of Tyr^{759} in gp130 results in recruitment and activation of the tyrosine phosphatase SHP-2 [Src homology region 2-containing protein tyrosine phosphatase 2; (24)]. In turn, SHP-2 then forms a complex with Grb2 (growth factor receptor-binding protein 2) and Sos (Son of sevenless), which activates the Ras/Raf/MAPK pathway (25), a hallmark of many haematopoietic cytokine receptors.

A non-redundant signaling pathway distinguishing OSMR from the other receptors in the gp130 family of cytokines is recruitment of the adapter protein Shc1 (Src homology and collagen 1) to Tyr^{861} (26, 27). Shc proteins are phosphotyrosine adapters which link activated transmembrane receptors to downstream signaling cascades (28). Four members of this family have been described, designated Shc1, Shc2, Shc3 and Shc4. Three isoforms of Shc1 protein generated by differential promoter usage (p66) or alternative translational initiation (p46, p52) have been discovered. Shc1 contains both phosphotyrosine binding domains (PTB) and SH2 domains and is able to recruit the Ras/Raf/MAPK adapter Grb2 to the SH2 domain. Phosphorylation of the OSMR on Tyr^{861} allows binding of activated Shc1 to the OSMR, recruitment of Grb2 and subsequent induction of a Ras-dependent kinase cascade, which results in activation of MAPK (26). This is different from the LIF-induced activation of MAPK, where recruitment of SHP-2 to the gp130 subunit in the LIFR mediates activation of MAPK (2). Since OSMR lacks the recruitment motif for SHP-2, activation of Shc1 substitutes for SHP-2 mediated activation of the MAPK caused by the closely related LIFR, but the functional relevance of OSMR-Shc1 in bone has not been investigated. Interestingly, activation of Shc1 has also recently been shown to potentiate STAT3 phosphorylation in breast cancer cells (29), but a role for the OSMR-Shc1-STAT3 axis in osteoblasts has not been assessed.

The aim of the present study was to investigate the importance of the Shc1-STAT3 signaling pathway in OSM-induced RANKL formation in osteoblasts and subsequent osteoclast formation.

MATERIALS AND METHODS

Materials

Recombinant mouse LIF, mouse OSM, bone morphogenetic protein-2 (BMP-2), macrophage colony-stimulating factor (M-CSF), RANKL (amino acids 158–316; cat. no. 462-TEC) and the ELISA kits for mouse RANKL and mouse OPG were purchased from R&D Systems, Abingdon, UK; bacterial collagenase type I from Worthington Biochemical Corp., Lakewood, NJ, USA; α-MEM, FBS, L-glutamine, and oligonucleotide

Abbreviations: AMV, avian myeloblastosis virus; BMM, bone marrow macrophages; BMC, bone marrow cells; BMP-2, bone morphogenetic protein-2; D3, 1,25$(OH)_2$-vitamin D3; EMSA, electrophoretic mobility shift assay; GAPDH, glyceraldehyde-3-phosphate dehydrogenase; gp130, glycoprotein 130; Grb2, Growth factor receptor-binding protein 2; IL, interleukin; JAK, Janus kinase; LIF, leukemia inhibitory factor; LIFR, LIF receptor; MAPK, mitogen-activated protein kinase; M-CSF, macrophage colony-stimulating factor; OPG, osteoprotegerin; OSM, oncostatin M; OSMR, OSM receptor; PTB, phosphotyrosine binding domain; PTH, parathyroid hormone; RANKL, receptor activator of NF-κB ligand; SH2, Src homology 2; Shc, Src homology and collagen; SHP-2, SH2 domain-containing tyrosine phosphatase 2; Sos, Son of sevenless; STAT, signal transducer and activator of transcription; TRAP, tartrate-resistant acid phosphatase; $TRAP^+$MuOCL, $TRAP^+$ multinucleated osteoclasts.

primers from Invitrogen, Stockholm, Sweden; RNAqueous®-4PCR RNA isolation kit from Ambion, Inc., Austin TX, USA; 1st strand cDNA synthesis Kit and PCR Core Kit from Roche, Mannheim, Germany; DYEnamic ET terminator cycle sequencing kit from GE Healthcare, Uppsala, Sweden; QIAquick PCR Purification kit was from Qiagen Ltd., Crawley, West Sussex, England; TaqMan Universal PCR Master Mix and TaqMan probes from Applied Biosystems, Foster City, CA, USA; all primary and secondary antibodies used are specified in **Supporting Information Table I**; anti-IgG-HRP secondary antibodies used for Western blot were from Santa Cruz Biotechnology, Inc., Santa Cruz, CA, USA; culture dishes and multi-well plates from Costar, Cambridge, MA, USA, or Nunc International Corp., Naperville, IL, USA. Indomethacin was kindly supplied by Merck, Sharp & Dohme, Haarlem, the Netherlands; the mouse bone marrow stromal cell line ST-2 from Riken BRC Cell Bank (www.brc.riken.go.jp).

Animals

CsA mice from the inbred colony at Umeå University, Swiss mice from the School of Dentistry at Araraquara and C57Bl/6 mice from the University of Gothenburg were used for isolation of calvarial osteoblasts, bone marrow cells or calvarial bone explants. The Institutional Animal Care and Ethics Committees at Umeå University, at the School of Dentistry, Araraquara and at the University of Gothenburg approved all experimental studies. The observation that OSM is a more robust stimulator than LIF of *Tnfsf11* (encoding RANKL) mRNA expression was made in cells from all three genotypes; OSM-induced phosphorylation of Shc1 was assessed in cells from CsA and Swiss mice and found to activate Shc1 in both strains.

Bone Resorption Bioassay

Bone resorption was assessed in organ culture of parietal bones from 6 to 7 days-old mice by analyzing the release of ^{45}Ca from prelabelled bones as previously described (30, 31). Release of isotope was expressed as the percentage release of the initial amount of isotope (calculated as the sum of radioactivity in medium and bone after culture). The data were recalculated and the results expressed as percent of control that was set at 100%, which allowed for accumulation of data from several experiments.

Isolation and Culture of Mouse Calvarial Osteoblasts

Bone cells were isolated from calvariae harvested from 2 to 5 days-old mice using bacterial collagenase in the modified time sequential enzyme-digestion technique (32). Cells from populations 6 to 10, showing an osteoblastic phenotype as assessed by their cyclic AMP-responsiveness to PTH, expression of alkaline phosphatase, osteocalcin and bone sialoprotein, as well as the capacity to form mineralized bone noduli (data not shown), were used. The cells were seeded in culture flasks containing α-MEM supplemented with 10% FBS, L-glutamine and antibiotics at 37°C in humidified air containing 5% CO_2. After 4 days, the cells were sub-cultured in culture dishes or multi-well plates.

Osteoclast Differentiation in Bone Marrow Cell Cultures

Bone marrow cells (BMC) were flushed from femur and tibiae from 6 week-old mice and seeded in 48 multi-well plates containing α-MEM/10% FBS and incubated overnight. The cells were then cultured in the same medium with or without test substances for 7–9 days. Cells staining positive for tartrate-resistant acid phosphatase (TRAP) and containing three or more nuclei were considered osteoclasts and the number of TRAP-positive multinucleated osteoclasts (TRAP$^+$ MuOCL) was counted.

Osteoclast Differentiation in Bone Marrow Macrophage Cultures

Bone marrow cells from 6 to 12 weeks old mice were isolated and incubated in the presence of M-CSF (30 ng/mL) for 3 days in culture dishes, to which stromal cells and lymphoid cells cannot adhere, as previously described (33, 34). The cells adherent to the bottom of the dishes are devoid of phenotypic markers for stromal cells, T- and B-cells, express CD115/c-Fms (75%) and CD11b/Mac-1 (100%), and were used as bone marrow macrophages (BMM). The BMM cells were seeded in 96 multi-well plates and then incubated in M-CSF (30 ng/mL) or M-CSF + RANKL (30 ng/mL + 4 ng/mL) with or without LIF (100 ng/mL) or OSM (100 ng/mL). Cells staining positive for TRAP and containing three or more nuclei were considered osteoclasts and the number of TRAP$^+$ MuOCL was counted.

Stromal Cells

The ST-2 cells were seeded in multi-well plates and incubated in α-MEM/10% FBS overnight. Following incubation, medium with and without test substances was added and the cells incubated for 24 h for subsequent gene expression analysis.

Gene Silencing in Osteoblasts Using Small Interfering RNA

Calvarial osteoblasts were seeded in multi-well plates with α-MEM supplemented with 10% FBS and antibiotics. For co-culture and gene expression experiments, 10^3 cells were seeded per well in 96-well plates, while for protein extraction, 5×10^4 cells/well were seeded in 12-well plates. After overnight attachment, silencing of *Osmr*, *Lifr*, *Il6st*, *Shc1* or *Stat3* was performed using Lipofectamine RNAiMAX and 30 nM of the appropriate siRNAs listed in **Supporting Information Table II.** Cells treated with a scrambled (siSCR) sequence served as controls. Forty-eight hours after the first silencing, the protocol was repeated. Twenty-four hours after the second silencing, the cells were incubated in medium containing either vehicle, LIF or OSM. At the end of cultures, RNA or protein was extracted. In some experiments, the osteoblasts were co-cultured with BMMs.

Osteoblast and Bone Marrow Macrophage Co-cultures

Following silencing of *Shc1* or *Stat3* in osteoblasts, 2×10^4 BMMs were added to each well in 96-well plates containing osteoblasts. The co-cultures were exposed to vehicle or OSM (100 ng/mL) and 3 days later, the cells were fixed with PBS-buffered 4% paraformaldehyde and stained for TRAP. The number of $TRAP^+$ MuOCL was counted in each well.

RNA Isolation and First-Strand cDNA Synthesis

Total RNA was extracted using commercially available RNA isolation kits (Ambion or Qiagen) by following the manufacturer's protocol. For quantitative real-time polymerase chain reactions, RNA was extracted from a single cell culture well, or from individual bones. For semi-quantitative polymerase chain reactions, RNA extracted from three wells was pooled per treatment group. RNA was reverse transcribed into single-stranded cDNA with a commercially available cDNA synthesis kit using.

Semi-quantitative Polymerase Chain Reaction

Polymerase chain reaction analyses were performed using a standard protocol. The reaction conditions were: denaturing at 94°C for 2 min, annealing for 40 s, and elongation at 72°C for 60 s; in subsequent cycles denaturing was performed at 94°C for 40 s. Reaction conditions for OPG and RANKL were as follows: denaturation at 94°C for 35 s, annealing at 65°C for 35 s, and elongation at 72°C for 60 s for 10 cycles. In subsequent cycles, the primer annealing temperature was decreased stepwise by 5°C every 5 cycles from 65 to 45°C. The primer sequences (forward and reverse, given in the 5′-3′ orientation), expected fragment lengths and annealing temperatures used in PCR are listed in **Supporting Information Table III**. The expressions of the target genes were compared at the logarithmic phase of the PCR reaction. No amplification was detected in samples where the RT reaction had been omitted (data not shown). The PCR products were electrophoretically size fractionated in 1.5% agarose gel and visualized using ethidium bromide. The identity of the PCR products was confirmed using a DYEnamic ET terminator cycle sequencing kit with sequences analyzed on an ABI 377 XL DNA Sequencer (PE Applied Biosystems, Foster City, CA).

Quantitative Real-Time Polymerase Chain Reaction

Quantitative real-time PCR analysis was performed using TaqMan kinetics. In each reaction, cDNA was amplified using a TaqMan Universal PCR Master Mix kit, 300 nmol/L of each primer and 100 nmol/L of probe on an ABI Prism 7900 HT Sequence Detection System (Applied Biosystems, Foster City, CA, USA) or predesigned Taqman Assays and Taqman Fast Advance Master Mix on a StepOnePlus Real-Time PCR system. The primers and probes used are listed in **Supporting Information Tables III, IV**. Gapdh (for BMM) or β-actin or 36B4 (for BMC and calvarial osteoblasts) were used as internal standard to correct for differences in starting mRNA concentrations.

Protein Analyses of RANKL and OPG

The protein levels of RANKL and OPG in calvarial bones were analyzed using commercially available ELISA kits. Calvarial cells were lysed using 0.2% Triton X-100 and the extracted samples were analyzed by following the manufacturer's protocol.

Preparation of Total Cell Lysates

Calvarial osteoblasts were seeded in 60 cm^2 dishes at a density of 2×10^4 cells/cm^2. After 3 days of culture with one media change, the cells were incubated in the absence (control) or presence of test substances for different time periods. Following incubation, the cells were washed twice in PBS before addition of lysis buffer (1% Igepal CA-630, 0.1% SDS, 2 mM EDTA, 50 mM NaF, 0.1 mg/mL PMSF, 10 µg/mL leupeptin, 10 µg/mL pepstatin A, in PBS). The dishes were kept on ice for 15 min followed by scraping and collection of cell lysates. Before use in Western blot, cell lysates were concentrated using Microcon centrifugal filter devices according to manufacturer's recommendations. Protein concentration of the cell lysates was measured using the BCA method with bovine albumin as standard.

Western Blot Analysis

For Western blot analysis, cell lysates pooled from three culture dishes were mixed with sample buffer (200 mM Tris-HCl, pH 6.7, 20% glycerol, 10% β-mercaptoethanol, 5% SDS, 0.01% Pyronin Y) and boiled for 3 min. Protein samples were then loaded on 4–12% Tris-HCl polyacrylamide gels and electrophoresis was performed according to the Laemmli method. Electrophoretically separated proteins were then blotted onto a PVDF membrane which was blocked (5% BSA in TBS) overnight. For detection, the membrane was incubated with primary antibody overnight in 1% BSA/PBS in dilutions specified in **Supporting Information Table I**. Three times 10 min of wash in TBS with 0.05% Tween-20 (TBST) was followed by incubation with HRP-conjugated secondary antibody (1:5,000 in 1% BSA, 0.05% Tween-20 in TBS) for 60 min at room temperature. Finally, the membrane was washed extensively with TBST and TBS followed by development using a chemiluminescence detection kit according to manufacturer's protocol.

Preparation of Nuclear Extracts

Calvarial osteoblasts were plated at a density of 2 x 10^4 cells/cm^2 in culture dishes (60 cm^2) containing α-MEM with 10% FBS, L-glutamine and antibiotics. After 4 days with one media change, the cells were incubated in the absence (control) or presence of test substances for 30 min. Following incubation, the cells were washed with ice cold PBS and scraped. Cell suspensions from two culture dishes were pooled and centrifuged briefly and pelleted cells homogenized in lysis buffer A (10 mM HEPES, pH 7.9, 0.1 mM EDTA, 10 mM KCl, 625 µg/mL spermidine, 625 µg/mL spermine, 0.5 mM DTT, 0.5 mM PMSF, 1 µg/mL leupeptin, 1 µg/mL pepstatin A). After 15 min on ice, Igepal CA-630 was added to a final concentration of 0.5%. The nuclei were collected by centrifugation at 12 000 x g for 2 min, and pelleted nuclei were lysed by incubation for 30 min on ice in lysis buffer B (20 mM HEPES, pH 7.9, 0.2 mM EDTA, 0.42 M NaCl, 25% glycerol, 625 µg/mL spermidine, 625 µg/mL spermine, 0.5 mM DTT, 0.5 mM PMSF, 1 µg/mL leupeptin, 1 µg/mL pepstatin A). Supernatants were collected by centrifugation at 16 000 x g for 10 min. The protein concentration of the samples was determined by the

Bradford method and aliquots were stored at −80°C until use in electrophoretic mobility shift assays (EMSAs).

EMSA

Consensus oligonucleotides including an AP-1 site (CGCTTG ATGACTCAGCCGGAA) and a κB site (AGTTGAGGGGAC TTTCCCAGGC) were end-labeled with [γ-^{32}P] ATP using T4 kinase according to manufacturer's instructions. Mutated forms of the AP-1 (CGCTTGATGACTCCGGAA) and NF-κB (AGT TGAGGGACTTTCCCAGGC) oligonucleotides were used in competition studies. Annealing of complementary strands of both labeled and unlabelled oligonucleotides was performed before used in electrophoretic mobility shift assay (EMSA). Reaction mixtures containing 8 μg of nuclear extract, 0.5–1 ng of probe (50 000 cpm), 4 μg poly(dI-dC)•poly(dI-dC), 20 nM DTT, and reaction buffer (50 mM Tris-HCl, pH 7.5, 0.25 M NaCl, 5 mM EDTA, 25% glycerol) were incubated at room temperature for 30 min. In antibody supershifts and competition studies, 2 mg/mL of antibody, or 50- or 100-fold excess of unlabelled probe, was pre-incubated with reaction mixture without probe for 30 min before addition of ^{32}P-labeled probe. After incubation for 30 min at room temperature, samples were loaded onto a non-denaturing polyacrylamide gel and electrophoresed, followed by drying of the gel and autoradiography.

Statistical Analysis

Statistical significance was determined by ANOVA using Levene's homogeneity test and Dunnett's 2-sided, Dunnett's T3 or Tukey's post hoc test. When comparing two groups, non-parametric Mann-Whitney U test, or two-sided Student's t-test was used, where applicable. A $P < 0.05$ was considered statistically significant. Statistical significance is presented as follows, $^{*}P < 0.05$, $^{**}P < 0.01$, and $^{***}P < 0.001$. Data are expressed as mean ± SEM. Numerical values are expressed as percent of unstimulated control, with controls presented as 100% or 1-fold, if not otherwise stated. We have used four wells or six bones (^{45}Ca release) per treatment group and then calculated a mean value and standard variation (SEM) for each group, which have been used for statistical analyses and to create the figures. The experiments have then been repeated using the same design and calculations 2–3 times with similar results.

RESULTS

OSM, in Contrast to LIF, Robustly Activates ERK and the AP-1 Complex in Calvarial Osteoblasts

Stimulation of calvarial osteoblasts with OSM (100 ng/mL) resulted in a robust, time-dependent activation of the MAP kinase ERK, as assessed by phosphorylation of Tyr^{204} (**Figure 1A**). OSM treatment also resulted in increased phosphorylation of the MAP kinase JNK on Tyr^{185} and Thr^{183}. In contrast, OSM did not stimulate phosphorylation of the p38 MAPK on Tyr^{182}. Treatment of the osteoblasts with LIF (100 ng/mL) caused a weak, rapidly transient activation of JNK, but did not affect phosphorylation of ERK or p38. Neither OSM nor LIF had any effect on total protein levels of p38, JNK or ERK (**Figure 1A**).

Activation of AP-1 is a consequence of MAPK activation and we, therefore, next studied the effects of OSM on transcriptional control of AP-1 subunits and DNA binding of AP-1, as assessed by semi-quantitative RT-PCR and EMSA, respectively.

OSM (100 ng/mL) increased the mRNA expression in mouse calvarial osteoblasts of *Fos* and *Jun* after 48 h treatment (**Figure 1B**), whereas *Fosb*, *Fosl1*, *Fosl2*, *Junb*, and *Jund* mRNA expressions were unaffected (**Figure 1B**). In contrast, LIF caused a marginal increase of *Fos* mRNA but did not affect the expression of the other AP-1 subunits (**Figure 1B**).

Incubation of calvarial osteoblasts with OSM for 30 min resulted in enhanced DNA binding of AP-1 as assessed by EMSA, whereas LIF had no effect (**Figure 1C**, left top panel). The binding specificity was evident by the complete displacement with a 50-fold excess of unlabelled (cold) homologous oligonucleotide (C), whereas a mutated homologous oligonucleotide (M) and a non-homologous oligonucleotide (NF-κB; NF) had no effect (**Figure 1C**, middle top panel). The antibody shift experiment demonstrated the involvement of both c-Jun (Jun) and c-Fos (Fos) in the AP-1 complex activated by OSM (**Figure 1C**, right top panel). In contrast to the enhanced AP-1 DNA binding activity by OSM, treatment with either OSM or LIF did not result in an effect on NF-κB DNA binding activity (**Figure 1C**, lower panel).

These observations demonstrated clear differences in signaling events downstream the OSM and LIF receptors in primary mouse calvarial osteoblasts, which are in line with observations made in the human osteoblastic MG-63 cell line showing a clear activation of ERK by OSM, but a weaker by LIF (35).

OSM Is a More Robust Activator Than LIF of STAT3 mRNA Expression and Phosphorylation

Stimulation of calvarial osteoblasts with OSM (100 ng/mL) increased expression of *Stat3* mRNA, whereas no such effect was observed after stimulation with LIF (**Figure 2A**).

Western blot analyses indicated that phosphorylation of the transcription factor STAT3 on Tyr^{705}, which is crucial for dimerization of STAT3 and subsequent DNA binding (36), was much greater after treatment with OSM than LIF (**Figure 2B**). No effect on total STAT3 protein by OSM or LIF was observed.

These findings show that OSM robustly activates STAT3, whereas LIF only causes a marginal activation of this transcription factor.

Activation by OSM of the Adapter Protein Shc1 in Calvarial Osteoblasts Is Crucial for STAT3 and ERK Activation

Having observed the differences in MAPK and STAT3 activation in osteoblasts stimulated with OSM and LIF, and knowing that only OSM has been reported to activate the adapter protein Shc1 in several other cell types, we next investigated the role of Shc adapters for the robust activation by OSM of ERK and STAT3 in

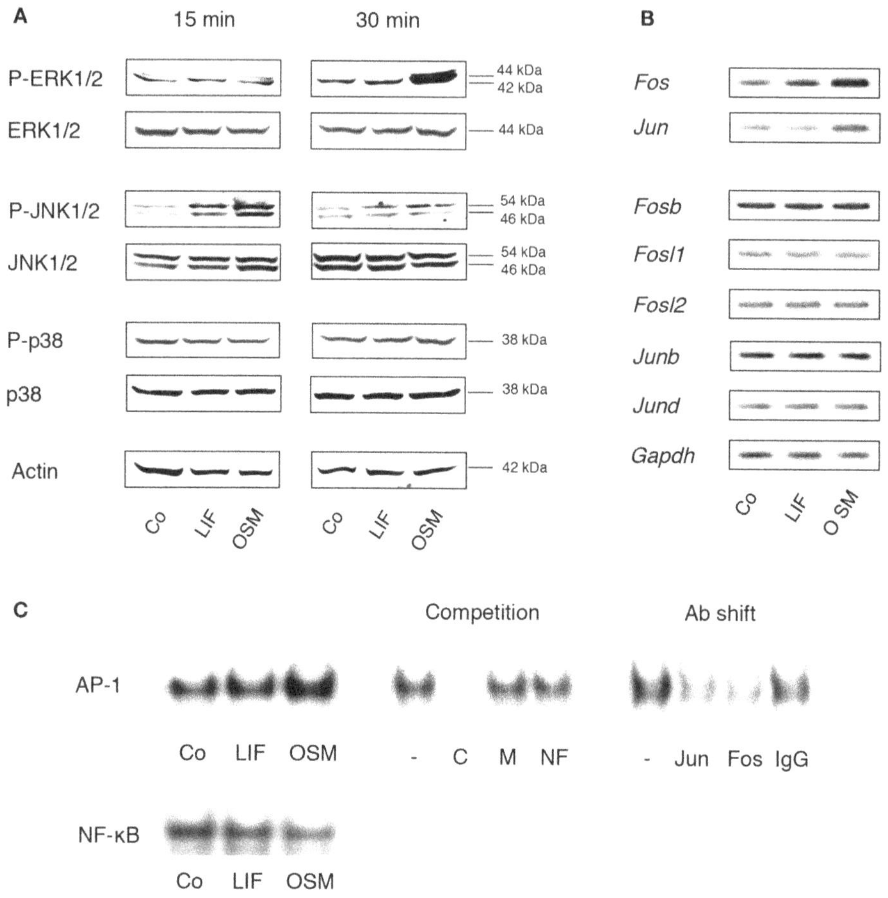

FIGURE 1 | MAP kinases and the AP-1 complex are differentially activated by OSM and LIF. **(A)** Mouse calvarial osteoblasts were cultured in the absence (Co) or presence of LIF or OSM (both at 100 ng/mL) for 15 and 30 min followed by cell lysis and Western blot analysis of total, as well as phosphorylated, ERK, JNK and p38. Actin served as the internal control for protein loading. **(B)** Semi-quantitative PCR analysis of AP-1 subunit mRNA expression after incubation without (Co) or with LIF or OSM (both at 100 ng/mL) for 48 h. *Gapdh* served as loading control. **(C)** EMSA analysis of nuclear extracts from cells incubated for 30 min in the absence (Co) or the presence of LIF or OSM (both at 100 ng/mL). Left upper panel, EMSA for nuclear extracts incubated with AP-1 consensus probe. Middle upper panel, competition studies on nuclear extracts from OSM-stimulated cells. From left: No competitor (–), homologous unlabelled (cold) AP-1 consensus probe (C), mutated AP-1 consensus probe (M), non-homologous probe (NF-κB; NF). Right upper panel, supershifts using antibodies against c-Jun (Jun), c-Fos (Fos), and unspecific IgG (IgG) of nuclear extracts from OSM-stimulated cells. Lower panel, EMSA for nuclear extracts incubated with NF-κB consensus probe.

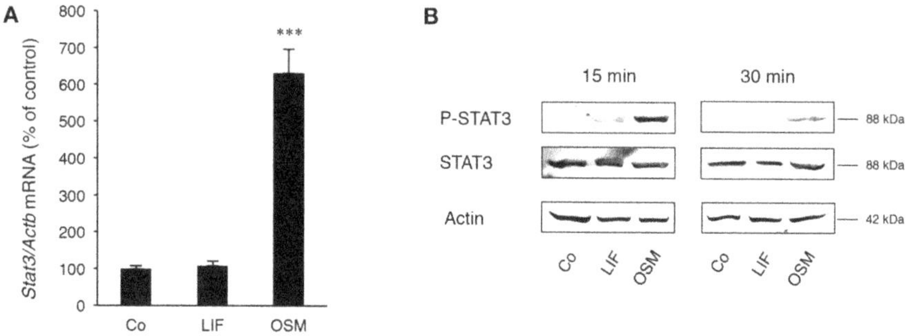

FIGURE 2 | STAT3 is differentially expressed and activated by OSM and LIF. Mouse calvarial osteoblasts were cultured in the absence (Co) or presence of LIF or OSM (both at 100 ng/mL) for 48 h to assess *Stat3* mRNA expression by RT-qPCR **(A)** or for 15 and 30 min to assess phosphorylated and total STAT3 protein levels by Western Blot **(B)**. Values in **(A)** represent means for four wells and SEM is shown as vertical bars. Significant differences compared to untreated cells (Co) is defined as $^{***}P < 0.001$ analyzed by one-way ANOVA followed by Dunnet's multiple comparison test vs. Co.

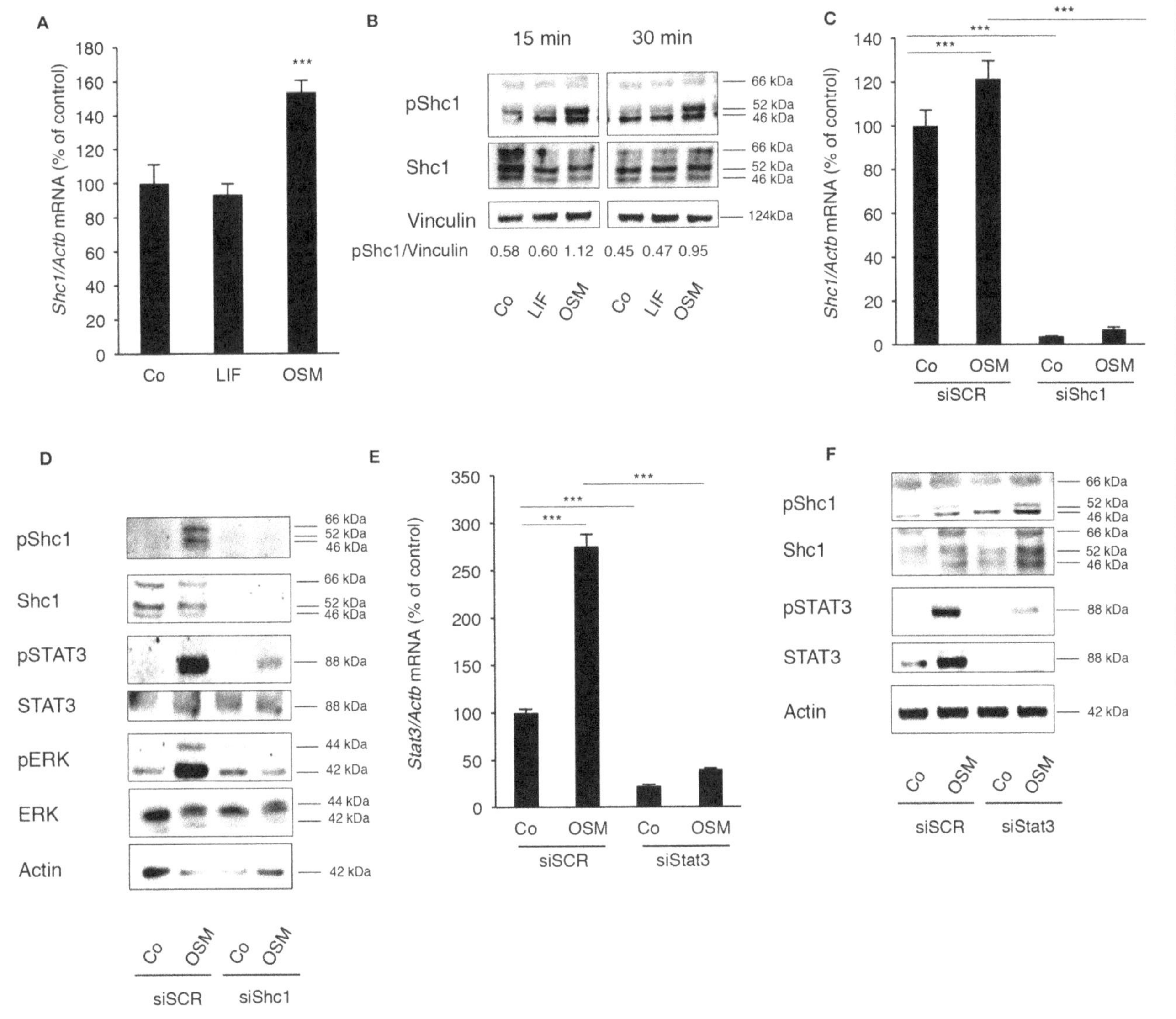

FIGURE 3 | OSM stimulates activation of STAT3 and ERK by phosphorylating the adapter protein Shc1. **(A)** Mouse calvarial osteoblasts were cultured in the absence (Co) or presence of LIF or OSM (both at 100 ng/mL) for 24 h and RNA was extracted for RT-qPCR analysis of *Shc1* mRNA. **(B)** The cells were exposed to LIF or OSM at 100 ng/mL for 15 and 30 min followed by cell lysis and Western blot for phosphorylated Shc1; the bands were quantified and normalized by vinculin. **(C)** Calvarial osteoblasts had the *Shc1* gene silenced by small interfering RNA and were exposed to LIF or OSM (both at 100 ng/mL) for 24 h before RNA extraction and analysis of *Shc1* mRNA expression by RT-qPCR; a scrambled sequence (siSCR) served as control. **(D)** Osteoblasts that had the *Shc1* gene knocked-down by siRNA and control cells exposed to scrambled sequence (siSCR) were exposed to OSM at 100 ng/mL or vehicle for 15 min and proteins were extracted for analysis of the phosphorylation of Shc1, STAT3 and ERK. **(E)** The *Stat3* gene was silenced in calvarial osteoblasts, which were subsequently exposed to OSM at 100 ng/mL or vehicle (Co) for 24 h before analysis of *Stat3* gene expression by RT-qPCR. **(F)** The effect of *Stat3* silencing on phosphorylation of STAT3 and Shc1 was analyzed by Western blot in osteoblasts treated with OSM for 15 min. **(A,C,E)** Values represent means for four wells and SEM is shown as vertical bars. **(A)** Significant differences compared to untreated cells (Co) at each time point are defined as $^{***}P < 0.001$; analyzed by one-way ANOVA followed by Dunnet's post *hoc-test*. **(C,E)** Significant differences are indicated by horizontal lines where $^{***}P < 0.001$ two-way ANOVA followed by Tukey post *hoc-test*. The difference in OSM-induced response with and without silencing analyzed by two-way ANOVA was statistically significant [interaction *P*-value in **C** ($P < 0.005$) and in **E** ($P < 0.0001$)]. OSM had no statistically significant effect ($P > 0.05$) on *Shc1* or *Stat3* mRNA expression in cells which had been silenced for *Shc1* or *Stat3*, respectively **(C,E)**.

osteoblasts. The expression of Shc proteins in osteoblasts had not been examined previously and to determine the role of Shc, the expression pattern of Shc proteins in calvarial osteoblasts treated with either OSM or LIF was evaluated.

Calvarial osteoblasts expressed *Shc1* (**Figure 3A**), but not *Shc2*, *Shc3* or *Shc4* mRNA (data not shown). Interestingly, *Shc1* mRNA was upregulated by OSM (**Figure 3A**). All three isoforms of Shc1 protein, p46, p52, and p66, were expressed by the osteoblasts (**Figure 3B**) and activation by OSM stimulated the phosphorylation of Shc1 (**Figure 3B**). OSM activated the phosphorylation of the p52 isoform in all experiments, but phosphorylation of the other isoforms was also observed in some experiments. In contrast to OSM, LIF did not affect *Shc1* mRNA expression or phosphorylation of Shc1 protein (**Figures 3A,B**).

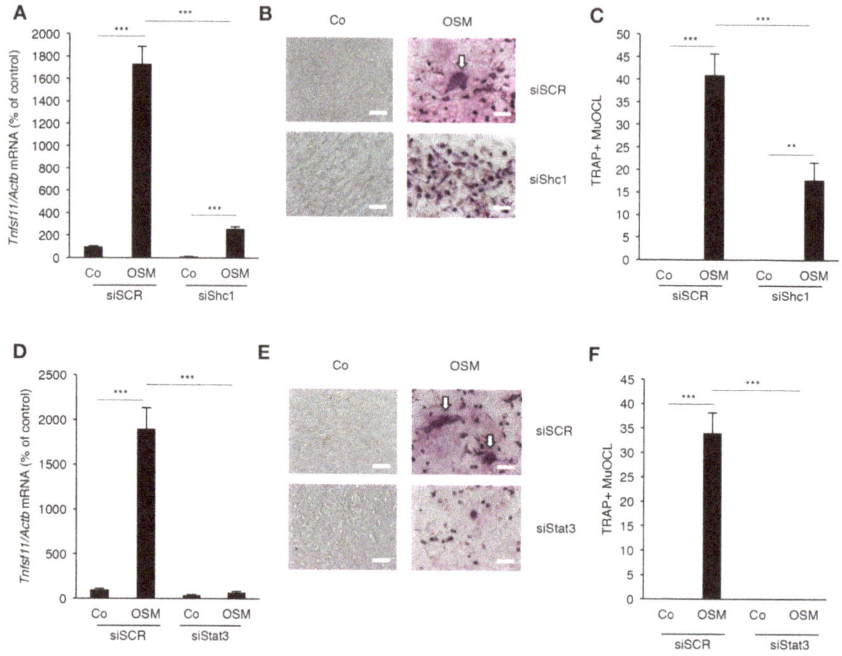

FIGURE 4 | Expression of RANKL in osteoblasts and osteoclastogenesis in co-cultures of bone marrow macrophages and calvarial osteoblasts induced by OSM are dependent on Shc1 and STAT3. Osteoblasts in which the *Shc1* gene **(A)** or the *Stat3* gene **(D)** was knocked-down by siRNA were treated with OSM at 100 ng/mL for 24 h before analysis of *Tnfsf11* gene expression. Osteoblasts transfected with scrambled RNA (siSCR) were similarly treated and analyzed. Osteoblasts in which *Shc1* **(B,C)** or *Stat3* **(E,F)** was knocked down (or siSCR as control) were exposed to OSM (100 ng/mL) or vehicle and co-cultured with BMMs for 3 days before TRAP staining and counting of TRAP$^+$ MuOCL **(A,C,D,F)**. Values represent means for four wells and SEM is shown as vertical bars. Significant differences are indicated by horizontal lines where $^{**}P < 0.01$; $^{***}P < 0.001$; analyzed by two-way ANOVA followed by Tukey post *hoc-test*. The difference in OSM-induced response with and without silencing analyzed by two-way ANOVA was statistically significant [interaction *P*-value in **A** (P<0.0001), **C** (P <0.005), **D** (P <0.0001) and **F** (P <0.0001)]. Scale bar in **(B,E)** is 50 μm.

The importance of Shc1 for OSM-induced STAT3 and ERK activation was then determined by silencing *Shc1* expression in the osteoblasts. The siRNA used decreased the mRNA expression of *Shc1* by 97% in control cells, as well as caused a significant decrease of *Shc1* mRNA in OSM-treated cells (**Figure 3C**). The silencing subsequently resulted in effective reductions of Shc1 protein expression and phosphorylation (**Figure 3D**). Decreased Shc1 activation substantially decreased OSM-induced phosphorylation of STAT3 and ERK, without affecting total protein levels of STAT3 and ERK (**Figure 3D**).

After observing a robust activation of STAT3 by OSM, the role of STAT3 phosphorylation in the OSM-induced activation of Shc1 was evaluated. Treatment of osteoblasts with OSM (100 ng/mL) resulted in a 2.8-fold increase of *Stat3* mRNA expression (**Figure 3E**). Silencing of *Stat3* expression decreased the mRNA expression of *Stat3* in untreated control cells by 80% and significantly decreased OSM-induced upregulation of *Stat3* mRNA (**Figure 3E**). Silencing of *Stat3* resulted in a decrease in STAT3 protein expression and OSM-induced STAT3 phohorylation, as expected, but did not affect phosphorylation of Shc1 (**Figure 3F**). The fact that silencing of *Shc1* resulted in impaired phosphorylation of STAT3 induced by OSM, whereas silencing of *Stat3* did not decrease the OSM-induced activation of Shc1 (**Figure 3F**), indicate that Shc1 activation is upstream of STAT3.

Activation of STAT3 and the Adapter Protein Shc1 by OSM Is Crucial for Stimulation of RANKL Expression and Osteoclastogenesis

Next, the importance of the Shc1-ERK and JAK-STAT3 pathways for stimulation of RANKL expression by OSM was evaluated. Silencing of *Shc1* significantly decreased the OSM-induced mRNA expression of *Tnfsf11* (encoding RANKL) (**Figure 4A**). Importantly, silencing of *Shc1* expression in osteoblasts decreased OSM-induced osteoclast formation in co-cultures of calvarial osteoblasts and BMM (**Figures 4B,C**). Silencing of *Stat3* also resulted in substantially decreased expression of OSM-induced T*nfsf11* mRNA expression (**Figure 4D**), and totally prevented formation of osteoclasts in OSM-stimulated co-cultures of calvarial osteoblasts and BMM (**Figures 4E,F**).

OSM Is a More Robust Stimulator of ^{45}Ca Release and Expression of RANKL in Mouse Calvarial Bones and Calvarial Osteoblasts

Having observed that OSM but not LIF receptors activate Shc1-dependent signaling, we next assessed the importance of this difference for bone resorption, RANKL production and osteoclastogenesis.

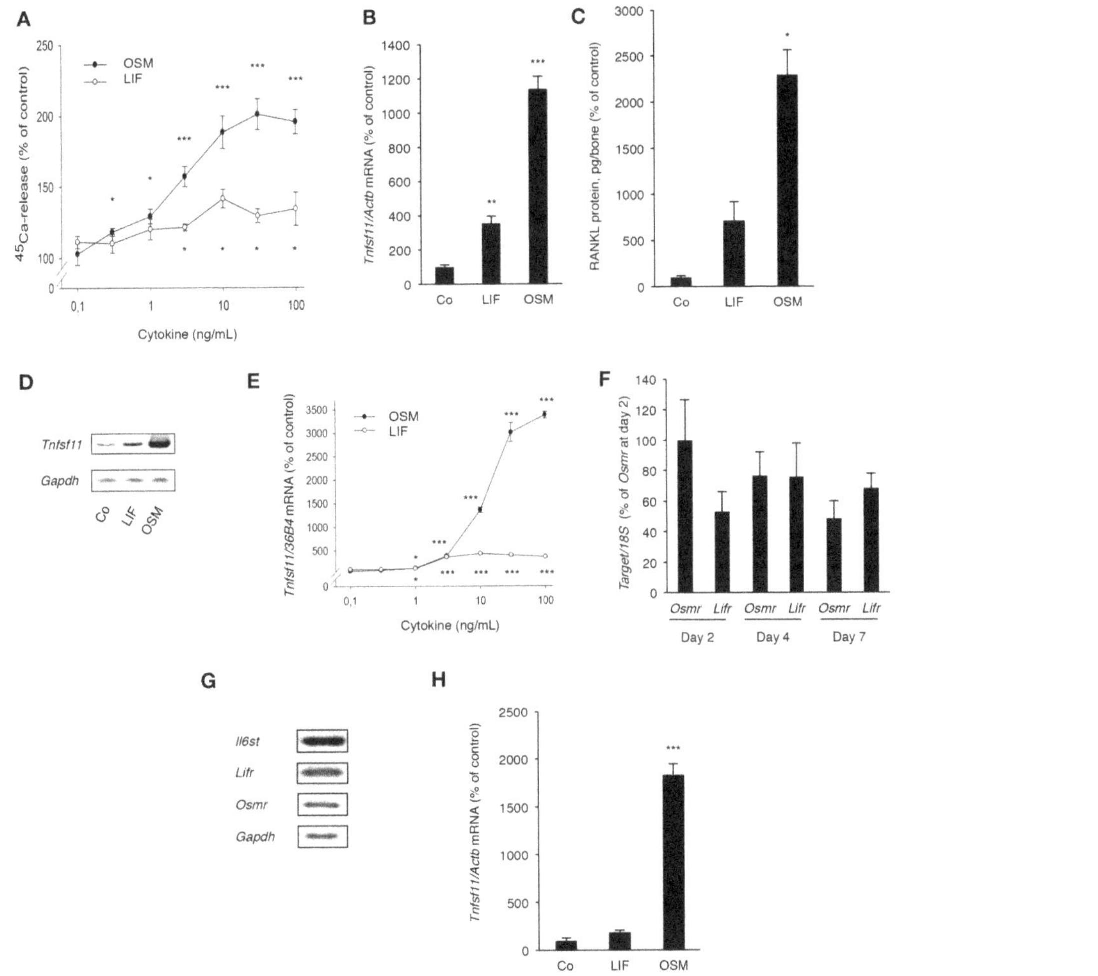

FIGURE 5 | OSM and, to a lesser extent, LIF stimulate bone resorption and RANKL production in calvarial bones, calvarial osteoblasts and stromal cells. **(A)** Mouse calvarial bones were cultured in the absence or the presence of LIF or OSM (both 0.1–100 ng/mL) and bone resorption was assessed by ^{45}Ca release after a 5-day culture period. **(B)** RT-qPCR was performed using mRNA extracted from calvarial bones treated with either LIF or OSM (both at 100 ng/mL) for 24 h to assess the expression of *Tnfsf11*. **(C)** Protein expression of RANKL after 48 h was also analyzed in calvarial bone treated with LIF or OSM (both at 100 ng/L). **(D)** Mouse calvarial osteoblasts were incubated in the absence (Co) or the presence of LIF (100 ng/mL) or OSM (100 ng/mL) for 48 h and expression of *Tnfsf11* was analyzed by semi-quantitative RT-PCR. **(E)** The expression of *Tnfsf11* mRNA in calvarial osteoblasts stimulated by LIF and OSM a different concentrations (0.1-100 ng/mL) was performed using quantitative RT-PCR. **(F)** The mRNA expression of *Osmr* and *Lifr* in osteoblasts was compared at three different time points. **(G)** The receptor components *Il6st, Lifr* and *Osmr* are expressed in ST-2 stromal cells as assessed by RT-PCR. **(H)** The mRNA expression of *Tnfsf11* in ST-2 cells cultured without (Co) or with LIF or OSM (both at 100 ng/mL) for 48 h was analyzed. Values represent means for six bones (calvarial bones) or four wells (cell culture experiments) and SEM is shown as vertical bars. *, **, and ***, indicate significant difference compared to untreated (Co) cells, *$P < 0.05$, **$P < 0.01$, and ***$P < 0.001$, respectively. Statistical significance was determined by ANOVA using Levene's homogeneity test followed by Dunnett's T3 *post-hoc* tests vs. Co. In **(F)**, Tukey *post-hoc* test was used to compare all groups and no statistical difference was observed.

Both OSM and LIF stimulated bone resorption, as assessed by ^{45}Ca release from neonatal mouse calvarial bone, in a concentration-dependent manner with OSM being a substantially more effective and potent stimulator than LIF (**Figure 5A**). The effects seen were statistically significant at and above 0.3 ng/mL (10 nM) OSM and 3 ng/mL (140 nM) LIF.

Quantitative PCR analysis revealed that OSM, and to a lesser extent LIF, increased mRNA expression of *Tnfsf11* in the calvarial bones (**Figure 5B**). This was in line with the finding that the protein level of RANKL in the mouse calvarial bones was increased 23-fold by OSM and 7-fold by LIF, respectively (**Figure 5C**).

Calvarial osteoblasts responded to LIF and OSM (both at 100 ng/mL) with enhanced *Tnfsf11* mRNA expression, with OSM clearly being the more effective stimulator (**Figure 5D**). Quantitative real-time PCR analysis showed that the difference in responsiveness between OSM and LIF could be observed over a wide range of concentrations with OSM treatment resulting in a more robust stimulatory effect on *Tnfsf11* mRNA expression (**Figure 5E**). The difference in response seemed not to be due

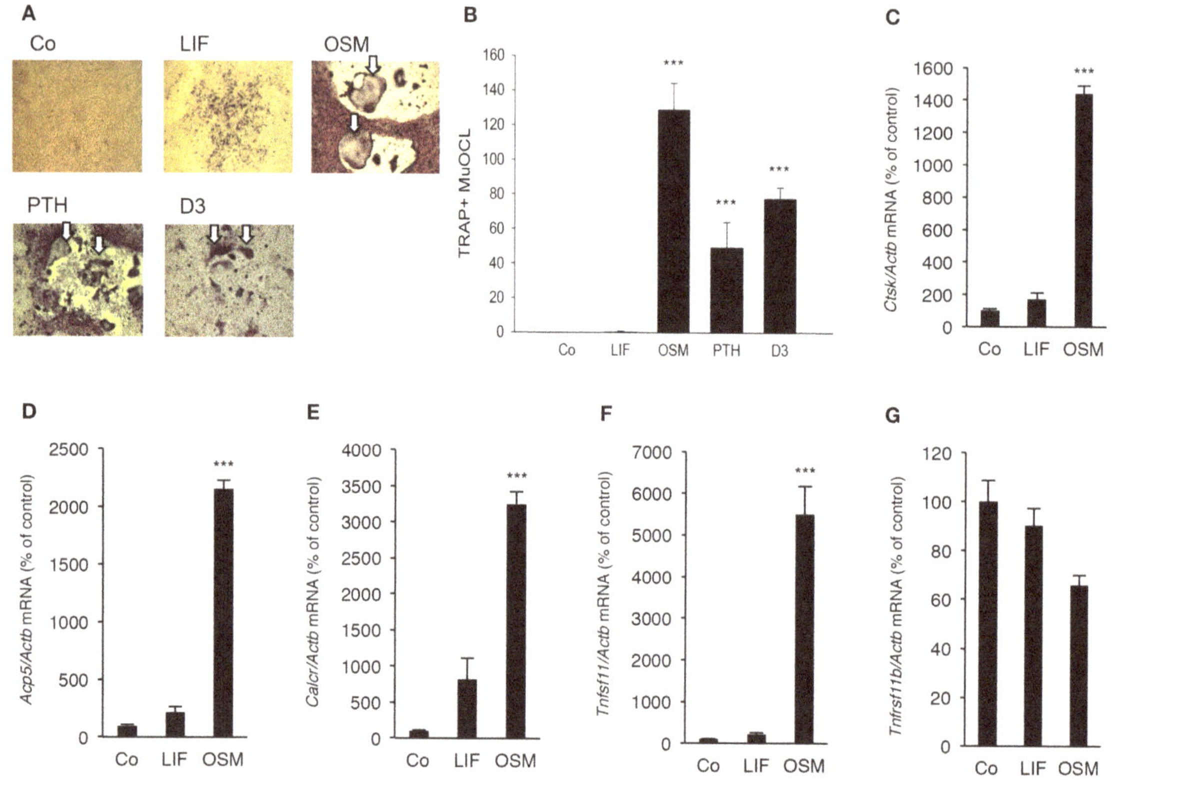

FIGURE 6 | OSM, but not LIF, stimulates osteoclastogenesis in bone marrow cell cultures. Mouse bone marrow cells (BMC) were cultured in the absence (Co) or the presence of LIF, or OSM (both at 100 ng/mL), PTH or 1,25(OH)$_2$-vitamin D3 (D3; both at 10^{-8} M) for 7 days before staining **(A)** and counting **(B)** of tartrate-resistant acid phosphatase (TRAP)-positive multinucleated osteoclasts (TRAP$^+$MuOCL). Quantitative real-time PCR analysis of mRNA expression of cathepsin K (*Ctsk*, **C**), TRAP (*Acp5*, **D**), calcitonin receptor (*Calcr*, **E**) RANKL (*Tnfsf11*, **F**) and OPG (*Tnfsf11b*, **G**) in BMC cultured without (Co) or with LIF or OSM (both at 100 ng/mL) for 7 days. Values represent means for four wells and SEM is shown as vertical bars. ***, indicates significant difference compared to untreated (Co) cells, ***$P < 0.001$. Statistical significance was determined by ANOVA using Levene's homogeneity test followed by Dunnett's 2-sided **(B–F)** or Dunnett's T3 **(G)** *post-hoc* test.

to differences in receptor expression, as assessed by the mRNA expression of *Osmr* and *Lifr* (**Figure 5F**).

The stimulatory effect of OSM on *Tnfsf11* mRNA in the calvarial osteoblasts was dependent on the expression of *Il6st* (encoding gp130) and *Osmr*, but independent of *Lifr* expression, as demonstrated by silencing of the expression of these three receptor components in the calvarial osteoblasts (**Supporting Information Figure S1**). These findings are in agreement with previously reported observations that mouse OSM did not induce *Tnfsf11* mRNA in osteoblasts from *Osmr*$^{-/-}$ mice (5).

The ST-2 stromal cells expressed mRNA for *Il6st*, *Lifr* and *Osmr* (**Figure 5G**) and responded to OSM with a robust 18-fold increase of *Tnfsf11* mRNA expression, whereas LIF did not cause any significant effect (**Figure 5H**).

OSM but Not LIF Stimulates Osteoclast Formation and Expression of RANKL in Mouse Bone Marrow Cultures

Addition of OSM (100 ng/mL) for 7 days to mouse bone marrow cell (BMC) cultures significantly stimulated the formation of TRAP$^+$ MuOCL (**Figures 6A,B**). The stimulation by OSM was more pronounced than stimulations caused by maximally effective concentrations of parathyroid hormone (PTH) and 1,25(OH)$_2$-vitamin D3. In contrast, treatment with LIF (100 ng/mL) only resulted in formation of a few osteoclasts (**Figures 6A,B**).

It was also found that OSM (100 ng/mL) caused a 14–32 fold enhancement of the mRNA expression of the osteoclastic markers *Ctsk* (encoding cathepsin K), *Acp5* (encoding TRAP, tartrate-resistant acid phosphatase) and *Calcr* (encoding calcitonin receptor), whereas LIF (100 ng/mL) only caused a small 2–8 fold stimulation of the mRNA expression of these genes which was not statistically significant (**Figures 6C–E**).

OSM upregulated *Tnfsf11* mRNA in the BMC cultures 22-fold but did not affect *Tnfrsf11b* mRNA (encoding OPG) (**Figures 6F,G**). No significant effect of LIF on *Tnfsf11* or *Tnfrsf11b* mRNA was observed in the BMC cultures (**Figures 6F,G**).

OSM and LIF Have No Direct Effect on Osteoclastogenesis

Analysis of BMM cultures revealed that neither LIF nor OSM stimulated formation of TRAP$^+$ MuOCL in M-CSF treated BMM

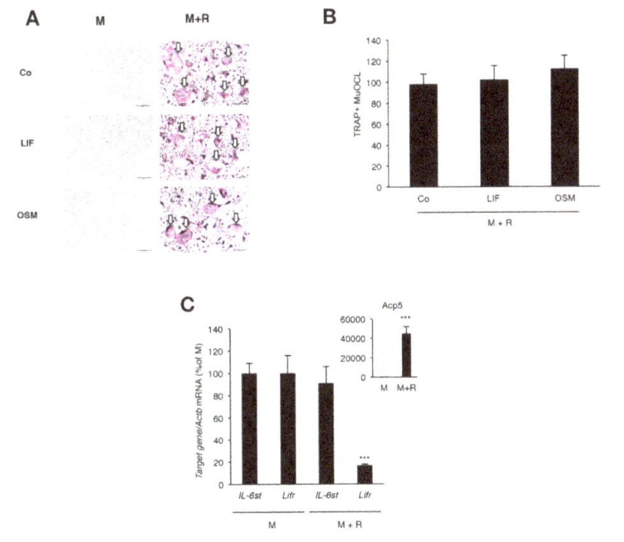

FIGURE 7 | Lack of effect by OSM and LIF on osteoclast formation in bone marrow macrophage cultures. **(A,B)** BMMs were cultured in M-CSF (30 ng/mL) or differentiated to osteoclasts by addition of M-CSF + RANKL (30 and 4 ng/mL, respectively) in the presence or absence of LIF or OSM (both at 100 ng/mL) for 3 days before staining for tartarate-resistant acid phosphatase (TRAP)-positive multinucleated osteoclasts (TRAP$^+$ MuOCL), which then were counted. No osteoclasts were formed in the absence of RANKL. **(C)** Quantitative PCR analyses of *Il6st*, *Lifr*, and *Acp5* in BMM cultured for 72 h with M-CSF (30 ng/ml) or M-CSF+RANKL (30 and 4 ng/ml, respectively). Values represent means for four wells and SEM is shown as vertical bars. In **(C)** ***, indicates significant difference compared to cells treated with M-CSF (M), $P < 0.001$. In **(B)** Statistical significance was determined one-way ANOVA followed by Tukey's *post-hoc* test and in **(C)**, Student's *t*-test was used for comparison between M and M + R groups for each gene.

(**Figure 7A**). The cytokines also did not affect osteoclastogenesis when the formation of TRAP$^+$ MuOCL in BMM was stimulated by M-CSF and RANKL (**Figures 7A,B**). In M-CSF- and M-CSF+RANKL-stimulated BMM, mRNA of *Il6st* (encoding gp130) and *Lifr* could be detected, but mRNA of *Osmr* was not detected (**Figure 7C**). RANKL-induced differentiation, as demonstrated by time-dependent upregulation of mRNA levels for *Acp5* (encoding TRAP), did not affect the expression of *Il6st* mRNA, but down-regulated *Lifr* mRNA expression (**Figure 7C**).

DISCUSSION

The present study shows that OSM is a more effective stimulator of bone resorption in mouse calvarial bones and a more potent stimulator of osteoclast differentiation and formation in mouse bone marrow cultures than is LIF. These effects were due to indirect effects mediated by osteoblasts/stromal cells rather than due to direct effects on osteoclast progenitor cells. Similarly, Tamura et al. found that LIF was a weaker stimulator of osteoclast formation than OSM in co-cultures of mouse osteoblasts and bone marrow cells (20). Other studies evaluating OSM and LIF have also noted a similar hierarchy of action for the two cytokines using mouse embryonic fibroblasts and rat hepatocytes (37), synovial fibroblasts (38, 39), NIH 3T3 fibroblasts and mouse lung fibroblasts (40). In the present study, we provide evidence that the difference in effects on osteoclastogenesis and bone resorption can be explained by recruitment of the adapter protein Shc1 to the OSMR. This recruitment results in a more robust activation of ERK/STAT3 signaling and expression of RANKL by OSM in comparison to LIFR-mediated signaling.

Heterodimerization of either OSMR:gp130 or LIFR:gp130 results in activation of both JAK/STAT and JAK/SHP-2/Grb2/Sos/Ras/Raf/MAPK signaling through docking of STATs and SHP-2 to different phosphorylated Tyr sites in the gp130 molecule (2, 6, 35, 41). The role of these pathways for bone mass has been assessed in "knock-in" mutant mice, one in which the C-terminal moiety of gp130 has been deleted ($gp130^{\Delta STAT \Delta STAT}$) to reduce STAT1/3 signaling, and another strain of mice in which a point mutation substituting Tyr^{757} (equivalent to Tyr^{759} in human gp130) with Phe^{757} ($gp130^{Y757F/Y757F}$) blocks signaling through the SHP-2/MAPK pathway (42). In a parallel study, mice with a knock-in of gp130 carrying a substitution of Tyr^{759} with Phe^{759} (designated $gp130^{F759/F759}$), which also results in defective SHP-2/MAPK signaling, have been used (43). These studies suggest that SHP-2/MAPK signaling, rather than STAT1/3 signaling, is important for basal bone remodeling and bone mass. However, the activation of downstream signaling pathways by specific cytokines in the gp130 family was not studied in these mice.

The fact that no difference in the mRNA expression of *Osmr* and *Lifr* in osteoblasts was observed indicate that the more robust stimulation of osteoclast formation by OSM is not likely to be due to differences in receptor numbers, but rather explained by differences in downstream signaling.

We found that OSM was a more robust stimulator than LIF of JNK (Tyr^{185}/Thr^{183}) and ERK (Tyr^{204}) in mouse calvarial osteoblasts. This is in agreement with the study by Walker et al. reporting that OSM activates ERK more robustly than LIF in primary osteoblasts. Activation of the transcription factor AP-1 is an important downstream event following MAPK activation and experiments were conducted to determine if OSM affected DNA binding of AP-1 in calvarial osteoblasts (5). In agreement with the activation of ERK by OSM, it was determined with EMSA analysis that increased DNA binding of AP-1 occurred with OSM in calvarial osteoblasts, but not with LIF. Gelshift studies showed that the bound AP-1 heterodimer consisted of c-Fos and c-Jun subunits. In contrast to the increased DNA binding of AP-1 by OSM, EMSA analysis did not show any effect on the DNA binding of NF-κB by OSM or LIF, an observation that is in agreement with EMSA analysis in OSM-stimulated human peritoneal mesothelial cells (44).

Activation of JAK/STAT signaling is a well documented signaling event for cytokines in the IL-6 family. It has previously been reported that OSM and LIF can activate STAT1, STAT3, and STAT5 in osteoblasts, and that signaling through OSMR results in more robust activation of these transcription factors (5). In agreement with these observations, we found that OSM is a more robust activator of STAT3 than LIF, observations which also are in agreement with Itoh et al., who found that OSM caused a more robust and prolonged phosphorylation of STAT3 than LIF in osteoblasts from wild type mice (43). These findings likely explain why OSM more effectively than LIF enhanced the mRNA and protein expression of RANKL in calvarial bone, calvarial osteoblasts and bone marrow stromal cells. Similarly, O'Brien et al. have demonstrated that OSM-induced *Tnfsf11* mRNA in the UAMS-32 cell line was decreased by transfection with a dominant negative *Stat3* retrovirus (18) and investigators have showed that that silencing of *Stat3* impairs up-regulation of *Tnfsf11* mRNA by OSM in ST2 cells (45, 46). The important role of STAT3 for OSM-induced signaling in osteoblasts has also been demonstrated by the finding that OSM-induced activation of cyclin-dependent kinase inhibitor $p21^{WAF1,CIP1,SDI1}$ in the human osteosarcoma cell line MG-63 can be inhibited by transfection with a dominant negative *Stat3* plasmid (47). Furthermore, OSM promotes the binding of STAT3 and RNA polymerase II to 5′ enhancer regions in the *Tnfsf11* promoter shared by PTH and 1,25-dihydroxyvitamin-D3 (48) and to a more distal enhancer region shared by IL-6 (45).

An explanation why OSM is a more robust activator of JAK/STAT and MAPK signaling in the osteoblasts compared to LIF may be that phosphorylated Tyr^{861} in the OSMR acts as a binding site for an SH2 domain in the adapter protein Shc1, which is not recruited to the LIFR:gp130 complex (26). The Shc family of adapter proteins is well known for its role in growth factor signaling, especially the Ras/MAPK pathway, but a role in RANKL expression and osteoclast formation has not been shown previously. Hermanns et al. have shown that mutation of OSMR Tyr^{861} in transfected COS-7 cells not only decreased Shc1 binding to the OSMR, but also decreased phosphorylation of ERK stimulated by OSM without affecting STAT phosphorylation (26). These data suggest that Shc1 plays a unique role in downstream signaling induced by OSM.

In this report, we show for the first time that Shc1 is expressed in osteoblasts and that OSM, but not LIF, upregulates the mRNA expression of *Shc1*. Furthermore, OSM, but not LIF, induced the phosphorylation of Shc1. Furthermore, OSM consistently induced phosphorylation of the p52 isoform, which is the isoform known to be important for activation of the Ras/MAPK pathway. By silencing the expression of *Shc1*, it was found that activations of both STAT3 and ERK elicited by OSM were substantially decreased. Activation of Shc1, however, was not affected by silencing of *Stat3*, indicating that STAT3 is acting downstream of Shc1 in osteoblasts. Although some reports have shown that Shc1 is not upstream of STAT3, a recent study in breast cancer cells expressing *Shc1* mutated in the domain containing Tyr^{239} and Tyr^{240} has also demonstrated that Shc1 is upstream of STAT3 (29). The present observations confirmed previous finding showing that activation of STAT3 is part of the downstream signaling which occurs following LIF and OSM

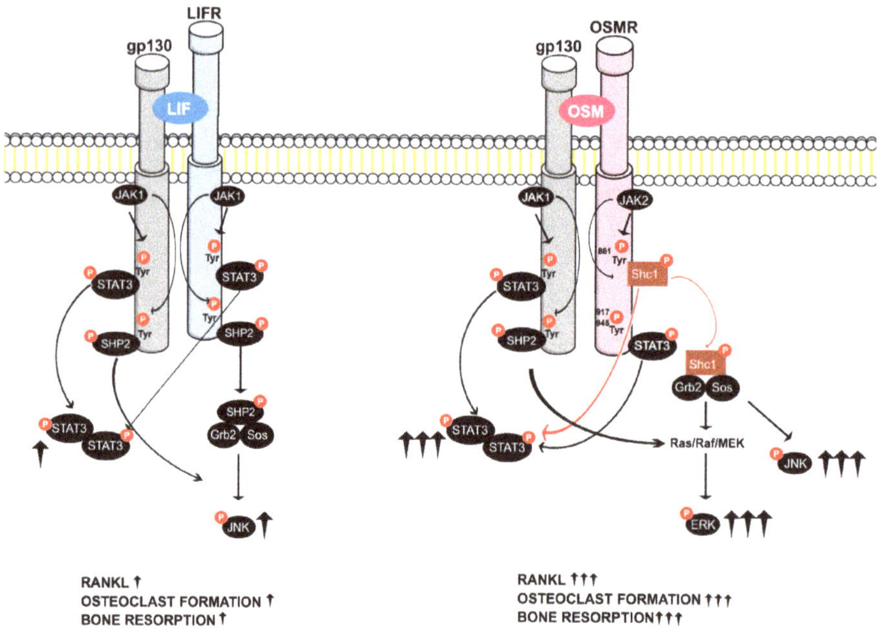

FIGURE 8 | Schematic drawing of the suggested intracellular signaling pathways of LIF and OSM receptors in osteoblasts mediating expression of osteoclastogenic factors, osteoclast formation and bone resorption. Common LIFR/OSMR signaling pathways induced by JAK-mediated phosphorylation of the signal transducer gp130 involve activation of STAT3, as well as activation of JNK through a possible SHP2/Ras/Raf/MAPK cascade **(Left)**. The figure indicates that LIF binds to the LIFR. As discussed in the Introduction section, 2nd paragraph, OSM can also bind to the LIFR to regulate sclerostin expression. In addition to the gp130-mediated pathways common for LIFR and OSMR, the OSM receptor has previously been shown to activate a Shc1-mediated pathway where phosphorylation of the OSMR on Tyr^{861} results in docking and phosphorylation of the adapter molecule Shc1 (26, 27). The activated pShc1 is recruited to the Grb2:SoS complex which in turn induces a Ras/Raf/MAPK cascade that ultimately activates ERK. The Shc1-mediated signaling pathway **(Right)** is suggested to explain the stronger effects by OSM on expression of osteoclastogenic factors, osteoclast formation and bone resorption in comparison to activation of the LIFR:gp130 complex by LIF.

receptor activations, but the more robust activation of STAT3 by OSM and the unique activation of ERK by OSM suggest that these particular effects are dependent on recruitment of Shcl to the OSMR. In addition, by using the siRNA approach to decrease the expression of *Shc1*, it was shown that recruitment of Shcl to the OSMR was a crucial downstream signaling event in the mechanism by which OSM induces *Tnfsf11* mRNA expression and osteoclast formation. Using the same technique, it was also found that induction of *Tnfsf11* mRNA expression in osteoblasts, and osteoclast formation in co-cultures stimulated by OSM, were critically dependent on the expression of *Stat3* mRNA.

In summary, when compared to LIF, OSM was found to be a more potent stimulator of calvarial bone resorption and osteoclast formation in bone marrow cultures. This was due to greater stimulation of RANKL expression in osteoblasts/stromal cells caused by enhanced activation of STAT3 and JNK by OSM and an ability of OSM to activate ERK that was not shared by LIF. These novel findings in the present study show that the robust and unique stimulatory effects of OSM are dependent on the recruitment of the activated adapter protein Shcl to the OSMR subunit of the OSMR:gp130 heterodimer, a recruitment that is absent in the LIFR:gp130 complex. From a clinical perspective, inhibition of Shcl could be a mechanism to decrease OSM-induced bone loss in inflammatory diseases. The suggested differences in signaling downstream of the OSMR and LIFR complexes are summarized in **Figure 8**.

Committees at Umeå University, at the School of Dentistry, Araraquara and at the University of Gothenburg guidelines. The protocol was approved by the Institutional Animal Care and Ethics Committees at Umeå University, at the School of Dentistry, Araraquara and at the University of Gothenburg.

AUTHOR CONTRIBUTIONS

EP and PS contributed equally. EP, PS, and UL designed the study. EP, PS, TF-M, and PH conducted the experiments. EP, PS, TF-M, PH, HC, and UL interpreted the data. EP, PS, and UL wrote the first draft of the manuscript which was edited and approved by all authors.

ACKNOWLEDGMENTS

Anita Lie and Anna Westerlund are acknowledged for excellent technical assistance. This work was supported by the Swedish Research Council, Swedish Rheumatism Association, Royal 80-Year Fund of King Gustav V, COMBINE, the Swedish state under the agreement between the Swedish government and the county councils, the ALF-agreement (#237551), the IngaBritt and Arne Lundberg Foundation, County Council of Västerbotten, grants #2014/05283-3 and 2015/00410-0, São Paulo Research Foundation (FAPESP) and by a scholarship to TF-M from the Coordenação de Aperfeiçoamento de Pessoal de Nível Superior–Brasil (CAPES)–Finance code 001 and grant #061/2013 (PVE080/2012).

REFERENCES

1. Zarling JM, Shoyab M, Marquardt H, Hanson MB, Lioubin MN, Todaro GJ. Oncostatin M: a growth regulator produced by differentiated histiocytic lymphoma cells. *Proc Natl Acad Sci USA.* (1986) 83:9739–43. doi: 10.1073/pnas.83.24.9739
2. Hermanns HM. Oncostatin M and interleukin-31: Cytokines, receptors, signal transduction and physiology. *Cytokine Growth Factor Rev.* (2015) 26:545–58. doi: 10.1016/j.cytogfr.2015.07.006
3. West NR, Hegazy AN, Owens BMJ, Bullers SJ, Linggi B, Buonocore S, et al. Oncostatin M drives intestinal inflammation and predicts response to tumor necrosis factor-neutralizing therapy in patients with inflammatory bowel disease. *Nat Med.* (2017) 23:579–89. doi: 10.1038/nm.4307
4. Su CM, Chiang YC, Huang CY, Hsu CJ, Fong YC, Tang CH. Osteopontin promotes oncostatin m production in human osteoblasts: implication of rheumatoid arthritis therapy. *J Immunol.* (2015) 195:3355–64. doi: 10.4049/jimmunol.1403191
5. Walker EC, McGregor NE, Poulton IJ, Solano M, Pompolo S, Fernandes TJ, et al. Oncostatin M promotes bone formation independently of resorption when signaling through leukemia inhibitory factor receptor in mice. *J Clin Invest.* (2010) 120:582–92. doi: 10.1172/JCI40568
6. Richards CD. The enigmatic cytokine oncostatin m and roles in disease. *ISRN Inflamm.* (2013) 2013:512103. doi: 10.1155/2013/512103
7. Sims NA. Cell-specific paracrine actions of IL-6 family cytokines from bone, marrow and muscle that control bone formation and resorption. *Int J Biochem Cell Biol.* (2016) 79:14–23. doi: 10.1016/j.biocel.2016.08.003
8. Tanaka M, Hirabayashi Y, Sekiguchi T, Inoue T, Katsuki M, Miyajima A. Targeted disruption of oncostatin M receptor results in altered hematopoiesis. *Blood.* (2003) 102:3154–62. doi: 10.1182/blood-2003-02-0367
9. Bolin C, Tawara K, Sutherland C, Redshaw J, Aranda P, Moselhy J, et al. Oncostatin m promotes mammary tumor metastasis to bone and osteolytic bone degradation. *Genes Cancer.* (2012) 3:117–30. doi: 10.1177/1947601912458284
10. Sterbova S, Karlsson T, Persson E. Oncostatin M induces tumorigenic properties in non-transformed human prostate epithelial cells, in part through activation of signal transducer and activator of transcription 3 (STAT3). *Biochem Biophys Res Commun.* (2018) 498:769–74. doi: 10.1016/j.bbrc.2018.03.056
11. Ayaub EA, Dubey A, Imani J, Botelho F, Kolb MRJ, Richards CD, et al. Overexpression of OSM and IL-6 impacts the polarization of pro-fibrotic macrophages and the development of bleomycin-induced lung fibrosis. *Sci Rep.* (2017) 7:13281. doi: 10.1038/s41598-017-13511-z
12. Mozaffarian A, Brewer AW, Trueblood ES, Luzina IG, Todd NW, Atamas SP, et al. Mechanisms of oncostatin M-induced pulmonary inflammation

and fibrosis. *J Immunol.* (2008) 181:7243–53. doi: 10.4049/jimmunol.181.10.7243

13. Simpson JL, Baines KJ, Boyle MJ, Scott RJ, Gibson PG. Oncostatin M (OSM) is increased in asthma with incompletely reversible airflow obstruction. *Experimental Lung Res.* (2009) 35:781–94. doi: 10.3109/01902140902906412
14. Pradeep AR, Garima G, Raju A. Serum levels of oncostatin M (a gp 130 cytokine): an inflammatory biomarker in periodontal disease. *Biomarkers.* (2010) 15:277–82. doi: 10.3109/13547500903573209
15. Lisignoli G, Piacentini A, Toneguzzi S, Grassi F, Cocchini B, Ferruzzi A, et al. Osteoblasts and stromal cells isolated from femora in rheumatoid arthritis (RA) and osteoarthritis (OA) patients express IL-11, leukaemia inhibitory factor and oncostatin M. *Clin Exp Immunol.* (2000) 119:346–53. doi: 10.1046/j.1365-2249.2000.01114.x
16. Torossian F, Guerton B, Anginot A, Alexander KA, Desterke C, Soave, S. et al. Macrophage-derived oncostatin M contributes to human and mouse neurogenic heterotopic ossifications. *JCI Insight.* (2017) 2:96034. doi: 10.1172/jci.insight.96034
17. Palmqvist P, Persson E, Conaway HH, Lerner UH. IL-6, leukemia inhibitory factor, and oncostatin M stimulate bone resorption and regulate the expression of receptor activator of NF-κB ligand, osteoprotegerin, and receptor activator of NF-κB in mouse calvariae. *J Immunol.* (2002) 169:3353–62. doi: 10.4049/jimmunol.169.6.3353
18. O'Brien CA, Gubrij I, Lin SC, Saylors RL, Manolagas SC. STAT3 activation in stromal/osteoblastic cells is required for induction of the receptor activator of NF-kappaB ligand and stimulation of osteoclastogenesis by gp130-utilizing cytokines or interleukin-1 but not 1,25-dihydroxyvitamin D3 or parathyroid hormone. *J Biol Chem.* (1999) 274:19301–8. doi: 10.1074/jbc.274.27.19301
19. Richards CD, Langdon C, Deschamps P, Pennica D, Shaughnessy SG. Stimulation of osteoclast differentiation *in vitro* by mouse oncostatin M, leukaemia inhibitory factor, cardiotrophin-1 and interleukin 6: synergy with dexamethasone. *Cytokine.* (2000) 12:613–21. doi: 10.1006/cyto.1999.0635
20. Tamura T, Udagawa N, Takahashi N, Miyaura C, Tanaka S, Yamada Y, et al. Soluble interleukin-6 receptor triggers osteoclast formation by interleukin 6. *Proc Natl Acad Sci USA.* (1993) 90:11924–8. doi: 10.1073/pnas.90.24.11924
21. Hermanns HM, Radtke S, Haan C, Schmitz-Van de Leur H, Tavernier J, Heinrich PC, et al. Contributions of leukemia inhibitory factor receptor and oncostatin M receptor to signal transduction in heterodimeric complexes with glycoprotein 130. *J Immunol.* (1999) 163:6651–8.
22. Hintzen C, Evers C, Lippok BE, Volkmer R, Heinrich PC, Radtke S, et al. Box 2 region of the oncostatin M receptor determines specificity for recruitment of Janus kinases and STAT5 activation. *J Biol Chem.* (2008) 283:19465–77. doi: 10.1074/jbc.M710157200
23. Schmitz J, Dahmen H, Grimm C, Gendo C, Muller-Newen G, Heinrich PC, et al. The cytoplasmic tyrosine motifs in full-length glycoprotein 130 have different roles in IL-6 signal transduction. *J Immunol.* (2000) 164:848–54. doi: 10.4049/jimmunol.164.2.848
24. Anhuf D, Weissenbach M, Schmitz J, Sobota R, Hermanns HM, Radtke S, et al. Signal transduction of IL-6, leukemia-inhibitory factor, and oncostatin M: structural receptor requirements for signal attenuation. *J Immunol.* (2000) 165:2535–43. doi: 10.4049/jimmunol.165.5.2535
25. Neel BG, Gu H, Pao L. The 'Shp'ing news: SH2 domain-containing tyrosine phosphatases in cell signaling. *Trends Biochem Sci.* (2003) 28:284–93. doi: 10.1016/S0968-0004(03)00091-4
26. Hermanns HM, Radtke S, Schaper F, Heinrich PC, Behrmann I. Non-redundant signal transduction of interleukin-6-type cytokines. The adapter protein Shc is specifically recruited to the oncostatin M receptor. *J Biol Chem.* (2000) 275:40742–8. doi: 10.1074/jbc.M005408200
27. Wang Y, Robledo O, Kinzie E, Blanchard F, Richards C, Miyajima A, et al. Receptor subunit-specific action of oncostatin M in hepatic cells and its modulation by leukemia inhibitory factor. *J Biol Chem.* (2000) 275:25273–85. doi: 10.1074/jbc.M002296200
28. Wills MK, Jones N. Teaching an old dogma new tricks: twenty years of Shc adaptor signalling. *Biochem J.* (2012) 447:1–16. doi: 10.1042/BJ20120769
29. Ahn R, Sabourin V, Bolt AM, Hebert S, Totten S, De Jay N, et al. The Shc1 adaptor simultaneously balances Stat1 and Stat3 activity to promote breast cancer immune suppression. *Nat Commun.* (2017) 8:14638. doi: 10.1038/ncomms14638
30. Lerner UH. Modifications of the mouse calvarial technique improve the responsiveness to stimulators of bone resorption. *J Bone Miner Res.* (1987) 2:375–83. doi: 10.1002/jbmr.5650020504
31. Ljunggren O, Ransjo M, Lerner UH. *In vitro* studies on bone resorption in neonatal mouse calvariae using a modified dissection technique giving four samples of bone from each calvaria. *J Bone Miner Res.* (1991) 6:543–50. doi: 10.1002/jbmr.5650060604
32. Granholm S, Henning P, Lindholm C, Lerner UH. Osteoclast progenitor cells present in significant amounts in mouse calvarial osteoblast isolations and osteoclastogenesis increased by BMP-2. *Bone.* (2013) 52:83–92. doi: 10.1016/j.bone.2012.09.019
33. Granholm S, Lundberg P, Lerner UH. Calcitonin inhibits osteoclast formation in mouse haematopoetic cells independently of transcriptional regulation by receptor activator of NF-{kappa}B and c-Fms. *J Endocrinol.* (2007) 195:415–27. doi: 10.1677/JOE-07-0338
34. Takeshita S, Kaji K, Kudo A. Identification and characterization of the new osteoclast progenitor with macrophage phenotypes being able to differentiate into mature osteoclasts. *J Bone Miner Res.* (2000) 15:1477–88. doi: 10.1359/jbmr.2000.15.8.1477
35. Bellido T, Borba VZ, Roberson P, Manolagas SC. Activation of the Janus kinase/STAT (signal transducer and activator of transcription) signal transduction pathway by interleukin-6-type cytokines promotes osteoblast differentiation. *Endocrinology.* (1997) 138:3666–76. doi: 10.1210/endo.138.9.5364
36. Heinrich PC, Behrmann I, Muller-Newen G, Schaper F, Graeve L. Interleukin-6-type cytokine signalling through the gp130/Jak/STAT pathway. *Biochem J.* (1998) 334:297–314. doi: 10.1042/bj3340297
37. Richards CD, Kerr C, Tanaka M, Hara T, Miyajima A, Pennica D, et al. Regulation of tissue inhibitor of metalloproteinase-1 in fibroblasts and acute phase proteins in hepatocytes *in vitro* by mouse oncostatin M, cardiotrophin-1, and IL-6. *J Immunol.* (1997) 159:2431–7.
38. Langdon C, Kerr C, Hassen M, Hara T, Arsenault AL, Richards CD. Murine oncostatin M stimulates mouse synovial fibroblasts *in vitro* and induces inflammation and destruction in mouse joints *in vivo*. *Am J Pathol.* (2000) 157:1187–96. doi: 10.1016/S0002-9440(10)64634-2
39. Langdon C, Leith J, Smith F, Richards CD. Oncostatin M stimulates monocyte chemoattractant protein-1- and interleukin-1-induced matrix metalloproteinase-1 production by human synovial fibroblasts *in vitro*. *Arthritis Rheumat.* (1997) 40:2139–46. doi: 10.1002/art.1780401207
40. Langdon C, Kerr C, Tong L, Richards CD. Oncostatin M regulates eotaxin expression in fibroblasts and eosinophilic inflammation in C57BL/6 mice. *J Immunol.* (2003) 170:548–55. doi: 10.4049/jimmunol.170.1.548
41. Nicola NA, Babon JJ. Leukemia inhibitory factor (LIF). *Cytokine Growth Factor Rev.* (2015) 26:533–44. doi: 10.1016/j.cytogfr.2015.07.001
42. Sims NA, Jenkins BJ, Quinn JM, Nakamura A, Glatt M, Gillespie MT, et al. Glycoprotein 130 regulates bone turnover and bone size by distinct downstream signaling pathways. *J Clin Invest.* (2004) 113:379–89. doi: 10.1172/JCI19872
43. Itoh S, Udagawa N, Takahashi N, Yoshitake F, Narita H, Ebisu S, et al. A critical role for interleukin-6 family-mediated Stat3 activation in osteoblast differentiation and bone formation. *Bone.* (2006) 39:505–12. doi: 10.1016/j.bone.2006.02.074
44. Hams E, Colmont CS, Dioszeghy V, Hammond VJ, Fielding CA, Williams AS, et al. Oncostatin M receptor-beta signaling limits monocytic cell recruitment in acute inflammation. *J Immunol.* (2008) 181:2174–80. doi: 10.4049/jimmunol.181.3.2174
45. Bishop KA, Meyer MB, Pike JW. A novel distal enhancer mediates cytokine induction of mouse RANKl gene expression. *Mol Endocrinol.* (2009) 23:2095–110. doi: 10.1210/me.2009-0209
46. Onal M, St. John HC, Danielson AL, Markert JW, Riley EM, Pike JW. Unique distal enhancers linked to the mouse Tnfsf11 gene direct tissue-specific and

inflammation-induced expression of RANKL. *Endocrinology.* (2016) 157:482–96. doi: 10.1210/en.2015-1788

47. Bellido T, O'Brien CA, Roberson PK, Manolagas SC. Transcriptional activation of the p21(WAF1,CIP1,SDI1) gene by interleukin-6 type cytokines. A prerequisite for their pro-differentiating and anti-apoptotic effects on human osteoblastic cells. *J Biol Chem.* (1998) 273:21137–44. doi: 10.1074/jbc.273.33.21137
48. Fu Q, Manolagas SC, O'Brien CA. Parathyroid hormone controls receptor activator of NF-κB ligand gene expression via a distant transcriptional enhancer. *Mol Cell Biol.* (2006) 26:6453–68. doi: 10.1128/MCB.00356-06

12

MicroRNAs: Key Regulators to Understand Osteoclast Differentiation?

Claire Lozano[1,2]*, Isabelle Duroux-Richard*[1]*, Hüseyin Firat*[3]*, Eric Schordan*[3] *and Florence Apparailly*[1*]

[1] *IRMB, Univ Montpellier, INSERM, CHU Montpellier, Montpellier, France,* [2] *Immunology Department, CHU Montpellier, Montpellier, France,* [3] *Firalis SA, Molecular Diagnostics, Huningue, France*

Correspondence:
Florence Apparailly
florence.apparailly@inserm.fr

MicroRNAs (miRNAs) are small non-coding single-stranded RNAs that represent important posttranscriptional regulators of protein-encoding genes. In particular, miRNAs play key roles in regulating cellular processes such as proliferation, migration, and cell differentiation. Recently, miRNAs emerged as critical regulators of osteoclasts (OCs) biology and have been involved in OCs pathogenic role in several disorders. OCs are multinucleated cells generated from myeloid precursors in the bone marrow, specialized in bone resorption. While there is a growing number of information on the cytokines and signaling pathways that are critical to control the differentiation of osteoclast precursors (OCPs) into mature OCs, the connection between OC differentiation steps and miRNAs is less well-understood. The present review will first summarize our current understanding of the miRNA-regulated pathways in the sequential steps required for OC formation, from the motility and migration of OCPs to the cell-cell fusion and the final formation of the actin ring and ruffled border in the functionally resorbing multinucleated OCs. Then, considering the difficulty of working on primary OCs and on the generation of robust data we will give an update on the most recent advances in the detection technologies for miRNAs quantification and how these are of particular interest for the understanding of OC biology and their use as potential biomarkers.

Keywords: microRNA, osteoclast, differentiation, regulation, detection, biomarker

INTRODUCTION

MicroRNAs (miRNAs) are key regulatory molecules that control cellular processes such as proliferation, migration and cell differentiation small. As shown in **Figure 1**, in the canonical pathway, miRNAs are transcribed by RNA polymerase II as large RNA precursors called primary (pri-) miRNAs that will be cleaved in the nucleus by the microprocessors complex into short hairpin precursors (pre-miRNAs) of about 70-nucleotides in length (1, 2). Pre-miRNAs are subsequently exported to the cytoplasm to be processed by DICER and yield mature miRNA duplexes (~22 nucleotides long) prior their loading onto the Argonaute-containing RNA-induced silencing complex (RISC). They bind through imperfect complementarity, mostly to the 3′-UTR regions of their target mRNAs, and lead to translation inhibition or degradation (3). These single-stranded RNAs thus modulate gene expression mostly at a posttranscriptional level. Current database describes more than 1,917 miRNA genes, which can contain 3 and 5p miRNAs. MiRNAs are recognized as crucial regulators of the expression of more than 60% of mammalian genes. The

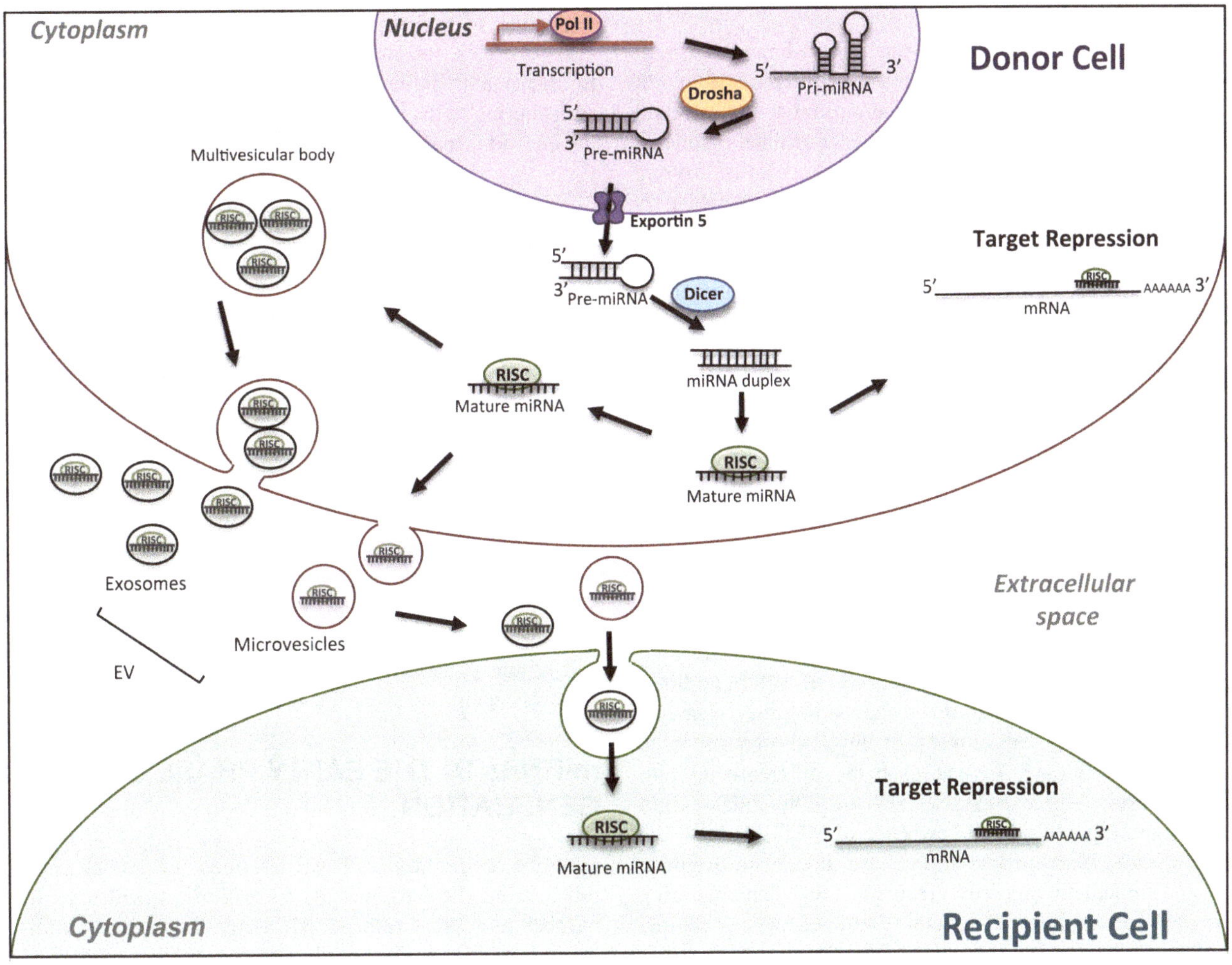

FIGURE 1 | Schematic miRNA biogenesis and mode of action. miRNA biogenesis begins in the nucleus with transcription of miRNA gene into a pri-miRNA, followed by the action of the enzyme Drosha to produce pre-miRNA hairpins. After exportation into the cytosol, pre-miRNA, are processed into an intermediary miRNA duplex by Dicer. One miRNA strand is loaded onto the RNA-induced silencing complex (RISC) to form mature miRNA, which can regulate the expression of target mRNAs. The miRNA/RISC complex can also be incorporated into extracellular vesicles such as exosomes or microvesicle bodies, to be released into extracellular space. Then, miRNAs can be found in body fluids and travel across the entire body till elimination, or can be incorporated into a recipient cell and specifically regulate the expression of target genes into this new cell. Drosha, RNase III-type endonuclease family protein; Dicer, endoribonuclease; RISC; RNA- used silencing complex; EV, extracellular vesicles.

number of encoded miRNAs is limited compared to mRNAs and proteins expressed; however, one miRNA may regulate hundreds of mRNAs/lncRNAs and, as a result, may have substantial effects on gene expression networks. Although a lot of miRNAs have conserved sequences between species, the targeted mRNA sequences may be poorly conserved and biological effects are difficult to predict. *In silico* analyses using updated databases are thus useful to screen for putative targets according to the species and to find the miRNA sequence homology. *In vitro* functional studies are however needed to validate the miRNA targets, which may provide clues on the biological effects of the miRNA. In addition, available and freely accessible algorithms have been designed to identify potential miRNA-promoter interactions conserved between species that could represent additional clues to further push toward experimental validation (4). *In vivo* studies add indeed robustness to the biological role of miRNA-mediated regulation in pathophysiological conditions.

As to many other biological processes, miRNAs act as fine modulators to maintain bone homeostasis. Key evidence that miRNAs are essential to osteoclastogenesis is provided by genetic studies deleting one enzyme essential for their biogenesis, DICER1. DICER deficient mouse and osteoclast-specific DICER gene deficiency both lead to impaired osteoclast (OC) formation and activity (5, 6). Since then, the field of bone biology has regularly reviewed the role of miRNAs in OC biology or bone remodeling, mostly in the context of osteoporosis (7–13). A growing interest in miRNA-based therapeutic strategies has also emerged in bone-related disorders [for review see (14)]. Although the role of miRNAs in the OC lineage and ontogeny is a current hot topic, it remains poorly studied.

OCs are multinucleated cells specialized in bone resorption and derived from myeloid precursors that differentiate *in situ* in the bone marrow (15). The commitment of myeloid precursors in osteoclastic differentiation is controlled by micro-environmental factors to maintain bone homeostasis. Among them, osteoblasts, osteocytes and bone marrow stromal cells stimulate OC differentiation through the production of receptor activator of nuclear factor kappa-B ligand (RANKL), which binds to its receptor RANK. The growth factor macrophage colony-stimulating factor (MCSF) is also required to initiate the differentiation of osteoclastic precursors by binding its receptor CSF1R (colony stimulating factor 1 receptor). The Wnt-5a ligand is another pro-osteoclastic factor secreted by osteoblasts and OCs themselves (16, 17). In addition to these pro-osteoclastogenic factors, there are several inhibitory regulators including the osteoprotegerin (OPG), a soluble protein secreted by stromal cells that binds soluble and membrane forms of RANKL, thus preventing the activation of the RANK/RANKL signaling pathway. Indirectly, estrogens repress bone resorption by stimulating the production of OPG. Other environmental factors such as cytokines and lipid mediators impact on the osteoclastogenesis (18, 19). In addition to these well-known regulatory mechanisms, other elements could influence the commitment of myeloid precursors to the osteoclastic lineage. Instead of being differentiated into OCs, the myeloid precursors can also be differentiated into macrophages, especially in the presence of MCSF. Indeed, the osteoclastic and macrophagic lineages are thought to originate from an immediate bipotent precursor (20), demonstrating their close proximity. OCs retain the phagocytic potential and the ability to present the antigen of macrophages (21) but are the only cells capable of bone resorption. Among critical regulators of the polarization toward the OC vs. macrophage lineage, the mitochondrial metabolism has been involved (22). Although the role of miRNAs in the commitment of hematopoietic (23) and osteoblastic (24) lineages has been reviewed, only few studies have addressed the involvement of miRNAs in the commitment of the osteoclastic lineage.

The initiation of osteoclastogenesis requires the major signaling pathways RANK/RANKL and CSF1R/MCSF. The transcription factor NFATC1 (nuclear factor of activated T cells 1) is the cornerstone of the early phase of osteoclastogenesis. An amplification loop of NFATC1 induces the expression of many genes of the late phase, such as ACP5 (acid phosphatase 5, tartrate resistant), CTSK (Cathepsin K), and DCSTAMP (dendrocyte expressed seven transmembrane protein) [reviewed in (25)].

Under physiological conditions, the selective expression of miRNAs promoting and repressing the generation of OCs relies on the regulation of their own promoter (a shared promoter in case of miRNA clusters) and is thus closely linked to the sequential signaling pathways involved in the different steps of OC differentiation. MiRNAs are thus essential in a lot of biological feedback loops, including in the regulation of the OC biology.

Our present review will focus on the miRNA-mediated regulation of the sequential steps of OC formation. We will also report on the most recent advances in technologies used for the quantification of miRNAs. Finally, we will discuss the contribution of these technologies to the field of OC biology and the questions that remain to be asked.

miRNAs AND THE COMMITMENT OF PROGENITORS TOWARD OCs

There are very few studies available on the miRNA-mediated regulation of OC commitment. Osteoclastogenesis is repressed by miR-155-mediated control of the transcription factor MITF (melanocyte inducing transcription factor) that is involved in the differentiation of monocytes toward macrophages (26). Conversely, miR-29 family (miR-29a, b, c) guides the commitment of bone marrow precursors toward the OC lineage by inhibiting GPR85 and CD93, two molecules involved in macrophage engagement (27). Authors showed that the transfection of the mouse monocytic cell line RAW264.7 with an inhibitor of miR-29 promotes macrophage differentiation, as evidenced by an up-regulation of the F4/80 surface marker and of the phagocytosis, even in presence of the major pro-osteoclastogenic cytokine RANKL.

miRNAs IN THE EARLY PHASE OF OCs GENERATION

Majority of the studies have described the global impact of miRNAs on the terminal OC formation, as evidenced by OC number and bone resorption activity. Few studies addressed beyond this final step which cellular processes are impacted. In **Figure 2**, we have summarized the miRNAs involved in the functional steps paving the generation of OCs, including cell survival, proliferation and motility of OC precursors. We also provide an updated list of their validated target genes (**Table 1**).

Pro-Osteoclastogenic miRNAs

In addition to its role in the OC commitment of precursors, miR-29 family may promote migration of precursors since miR-29 neutralization inhibits the migration RAW264.7 cells (27). Furthermore, miR-29 family is involved in early phase of osteoclastogenesis by targeting NFIA (nuclear factor I A), a negative regulator of CSF1R (27). CSF1R is also indirectly induced by miR-223 through NFIA targeting as a positive feedback loop enhanced by the transcription factor PU.1 induced downstream of the MCSF/CSF1R (5). Same authors however previously reported contradictory findings using the same RAW264.7 cell line, as overexpression of miRNA-223 suppressed TRAP-positive OC formation (28). These later data were in agreement with a work performed on human peripheral blood mononuclear cells (PBMCs) (29). Bone loss is enhanced in arthritic condition due to activation of OC differentiation, and miR-223 is intensely expressed in rheumatoid arthritis (RA) synovium, particularly in monocyte/macrophage and $CD4^+$ T-cell subsets (29). All these findings suggest an important role of

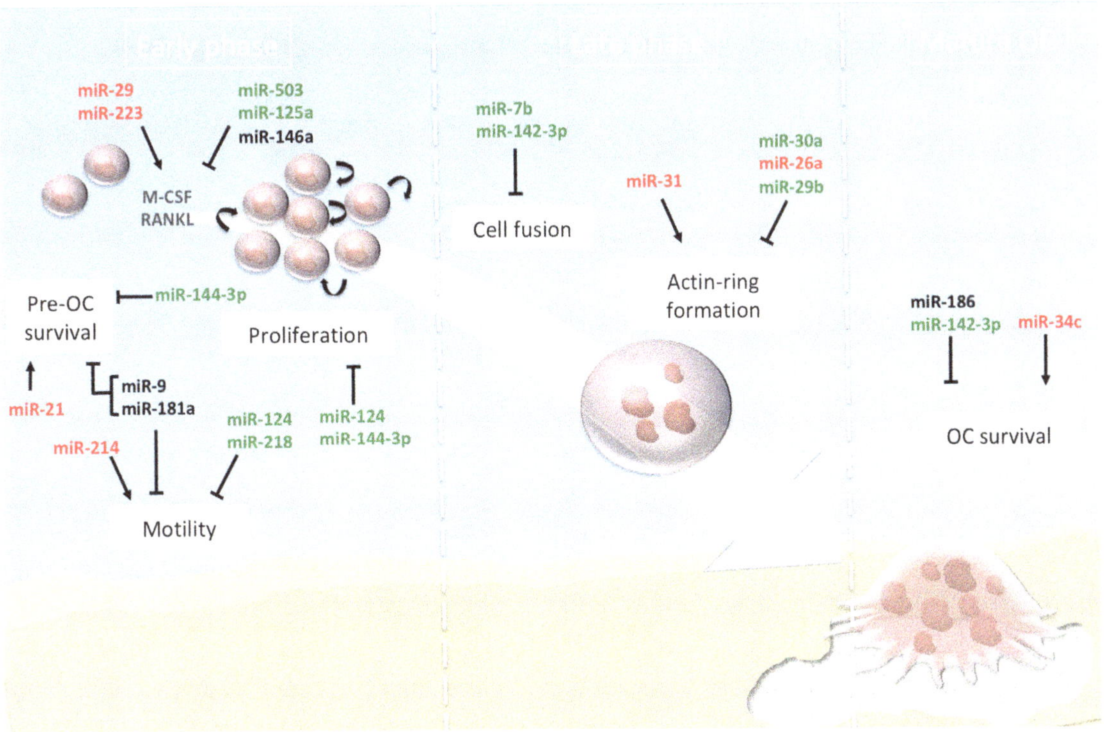

FIGURE 2 | miRNA regulation of osteoclast differentiation. Illustration of the 3 phases of osteoclastogenesis. The early phase is associated with pre-osteoclast (OC) survival, motility, and proliferation; the late phase focused on pre-OC cell fusion and OC acting-ring formation; and the mature OC phase consists in the degradation of the mineralized matrix by mature OC. Green, red and black colors indicate down, up and normal miRNA expression, respectively. Arrows and bars indicate positive or negative effects on osteoclastogenesis respectively. M-CSF, macrophage colony-stimulating factor; RANKL, Receptor activator of NF-κB ligand.

miR-223 in the early phase of osteoclastogenesis, but an in-depth evaluation of the expression level of miR-223 under physiological osteoclastogenesis requires further studies.

The early phase of OC generation triggers increased NFATC1 expression, together with reduced expression of its three negative regulators MAFB (MAF bZIP transcription factor B), IRF8 (interferon regulatory factor 8), and BCL6 (BCL6, transcription repressor) (25). MAFB is a relevant target of miRNAs in OC precursors. Up-regulation of miR-199a-5p and miR-148a promotes the amplification loop of NFATC1 and the formation of resorbing OCs by targeting MAFB in RAW264.7 cells (30) and in $CD14^+$ PBMCs (31), respectively. MiR-9718 is a newly described miRNA specifically expressed in the OC lineage, which promotes OC differentiation by targeting PIAS3 (protein inhibitor of activated STAT3) (32), another negative modulator of NFATC1 (33). Finally, the injection of molecules neutralizing miR-148a or miR-9718 in ovariectomy-induced osteoporotic mice increases total bone mass and decreases the OC number and activity (31, 32).

Among the other miRNAs up-regulated in OCs, the pro-osteoclastogenic role of miR-21 was demonstrated *in vivo* using the miR-21 KO mouse that display a slight increase in the trabecular bone mass and a reduced OC number and bone resorption (34). The expression of miR-21 is induced by c-Fos, which activation upon RANKL treatment of mouse bone marrow-derived macrophages (BMMs) operates a positive feedback loop by targeting the programmed cell death protein 4 (PDCD4) (35). The binding of c-Fos to miR-21 promoter is strikingly diminished by estrogen E2 treatment in RANKL-induced osteoclastogenesis. Estrogen attenuate miR-21 biogenesis, leading to increased FasL protein level and caspase-3 activity in mouse BMMs precursors (36). These results suggest that miR-21 expression is important in the development of OCs, particularly by controlling pre-osteoclast survival.

The activation of mitogen activated protein kinases (MAPKs) downstream of the early RANKL pro-osteoclastogenic signaling cascade is supported by the reactive oxygen species (ROS) produced by RANK-NADPH oxidase 1-dependant pathway (25). ROS production by mouse BMMs is regulated by heme oxygenase 1 (HMOX1), which attenuates osteoclastogenesis, specifically during the early phase of OC formation (37). MiR-183 is up-regulated by RANKL and targets HMOX1, thus promoting the early phase of osteoclastogenesis (38).

The PI3K/AKT pathway is induced by RANKL signaling and promotes cell survival (39). By reversing the action of PI3K (phosphoinositide 3-kinase), PTEN (phosphatase and tensin homolog) negatively impacts on OC precursor motility in the early phase of osteoclastogenesis (40). It was shown that miR-214 enhances the OC precursor differentiation via the PTEN/PI3K/AKT pathway, downstream of RANK signaling in RAW264.7 and primary mouse BMMs. *In vivo*, OC-specific miR-214 transgenic mice exhibit reduced expression of PTEN,

TABLE 1 | MiRNAs involved in the early phase of OC generation.

miRNAs	Species	Up/Down	Overall impact	Targets	Early steps impacted	References
miR-21	Mouse[a,b]	Up	Positive	PDCD4 FASLG	Survival	(34–36)
miR-29 family	Mouse[a]	Up	Positive	NFIA CDC42 SRGAP2	ND	(27)
miR-148a	Human[a] Mouse [a,b]	Up	Positive	MAFB	ND	(31)
miR-183	Mouse[a]	Up	Positive	HMOX1	ND	(38)
miR-199a-5p	Mouse[a]	Up	Positive	MAFB	ND	(30)
miR-214	Mouse[a,b]	Up	Positive	PTEN	Motility	(41)
miR-223	Mouse[a,b]	Up	Pos/neg	NFIA	ND	(5)
miR-9718	Mouse[a,b]	Up	Positive	PIAS3	ND	(32)
miR-34a	Mouse[a,b] Human [a]	Down	Negative	TGIF2	NS (survival, proliferation)	(54)
miR-124	Mouse[a] Rat [a,b]	Down	Negative	NFATC1	Proliferation, motility	(67, 68)
miR-125a	Human[a]	Down	Negative	TRAF6	ND	(48)
miR-141	Monkey[a,b]	Down	Negative	EPHA2 CALCR	ND	(56)
miR-144-3p	Human[a]	Down	Negative	RANK	Survival, proliferation	(47)
miR-145	Mouse[a,b]	Down	Negative	SMAD3	ND	(58)
miR-155	Mouse[a]	Down	Negative	SOCS1 MITF	ND	(61)
miR-155	Mouse[a]	Down	Positive	TAB2	ND	(63)
miR-218	Mouse[a]	Down	Negative	ND	Motility	(52)
miR-218	Mouse[a]	Down	Negative	TNFRSF1A	ND	(53)
miR-340	Mouse[a]	Down	Negative	MITF	ND	(65)
miR-503	Human[a] Mouse [a,b]	Down	Negative	RANK	ND	(46)
miR-9; miR-181a	Mouse[a]	ND	Negative	CBL	Survival, motility	(45)
miR-146a	Human[a] Mouse [a,b]	ND	Negative	TRAF6	ND	(50, 51)

Species and experimental context of the model used are indicated (a, in vitro). Up- or down-regulation of respective miRNAs during OC generation and the overall impact on OC differentiation are given. We detailed steps impacted in OC precursors (pre-OC) such as cell survival, proliferation and motility. Validated targets are also listed. PDCD4, programmed cell death protein 4; FASLG, Fas ligand; NFIA, nuclear factor I A; CDC42, cell division cycle 42; SRGAP2, SLIT-ROBO Rho GTPase activating protein 2; MAFB, MAF bZIP transcription factor B; HMOX1, heme oxygenase 1; PTEN, phosphatase and tensin homolog; PIAS3, protein inhibitor of activated STAT3; TGIF2, TGFB induced factor homeobox 2; NFATC1, nuclear factor of activated T cells 1; TRAF6, TNF receptor associated factor 6; EphA2: EPH receptor A2; CALCR, calcitonin receptor; RANK, receptor activator of nuclear factor kappa-B; SMAD3, SMAD family member 3; SOCS1, suppressor of cytokine signaling 1; MITF, melanocyte inducing transcription factor; TAB2, TGF-beta activated kinase 1 binding protein 2; TNFRSF1A, TNF receptor superfamily member 1A; CBL, Cbl proto-oncogene. ND, not determined; NS, not significant.

increased OC resorption activity, and reduced bone mineral density (41). Since a miR-214/PTEN axis has been involved in cell proliferation and invasion of various cancer cells (42–44), it would be of particular interest to investigate the specific role of miR-214 on cell proliferation, survival and motility in the context of OC lineage.

The over-expression of miR-9 and miR-181a diminishes the migration of RAW264.7 cells and primary mouse OC survival by repressing the expression of the proto-oncogene Cbl, which enhances the amount of the pro-apoptotic protein Bim (45). This was the first study reporting a functional role for miR-9 and miR-181a by targeting proteins belonging to the apoptosis pathway. Further experiments are needed to confirm the potential role of these miRNAs on the precursor survival during osteoclastogenesis.

miRNAs With an Inhibitory Role on OC Precursors

The initiation of the OC precursor differentiation is largely mediated by RANK/RANKL signaling. The expression density of RANK at the cell surface conditions the efficacy of RANK trimerization and downstream signal transduction. In human $CD14^+$ precursors, miR-503 targets RANK mRNA in the coding sequence (CDS) region, leading to reduced RANK protein level, OC numbers and cell density *in vitro* (46). *In vivo*, treatment of OVX mice with anti-miR-503 reduced bone resorption (46). The 3′ untranslated region (UTR) of RANK is also targeted by miR-144-3p in $CD14^+$ precursors, controlling OC formation, proliferation and survival of OC precursors (47).

The binding of RANKL to RANK induces the recruitment of the adaptor protein TRAF6 (TNF Receptor Associated

Factor 6). This important signaling adaptor for RANK is targeted by miR-125a and miR-146a in human PBMCs (48, 49). The expression of miR-125a is controlled by NFATC1, which directly binds to the promoter of miR-125a during osteoclastogenesis and reduces its expression (48). MiR-146a has been extensively studied in monocytes in pathological conditions, including pathologies associated with bone erosion such as RA. The expression of miR-146a is induced by LPS, TNFα, or IL1β signaling cascades, through the activation of NF-κB (nuclear factor kappa B), which directly binds to the miR-146 promoter (49). It was shown that miR-146a inhibits OC formation from human PBMCs in a dose-dependent manner and that the treatment of collagen-induced arthritic mice with miR-146 mimics attenuates bone resorption (50). We recently demonstrated that the reduced expression of miR-146a in the Ly6C^{high} monocyte subset of arthritic mice is involved in the pathogenic bone erosion, and that it can be rescued by specific delivery of miR-146 mimics to Ly6C^{high} monocytes (51). Taken together, these findings evidence a negative regulation of osteoclastogenesis by NFκB-induced miR-146a to partly counterbalance the deregulated differentiation of OC precursors in inflammatory disorders.

The RANK/TRAF6 signaling cascade activates the NFκB and MAPK pathways, which may represent additional miRNA targets. Indeed, miR-218 over-expression inhibits osteoclastogenesis by controling the p38MAPK pathway in mouse BMMs (52). Interestingly, miR-218 negatively impacts on the migration of RANKL-treated BMMs. Although authors also reported a decrease of actin-ring formation, it was most probably a consequence than a cause of the decreased OC number. The putative targets of miR-218 were not explored in this study. A recent study confirmed the negative regulation of osteoclastogenesis by miR-218, and show that it was mediated by targeting TNFRSF1A (TNF receptor superfamily member 1A), which leads to the inhibition of the NFκB pathway activation in RAW264.7 cells (53). Overall, miR-218 may act on both NFκB and MAPK pathways in OC precursors to control OC precursor differentiation, and further studies are required to unravel the molecular mechanisms involved.

The early RANKL signaling is mediated by two transcription factors, NFκB and AP1, which are essential to the initiation of the NFATC1 amplification loop. AP1 components such as c-Jun and c-Fos could be critical targets to modulate NFATC1 activation in OC precursors. The transcriptional regulator TGIF2 (TGFB induced factor homeobox 2) is induced by NFATC1, c-Fos and c-Jun and potentiates the activity of NFATC1 and c-Jun in turn, promoting the osteoclastogenesis in a positive feedback loop (54). Interestingly, TGIF2 is a direct target of miR-34a, and OC-specific miR-34a transgenic mice exhibit lower bone resorption and higher bone mass, with no alteration of OC precursor survival and proliferation (54). Finally, miR-34a seems to negatively regulate the NFATC1 pathway during OC differentiation, mostly in the early phase upon RANKL signaling.

RANKL signaling enhances another co-stimulatory signal mediated by the ephrinA2-EphA2 interaction at the cell surface of OC precursors. EphrinA2 expression is rapidly induced in a c-Fos-dependent manner and cleaved by metalloproteinases to release an active soluble form able to interact with its receptor EphA2, enhancing osteoclastogenesis (55). In rhesus monkey BMMs EphA2 is a potential target of miR-141 (56). OC differentiation and bone resorption are suppressed *in vitro* by miR-141, and *in vivo* using repeated injections of an OC-targeted delivery system into aged monkeys (56). The calcitonin receptor (CALCR) is also a target of miR-141 in rhesus OCs. A down-regulation of CALCR is however expected to suppress the negative effect of calcitonin on OC differentiation and to enhance bone resorption, whereas miR-141 globally inhibits OC differentiation and activity, both *in vitro* and *in vivo*. One can speculate that the targeting of CALCR by miR-141 may represent a minor part of the effects of miR-141 functions in rhesus OCs.

Another critical interaction in RANKL-induced osteoclast ogenesis is the cooperation between Smad complex and c-Fos, which leads to NFATC1 transcription (57). Recently, miR-145 was shown to target Smad3, thus reducing the formation of p-Smad2/3 complex, repressing c-Fos and NFATC1 transcription in mouse OC precursors, and decreasing OC number (58). Smad proteins are induced by members of the transforming growth factor beta (TGFβ) super family, and Smad pathway has become of particular interest in inflammatory disorders [reviewed in (59)]. TGFβ1/Smad4 signaling directly induces miR-155 expression, a negative regulator of osteoclastogenesis (60). In addition, miR-155 is induced by interferon (IFN)-β and mediates its suppressive effect on OC differentiation by targeting the pro-osteoclastogenic gene SOCS1 (suppressor of cytokine signaling 1) in OC precursors (61). These data were suggestive of a suppressive role of miR-155 in osteoclastogenesis. In physiological condition, miR-155 is downregulated during osteoclastogenesis. Nevertheless, miR-155 is up-regulated in activated immune cells, such as lymphocyte B-cells, T-cells and dendritic cells, promoting the inflammatory response and thus aggravating the inflammatory-induced arthritis and bone erosion *in vivo* through the indirect immune-mediated activation of OCs [reviewed in (62)]. In lipopolysaccharide (LPS)-induced inflammatory condition, miR-155 directly induces autophagy in OCs as well as OC differentiation and activity by targeting TGFβ-activated kinase 1-binding protein 2 (TAB2) (63). A fine modulation of the TAB2 expression level may promote the destabilization of the inactive complex TAB2/Beclin1, leading to (i) the release of Beclin1 and induction of autophagy and (ii) the interaction of the adaptor proteins TAB2 and TAK1 that activates the RANK/TRAF6/NFκB pathway. These findings illustrate the variable role of miR-155 in osteoclastogenesis depending on the microenvironment, i.e., according to the presence of LPS, IFNβ, or TGFβ-mediated inflammatory signals. To make things even more complex, miR-155 also targets the transcription factor MITF that is up-regulated upon RANKL signaling (60, 61). MITF plays a critical role in the OC differentiation by collaborating with NFATC1 in the early phase of osteoclastogenesis (64). In summary, miR-155 seems to globally inhibit the OC generation in physiological condition by acting both in the commitment of myeloid precursors (26) and in osteoclastogenesis (61) through

TABLE 2 | MiRNAs involved in the late phase of OC generation.

miRNAs	Species	Up/Down	Overall impact	Targets	Late steps impacted	References
miR-26a	Mouse[a]	Up	Negative	CTGF	Actin ring formation	(82)
miR-31	Mouse[a]	Up	Positive	RHOA	Actin ring formation	(70)
miR-34c	Mouse[a]	Up	Positive	LGR4	OC survival	(74)
miR-7b	Mouse[a]	Down	Negative	DCSTAMP	Cell fusion	(79)
miR-29b	Human[a]	Down	Negative	FOS MMP2	Actin ring formation	(77)
miR-30a	Mouse[a]	Down	Negative	DCSTAMP	Actin ring formation	(80)
miR-124	Mouse[a]	Down	Negative	RAB27A	ND	(69)
miR-142-3p	Human[a]	Down	Negative	PRKCA	Cell fusion, OC survival	(83)
miR-186	Mouse[a]	ND	Negative	CTSK	OC survival	(84)

Species of model used are indicated; whether experiments were performed in vitro (a) or in vivo (b) is specified with superscript letters. Up- or down-regulation of respective miRNAs during OC generation and the overall impact on OC differentiation are given. We detailed steps impacted in the late phase such as cell fusion, actin ring formation and the survival of mature OCs. Validated targets are also listed. CTGF, connective tissue growth factor; RHOA, ras homolog family member A; LGR4, leucine rich repeat containing G protein-coupled receptor 4; DCSTAMP, dendrocyte expressed seven transmembrane protein; FOS, Fos proto-oncogene, AP-1 transcription factor subunit; MMP2, matrix metallopeptidase 2; RAB27A, RAB27A, member RAS oncogene family; PRKCA, protein kinase C alpha; CTSK, cathepsin K. ND, not determined; NS, not significant.

the regulation of MITF expression. MITF is also targeted by miR-340, which inhibits the OC differentiation of mouse BMMs (65). This reinforces the idea that MITF is a key target for miRNAs in osteoclastogenesis.

Finally, NFATC1 has hardly been described as a direct target of miRNAs so far. The activity of NFATC1 is regulated by phosphorylation, which retains NFATC1 in the cytosol compartment and inhibits its translocation into the nucleus. Epigenetic controls of the NFATC1 gene have been reported [reviewed in (66)]. To date, only miR-124 is predicted to bind NFATC1 in its 3′ UTR in OC precursors (67). The targeting of the 3′UTR of both rat and human NFATC1 mRNAs by miR-124 was confirmed using luciferase reporter assays (68). Functionally, miR-124 represses NFATC1 expression in mouse BMMs and diminishes the migration and proliferation of OC precursors (67), without impact on their survival (69).

miRNAs IN THE LATE PHASE OF OC GENERATION

To achieve OC maturation, the key transcription factors MITF, PU.1, and NFATC1 lead to the expression of several osteoclastogenic genes involved in the cytoskeleton organization, the cell fusion and actin-ring formation. MiRNAs also regulate the late stage of OC formation by targeting Rho GTPases, DCSTAMP, CSTK, and the RANKL-receptor inhibitor LGR4 (**Table 2**).

Pro-Osteoclastogenic miRNAs

One of the most up-regulated miRNAs during osteoclastogenesis in mouse BMMs is miR-31. It specifically acts on the actin-ring formation (70). Neutralization of miR-31 impairs the matrix resorption and the ring-shaped OC formation, while cell-fusion is conserved. Increased RhoA activity and protein expression level are also observed in miR-31-deficient OC precursors, suggesting that RhoA is targeted by miR-31 in the OC lineage (70). Small GTPases of the Rho family (Rac1, Rac2, CDC42, RhoA, and RhoU) play important roles in the cell-fusion of OC precursors, podosome organization, migration, and polarization of mature OCs [reviewed in (71)]. RhoA controls the polymerization of actin, the turnover of podosomes, and the migration of OCs through the bone matrix (72). While a moderate level of RhoA activity is required to allow both stability of the sealing zone and bone resorption, RhoA over-activation or inhibition cause disassembly of the podosomes and thus impair the OC activity [reviewed in (73)]. Finally, miR-31 seems essential to OC maturation by finely modulating RhoA activity.

Another relevant miRNA in mature OC biology is miR-34c, which promotes the OC survival at the end of maturation by targeting the R-spondins receptor LGR4 (leucine rich repeat containing G protein-coupled receptor 4), also known as GPR48 (74). During the OC maturation, NFATC1 induces the expression of LGR4 at the cell surface to negatively regulate RANK/RANKL-signaling by a direct competition with RANK. The binding of RANKL to LGR4 activates the NFκB-inhibitor GSK3β, which results in OC apoptosis (75). These data suggest that miR-34c sustains the OC formation.

miRNAs Displaying an Inhibitory Role in OC Maturation

Based on the study of Franceschetti et al. (27), we reviewed above the role of miR-29 family in the OC commitment and in the early phase of OC generation. The authors however also showed a late up-regulation of miR-29 (a, b, c) family members at the third day of RANKL-induced OC differentiation of mouse BMMs, suggesting another predominant role of miR-29 in the late phase of osteoclastogenesis. They found two targets involved in the cytoskeleton organization, CDC42 and SRGAP2 (SLIT-ROBO Rho GTPase Activating Protein 2), which present opposite effects. Indeed, SRGAP2 belongs to GAP family, which inactivates Rho GTPases such as CDC42 by increasing the intrinsic GTPase activity of Rho proteins (76). Rho GTPases are essential in the polarization and the podosome belt/sealing zone formation of functional OCs [reviewed in (17, 71)].The neutralization of miR-29 family has no effect on the formation of the actin-ring in mature RAW-derived OCs. A role for miR-29 family in the OC maturation remains thus questionable. Another study showed a down-regulation of miR-29b during OC generation, and demonstrated an inhibitory role of miR-29b in resorption and actin-ring formation in human CD14^{+}-derived OCs (77). Considering only the multinucleated cells for their analysis, authors observed disarranged nodular actin spots in OCs over-expressing miR-29b, leading to a failure to form actin-rings. Although the authors did not perform a validation of the known targets of miR-29b in the OC lineage, they observed a significant down-regulation of c-Fos and MMP2 expression in miR-29b-transfected OCs at the end of the differentiation. The apparent discrepancies on the role of miR-29 family members and miR-29b could be partially explained by the chosen approach in the different studies, which rely either on gain-of function of miR-29b (77) or loss-of function of miR-29 family (27), as well as on the nature of OC precursors used (cell line vs. primary cells).

In addition to its negative effect on cell proliferation and motility in the early phase of osteoclatogenesis (67), miR-124 seems to act on the late phase of the differentiation by targeting Rab27a (69), a protein belonging to the small Rab GTPase family and involved in vesicle trafficking and resorbing activity of OCs (78). Notably, miR-124 is under-expressed in the OVX mouse model, which displays a deregulated resorbing activity (69).

DCSTAMP is a key protein involved in cell fusion. DCSTAMP is targeted by miR-7b and miR-30a in mouse BM precursors (79, 80). Mimics of miR-7b and miR-30a repress the expression level of DCSTAMP, decrease the OC number and inhibit matrix resorption. Conversely, anti-miR-7b promotes the OC formation and increase nuclei number in mature OC, suggesting an increase of cell fusion events (79). By measuring the membrane merge rate, the authors confirmed that overexpression of miR-7b in mouse BMMs significantly abrogates OC fusion (81). Anti-miR-30a enhances the actin-ring formation (80). Similarly, miR-26a attenuates the actin-ring formation and resorption in mouse BMMs. MiR-26a targets the connective tissue growth factor (CTGF), which induces and interacts with DCSTAMP (82). Contrary to miR-7b and miR-30a, miR-26a is upregulated in the late phase of osteoclastogenesis, suggesting a physiological regulation of multinucleation in the OC lineage. Thus, it will be of particular interest to evaluate the role of miR-30a and miR-26a on cell fusion.

During OC formation from human CD14^{+} progenitors, the enforced expression of miR-142-3p inhibits cell-to-cell contact, clustering and fusion events associated with the induction of OC apoptosis upon RANKL stimulation (83). The negative effect of miR-142-3p on OC fusion could be partially explained by the silencing of PKCα. Indeed, PKCα is involved in the microtubule and actin networks and is predicted as a putative target of miR-142-3p by prediction software. A decreased expression of anti-apoptotic factors downstream of PKCα might also explain the induction of cell death (83), however it has not been functionally explored yet.

Finally, miR-186 was newly described as a negative regulator of mature OC survival. Mimics of miR-186 induce caspase-3/7 activity and OC apoptosis in transfected RAW264.7-derived mature OCs (84). Moreover, miR-186 targets the CTSK gene (84) and probably represses the resorbing function of OCs, although it remains to be explored in functional assays.

ADVANCES IN TECHNOLOGIES FOR THE QUANTIFICATION OF miRNAs IN BIOLOGICAL TISSUES

MiRNAs are classically studied from the total mRNA (including small RNAs) extracted from the tissue of interest. As miRNAs are expressed in various cell types and tissues, it is necessary to well define the targeted sample and to control the purity of the elicited source of miRNAs. The study of miRNAs in primary OCs is challenging because of the localization of OCs into bone cavities, and thus a purified extract of primary OCs is very hard. Finally, primary OC precursors from blood sample or bone marrow are used to derive OCs in *in vivo* experiments. Nevertheless, the OC differentiation in culture is only partial without reaching a pure OC population. The obtained population includes all stages from the precursor to the mature OC. The study of miRNAs in such heterogeneous cell culture is not satisfactory and gives a lot of variations between samples that could impact on the reliability of the results, particularly in "end-point" studies without a kinetic expression of miRNAs during the OC differentiation. Some studies are based on purified OCs using chemical methods to eliminate non- and poor-adherent cells, as mature OCs are extremely adherent. Very recently, a novel method of purification based on the OC sorting has been described, allowing a standardized approach to better characterize the miRNA profiling in mature OCs (85).

Other biological tissues are become novel sources of study in the OC biology and the bone remodeling. Indeed, miRNAs can be exported from a donor cell to a recipient *via* exosomes and microvesicles (**Figure 1**), and thus participate to the cell communication between osteocytes, osteoblasts and osteoclasts in the bone micro-environment (86–89). Circulating miRNAs can also be used as biomarkers in pathophysiological conditions, reaching liquid biopsies as potential interesting samples in clinical application.

Molecular technologies are used to detect and quantify miRNAs, and some panels were developed to determine the miRNA profiling. Here we provide a global and detailed view of these technologies and their application in the quantification of miRNAs in biological tissues.

Screening Methods for the miRNA Profiling

In recent years, technological advances in research tools including qPCR, microarrays, and next generation sequencing (NGS), have enabled sensitive detection of miRNAs. Typically, miRNA biomarkers are measured with quantitative polymerase chain reaction (qPCR) after RNA extraction and conversion into complementary DNA (cDNA). Many other methods are available for large screening of the miRNome to understand pathologies or discovery of biomarkers. Mestdagh et al., have extensively analyzed analytical parameters of many solutions available for miRNA measurement based on qPCR, hybridization platforms and sequencing technologies (90). Recently, new technologies for miRNAs measurement or optimization of existing methods have emerged. Currently, the miRbase 22 includes 1917 miRNA genes. With the constant evolution of the miRbase, the different miRNA detection platforms need to adapt their product. This flexibility however depends on the technic used. New technologies that are more sensitive, or extraction free chemistry, are definitively modifying the miRNA measurement landscape (**Table 3**).

Among these technologies, we will focus on the most innovative technologies for miRNA detection. These technologies provide real advance and alternative with the direct use of matrices avoiding preprocessing step or optimized library preparation for RNA-Seq method for the profiling of miRNAs. For the measurement of single miRNAs, new methods using microfluidic detection by laminar flow (91) or absolute quantification of signal by RCA-FRET technology (92) are in development. These last technologies may simplify the adoption of miRNA testing in clinical laboratories.

Screening methods such as the microarrays of Affymetrix (version 4.1) and Agilent (v21) now include 2,578 and 2,549 miRNAs, respectively, thus offering a more comprehensive dataset. In addition to these updated microarray versions, the company Takara Bio have recently developed the SMARTer miRNA-Seq kit, which uses Mono-Adapter ligation and Intramolecular Circularization (MAGIC) technology to efficiently capture miRNA species with reduced bias inherent to other approaches. Measurement of equimolar mixture of 963 miRNAs shows that >70% of the miRNAs are accurately represented, whereas other competitors have 49–79% of the miRNAs underrepresented Nevertheless, besides having less bias than the competitors (including TruSeq and NEXTFlex), this kit also produces large amounts of side products and as a result did not perform better for the detection of biological miRNAs (93). Since several years now, a new technology of HTG Molecular (High Throughput Genomic) called EdgeSeq provides miRNAs measurement without RNA extraction. The technology is a combination of hybridization with nuclease protection assay and next generation sequencing. Based on an extraction free chemistry, the technology[1] allows the direct measurement of miRNAs from as little as 15 μl of body fluid. This last critical point avoids biases associated to the extraction protocols (94) and increases the sensitivity of the measure. Correlation between replicates is very similar to those shown previously (90) for hybridization and sequencing technologies, whereas accuracy of the gradient of miRNA measure is superior to other hybridization and sequencing platform[2]. Nevertheless, cross reactivity is higher compared to qPCR assays[2]. It has been shown that HTG EdgeSeq results were closest to the RNASeq results with >95% concordance on tissue samples (95). The technology also shows very good correlation with the PCR on plasma samples, with Pearson's coefficient of 0.93 and 0.94 for qPCR and digital PCR (dPCR) data, respectively (96).

Circulating miRNAs as Biomarkers

In the past decade, the search for circulating miRNA for functional studies and biomarkers research has yielded numerous associations between miRNAs and different types of disease. However, many of these relations could not be replicated in subsequent studies under similar experimental conditions. Although this lack of reproducibility may be explained by variations in experimental design and analytical methods, guidelines of the most appropriate design and methods of analysis are scarce. MiRNAs have significant promise as biomarkers for diseases, due to their regulatory role in many cellular processes, and their stability in samples such as plasma and serum. Circulating miRNAs are moreover easily accessible. Biomarker experiments generally consist of a discovery phase and a validation phase. In the discovery phase, typically hundreds of miRNAs are simultaneously measured to identify candidates. Because of the costs of such high-throughput experiments, numbers of subjects are often too small, which can lead to false positives and negatives. In validation phase, a small number of identified candidates are measured in a large cohort, generally using quantitative PCR (qPCR). Although qPCR is a sensitive method to measure miRNAs in the circulation, experimental design, and qPCR data analysis remain challenging with many sources of biases. The MIQE guidelines are useful to stress on the most important biases in qPCR experiments and to give some elements to improve experimental practice (97). There is still a need for standardization or development of new methods to reach the clinic. Thus, choosing the right tools is critical for a successful miRNA-based experiment.

Despite new advances and evolution of technologies, many challenges remain unmet. For example, the impact of RNA isolation, which is known to induce biases (94), but also the lack of standardization of miRNA measurement or normalization of miRNAs data from plasma/serum samples, are key factors of variation, making more challenging the translation of biomarker discovery to diagnostic tool. Indeed, while many reports are describing miRNAs as potential biomarkers since many years, miRNA-based diagnostics have many difficulties to enter to the clinic and to get IVD approval. Moreover, these kinds of tests are likely best suited to a companion role. In contrast to RNA or DNA-based tests, especially that indicate the presence of SNP or a specific expression profile (98), miRNA tests produce results that are more difficult to interpret. While many miRNAs were reported as biomarkers in many reports (99), most miRNAs are expressed widely in a non-cell-specific manner, and their levels of expression are not differing drastically between patients' group and controls. For liquid biopsies such as blood, urine, or other body fluids, miRNA levels are very sensitive to pre-processing and post-processing factors. As a result, despite being very stable, miRNA-based tests are often based on a combination of miRNAs associated with an algorithm, and strict standardization of the entire process, from obtaining and processing the sample to results reporting, is mandatory and is key for reproducible results, no matter what technology is used.

Point of care diagnostics requires short detection time, small sample volume and portability of the device. These requests are often not compatible with miRNA measurement technologies since they are requesting many steps and devices. New methods based on microfluidic chip and laminar flow assisted dentritic amplification is currently under development, with a promise of time to result of only 20 min (91). Sensitivity and accuracy have still to be increased, but this attractive solution could potentially allow the compatibility of miRNAs to short diagnostic

[1] From www.takarabio.com/learning-centers/next-generation-sequencing/technical-notes/accurate-mirna-representation-in-microrna-seq,2018

[2] From the poster presented at ESHG, 2017, available on https://www.htgmolecular.com/assets/htg/publications/PO-17-Aissaoui-EHSG-miRNA-Metrics.pdf

TABLE 3 | Technologies of miRNA profiling.

	Exiqon qiagen LNA	Open array (Taqman)	Takara smarter microRNA-Seq kit	Illumina TruSeq	IonTorrent	Affymetrix miRNA 4.1	Agilent miRNA microarray (21.0)	Nanostring ncounter	HTG molecular
Technology	qPCR	qPCR	NGS	NGS	NGS	Hybrid.	Hybrid.	Hybrid.	Hybrid. and NGS
Input RNA	40 ng	100 ng	100 ng	1000 ng	1000 ng	130 ng	100 ng	100 ng	15 μl/25 ng
Extraction	Yes	Yes	Yes	Yes	Yes	Yes	Yes	Yes	No
miRNAs in the assay	752	754	miRNome*	miRNome*	miRNome*	2,578	2,549	800	2,083

LNA, locked nucleic acid; HTG, high throughput genomic; qPCR, quantitative polymerase chain reaction; NGS, next generation sequencing; Hybrid, hybridization.
**Based on current database miRBase 22 with 1,917 entries.*

delay. Without such solution able to reduce time to results, use of miRNAs in diagnostic is only possible for non-urgent test. Most used platforms remain qPCR, with various technologies available such as LNA/Taqman/SybrGreen PCR, which request high level of standardization to provide accurate and stable results. Another novel technology that could facilitate miRNA transfer to clinic is called RCA-FRET, which is a combination of rolling circle amplification (RCA) and Förster resonance energy transfer (FRET) (92). Key advantage of the technology is a simple workflow, device needed and material for absolute quantification results. This last point is of key importance since normalization of miRNA data is a true hurdle.

Indeed, accurate quantification of miRNAs using qPCR is largely dependent on proper normalization techniques, the absence of which can lead to misinterpretation of data and incorrect conclusions (100). The goal of most miRNA experiments using qPCR is to identify differences in expression between two groups of samples. In this case, cell-free miRNAs from biofluids are emerging as important noninvasive biomarkers because of their stability. Many works are describing miRNAs as potential blood biomarkers. One challenge in studying miRNAs from serum and plasma is their relatively low abundance and lack of reliable endogenous controls. It has been shown that hsa-miR-24, hsamiR-126, hsa-miR-484 (101), hsa-miR-16-5p, hsa-miR-93-5p (102), hsamiR-484, and hsa-miR-191-5p (103) are stable normalizers in serum. Nevertheless, some reports indicate also these miRNAs not as normalizers but as biomarkers, as for miR-16-5p described in the progression of gastric cancer for example (104). In the absence of reliable endogenous controls in serum/plasma, exogenous or spike-in controls can be used to normalize miRNA expression data. Exogenous controls can also be used to monitor extraction efficiency or sample input amount for difficult samples (e.g., serum, plasma, or other biofluids).

In addition to most common used matrices, extracellular vesicles (EVs) are emerging and even more challenging to get reliable results. EVs are nanometer-scale particles, which include exosomes, microvesicles, and apoptotic bodies. EVs are intercellular communicators released by most cell types with key functions in physiological and pathological processes (86, 105). EVs deliver specific proteins, microRNAs and other cellular components. One of the most important aspects of EV research is analyzing their nucleic acid cargo, particularly miRNAs. These are commonly quantified by RT-qPCR or, increasingly, by comprehensive transcriptomic profiling using NGS or hybridization technologies. One critical issue is the methods for RNA extraction that can influence downstream analyses by yielding non-identical, kit-specific results. This is of particular challenge since typical concentration of this type of sample is low, RNA integrity is decreased and associated to high individual variability. Several kits are on the market and tested (106) but optimal isolation methodology is mainly dependent on the respective research setting and downstream analyses.

Overall, it is not easy to give a simple answer to a complex problem. Many methods are available for miRNAs measurement and generate complex data that need to be validated. Real efforts have to be done on standardization and analytical validation until one can consider to successfully translate biomarker discovery to the clinic.

CONCLUSION

In the present review we have shown the complexity of understanding OC biology and pointed out key miRNAs that have been involved in OC differentiation as key regulators, with very specific roles in the different phases progressing from early progenitors toward fully mature OC. We also stressed the challenge to get reliable data from miRNA measurement either for supporting the knowledge of OC regulation or the translation into biomarker tools for clinical application.

AUTHOR CONTRIBUTIONS

CL, ID-R, HF, ES, and FA wrote the review. CL, ID-R, and ES designed the figures and tables.

REFERENCES

1. Fire A, Xu S, Montgomery MK, Kostas SA, Driver SE, Mello CC. Potent and specific genetic interference by double-stranded RNA in *Caenorhabditis elegans*. *Nature*. (1998) 391:806–11. doi: 10.1038/35888
2. Winter J, Jung S, Keller S, Gregory RI, Diederichs S. Many roads to maturity: microRNA biogenesis pathways and their regulation. *Nat Cell Biol.* (2009) 11:228–34. doi: 10.1038/ncb0309-228
3. Ha M, Kim VN. Regulation of microRNA biogenesis. *Nat Rev Mol Cell Biol.* (2014) 15:509–24. doi: 10.1038/nrm3838
4. Piriyapongsa J, Bootchai C, Ngamphiw C, Tongsima S. microPIR2: a comprehensive database for human-mouse comparative study of microRNA-promoter interactions. *Database.* (2014) 2014:bau115. doi: 10.1093/database/bau115
5. Sugatani T, Hruska KA. Impaired Micro-RNA pathways diminish osteoclast differentiation and function. *J Biol Chem.* (2009) 284:4667–78. doi: 10.1074/jbc.M805777200
6. Mizoguchi F, Izu Y, Hayata T, Hemmi H, Nakashima K, Nakamura T, et al. Osteoclast-specific Dicer gene deficiency suppresses osteoclastic bone resorption. *J Cell Biochem.* (2010) 109:866–75. doi: 10.1002/jcb.22228
7. Xia Z, Chen C, Chen P, Xie H, Luo X. MicroRNAs and their roles in osteoclast differentiation. *Front Med.* (2011) 5:414–9. doi: 10.1007/s11684-011-0168-0
8. Tang P, Xiong Q, Ge W, Zhang L. The role of microRNAs in osteoclasts and osteoporosis. *RNA Biol.* (2014) 11:1355–63. doi: 10.1080/15476286.2014.996462
9. Chen J, Qiu M, Dou C, Cao Z, Dong S. MicroRNAs in bone balance and osteoporosis. *Drug Dev Res.* (2015) 76:235–45. doi: 10.1002/ddr.21260
10. Sun M, Zhou X, Chen L, Huang S, Leung V, Wu N, et al. The regulatory roles of MicroRNAs in bone remodeling and perspectives as biomarkers in osteoporosis. *Biomed Res Int.* (2016) 2016:1652417. doi: 10.1155/2016/1652417
11. Ji X, Chen X, Yu X. MicroRNAs in osteoclastogenesis and function: potential therapeutic targets for osteoporosis. *Int J Mol Sci.* (2016) 17:349. doi: 10.3390/ijms17030349
12. Gennari L, Bianciardi S, Merlotti D. MicroRNAs in bone diseases. *Osteoporos Int.* (2017) 28:1191–13. doi: 10.1007/s00198-016-3847-5
13. Feng Q, Zheng S, Zheng J. The emerging role of microRNAs in bone remodeling and its therapeutic implications for osteoporosis. *Biosci Rep.* (2018) 38:BSR20180453. doi: 10.1042/BSR20180453
14. Yang Y, Fang S. Small non-coding RNAs-based bone regulation and targeting therapeutic strategies. *Mol Cell Endocrinol.* (2017) 456:16–35. doi: 10.1016/j.mce.2016.11.018
15. Boyle WJ, Simonet WS, Lacey DL. Osteoclast differentiation and activation. *Nature.* (2003) 423:337–42. doi: 10.1038/nature01658
16. Maeda K, Kobayashi Y, Udagawa N, Uehara S, Ishihara A, Mizoguchi T, et al. Wnt5a-Ror2 signaling between osteoblast-lineage cells and osteoclast precursors enhances osteoclastogenesis. *Nat Med.* (2012) 18:405–12. doi: 10.1038/nm.2653
17. Uehara S, Udagawa N, Kobayashi Y. Non-canonical Wnt signals regulate cytoskeletal remodeling in osteoclasts. *Cell Mol Life Sci.* (2018) 75:3683–92. doi: 10.1007/s00018-018-2881-1
18. Oikawa T, Kuroda Y, Matsuo K. Regulation of osteoclasts by membrane-derived lipid mediators. *Cell Mol Life Sci.* (2013) 70:3341–53. doi: 10.1007/s00018-012-1238-4
19. Amarasekara DS, Yun H, Kim S, Lee N, Kim H, Rho J. Regulation of osteoclast differentiation by cytokine networks. *Immune Netw.* (2018) 18:e8. doi: 10.4110/in.2018.18.e8
20. Xiao Y, Palomero J, Grabowska J, Wang L, de Rink I, van Helvert L, et al. Macrophages and osteoclasts stem from a bipotent progenitor downstream of a macrophage/osteoclast/dendritic cell progenitor. *Blood Adv.* (2017) 1:1993–2006. doi: 10.1182/bloodadvances.2017008540
21. Li H, Hong S, Qian J, Zheng Y, Yang J, Yi Q. Cross talk between the bone and immune systems: osteoclasts function as antigen-presenting cells and activate CD4+ and CD8+ T cells. *Blood.* (2010) 116:210–7. doi: 10.1182/blood-2009-11-255026
22. Jin Z, Wei W, Yang M, Du Y, Wan Y. Mitochondrial complex I activity suppresses inflammation and enhances bone resorption by shifting macrophage-osteoclast polarization. *Cell Metab.* (2014) 20:483–98. doi: 10.1016/j.cmet.2014.07.011
23. Undi RB, Kandi R, Gutti RK. MicroRNAs as haematopoiesis regulators. *Adv Hematol.* (2013) 2013:695754. doi: 10.1155/2013/695754
24. Valenti MT, Dalle Carbonare L, Mottes M. Role of microRNAs in progenitor cell commitment and osteogenic differentiation in health and disease (Review). *Int J Mol Med.* (2018) 41:2441–9. doi: 10.3892/ijmm.2018.3452
25. Park JH, Lee NK, Lee SY. Current understanding of RANK signaling in osteoclast differentiation and maturation. *Mol Cells.* (2017) 40:706–13. doi: 10.14348/molcells.2017.0225
26. Mann M, Barad O, Agami R, Geiger B, Hornstein E. miRNA-based mechanism for the commitment of multipotent progenitors to a single cellular fate. *Proc Natl Acad Sci USA.* (2010) 107:15804–9. doi: 10.1073/pnas.0915022107
27. Franceschetti T, Kessler CB, Lee S-K, Delany AM. miR-29 promotes murine osteoclastogenesis by regulating osteoclast commitment and migration. *J Biol Chem.* (2013) 288:33347–60. doi: 10.1074/jbc.M113.484568
28. Sugatani T, Hruska KA. MicroRNA-223 is a key factor in osteoclast differentiation. *J Cell Biochem.* (2007) 101:996–9. doi: 10.1002/jcb.21335
29. Shibuya H, Nakasa T, Adachi N, Nagata Y, Ishikawa M, Deie M, et al. Overexpression of microRNA-223 in rheumatoid arthritis synovium controls osteoclast differentiation. *Mod Rheumatol.* (2013) 23:674–85. doi: 10.3109/s10165-012-0710-1
30. Guo K, Zhang D, Wu H, Zhu Q, Yang C, Zhu J. MiRNA-199a-5p positively regulated RANKL-induced osteoclast differentiation by target Mafb protein. *J Cell Biochem.* (2018). doi: 10.1002/jcb.27968. [Epub ahead of print].
31. Cheng P, Chen C, He H-B, Hu R, Zhou H-D, Xie H, et al. miR-148a regulates osteoclastogenesis by targeting V-maf musculoaponeurotic fibrosarcoma oncogene homolog B. *J Bone Miner Res.* (2013) 28:1180–90. doi: 10.1002/jbmr.1845
32. Liu T, Qin A-P, Liao B, Shao H-G, Guo L-J, Xie G-Q, et al. A novel microRNA regulates osteoclast differentiation via targeting protein inhibitor of activated STAT3 (PIAS3). *Bone.* (2014) 67:156–65. doi: 10.1016/j.bone.2014.07.004
33. Kim K, Lee J, Kim JH, Jin HM, Zhou B, Lee SY, et al. Protein inhibitor of activated STAT 3 modulates osteoclastogenesis by down-regulation of NFATc1 and osteoclast-associated receptor. *J Immunol.* (2007) 178:5588–94. doi: 10.4049/jimmunol.178.9.5588
34. Hu C-H, Sui B-D, Du F-Y, Shuai Y, Zheng C-X, Zhao P, et al. miR-21 deficiency inhibits osteoclast function and prevents bone loss in mice. *Sci Rep.* (2017) 7:43191. doi: 10.1038/srep43191
35. Sugatani T, Vacher J, Hruska KA. A microRNA expression signature of osteoclastogenesis. *Blood.* (2011) 117:3648–57. doi: 10.1182/blood-2010-10-311415
36. Sugatani T, Hruska KA. Down-regulation of miR-21 biogenesis by estrogen action contributes to osteoclastic apoptosis. *J Cell Biochem.* (2013) 114:1217–22. doi: 10.1002/jcb.24471
37. Florczyk-Soluch U, Józefczuk E, Stępniewski J, Bukowska-Strakova K, Mendel M, Viscardi M, et al. Various roles of heme oxygenase-1 in response of bone marrow macrophages to RANKL and in the early stage of osteoclastogenesis. *Sci Rep.* (2018) 8:10797. doi: 10.1038/s41598-018-29122-1
38. Ke K, Sul O-J, Rajasekaran M, Choi H-S. MicroRNA-183 increases osteoclastogenesis by repressing heme oxygenase-1. *Bone.* (2015) 81:237–46. doi: 10.1016/j.bone.2015.07.006
39. Teitelbaum SL, Ross FP. Genetic regulation of osteoclast development and function. *Nat Rev Genet.* (2003) 4:638–49. doi: 10.1038/nrg1122
40. Sugatani T, Alvarez U, Hruska KA. PTEN regulates RANKL- and osteopontin-stimulated signal transduction during osteoclast differentiation and cell motility. *J Biol Chem.* (2003) 278:5001–8. doi: 10.1074/jbc.M209299200
41. Zhao C, Sun W, Zhang P, Ling S, Li Y, Zhao D, et al. miR-214 promotes osteoclastogenesis by targeting Pten/PI3k/Akt pathway. *RNA Biol.* (2015) 12:343–53. doi: 10.1080/15476286.2015.1017205

42. Penna E, Orso F, Taverna D. miR-214 as a key hub that controls cancer networks: small player, multiple functions. *J Invest Dermatol.* (2015) 135:960–9. doi: 10.1038/jid.2014.479
43. Xin R, Bai F, Feng Y, Jiu M, Liu X, Bai F, et al. MicroRNA-214 promotes peritoneal metastasis through regulating PTEN negatively in gastric cancer. *Clin Res Hepatol Gastroenterol.* (2016) 40:748–54. doi: 10.1016/j.clinre.2016.05.006
44. Liu J, Chen W, Zhang H, Liu T, Zhao L. miR-214 targets the PTEN-mediated PI3K/Akt signaling pathway and regulates cell proliferation and apoptosis in ovarian cancer. *Oncol Lett.* (2017) 14:5711–8. doi: 10.3892/ol.2017.6953
45. Wang S, Tang C, Zhang Q, Chen W. Reduced miR-9 and miR-181a expression down-regulates Bim concentration and promote osteoclasts survival. *Int J Clin Exp Pathol.* (2014) 7:2209–18.
46. Chen C, Cheng P, Xie H, Zhou H-D, Wu X-P, Liao E-Y, et al. MiR-503 regulates osteoclastogenesis via targeting RANK. *J Bone Miner Res.* (2014) 29:338–47. doi: 10.1002/jbmr.2032
47. Wang C, He H, Wang L, Jiang Y, Xu Y. Reduced miR-144-3p expression in serum and bone mediates osteoporosis pathogenesis by targeting RANK. *Biochem Cell Biol.* (2018) 96:627–35. doi: 10.1139/bcb-2017-0243
48. Guo L-J, Liao L, Yang L, Li Y, Jiang T-J. MiR-125a TNF receptor-associated factor 6 to inhibit osteoclastogenesis. *Exp Cell Res.* (2014) 321:142–52. doi: 10.1016/j.yexcr.2013.12.001
49. Taganov KD, Boldin MP, Chang K-J, Baltimore D. NF-kappaB-dependent induction of microRNA miR-146, an inhibitor targeted to signaling proteins of innate immune responses. *Proc Natl Acad Sci USA.* (2006) 103:12481–6. doi: 10.1073/pnas.0605298103
50. Nakasa T, Shibuya H, Nagata Y, Niimoto T, Ochi M. The inhibitory effect of microRNA-146a expression on bone destruction in collagen-induced arthritis. *Arthritis Rheum.* (2011) 63:1582–90. doi: 10.1002/art.30321
51. Ammari M, Presumey J, Ponsolles C, Roussignol G, Roubert C, Escriou V, et al. Delivery of miR-146a to Ly6C ^{high} monocytes inhibits pathogenic bone erosion in inflammatory arthritis. *Theranostics.* (2018) 8:5972–85. doi: 10.7150/thno.29313
52. Qu B, Xia X, Yan M, Gong K, Deng S, Huang G, et al. miR-218 is involved in the negative regulation of osteoclastogenesis and bone resorption by partial suppression of p38MAPK-c-Fos-NFATc1 signaling: potential role for osteopenic diseases. *Exp Cell Res.* (2015) 338:89–96. doi: 10.1016/j.yexcr.2015.07.023
53. Wang W, Yang L, Zhang D, Gao C, Wu J, Zhu Y, et al. MicroRNA-218 negatively regulates osteoclastogenic differentiation by repressing the nuclear factor-κB signaling pathway and targeting tumor necrosis factor receptor 1. *Cell Physiol Biochem.* (2018) 48:339–47. doi: 10.1159/000491740
54. Krzeszinski JY, Wei W, Huynh H, Jin Z, Wang X, Chang T-C, et al. miR-34a blocks osteoporosis and bone metastasis by inhibiting osteoclastogenesis and Tgif2. *Nature.* (2014) 512:431–5. doi: 10.1038/nature13375
55. Irie N, Takada Y, Watanabe Y, Matsuzaki Y, Naruse C, Asano M, et al. Bidirectional signaling through ephrinA2-EphA2 enhances osteoclastogenesis and suppresses osteoblastogenesis. *J Biol Chem.* (2009) 284:14637–44. doi: 10.1074/jbc.M807598200
56. Yang S, Zhang W, Cai M, Zhang Y, Jin F, Yan S, et al. Suppression of bone resorption by miR-141 in aged rhesus monkeys. *J Bone Miner Res.* (2018) 33:1799–812. doi: 10.1002/jbmr.3479
57. Omata Y, Yasui T, Hirose J, Izawa N, Imai Y, Matsumoto T, et al. Genomewide comprehensive analysis reveals critical cooperation between Smad and c-Fos in RANKL-induced osteoclastogenesis. *J Bone Miner Res.* (2015) 30:869–77. doi: 10.1002/jbmr.2418
58. Yu F, Xie C, Sun J, Peng W, Huang X. Overexpressed miR-145 inhibits osteoclastogenesis in RANKL-induced bone marrow-derived macrophages and ovariectomized mice by regulation of Smad3. *Life Sci.* (2018) 202:11–20. doi: 10.1016/j.lfs.2018.03.042
59. Fennen M, Pap T, Dankbar B. Smad-dependent mechanisms of inflammatory bone destruction. *Arthritis Res Ther.* (2016) 18:279. doi: 10.1186/s13075-016-1187-7
60. Zhao H, Zhang J, Shao H, Liu J, Jin M, Chen J, et al. Transforming growth factor β1/Smad4 signaling affects osteoclast differentiation via regulation of miR-155 expression. *Mol Cells.* (2017) 40:211–21. doi: 10.14348/molcells.2017.230
61. Zhang J, Zhao H, Chen J, Xia B, Jin Y, Wei W, et al. Interferon-β-induced miR-155 inhibits osteoclast differentiation by targeting SOCS1 and MITF. *FEBS Lett.* (2012) 586:3255–62. doi: 10.1016/j.febslet.2012.06.047
62. Su L-C, Huang A-F, Jia H, Liu Y, Xu W-D. Role of microRNA-155 in rheumatoid arthritis. *Int J Rheum Dis.* (2017) 20:1631–7. doi: 10.1111/1756-185X.13202
63. Sul O-J, Sung Y-B, Rajasekaran M, Ke K, Yu R, Back S-H, et al. MicroRNA-155 induces autophagy in osteoclasts by targeting transforming growth factor β-activated kinase 1-binding protein 2 upon lipopolysaccharide stimulation. *Bone.* (2018) 116:279–89. doi: 10.1016/j.bone.2018.08.014
64. Lu S-Y, Li M, Lin Y-L. Mitf regulates osteoclastogenesis by modulating NFATc1 activity. *Exp Cell Res.* (2014) 328:32–43. doi: 10.1016/j.yexcr.2014.08.018
65. Zhao H, Zhang J, Shao H, Liu J, Jin M, Chen J, et al. miRNA-340 inhibits osteoclast differentiation via repression of MITF. *Biosci Rep.* (2017) 37:BSR20170302. doi: 10.1042/BSR20170302
66. Kim JH, Kim N. Regulation of NFATc1 in osteoclast differentiation. *J Bone Metab.* (2014) 21:233–41. doi: 10.11005/jbm.2014.21.4.233
67. Lee Y, Kim HJ, Park CK, Kim Y-G, Lee H-J, Kim J-Y, et al. MicroRNA-124 regulates osteoclast differentiation. *Bone.* (2013) 56:383–9. doi: 10.1016/j.bone.2013.07.007
68. Nakamachi Y, Ohnuma K, Uto K, Noguchi Y, Saegusa J, Kawano S. MicroRNA-124 inhibits the progression of adjuvant-induced arthritis in rats. *Ann Rheum Dis.* (2016) 75:601–8. doi: 10.1136/annrheumdis-2014-206417
69. Tang L, Yin Y, Liu J, Li Z, Lu X. MiR-124 attenuates osteoclastogenic differentiation of bone marrow monocytes via targeting Rab27a. *Cell Physiol Biochem.* (2017) 43:1663–72. doi: 10.1159/000484027
70. Mizoguchi F, Murakami Y, Saito T, Miyasaka N, Kohsaka H. miR-31 controls osteoclast formation and bone resorption by targeting RhoA. *Arthritis Res Ther.* (2013) 15:R102. doi: 10.1186/ar4282
71. Strzelecka-Kiliszek A, Mebarek S, Roszkowska M, Buchet R, Magne D, Pikula S. Functions of Rho family of small GTPases and Rho-associated coiled-coil kinases in bone cells during differentiation and mineralization. *Biochim Biophys Acta Gen Subj.* (2017) 1861:1009–23. doi: 10.1016/j.bbagen.2017.02.005
72. Chellaiah MA, Soga N, Swanson S, McAllister S, Alvarez U, Wang D, et al. Rho-A is critical for osteoclast podosome organization, motility, and bone resorption. *J Biol Chem.* (2000) 275:11993–2002. doi: 10.1074/jbc.275.16.11993
73. Georgess D, Machuca-Gayet I, Blangy A, Jurdic P. Podosome organization drives osteoclast-mediated bone resorption. *Cell Adh Migr.* (2014) 8:191–204. doi: 10.4161/cam.27840
74. Cong F, Wu N, Tian X, Fan J, Liu J, Song T, et al. MicroRNA-34c promotes osteoclast differentiation through targeting LGR4. *Gene.* (2017) 610:1–8. doi: 10.1016/j.gene.2017.01.028
75. Luo J, Yang Z, Ma Y, Yue Z, Lin H, Qu G, et al. LGR4 is a receptor for RANKL and negatively regulates osteoclast differentiation and bone resorption. *Nat Med.* (2016) 22:539–46. doi: 10.1038/nm.4076
76. Heasman SJ, Ridley AJ. Mammalian Rho GTPases: new insights into their functions from *in vivo* studies. *Nat Rev Mol Cell Biol.* (2008) 9:690–701. doi: 10.1038/nrm2476
77. Rossi M, Pitari MR, Amodio N, Di Martino MT, Conforti F, Leone E, et al. miR-29b negatively regulates human osteoclastic cell differentiation and function: implications for the treatment of multiple myeloma-related bone disease. *J Cell Physiol.* (2013) 228:1506–15. doi: 10.1002/jcp.24306
78. Shimada-Sugawara M, Sakai E, Okamoto K, Fukuda M, Izumi T, Yoshida N, Tsukuba T. Rab27A regulates transport of cell surface receptors modulating multinucleation and lysosome-related organelles in osteoclasts. *Sci Rep.* (2015) 5:9620. doi: 10.1038/srep09620
79. Dou C, Zhang C, Kang F, Yang X, Jiang H, Bai Y, et al. MiR-7b directly targets DC-STAMP causing suppression of NFATc1 and c-Fos signaling during osteoclast fusion and differentiation. *Biochim Biophys Acta.* (2014) 1839:1084–96. doi: 10.1016/j.bbagrm.2014.08.002
80. Yin Y, Tang L, Chen J, Lu X. MiR-30a attenuates osteoclastogenesis via targeting DC-STAMP-c-Fos-NFATc1 signaling. *Am J Transl Res.* (2017) 9:5743–53.

81. Dou C, Ding N, Luo F, Hou T, Cao Z, Bai Y, et al. Graphene-based MicroRNA transfection blocks preosteoclast fusion to increase bone formation and vascularization. *Adv Sci.* (2018) 5:1700578. doi: 10.1002/advs.201700578
82. Kim K, Kim JH, Kim I, Lee J, Seong S, Park Y-W, et al. MicroRNA-26a regulates RANKL-induced osteoclast formation. *Mol Cells.* (2015) 38:75–80. doi: 10.14348/molcells.2015.2241
83. Fordham JB, Guilfoyle K, Naqvi AR, Nares S. MiR-142-3p is a RANKL-dependent inducer of cell death in osteoclasts. *Sci Rep.* (2016) 6:24980. doi: 10.1038/srep24980
84. Ma Y, Yang H, Huang J. Icariin ameliorates dexamethasone-induced bone deterioration in an experimental mouse model via activation of microRNA-186 inhibition of cathepsin K. *Mol Med Rep.* (2018) 17:1633–41. doi: 10.3892/mmr.2017.8065
85. Madel M-B, Ibáñez L, Rouleau M, Wakkach A, Blin-Wakkach C. A novel reliable and efficient procedure for purification of mature osteoclasts allowing functional assays in mouse cells. *Front Immunol.* (2018) 9:2567. doi: 10.3389/fimmu.2018.02567
86. Liu M, Sun Y, Zhang Q. Emerging role of extracellular vesicles in bone remodeling. *J Dent Res.* (2018) 97:859–68. doi: 10.1177/0022034518764411
87. Xie Y, Chen Y, Zhang L, Ge W, Tang P. The roles of bone-derived exosomes and exosomal microRNAs in regulating bone remodelling. *J Cell Mol Med.* (2017) 21:1033–41. doi: 10.1111/jcmm.13039
88. Yuan F-L, Wu Q-Y, Miao Z-N, Xu M-H, Xu R-S, Jiang D-L, et al. Osteoclast-derived extracellular vesicles: novel regulators of osteoclastogenesis and osteoclast-osteoblasts communication in bone remodeling. *Front Physiol.* (2018) 9:628. doi: 10.3389/fphys.2018.00628
89. Tao S-C, Guo S-C. Extracellular vesicles in bone: "dogrobbers" in the "eternal battle field." *Cell Commun Signal.* (2019) 17:6. doi: 10.1186/s12964-019-0319-5
90. Mestdagh P, Hartmann N, Baeriswyl L, Andreasen D, Bernard N, Chen C, et al. Evaluation of quantitative miRNA expression platforms in the microRNA quality control (miRQC) study. *Nat Methods.* (2014) 11:809–15. doi: 10.1038/nmeth.3014
91. Ishihara R, Hasegawa K, Hosokawa K, Maeda M. Multiplex MicroRNA detection on a power-free microfluidic chip with laminar flow-assisted dendritic amplification. *Anal Sci.* (2015) 31:573–6. doi: 10.2116/analsci.31.573
92. Wu X, Zhu S, Huang P, Chen Y. Highly specific quantification of microRNA by coupling probe-rolling circle amplification and Förster resonance energy transfer. *Anal Biochem.* (2016) 502:16–23. doi: 10.1016/j.ab.2016.03.001
93. Dard-Dascot C, Naquin D, d'Aubenton-Carafa Y, Alix K, Thermes C, van Dijk E. Systematic comparison of small RNA library preparation protocols for next-generation sequencing. *BMC Genomics.* (2018) 19:118. doi: 10.1186/s12864-018-4491-6
94. Rice J, Roberts H, Burton J, Pan J, States V, Rai SN, et al. Assay reproducibility in clinical studies of plasma miRNA. *PLoS ONE.* (2015) 10:e0121948. doi: 10.1371/journal.pone.0121948
95. Yeri A, Courtright A, Danielson K, Hutchins E, Alsop E, Carlson E, et al. Evaluation of commercially available small RNASeq library preparation kits using low input RNA. *BMC Genomics.* (2018) 19:331. doi: 10.1186/s12864-018-4726-6
96. Songia P, Chiesa M, Valerio V, Moschetta D, Myasoedova VA, D'Alessandra Y, et al. Direct screening of plasma circulating microRNAs. *RNA Biol.* (2018) 15:1268–72. doi: 10.1080/15476286.2018.1526538
97. Bustin SA, Benes V, Garson JA, Hellemans J, Huggett J, Kubista M, et al. The MIQE guidelines: minimum information for publication of quantitative real-time PCR experiments. *Clin Chem.* (2009) 55:611–22. doi: 10.1373/clinchem.2008.112797
98. Deng MC. The AlloMap^{TM} genomic biomarker story: 10 years after. *Clin Transplant.* (2017) 31:e12900. doi: 10.1111/ctr.12900
99. Haider BA, Baras AS, McCall MN, Hertel JA, Cornish TC, Halushka MK. A critical evaluation of microRNA biomarkers in non-neoplastic disease. *PLoS ONE.* (2014) 9:e89565. doi: 10.1371/journal.pone.0089565
100. Peltier HJ, Latham GJ. Normalization of microRNA expression levels in quantitative RT-PCR assays: identification of suitable reference RNA targets in normal and cancerous human solid tissues. *RNA.* (2008) 14:844–52. doi: 10.1261/rna.939908
101. Marabita F, de Candia P, Torri A, Tegnér J, Abrignani S, Rossi RL. Normalization of circulating microRNA expression data obtained by quantitative real-time RT-PCR. *Brief Bioinform.* (2016) 17:204–12. doi: 10.1093/bib/bbv056
102. Song J, Bai Z, Han W, Zhang J, Meng H, Bi J, et al. Identification of suitable reference genes for qPCR analysis of serum microRNA in gastric cancer patients. *Dig Dis Sci.* (2012) 57:897–904. doi: 10.1007/s10620-011-1981-7
103. Hu Z, Dong J, Wang L-E, Ma H, Liu J, Zhao Y, et al. Serum microRNA profiling and breast cancer risk: the use of miR-484/191 as endogenous controls. *Carcinogenesis.* (2012) 33:828–34. doi: 10.1093/carcin/bgs030
104. Zhang J, Song Y, Zhang C, Zhi X, Fu H, Ma Y, et al. Circulating MiR-16-5p and MiR-19b-3p as two novel potential biomarkers to indicate progression of gastric cancer. *Theranostics.* (2015) 5:733–45. doi: 10.7150/thno.10305
105. Luo H, Li X, Li T, Zhao L, He J, Zha L, et al. Exosomes/microvesicles microRNA-423-3p derived from cardiac fibroblasts mediates the cardioprotective effects of ischemic postconditioning. *Cardiovasc Res.* (2018) doi: 10.1093/cvr/cvy231. [Epub ahead of print].
106. Buschmann D, Kirchner B, Hermann S, Märte M, Wurmser C, Brandes F, et al. Evaluation of serum extracellular vesicle isolation methods for profiling miRNAs by next-generation sequencing. *Extracell Vesicles.* (2018) 7:1481321. doi: 10.1080/20013078.2018.1481321

13

Investigation of NF-κB-94ins/del ATTG and CARD8 (rs2043211) Gene Polymorphism in Acute Lymphoblastic Leukemia

Chen Zhang [1], Fengjiao Han [1], Jie Yu [1], Xiang Hu [1], Mingqiang Hua [1], Chaoqin Zhong [1], Ruiqing Wang [1], Xueyun Zhao [1], Yufeng Shi [2], Chunyan Ji [1,3] and Daoxin Ma [1]*

[1] Department of Hematology, Qilu Hospital of Shandong University, Jinan, China, [2] Institute for Financial Studies and School of Mathematics, Shandong University, Jinan, China, [3] Shandong Provincial Key Laboratory of Immunohematology, Qilu Hospital of Shandong University, Jinan, China

***Correspondence:**
Daoxin Ma
daoxinma@sdu.edu.cn

NLRP3 inflammasome has been widely implicated in the development and progression of various hematological diseases. However, how NLRP3 inflammasome contributes to the pathogenesis and clinical features of acute lymphoblastic leukemia (ALL) is still unknown. Here, in ALL patients' bone marrow, we investigated the single-nucleotide polymorphisms (SNPs) and expression of NLRP3 inflammasome related genes, NF-κB, NLRP3, IL-1β, IL-18, Caspase-1, and ASC. A total of 308 ALL patients and 300 healthy participants were included in this study. D allele and DD genotype under codominant model of NF-κB-94ins/del ATTG were showed as a protective factor in susceptibility of ALL. As for CARD8 (rs2043211), AT/TT genotype under dominant model and TT genotype under codominant model greatly increased the ALL susceptibility. We further studied the relationship between NLRP3 inflammasome genetic polymorphisms and clinical relevance. The results showed that DD genotype of NF-κB-94 ins/del ATTG and AT/TT genotype of CARD8 (rs2043211) contributed to lower WBC count and T-cell immunophenotype, respectively. Moreover, we also found that AT and TT genotypes of CARD8 (rs2043211), GT and TT genotypes of IL-1β (rs16944), and TT genotype of IL-18 (rs1946518) were associated with higher mRNA expression of NLRP3 inflammasome related genes and secretion of downstream cytokines. In conclusion, NF-κB-94 ins/del ATTG and CARD8 (rs2043211) genotypes might serve as novel biomarkers and potential targets for ALL.

Keywords: NLRP3, polymorphism, NF-κB, CARD8, acute lymphoblastic leukemia

INTRODUCTION

Acute lymphoblastic leukemia (ALL) is a clonal disorder driven by accumulation of progenitor cells in the peripheral blood and bone marrow (1, 2). Although adult ALL accounts for only 20% of leukemia, it is more common in childhood acute leukemia (80% of cases). Nowadays, through traditional chemotherapy, the cure rate of ALL can only reach about 20–40% in adults compared to 80% in children (3, 4). Adult patients present higher risk features at diagnosis, more likely to come up with chemotherapy resistance and higher relapse rate after complete remission (CR) (5). Multiple studies reported that the genetic variants of some metabolism and inflammation related genes contribute to ALL pathogenesis and prognosis (6, 7).

Inflammasomes are large cytosolic multiprotein complexes that assemble in response to infection or stress-associated stimuli and lead to the activation of caspase-1-mediated innate immune responses (8). The NOD-like receptor family was the first family of sensor proteins discovered to form inflammasomes. Among the inflammasomes, the NLRP3 inflammasome has been the most thoroughly studied. NLRP3 inflammasome is composed of NLRP3, the adaptor protein ASC (apoptosis-associated speck-like protein containing a CARD) and caspase-1 (9). NLRP3 inflammasome can be activated by exogenous pathogen invasion or *in vivo* cell damage and death, and then lead to the interaction of the PYD domain in NLRP3 and ASC proteins. Assembled inflammasome triggers the cleavage of dormant procaspase-1 into its active form, which turns the inactive proinflammatory cytokines pro-IL-1β and pro-IL-18 into mature and biologically active IL-1β and IL-18, respectively (10, 11). Caspase recruitment domain-containing protein (CARD) 8 interacts with cleaved caspase-1 and then triggers downstream inflammatory response through nuclear factor (NF)-κB pathway (12). NLRP3 inflammasome could modulate cellular levels of the glucocorticoid receptor and affect glucocorticoid resistance of ALL patients (13). However, it is still unknown whether and how NLRP3 inflammasome contributes to the pathogenesis and clinical features of ALL.

Nowadays, the advanced high-throughput techniques have boosted the discovery of genetic variations including copy number variants (CNVs), indels (deletions or insertions), structural variants and single nucleotide polymorphisms (SNPs) (14). SNPs of NLRP3 greatly influence pathogenic challenges and lead to disease outcome, such as autoimmune diseases (15), cardiovascular diseases (16), and malignant tumors (17). The SNP of CARD8 rs2043211 polymorphism has been confirmed to be associated with cardiovascular diseases according to a meta-analysis (18). Accumulating evidences have revealed that NF-κB-94 ins/del ATTG polymorphism is associated with cancer risk such as gastric cancer, hepatocellular carcinoma, and lung cancer (19–21). The polymorphism rs1946518 of NLRP3 effector molecule IL-18 has been shown to influence periodontitis (22) and hepatocellular carcinoma (23). The SNP rs16944 of the other NLRP3 effector molecule IL-1β has been reported contributing to cervical carcinoma (24) and gastritis risk (25). Thus, polymorphism of NLRP3 inflammasome related genes showed strong relevance with malignant tumors, but the regulatory role of the SNP of NLRP3 inflammasome related genes in the ALL bone marrow microenvironment has not been reported until now.

Therefore, to determine the susceptibility and clinical significance of the NLRP3 inflammasome in ALL, we examined the SNPs of four NLRP3 inflammasome related genes, including NF-κB-94ins/del ATTG, CARD8 (rs2043211), IL-18 (rs1946518), and IL-1β (rs16944). We are looking forward to provide evidences for clinical management of ALL.

MATERIALS AND METHODS

Study Subjects and Sample Collection

A total of 308 ALL patients and 300 sex- and age-matched healthy controls were included in this study. The diagnosis of enrolled ALL was based on NCCN Guidelines for acute lymphoblastic leukemia (ALL) (26). The demographic and clinical characteristics of these subjects were shown in **Table 1**. The protocol was approved by the Medical Ethics Committee of Qilu Hospital of Shandong University. Informed consents were obtained from the participants.

TABLE 1 | The demographic and clinical characteristics of ALL patients and controls.

	ALL patients	Controls
No.	308	300
Age, mean ± SD	38.76 ± 17.02	40.06 ± 12.98
Gender (M/F)	184/124	167/133
WBC count (<30*10^9/L / >30*10^9/L)	240/68	NA
Hb (<60 g/L/ > 60 g/L)	250/58	NA
Cr (<115 g/L/ > 115 g/L)	298/10	NA
Spleen (Splenomegaly/Non-Splenomegaly)	248/60	NA
AST (<125 g/L/>125 g/L)	291/17	NA
Fasting blood-glucose (normal/abnormal)	242/66	NA
Immunophenotype (T/B)	66/242	NA
Ph(Ph+/Ph–)	235/73	NA

For determination of polymorphisms, we collected anti-coagulated bone marrow or peripheral blood from ALL patients or peripheral blood from healthy controls. For testing the association of NLRP3 molecules mRNA expression or plasma levels with the genetic polymorphisms, we used bone marrow samples from newly-diagnosed ALL patients. Bone marrow or peripheral blood samples were centrifuged at 430 g for 5 min, and the plasma supernatants were frozen at −80°C for the determination of cytokines by ELISA. The mononuclear cells were isolated by Ficoll-Hypaque density gradient centrifugation, and re-suspended in sterile PBS and centrifuged again for 5 min at 430 g to remove remaining Ficoll solution. The mononuclear cells were stored −20°C for DNA and RNA extraction.

DNA Extraction and Genotyping

DNA was extracted using TIANamp Genomic DNA Kit (Tiangen, Beijing, China) according to the supplier's recommendations. The concentration and purity of DNA were accessed at 260/280 absorbance using NanoDrop spectrophotometer. The genotype of CARD8 (rs2043211), IL-18 (rs1946518), or IL-1β (rs16944) was performed using TaqMan® allelic discrimination assay (Cat# 4351379; Thermo Fisher Scientific, USA) in accordance with the manufacturer's instruction. Followed the standard protocol, 3 μl TaqMan Universal PCR Master Mix (2×), 0.15 μl pre-designed primers and probes (40×), 1 μl (100 ng/μl) of DNA and 1.85 μl ddH_2O make up the 6 μl volume reaction system. The NF-κB-94 ins/del ATTG polymorphism was examined by using the forward primer: 5′-CCG TGC TGC CTG CGT T-3′, reverse primer: 5′-GCT GGA GCC GGT AGG GAA-3′, and probe 1: 5′-VIC-ACC ATT GAT TGG GCC -MGB-3′ and probe 2: 5′-FAM-CGA CCA TTG GGC C -MGB-3′. A total 10 μl volume reaction system was composed of 5 μl TaqMan Universal PCR Master Mix (2×), 0.8 μl (10 μM) forward primer, 0.8 μl (10 μM) reverse

TABLE 2 | The primer sequences of real-time quantitative PCR.

Gene	Forward (5′-3′)	Reverse (5′-3′)
NF-κB	TCC AGA CCA ACA ACA ACC CC	GAT CTT GAG CTC GGC AGT GT
NLRP3	CAG ACT TCT GTG TGT GGG ACT GA	TCC TGA CAA CAT GCT GAT GTG A
IL-1β	GCC CTA AAC AGA TGA AGT GCT C	GAA CCA GCA TCT TCC TCA G
IL-18	GCT TGA ATC TAA ATT ATC AGT C	GAA GAT TCA AAT TGC ATC TTA T
Caspase-1	AAA TCT CAC TGC TTC GGA CAT G	GGA ACT TGC TGT CAG AGG TCT T
ASC	TGG ATG CTC TGT ACG GGA AG	CCA GGC TGG TGT GAA ACT GAA
GAPDH	GCT CTC TGC TCC TCC TGT TC	GTT GAC TCC GAC CTT CAC CT

TABLE 3 | The association between selected SNPs and susceptibility of ALL.

SNP	Model/Allele	Genotype/Allele	Controls		ALL patients		P value
			Count	%	Count	%	
NF-kB 94ins/delATTG	Allele	W	339	56.5	383	62.2	
		D	261	43.5	233	37.8	0.047
	Codominant	WW	98	32.7	119	38.6	
		WD	143	47.7	145	47.1	
		DD	59	19.6	44	14.3	0.027
CARD 8rs2043211	Dominant	AA	93	31	62	20.1	
		AT+TT	207	69	246	79.9	0.002
	Codominant	AA	93	31	62	20.1	
		AT	134	44.7	172	55.8	
		TT	73	24.3	74	24	0.004

primer, 0.2 μl (10 μM) probe 1, 0.2 μl (10 μM) probe 2, 2.0 μl ddH_2O and 1 μl (100 ng/μl) of DNA. ABI7500 Real-Time PCR system (Applied Biosystems, Foster City, CA, USA) was applied for TaqMan SNP genotyping assay, conditions as followed: 50°C for 2 min, 95°C for 10 min, and then 40 cycles of amplification (92°C denaturation for 15 s, 62°C annealing/extension for 60 s). ABI7500 software v 1.3 and TaqMan Genotyper software were used to analyze the genotyping.

Real-Time Quantitative PCR Detection for NF-κB, NLRP3, IL-1β, IL-18, Caspase-1, and ASC

We determined the mRNA expression of NF-κB, NLRP3, IL-1β, IL-18, Caspase-1, and ASC by real-time quantitative PCR. RNA was extracted using TRIzol reagent (Invitrogen Life Technologies, Carlsbad, CA). A total of 1 μg RNA was used for reverse transcription of total 10 μl volume by applying the PrimeScript RT reagent Kit Perfect Real Time (Takara Bio, Japan). The quantitative PCR was performed on the LightCycler 480II real-time PCR system (Roche, Switzerland) according to standard protocol. The primers were shown in **Table 2**. The quantitative PCR is a 10 μl volume, comprised of 5 μl of 2× SYBR Green Real-time PCR Master Mix, 1 μl of cDNA, 0.8 μl of the forward and reverse primers, and 3.2 μl ddH_2O. The results were expressed relative to the number of GAPDH transcripts used as an internal control.

ELISA for IL-18 and IL-1β

The levels of IL-18 and IL-1β in plasma were determined with a quantitative sandwich enzyme-linked immunosorbent assay (ELISA) in accordance with the manufacturer's recommendations (lower detection limits were 62.5 pg/ml for IL-18 and 3.9 pg/ml for IL-1β; IL-18 ELISA kit was bought from Abcam and IL-1β ELISA kit was bought from R&D systems, USA).

Statistical Analysis

The *p* value of the Hardy–Weinberg equilibrium (HWE) was calculated using the calculator available at the Helmholtz Center Munich website. In addition to allelic frequencies, we analyzed genotypic frequencies under three genetic models, specifically, the codominant, dominant, and recessive models. Association between the SNPs and ALL susceptibility was calculated by a chi-squared ($\chi 2$) test or a Fisher's exact test. Univariate logistic regression analysis was used to analyze *p* values and odds ratios (ORs) with a corresponding 95% confidence interval (95% CI). A two-tailed $p < 0.05$ was considered statistically significant. All statistical analysis was performed using SPSS 22.0 software (SPSS Inc., Chicago, IL, USA).

RESULTS

The Polymorphisms of NF-κB-94 ins/del ATTG and CARD8 (rs2043211) Contribute to the Susceptibility of All

We examined SNPs of NLRP3 inflammasome related genes: NF-κB (-94 ins/del ATTG), CARD8 (rs2043211), IL-18 (rs1946518), and IL-1β (rs16944) in 308 ALL patients and 300 healthy controls. The distribution of AT/TT genotype under dominant and TT genotype under codominant models for rs2043211 in CARD8 were found significantly different between ALL patients and controls. In addition, both the D allele in allelic frequencies and DD genotype under the codominant model of NF-κB−94 ins/del ATTG were significantly associated with the susceptibility to ALL ($p < 0.05$; **Table 3**).

Univariate logistic regression analysis was used for analyzing NF-κB and CARD8. For 94 ins/del ATTG in NF-κB, the frequency of D allele was lower in ALL patients compared to controls (37.8 vs. 43.5%), and it was significantly associated with ALL susceptibility (OR = 0.790, 95% CI 0.628–0.994, p = 0.044). Furthermore, the frequency of the DD genotype of NF-κB (14.3 vs. 19.6%) was obviously lower in ALL rather than homozygote insertion or wildtype (WW) genotype under codominant model, which hinted a significant association with ALL susceptibility (OR = 0.641, 95% CI 0.383–0.946, p = 0.043). For CARD8 under dominant model, the AT/TT genotype was significantly higher in ALL patients compared to controls (79.9 vs. 69.0%), and was associated with ALL susceptibility (OR = 1.783, 95% CI 1.230–2.583, p = 0.002). As for codominant model, both AT and TT genotypes of CARD8 (55.8 vs. 44.7%; 24.0 vs. 24.3%, respectively) were much higher in ALL compared to controls, and it significantly contributed to ALL susceptibility rather than AA genotype (OR = 1.925, 95% CI 1.300–2.583, p = 0.001; OR = 1.521, 95% CI 0.964–2.399, p = 0.072, respectively; **Table 4**). Interestingly, the distribution of CARD8 rs2043211 and NF-κB-94 ins/del ATTG was found different between ALL patients and controls. NF-κB polymorphism demonstrated a protective effect, while AT/TT genotype of CARD8 (rs2043211) greatly increased the ALL susceptibility.

DD Genotype of NF-κB-94 ins/del ATTG and AT/TT Genotype of CARD8 (rs2043211) Contribute to Lower WBC Count and T-Cell Immunophenotype, Respectively

According to NCCN Guidelines for ALL, several prognostic indicators are listed to indicate the prognosis. Our study analyzed the associations between these prognostic indicators and four SNPs of NLRP3 inflammasome genes, aimed to figure out

TABLE 4 | NF-κB-94 ins/del ATTG and CARD8 (rs2043211) contribute to susceptibility of ALL.

SNP	Model/Allele	Genotype/Allele	Controls		ALL patients		OR (95%CI)	*P* value
			Count	%	Count	%		
NF-kB 94ins/delATTG	Allele	W	339	56.5	383	62.2	1.000	
		D	261	43.5	233	37.8	0.790 (0.628–0.994)	0.044
	Codominant	WW	98	32.7	119	38.6	1.000	
		WD	143	47.7	145	47.1	0.835 (0.568–1.189)	0.317
		DD	59	19.6	44	14.3	0.614 (0.383–0.986)	0.043
CARD8rs2043211	Dominant	AA	93	31	62	20.1	1.000	
		AT+TT	207	69	246	79.9	1.783 (1.230–2.583)	0.002
	Codominant	AA	93	31	62	20.1	1.000	
		AT	134	44.7	172	55.8	1.925 (1.300–2.852)	0.001
		TT	73	24.3	74	24	1.521 (0.964–2.399)	0.072

TABLE 5 | The polymorphisms of NF-κB-94 ins/del ATTG and CARD8 (rs2043211) were associated with prognosis characteristics of ALL.

SNP	Model/Allele	Genotype/Allele	Clinical characteristic				OR (CI95%)	*P* value
			Count	%	Count	%		
NF-kB 94ins/del ATTG	Recessive		WBC Count<30		>30			
		WW+WD	192	80	64	94.1	1.000	
		DD	48	20	4	5.9	0.250 (0.087–0.721)	0.010
	Codominant		WBC Count<30		>30			
		WW	91	37.9	28	41.2	1.000	
		WD	109	45.4	36	52.9	1.073 (0.609–1.892)	0.807
		DD	40	16.7	4	5.9	0.325 (0.107–0.998)	0.048
CARD8 rs2043211	Dominant		IPT (B-cell)		IPT (T-cell)			
		AA	55	22.7	7	10.6	1.000	
		AT+TT	187	77.3	59	89.4	2.479 (1.071–5.738)	0.034
	Codominant		IPT (B-cell)		IPT (T-cell)			
		AA	55	22.7	7	10.6	1.000	
		AT	127	52.5	45	68.2	2.748(1.182–6.559)	0.019
		TT	60	24.8	14	21.2	1.833(0.689–4.876)	0.225

the correlation between NLRP3 genetic polymorphisms and prognosis of ALL.

We found that NF-κB-94 ins/del ATTG was significantly associated with the lower white blood cells (WBC) count, which is supposed to be a poor prognostic indicator as long as WBC count over $30*10^9$ /L. After univariate logistic regression analysis, compared with WD/WW genotype of NF-κB under recessive model, DD genotype significantly associated with a lower WBC count (20.0 vs. 5.9%; OR = 0.250, 95% CI 0.087–0.721, $p = 0.010$). Under codominant model, DD genotype also associated with a lower WBC count compared to WW genotype (16.7 vs. 5.9%; OR = 0.325, 95% CI 0.403–0.998, $p = 0.048$). NF-κB-94 ins/del ATTG under both recessive and codominant model, patients with DD genotype tend to have a lower WBC count (**Table 5**).

Furthermore, CARD8 (rs2043211) was also found to be correlated with immunophenotype of ALL, which primary divided into T-cell immunophenotype and B-cell immunophenotype. According to NCCN Guideline for ALL, immunophenotype is a strong prognostic indicator. Compared with AA genotype under dominant model, AT/TT genotype was associated with T-cell immunophenotype (77.3 vs. 89.4%; OR = 2.479, 95% CI 1.071–5.738, $p = 0.034$). Under codominant model, AT genotype was also associated with T-cell immunophenotype compared to AA genotype (52.5 vs. 68.2%; OR = 2.748, 95% CI 1.182–6.559, $p = 0.019$; **Table 5**). Thus, DD genotype of NF-κB-94 ins/del ATTG was showed as a protective factor, while AT/TT genotype of CARD8 (rs2043211) associated with a poor prognosis.

NF-κB-94 ins/del ATTG, IL-18 (rs1946518) and IL-1β (rs16944) Contribute to Clinical Characteristics of All Patients

The NLRP3 inflammasome genetic polymorphisms are also correlated with other clinical indicators of diagnosis, treatment approaches, and complication management. For NF-κB-94 ins/del ATTG, univariate logistic regression analysis revealed that DD genotype ($p = 0.046$) was

TABLE 6 | The association between selected SNPs and clinical characteristics of ALL patients.

SNP	Model/Allele	Genotype/Allele	Clinical characteristics				OR (CI95%)	*P* value
			Count	%	Count	%		
NF-kB	Recessive		Hb<60		>60			
94ins/delATTG		WW+WD	43	74.1	213	85.2	1.000	
		DD	15	25.9	37	14.8	0.498 (0.251–0.986)	0.046
			Splenomegaly		Non-Splenomegaly			
	Codominant	WW	99	39.9	20	33.3	1.000	
		WD	120	48.4	25	41.7	1.031 (0.541–1.966)	0.926
		DD	29	11.7	15	25	2.560 (1.165–5.625)	0.019
	Allele		Splenomegaly		Non-Splenomegaly			
		W	318	64.1	65	54.2	1.000	
		D	178	35.9	55	45.8	1.512 (1.010–2.262)	0.045
IL-18 rs1946518	Recessive		Splenomegaly		Non-Splenomegaly			
		GG+GT	194	78.2	38	63.3	1.000	
		TT	54	21.8	22	36.7	2.080 (1.135–3.811)	0.018
			AST<125		>125			
		GG+GT	223	76.6	9	52.9	1.000	
		TT	68	23.4	8	47.1	2.915 (1.083–7.848)	0.034
	Codominant		Glu<6.1		>6.1			
		GG	59	24.4	22	33.3	1.000	
		GT	121	50	34	51.5	0.754 (0.405–1.401)	0.371
		TT	62	25.6	10	15.2	0.433 (0.189–0.990)	0.047
	Allele		Glu<6.1		>6.1			
		G	239	49.4	78	59.1	1.000	
		T	245	50.6	54	40.9	0.675 (0.457–0.998)	0.049
IL-1β rs16944	Recessive		Cr<115		>115			
		GG+GT	219	73.5	4	40	1.000	
		TT	79	26.5	6	60	4.158 (1.143–15.122)	0.031
	Allele		Cr<115		>115			
		A	302	50.7	5	25	1.000	
		G	294	49.3	15	75	3.082 (1.106–8.587)	0.031

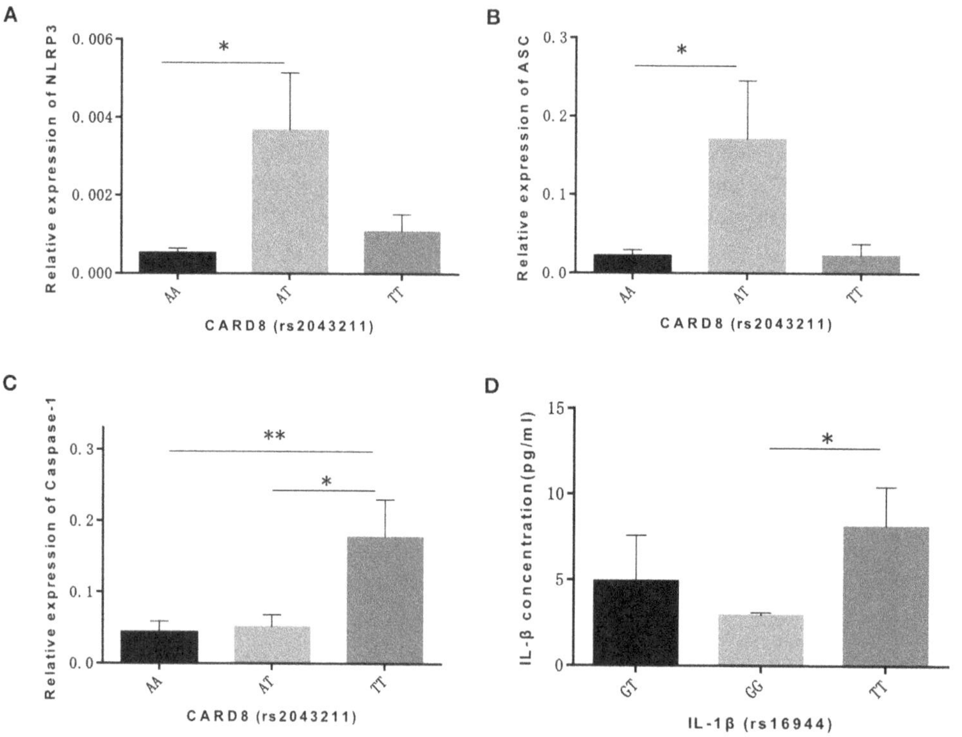

FIGURE 1 | CARD8 polymorphisms (rs2043211) was associated with the mRNA expression ofNLRP3 inflammasome related genes and its effective cytokines in ALL patients bone marrow microenvironment. AT genotype was correlated with higher mRNA expression ofNLRP3 **(A)** and ASC **(B)** compared to AA genotype, while TT genotype was correlated with higher caspase-1 **(C)** mRNA expression capared with AA and AT genotypes. TT genotype also contributed to the higher IL-18 concentration **(D)** in ALL patients bone marrow microenvironment. $^{*}p < 0.05$; $^{**}p < 0.01$.

statistically associated with hemoglobin (Hb) compared to WW/WD genotype under recessive model. Under codominant model, DD genotype ($p = 0.019$) was significantly associated with splenomegaly in contrast to WW genotype. As for the frequency of allele, compared with the−94insATTG (W) allele, the minor allele homozygotes were also associated with splenomegaly ($p = 0.045$; **Table 6**).

Under recessive model, TT genotype of IL-18 (rs1946518) was statistically correlated with both splenomegaly and AST concentration in serum compared with GG/GT genotype ($p = 0.018$, $p = 0.034$, respectively). In addition, TT genotype was also found to be related to the fasting blood-glucose under codominant model compared to GG genotype ($p = 0.047$). As for the frequency of allele, compared with the G allele, the T allele homozygote was also associated with the fasting blood-glucose ($p = 0.049$; **Table 6**).

Furthermore, the polymorphism in IL-1β rs16944 was supposed to have connection with creatinine concentration. Under recessive model, TT genotype ($p = 0.031$) was significantly associated with creatinine concentration by the contrast to GG/GT genotype. As for the frequency of allele, the G allele was also associated with creatinine concentration ($p = 0.031$; **Table 6**).

Association Between the Polymorphisms and the Expression of NLRP3 Inflammasome Related Genes

The pathogenesis and development of ALL involves a dysregulated immune microenvironment, which contains the production of multiple immunological effector proteins and the activation of the downstream pathways. To further comprehend the relationship between NLRP3 inflammasome related gene polymorphisms and its effective proteins, we use RT-PCR to examine NLRP3 inflammasome related gene expression at mRNA level, and ELISA to detect the secretion of effective proteins.

As for CARD8 (rs2043211), AT genotype showed a significant association with the higher mRNA expression levels of NLRP3 and ASC compared to AA genotype ($p = 0.017$, $p = 0.024$, respectively; **Figures 1A,B**). We also found that TT genotype was correlated with higher caspase-1 mRNA level when compared to both AA and AT genotype ($p = 0.009$, $p = 0.039$, respectively; **Figure 1C**). Moreover, TT genotype in CARD8 polymorphism was also found to be associated with IL-18 concentration in ALL bone marrow microenvironment compared to AA genotype (**Figure 1D**).

As for IL-1β (rs16944) polymorphism, GT genotype was significantly associated with IL-18 expression compared with

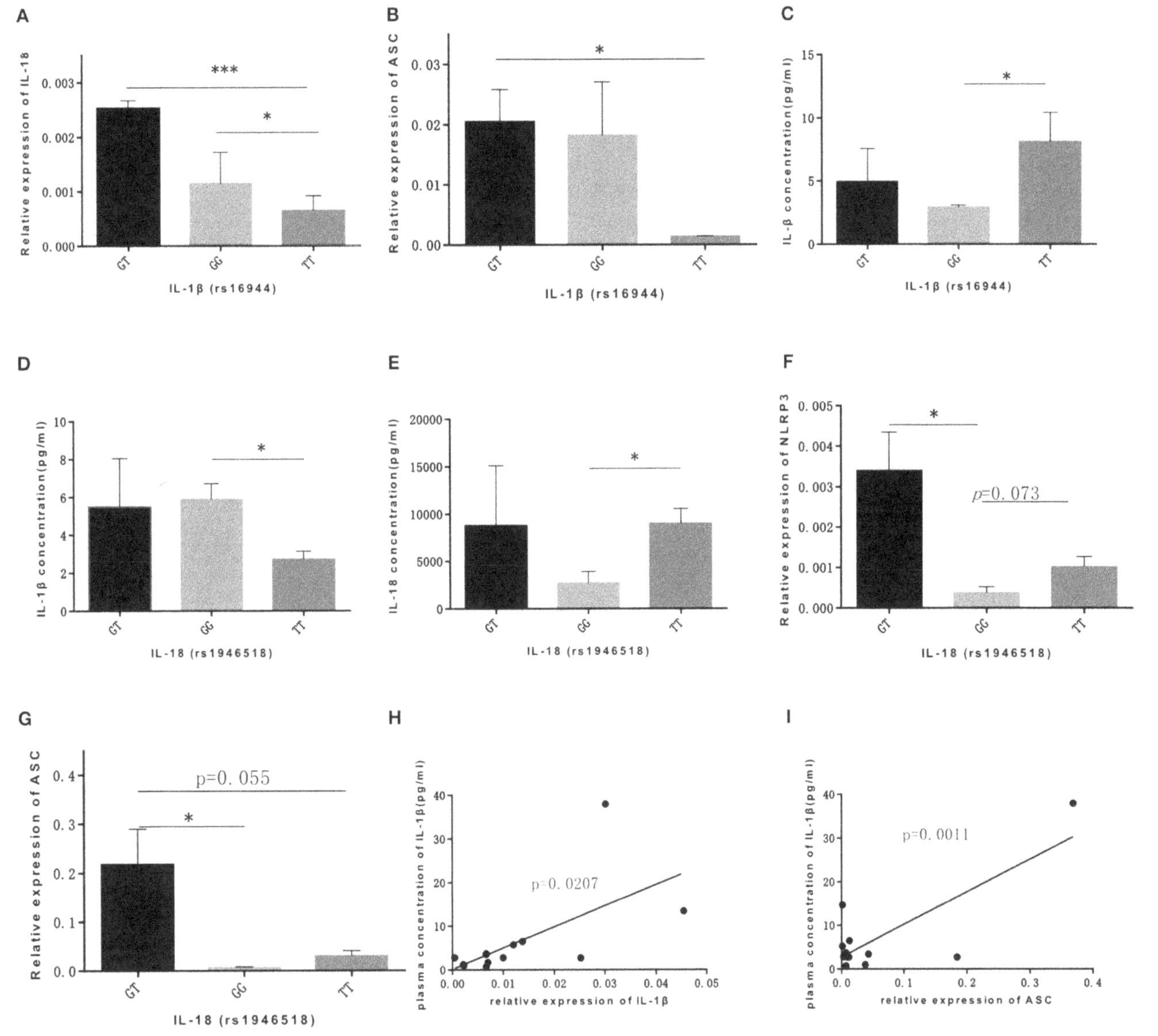

FIGURE 2 | IL-IP (rsl6944) and IL-18 (rsl946518) were associated with higher mRNA expression ofNLRP3 related genes and secreted cytokines. GT and GG genotypes of IL-IP (rsl6944) were associated with mRNA expression levels ofiL-18 **(A)** and ASC **(B)** compared to TT genotype. IL-I p concentration **(C)** was higher in ALL patients bone marrow with TT genotype. IL-I p concentration **(D)** or IL-18 concentration **(E)** were higher in GG or TT genotype of IL-18 (rs1946518) polymorphisms. NLRP3 **(F)** and ASC **(G)** mRNA expression levels were significant high in GT genotype ofiL-18 (rsl946518) polymorphisms. IL-IP concentration correlated with mRNA expression of IL-I p **(H)** and ASC **(I)**. *$p < 0.05$; ***$p < 0.001$.

GG and TT genotype ($p = 0.021$, $p = 0.000$, respectively; **Figure 2A**), and was also associated with ASC expression compared with TT genotype ($p = 0.045$; **Figure 2B**). Our data showed that TT genotype was correlated with IL-1β concentration ($p = 0.044$; **Figure 2C**). With the similar trend, TT genotype in IL-18 (rs1946518) polymorphism was also associated with both IL-1β and IL-18 concentration compared to GG genotype ($p = 0.029$, $p = 0.022$, respectively; **Figures 2D,E**). However, GT genotype in IL-18 polymorphism was related to a higher level of NLRP3 and ASC ($p = 0.034$, $p = 0.048$, respectively; **Figures 2F,G**). Besides, we also found significant correlation between concentration of IL-1β in bone marrow microenvironment and mRNA expression level of IL-1β and ASC ($p = 0.020$, $p = 0.001$, respectively; **Figures 2H,I**). Thus, AT and TT genotype of CARD8 (rs2043211), GT and TT genotype of IL-1β (rs16944) and TT genotype of IL-18 (rs1946518) were associated with higher mRNA expression of NLRP3 related genes and secreted cytokines.

DISCUSSION

ALL is a malignant blood disease with origins from somatic genetic alterations in bone marrow microenvironment (27). Though traditional chemotherapy has made a great progress in the last decade, ALL patients still have a poor prognosis. Compared with 90% 5-year overall survival in children, it is merely 30–40% in adult ALL. NLRP3 inflammasome systematically exists in human organism, and its activation has been identified as initiation of numerous diseases, such as immune diseases (28), cardiovascular diseases (29), gut homeostasis (30), and even malignant cancers (31). In hematological diseases, genetic polymorphisms of the NLRP3 have been reported to contribute to the pathogenesis of multiple myeloma (32) and lymphoma (33). But what is the correlation between NLRP3 inflammasome and ALL is still unknown. Therefore, our study mainly focused on the relationship between NLRP3 inflammasome and ALL in order to depict the internal communication between them.

We found that the DD genotype and D allele in NF-κB-94 ins/del ATTG was associated with a decreased risk of ALL, and had been considered as a protective factor. With the similar trend, under both recessive mode and codominant model, DD genotype exhibits as a protective factor on WBC count and Hb concentration. NF-κB-94 ins/del ATTG is considered as a protective factor for ALL patients. NF-κB is not only the downstream of NLRP3 inflammasome, but also is involved in many immune and inflammatory responses. In the resting state, NF-κB was found in cytoplasm, combined with several regulatory proteins, which inhibit its function (34, 35). After stimulating factors activate inflammatory responses, it moves into nucleus and binds to specific DNA sequences to modulate apoptosis and proliferation related genes (36). As NF-κB-94 ins/del ATTG polymorphism was determined as a protective factor in our study, this gene polymorphism may result in low affinity to nucleus; however, further studies need to be performed to illuminate its mechanisms.

On the contrary, CARD8 (rs2043211), another polymorphism we focused on, seems to increase the risk for ALL according to our study. It should be noted that TT genotype under codominant model increased the susceptibility of ALL, showed strong positive correlation with caspase-1 mRNA expression and the concentration of IL-18 in bone marrow microenvironment. CARD8 polymorphism was supposed to positively enhanced the NLRP3 inflammasome activation and the susceptibility of ALL.

Since we are aimed to provide new horizons for clinical management of ALL patients, we focused on several clinical indicators that may be related to prognosis. Though there were still many indicators we studied not listed in NCCN Guideline of prognostic indicators, they are significantly related to complications or the survival quality of ALL patients. According to our study, polymorphisms of IL-18 and IL-1β should be significantly associated with blood routine index, biochemical criterion.

In conclusion, our investigation found that NLRP3 inflammasome-related SNPs, especially NF-κB-94ins/del ATTG and CARD8 (rs2043211) genotype might serve as a novel biomarker and potential targets for ALL. Furthermore, IL-1 (rs16944) and IL-18 (rs1946518) polymorphism are able to predict the prognosis and guide the treatment of ALL. Further research with a larger sample size and in-depth mechanism study is required to validate the clinical potential of IL-1β (rs16944) and IL-18 (rs1946518) polymorphism.

AUTHOR CONTRIBUTIONS

DM and CJ conceived and designed the experiments. CZha performed the experiments. RW and FH analyzed the data. YS, CZho, and MH contributed reagents, materials, and analysis tools. XH and XZ wrote the paper. All authors read the manuscript critically and approved the submitted version.

FUNDING

This work was supported by grants from National Natural Science Foundation of China (No. 91642110, 81873439, 81470319), Shandong Key Research and Development Program (2017GSF218050), the Fundamental Research Funds of Shandong University (2018JC018), and grants from Taishan Scholars Program.

REFERENCES

1. Stock W, Johnson JL, Stone RM, Kolitz JE, Powell BL, Wetzler M, et al. Dose intensification of daunorubicin and cytarabine during treatment of adult acute lymphoblastic leukemia. *Cancer.* (2013) 119:90–8. doi: 10.1002/cncr.27617
2. Thomas DA, O'Brien S, Faderl S, Garcia-Manero G, Ferrajoli A, Wierda W, et al. Chemoimmunotherapy with a modified hyper-CVAD and rituximab regimen improves outcome in de novo Philadelphia chromosome-negative precursor B-lineage acute lymphoblastic leukemia. *J Clin Oncol.* (2010) 28:3880–9. doi: 10.1200/JCO.2009.26.9456
3. Kantarjian H, Thomas D, O'Brien S, Cortes J, Giles F, Jeha S, et al. Long-term follow-up results of hyperfractionated cyclophosphamide, vincristine, doxorubicin, and dexamethasone (Hyper-CVAD), a dose-intensive regimen, in adult acute lymphocytic leukemia. *Cancer-Am Cancer Soc.* (2004) 101:2788–801. doi: 10.1002/cncr.20668
4. Sive JI, Buck G, Fielding A, Lazarus HM, Litzow MR, Luger S, et al. Outcomes in older adults with acute lymphoblastic leukaemia (ALL): results from the international MRC UKALL XII/ECOG2993 trial. *Br J Haematol.* (2012) 157:463–71. doi: 10.1111/j.1365-2141.2012.09095.x
5. Hoelzer D, Walewski J, Dohner H, Viardot A, Hiddemann W, Spiekermann K, et al. Improved outcome of adult Burkitt lymphoma/leukemia with rituximab and chemotherapy: report of a large prospective multicenter trial. *Blood.* (2014) 124:3870–9. doi: 10.1182/blood-2014-03-563627
6. Milosevic G, Kotur N, Krstovski N, Lazic J, Zukic B, Stankovic B, et al. Variants in TPMT, ITPA, ABCC4 and ABCB1 genes as predictors of 6-mercaptopurine induced toxicity in children with acute lymphoblastic leukemia. *J Med Biochem.* (2018) 37:320–7. doi: 10.1515/jomb-2017-0060

7. Zehra A, Zehra S, Ismail M, Azhar A. Glutathione S-Transferase M1 and T1 gene deletions and susceptibility to acute lymphoblastic leukemia (all) in adults. *Pak J Med Sci.* (2018) 34:666–70. doi: 10.12669/pjms.343.14911
8. Franchi L, Munoz-Planillo R, Nunez G. Sensing and reacting to microbes through the inflammasomes. *Nat Immunol.* (2012) 13:325–32. doi: 10.1038/ni.2231
9. Lamkanfi M, Dixit VM. The inflammasomes. *PLoS Pathog.* (2009) 5:e1000510. doi: 10.1371/journal.ppat.1000510
10. Martinon F, Burns K, Tschopp J. The inflammasome: a molecular platform triggering activation of inflammatory caspases and processing of proIL-beta. *Mol Cell.* (2002) 10:417–26. doi: 10.1016/S1097-2765(02)00599-3
11. Wang L, Manji GA, Grenier JM, Al-Garawi A, Merriam S, Lora JM, et al. PYPAF7, a novel PYRIN-containing Apaf1-like protein that regulates activation of NF-kappa B and caspase-1-dependent cytokine processing. *J Biol Chem.* (2002) 277:29874–80. doi: 10.1074/jbc.M2039 15200
12. Strowig T, Henao-Mejia J, Elinav E, Flavell R. Inflammasomes in health and disease. *Nature.* (2012) 481:278–86. doi: 10.1038/nature10759
13. Paugh SW, Bonten EJ, Savic D, Ramsey LB, Thierfelder WE, Gurung P, et al. NALP3 inflammasome upregulation and CASP1 cleavage of the glucocorticoid receptor cause glucocorticoid resistance in leukemia cells. *Nat Genet.* (2015) 47:607–14. doi: 10.1038/ng.3283
14. Lander ES, Linton LM, Birren B, Nusbaum C, Zody MC, Baldwin J, et al. Initial sequencing and analysis of the human genome. *Nature.* (2001) 409:860–921. doi: 10.1038/35057062
15. Villani AC, Lemire M, Fortin G, Louis E, Silverberg MS, Collette C, et al. Common variants in the NLRP3 region contribute to Crohn's disease susceptibility. *Nat Genet.* (2009) 41:71–6. doi: 10.1038/ng.285
16. Grezzana GB, Vieira JL, Portal VL. Single-nucleotide polymorphisms: a perspective of cardiovascular prevention. *Rev Assoc Med Bras.* (2015) 61:458–68. doi: 10.1590/1806-9282.61.05.458
17. Howell WM, Rose-Zerilli MJ. Cytokine gene polymorphisms, cancer susceptibility, and prognosis. *J Nutr.* (2007) 137:194S–9S. doi: 10.1093/jn/137.1.194S
18. Huang H, Bi Q, Wei H, Luo B, He Y. Association between caspase recruitment domain-containing protein 8 rs2043211 polymorphism and cardiovascular disease susceptibility: a systematic review and meta-analysis. *Anatol J Cardiol.* (2018) 20:70–6. doi: 10.14744/AnatolJCardiol.2018.32650
19. Ungerback J, Belenki D, Jawad UA, Fredrikson M, Fransen K, Elander N, et al. Genetic variation and alterations of genes involved in NFkappaB/TNFAIP3- and NLRP3-inflammasome signaling affect susceptibility and outcome of colorectal cancer. *Carcinogenesis.* (2012) 33:2126–34. doi: 10.1093/carcin/bgs256
20. Cheng CW, Su JL, Lin CW, Su CW, Shih CH, Yang SF, et al. Effects of NFKB1 and NFKBIA gene polymorphisms on hepatocellular carcinoma susceptibility and clinicopathological features. *PLoS ONE.* (2013) 8:e56130. doi: 10.1371/journal.pone.0056130
21. Oltulu YM, Coskunpinar E, Ozkan G, Aynaci E, Yildiz P, Isbir T, et al. Investigation of NF-kappaB1 and NF-kappaBIA gene polymorphism in non-small cell lung cancer. *Biomed Res Int.* (2014) 2014:530381. doi: 10.1155/2014/530381
22. Tanaka K, Miyake Y, Hanioka T, Furukawa S, Miyatake N, Arakawa M. The IL18 promoter polymorphism, rs1946518, is associated with the risk of periodontitis in japanese women: the kyushu okinawa maternal and child health study. *Tohoku J Exp Med.* (2017) 243:159–64. doi: 10.1620/tjem.243.159
23. Zhu SL, Zhao Y, Hu XY, Luo T, Chen ZS, Zhang Y, et al. Genetic polymorphisms−137 (rs187238) and−607 (rs1946518) in the interleukin-18 promoter may not be associated with development of hepatocellular carcinoma. *Sci Rep.* (2016) 6:39404. doi: 10.1038/srep39404
24. Dutta S, Chakraborty C, Mandal RK, Basu P, Biswas J, Roychoudhury S, et al. Persistent HPV16/18 infection in Indian women with the A-allele (rs6457617) of HLA-DQB1 and T-allele (rs16944) of IL-1beta−511 is associated with development of cervical carcinoma. *Cancer Immunol Immunother.* (2015) 64:843–51. doi: 10.1007/s00262-015-1693-5
25. Sun X, Cai H, Li Z, Li S, Yin W, Dong G, et al. Association between IL-1β polymorphisms and gastritis risk: a meta-analysis. *Medicine.* (2017) 96:e6001. doi: 10.1097/MD.0000000000006001
26. Brown PA, Shah B, Fathi A, Wieduwilt M, Advani A, Aoun P, et al. NCCN guidelines insights: acute lymphoblastic leukemia, Version 1.2017. *J Natl Compr Canc Netw.* (2017) 15:1091–102. doi: 10.6004/jnccn.2017.0147
27. Hunger SP, Mullighan CG. Acute lymphoblastic leukemia in children. *N Engl J Med.* (2015) 373:1541–52. doi: 10.1056/NEJMra1400972
28. Zhong Z, Sanchez-Lopez E, Karin M. Autophagy, NLRP3 inflammasome and auto-inflammatory/immune diseases. *Clin Exp Rheumatol.* (2016) 34:12–16.
29. Liu D, Zeng X, Li X, Mehta JL, Wang X. Role of NLRP3 inflammasome in the pathogenesis of cardiovascular diseases. *Basic Res Cardiol.* (2017) 113:5. doi: 10.1007/s00395-017-0663-9
30. Zambetti LP, Mortellaro A. NLRPs, microbiota, and gut homeostasis: unravelling the connection. *J Pathol.* (2014) 233:321–30. doi: 10.1002/path.4357
31. Karki R, Man SM, Kanneganti TD. Inflammasomes and Cancer. *Cancer Immunol Res.* (2017) 5:94–9. doi: 10.1158/2326-6066.CIR-16-0269
32. Zhao X, Hua M, Yan S, Yu J, Han F, Zhong C, et al. The genetic polymorphisms of NLRP3 inflammasome associated with t helper cells in patients with multiple myeloma. *J Immunol Res.* (2018) 2018:7569809. doi: 10.1155/2018/7569809
33. Zhao X, Zhang C, Hua M, Wang R, Zhong C, Yu J, et al. NLRP3 inflammasome activation plays a carcinogenic role through effector cytokine IL-18 in lymphoma. *Oncotarget.* (2017) 8:108571–83. doi: 10.18632/oncotarget.21010
34. DiDonato J, Mercurio F, Rosette C, Wu-Li J, Suyang H, Ghosh S, et al. Mapping of the inducible IkappaB phosphorylation sites that signal its ubiquitination and degradation. *Mol Cell Biol.* (1996) 16:1295–304. doi: 10.1128/MCB.16.4.1295
35. Chen ZJ, Parent L, Maniatis T. Site-specific phosphorylation of IkappaBalpha by a novel ubiquitination-dependent protein kinase activity. *Cell.* (1996) 84:853–62. doi: 10.1016/S0092-8674(00)81064-8
36. Arenzana-Seisdedos F, Thompson J, Rodriguez MS, Bachelerie F, Thomas D, Hay RT. Inducible nuclear expression of newly synthesized I kappa B alpha negatively regulates DNA-binding and transcriptional activities of NF-kappa B. *Mol Cell Biol.* (1995) 15:2689–96. doi: 10.1128/MCB.15. 5.2689

14

Inhibition of JAK1/2 Tyrosine Kinases Reduces Neurogenic Heterotopic Ossification After Spinal Cord Injury

Kylie A. Alexander[1†], Hsu-Wen Tseng[1†], Whitney Fleming[1], Beulah Jose[1], Marjorie Salga[1,2], Irina Kulina[1], Susan M. Millard[1], Allison R. Pettit[1], François Genêt[2,3] and Jean-Pierre Levesque[1]*

[1] Mater Research Institute – The University of Queensland, Translational Research Institute, Woolloongabba, QLD, Australia, [2] CIC-IT 1429, Service de Médecine Physique et de Réadaptation, Raymond Poincaré University Hospital, AP-HP, Garches, France, [3] Université de Versailles Saint Quentin en Yvelines, END:ICAP Inserm U1179, Montigny le Bretonneux, France

***Correspondence:**
Jean-Pierre Levesque
jp.levesque@mater.uq.edu.au

† These authors share first authorship

Neurogenic heterotopic ossifications (NHO) are very incapacitating complications of traumatic brain and spinal cord injuries (SCI) which manifest as abnormal formation of bone tissue in periarticular muscles. NHO are debilitating as they cause pain, partial or total joint ankylosis and vascular and nerve compression. NHO pathogenesis is unknown and the only effective treatment remains surgical resection, however once resected, NHO can re-occur. To further understand NHO pathogenesis, we developed the first animal model of NHO following SCI in genetically unmodified mice, which mimics most clinical features of NHO in patients. We have previously shown that the combination of (1) a central nervous system lesion (SCI) and (2) muscular damage (via an intramuscular injection of cardiotoxin) is required for NHO development. Furthermore, macrophages within the injured muscle play a critical role in driving NHO pathogenesis. More recently we demonstrated that macrophage-derived oncostatin M (OSM) is a key mediator of both human and mouse NHO. We now report that inflammatory monocytes infiltrate the injured muscles of SCI mice developing NHO at significantly higher levels compared to mice without SCI. Muscle infiltrating monocytes and neutrophils expressed OSM whereas mouse muscle satellite and interstitial cell expressed the OSM receptor (OSMR). *In vitro* recombinant mouse OSM induced tyrosine phosphorylation of the transcription factor STAT3, a downstream target of OSMR:gp130 signaling in muscle progenitor cells. As STAT3 is tyrosine phosphorylated by JAK1/2 tyrosine kinases downstream of OSMR:gp130, we demonstrated that the JAK1/2 tyrosine kinase inhibitor ruxolitinib blocked OSM driven STAT3 tyrosine phosphorylation in mouse muscle progenitor cells. We further demonstrated *in vivo* that STAT3 tyrosine phosphorylation was not only significantly higher but persisted for a longer duration in injured muscles of SCI mice developing NHO compared to mice with muscle injury without SCI. Finally, administration of ruxolitinib for 7 days post-surgery significantly reduced STAT3 phosphorylation in injured muscles *in vivo* as well as NHO volume at all analyzed time-points up to 3 weeks post-surgery. Our results identify the JAK/STAT3 signaling pathway as a potential therapeutic target to reduce NHO development following SCI.

Keywords: spinal cord injury complications, heterotopic ossification, JAK- STAT signaling pathway, ruxolitinib, oncostatin M receptor

INTRODUCTION

Neurogenic heterotopic ossification (NHO) is the abnormal formation of extra-skeletal bones in muscles (1), mostly periarticular (2), and is a frequent and very incapacitating complication in patients with spinal cord injury (SCI) (15–25%) and traumatic brain injuries (5–12%) (3, 4). NHO prevalence is higher in combat-inflicted trauma particularly in victims of explosive blasts with associated SCI or TBI where NHO prevalence is over 60% (5, 6). NHOs are debilitating due to their size (up to 2 kg), causing significant pain and gradual reduction in the range of motion of affected limbs, often progressing to complete joint ankylosis. This exacerbates functional disabilities by increasing difficulty in sitting, eating and dressing (7). NHO growth can also cause nerve, blood vessel compression, and irreversibly damage the affected joint further increasing patient morbidity (8). Despite knowing this pathology for 100 years, treatment is currently limited to surgical resection after NHO have matured and become symptomatic (2, 7, 9–11). The surgical procedure is challenging, particularly when ossifications entrap joints, large blood vessels and nerves. Furthermore, even after resection, NHO recurrence is observed in at least 6% patients (1, 2, 9, 12). The development of improved treatments for NHO has been slow and trials of pharmacological interventions have continued to show limited effectiveness, reflecting the current limited knowledge on the etiology and pathophysiology of NHO. Identification of therapeutic targets to block NHO development in SCI/TBI patients remains a priority in order to decrease the prevalence and morbidity of this pathology (5).

We have developed the first clinically relevant animal model of NHO following SCI in genetically unmodified mice (13). In this model the combination of two injuries is necessary to trigger NHO development in the muscle: a severe lesion of the central nervous system such as a SCI in combination with a muscle injury (13). Development of NHO following spinal cord transection in this model was triggered by macrophages infiltrating damaged muscles exclusively in the context of a complete SCI (13, 14). More recently we established that the inflammatory cytokine oncostatin M (OSM) secreted in part by macrophages infiltrating the inflamed muscle contribute to both human and mouse NHO development (15). This is consistent with the pleiotropic role of OSM in regulating skeletal bone formation and resorption (16, 17) and the previous demonstration that macrophage-derived OSM can promote mesenchymal stem cell osteogenic differentiation (18) and intramembranous bone formation (19). OSM was shown to be elevated in the serum of patients developing NHO and OSM produced by activated macrophages isolated from NHO biopsies promoted osteoblastic differentiation and mineralization of human muscle-derived stromal cells extracted from NHOs (15). Likewise in mice, SCI caused the abnormal and persistent expression of OSM in the injured muscles. Importantly, mice defective for the OSM receptor (OSMR) α chain gene *Osmr* had significantly reduced NHO volumes in response to SCI and muscle injury (15). Overall our results provide strong evidence that macrophages contribute to NHO formation in part through the osteogenic action of OSM on muscle cells suggesting that OSM/OSMR signaling could be a suitable therapeutic target for NHO.

OSM is a member of the interleukin (IL)-6 family of cytokines which include IL-6, IL-11, leukemia inhibitory factor (LIF), cardiotrophin-1, and ciliary neurotrophic factor. These cytokines bind to diverse heteromeric receptors with a common glycoprotein 130 (Gp130) chain. Binding of IL-6 family cytokines to their cognate receptors, all of which comprise a common gp130 subunit, causes the activation of Janus tyrosine kinase (JAK)-1 and JAK2 which in turn tyrosine phosphorylate signal transducer and activator of transcription (STAT)-1 and STAT3 (20, 21). Once tyrosine phosphorylated (p), pSTAT1, and pSTAT3 translocate to the nucleus and activate the transcription of a large array of genes depending on the cell type. Mouse OSM binds with a strong affinity to the OSMR:gp130 complex and with a 30-fold lower affinity to the leukemia inhibitory factor receptor (LIFR):gp130 complex (22). Typically, OSM binding to the OSMR:gp130 complex causes the phosphorylation and activation of both STAT1 and STAT3 via JAK1/2 (23, 24) which in turns leads the transcription of a large range of genes that include suppressor of cytokine signaling (SOCS)-3. A negative feed-back loop is triggered by SOCS3, which binds to both gp130 and activated JAKs, suppressing this signaling cascade and STAT1 and STAT3 activation (25, 26).

Since OSM and OSMR play an important role in NHO pathogenesis following SCI (15), we further examined STAT3 activation status in mouse muscles during NHO development. We confirmed that muscle satellite and interstitial cells isolated from mouse muscles express OSMR, with JAK1/2-dependant tyrosine phosphorylation of STAT3 in response to OSM. In addition, we found higher and persistent STAT3 tyrosine phosphorylation in injured muscles of SCI mice developing NHO. We show that this persistent STAT3 phosphorylation and activation in the injured muscle is an important driver of NHO as administration of ruxolitinib, a small synthetic inhibitor of JAK1/2 tyrosine kinases used to treat myelofibrosis and polycythemia vera caused by activating mutations of JAK2 (27, 28), significantly reduced STAT3 phosphorylation in the injured muscles of mice. Importantly, ruxolitinib administration also significantly reduced NHO development following SCI.

MATERIALS AND METHODS

Animals

C57BL/6 mice were obtained from Animal Resource Center (Perth, Australia). All mouse procedures were approved by the Health Sciences Animal Ethics Committee of The University of Queensland and performed in accordance with the Australian Code of Practice for the Care and Use of Animals for Scientific Purposes.

NHO Mouse Model

NHO mouse model was carried out as previously described (15) by performing a spinal cord transection between T11 and T13 together with intramuscular injection (i.m.) of cardiotoxin (CDTX) purified from the venom of Naja pallida (Latoxan) at 0.32 mg/kg in the hamstring muscles under general anesthesia

(100 mg/kg Ketamine, 10 mg/kg xylazine, and 1% isofluorane). Control mice underwent sham-surgery and/or intramuscular injection of equal volume of phosphate buffered saline (PBS). In this model, NHO develop in the CDTX-injected muscle within 1–3 weeks (13, 15). Post-surgery, mice were administered ruxolitinib phosphate (LC Laboratories) 60 mg/kg by oral gavage twice daily from day 0 to day 7 post-surgery. Ruxolitinib phosphate powder was first dissolved as a 4X stock in dimethyl sulfoxide (DMSO) then diluted to 1X in vehicle (5 mg/ml hydroxypropyl methylcellulose, 0.1% Tween 20 in water). Control mice were gavaged with 25% DMSO in vehicle.

Tissue Collection

At 1–3 weeks post-surgery mice were euthanized by CO_2 asphyxiation. For histological analysis, the hind limbs were fixed in PBS with 4% paraformaldehyde as previously described (15). For western blots, muscle samples were harvested at specified time points and immediately placed in ice-cold protein extraction buffer (300 mM NaCl, 30 mM Tris-HCl, 1% Triton-X 100) containing a house made cocktail of phosphatase inhibitors (10 mM EDTA, 0.1% NaN_3, 20 mM NaF, 1 mM Na_3VO_4, 10 mM β-glycerophosphate, 10 mM levamisole) buffered at pH 7.4 and supplemented with 1X protease inhibitor cocktail (Complete™ ULTRA Tablets, Roche) and snap frozen in liquid nitrogen until extraction.

Muscle Cell Isolation, Sorting, and Culture

Isolation, sorting and culture of muscle $CD45^-Ter119^-CD31^-CD34^+Sca1^-$ satellite cells and $CD45^-Ter119^-CD31^-CD34^+Sca1^+$ interstitial cells was carried out as previously described (15). For pSTAT3 phos-flow analysis, cultured muscle satellite cells, interstitial cells, and the mouse mesenchymal progenitor cell line Kusa4b10 cells (29, 30) were detached by incubating cell monolayers in PBS plus 4 mM EDTA for 5 min at 37°C. Once in suspension, cells were washed in Dulbecco modified essential medium (DMEM, Gibco, Life Technologies), centrifuged and resuspended in DMEM. Cell aliquots (1×10^6) were then preincubated with or without 1 μM ruxolitinib (LC Laboratories), for 30 min at 37°C and subsequently stimulated by addition of 25 ng/mL recombinant mouse OSM (R&D Systems) for 10 min. Cells were then immediately washed in 10 mL ice cold Tris-buffered saline pH 7.4 containing 1 mM Na_3VO_4, centrifuged, and cell pellets resuspended for fixation and permeabilization (BD Cytofix, Perm buffer IV, BD Biosciences) for 10 and 30 min respectively, cells were then stained with AlexaFluor647-conjugated mouse anti-pSTAT3 (pY705) monoclonal antibody (BD Biosciences, catalog # 557815) for 30 min on ice, cells were then washed and subsequently run on a LSR Fortessa x20 flow cytometer (BD Biosciences). Files were subsequently analyzed with Flow Jo software version 10.4.

Protein Extraction and Western Blot

Frozen muscle samples were thawed and homogenized using a TissueRuptor (Qiagen), in ice cold protein extraction buffer for 3 rounds of 20 s at top speed, incubated on a horizontal rotator at 4°C for 15 min. Tissue debris were removed by centrifugation at 15,000 g at 4°C for 20 min. Supernatants were taken and protein concentrations measured using a BCA assay (ThermoFisher). Muscle lysates (25 μg protein per lane, one separate mouse per lane) were loaded on a 4–12% acrylamide Bis-Tris pre-cast gel (ThermoFisher), and subsequently wet transferred onto a Hybond C Extra membrane (Amersham Biosciences) and blocked with Odyssey Blocking Buffer. Primary antibodies included an anti-total-STAT3 rabbit monoclonal antibody (mAb) clone 79D7 diluted at 1/2,000 (Cell Signaling), anti-phospho-STAT3 (Tyr705) XP® rabbit mAb clone D3A7 (Cell Signaling) diluted 1/1,000. IRDye® 800CW-conjugated donkey anti-rabbit IgG (H+L) (LI-COR Biosciences) was used to detect primary antibodies using an Odyssey scanner (LI-COR Biosciences). Western blot zip files were uploaded onto Image Studio Lite Software (Version 5.2). Boxes were drawn around the bands with background boarder width set at 2 value for above and below the box. Intensity values minus background of pSTAT3 were divided by the values obtained for total STAT3, normalized to the average value obtained in control mice (SHAM+PBS) at the defined time-point, plotted, and significance calculated.

Mouse Muscle Monocyte Isolation

All leukocytes were isolated from either SHAM-operated or SCI mice with an intramuscular injection of CDTX as described above. Injected hamstrings were harvested at 4 days post-surgery and muscle monocyte populations were isolated using a skeletal muscle dissociation kit (Miltenyi Biotech). In brief, hamstrings were cut into 1 mm pieces and up to 0.5 g of tissue was used per dissociation sample as per manufactures instructions. Total muscle leukocytes were subsequently separated into multiple populations using a Beckman Coulter Life Sciences CytoFLEX benchtop flow cytometer using the following antibodies (Biolegend); PerCP/Cyanine (CY) 5.5 anti-mouse/human CD11b (clone M1/70), FITC anti-mouse CD48 (clone HM48-1), APC anti-mouse F4/80 (clone BM8), Pacific Blue™ anti-mouse Ly-6C (clone HK1.4), APC/Cy7 anti-mouse Ly-6G (clone 1A8), and Zombie Aqua™ Fixable Viability Kit. Subsequently total muscle leukocytes were also sorted into multiple populations using a BD FACS Aria Fusion using the following antibodies (Biolegend): Brilliant Violet 785™ anti-mouse CD45 (clone 30-F11), FITC anti-mouse TER-119/Erythroid Cells (clone TER-119), FITC anti-mouse/human CD45R/B220 (clone RA3-6B2), FITC anti-mouse CD3ε (clone 145-2C11), APC anti-mouse F4/80 (clone BM8), Brilliant Violet 510™ anti-mouse/human CD11b (clone M1/70), PE anti-mouse Ly-6G (clone 1A8), APC/Cy7 anti-mouse CD48 (clone HM48-1), Pacific Blue™ anti-mouse Ly-6C (clone HK1.4), and 7-aminoactinomycin D (Life Technologies). Files were subsequently analyzed with Flow Jo software version 10.4. Muscle monocyte populations were sorted directly into trizol LS (ThermoFisher) and frozen until extraction.

mRNA Extraction and qRT-PCR Analysis

For RNA isolation, frozen muscle was homogenized using a TissueRuptor (Qiagen), directly in Trizol (Life Technologies). After chloroform separation, RNA was isolated from aqueous phase. mRNA of sorted and cultured cells was isolated using chloroform separation followed by GeneJET RNA cleanup and concentration micro kit (ThermoFisher). Reverse transcription was performed using the iScript cDNA kit (BioRad) as per manufacturer's instructions. Analysis of mRNA expression for *Osm, Osmr, and Hprt* and was carried out using the Taqman Fast Advanced Master Mix and primer / probe sets (ThermoFisher): *Osmr* (Mm01307326_m1), *Osm* (Mm01193966_m1), and *Hprt* (Mm03024075_m1) on ViiA 7 Real-Time PCR System (Life Technologies) with PCR setting: 20 s at 95°C, then 40 cycles of 95°C (1 s) and 60°C (20 s). Results were normalized relative to *Hprt* mRNA expression.

Micro-Computerized Tomography (μCT) and NHO Volume Quantification

NHO volume was measured *in vivo* or *ex vivo* using the Inveon positron emission tomography/computed tomography (PET-CT) multimodality system (Siemens Medical Solutions Inc.) as previously described (15). In brief, parameters were as follows: 360° rotation, 180 projections, 500 ms exposure time, 80 kV voltage, 500 μA current, and effective pixel size 36 μm. 3D reconstitutions were performed with the Inveon Research Workplace (Siemens Medical Solutions). To calculate NHO volumes, the region of interest (ROI) was drawn around the muscles containing NHO, and was carefully checked from three dimensions. After defining the ROI, the NHO region was defined by setting the threshold Hounsfield units (HU) to 450 HU.

Histology

Fixed hind limbs were decalcified and processed as previously described (15). Five μm sections were cut and stained using Masson's Trichrome. In brief sections were deparaffinized and rehydrated then stained for 10 min in Weigert's iron hematoxylin, rinsed under tap water for 10 min, differentiated in 1% acid alcohol (1% hydrochloric acid) for 15–30 s, rinsed in tap water (3 min) then distilled water, followed by staining in Biebrich scarlet-acid fuchsine solution for 10–15 min (Biebrich scarlet, 1% aqueous, Acid fuchsine, 1% aqueous, glacial acetic acid), slides are then washed in distilled water and differentiated in 5% phosphomolybdic −5% phosphotungstic acid solution for 10–15 min or until collagen is not red. Slides were transferred into aniline blue solution for 5–10 min and rinsed in 1% acetic acid for 2–5 min, dehydrated, and mounted in resinous mounting medium. Immunohistochemistry was performed as previously described (15). Primary antibodies used were: rat anti-mouse F4/80 mAb (clone CI:A3-1, Abcam), rabbit anti-mouse Osterix/Sp7 polyclonal IgG (ab22552, Abcam), rabbit anti-mouse collagen type 1 polyclonal IgG (C7510-13, US Biological), or relevant isotype control antibodies; ratIgG2b (400602, Biolegend), or rabbit IgG (ab27478, Abcam). A 3-step procedure was employed using biotinylated F(ab)2 secondary antibodies (biotinylated goat anti-rat IgG and goat anti-rabbit IgG antibodies, Vector Labs) and VECTASTAIN Elite ABC -Peroxidase Kit (Vector Labs), was used to detect primary antibodies. Slides were viewed using an Olympus BX50 microscope with an attached DP26 camera and imaged using Olympus CellSens standard 1.7 imaging software (Olympus).

Quantification of F4/80 Immunohistochemistry

Immunohistochemistry staining for the pan macrophage marker F4/80 was imaged using an Olympus VS120 (Olympus) at 40X magnification. Automated digital image analysis was subsequently performed using the Visiopharm Integrator System (Visiopharm, Hoersholm, Denmark). In each sample, at each sectional depth (4 depths analyzed with each depth at least 50 μm apart), ROIs were generated which contained all damaged muscle. Automated analysis was performed from the ROIs and the data was calculated as percent of F4/80$^+$ staining per total area of injured muscle. All cases were visually reviewed to ensure accuracy. Data was represented separately at each sectional depth as the area of damaged tissue is not uniform throughout each hamstring.

Statistical Analysis

Statistically significant differences were determined using ANOVA with *post-hoc* Tukey's multiple comparison test or Mann-Whitney test using PRISM 6 or 7 (GraphPad software, La Jolla, CA, USA).

RESULTS

Increased Ly6C^{high} Monocyte Infiltration in Injured Muscles of Mice Following SCI

We have previously reported that systemic depletion of phagocytic macrophages and monocytes by injections of clodronate-loaded liposomes significantly reduces NHO development (13). Therefore, we further characterized the macrophage/monocyte populations present within the muscles of mice developing NHO by flow cytometry. In this model, only mice that undergo both SCI + i.m. CDTX injection develop NHO exclusively in the CDTX injected muscle (13, 15). Mice underwent SCI or SHAM surgery followed by an intramuscular injection of CDTX to cause muscle injury or a control PBS injection. At 4 days post-surgery leukocytes were extracted from the hamstrings of all mice and isolated into four subsets based on forward scatter, side scatter as well as zombie aqua negativity (viable cells), F4/80, Ly6G, CD11b, and Ly6C expression (**Figure 1A**). Preliminary flow cytometry analysis confirmed that CDTX-induced intramuscular injury caused a large and significant accumulation of total F4/80$^+$ monocyte/macrophages (**Figure 1Bi** $p < 0.0001$) in SCI+CDTX and SHAM+CDTX groups compared to control groups (SCI+PBS and SHAM+PBS). When the total F4/80$^+$ population was sub-gated based on expression of Ly6C, we observed a significantly higher frequency of Ly6C^{high} 'inflammatory monocytes/macrophages' (CD11b$^+$F4/80$^+$Ly6G$^-$Ly6C^{hi}) in the mice that develop NHO (SCI+CDTX), compared to SHAM+CDTX mice (**Figure 1Bii** $p = 0.0002$). Minimal Ly6C^{hi} monocyte/macrophages were noted in the SCI+PBS and SHAM+PBS groups. The frequencies of Ly6C$^{mid/lo}$ monocyte/macrophages (CD11b$^+$F4/80$^+$Ly6G$^-$Ly6C^{mid}/^{lo}) was unchanged between SCI+CDTX and SHAM+CDTX groups (**Figure 1Biii**). We also observed the presence of

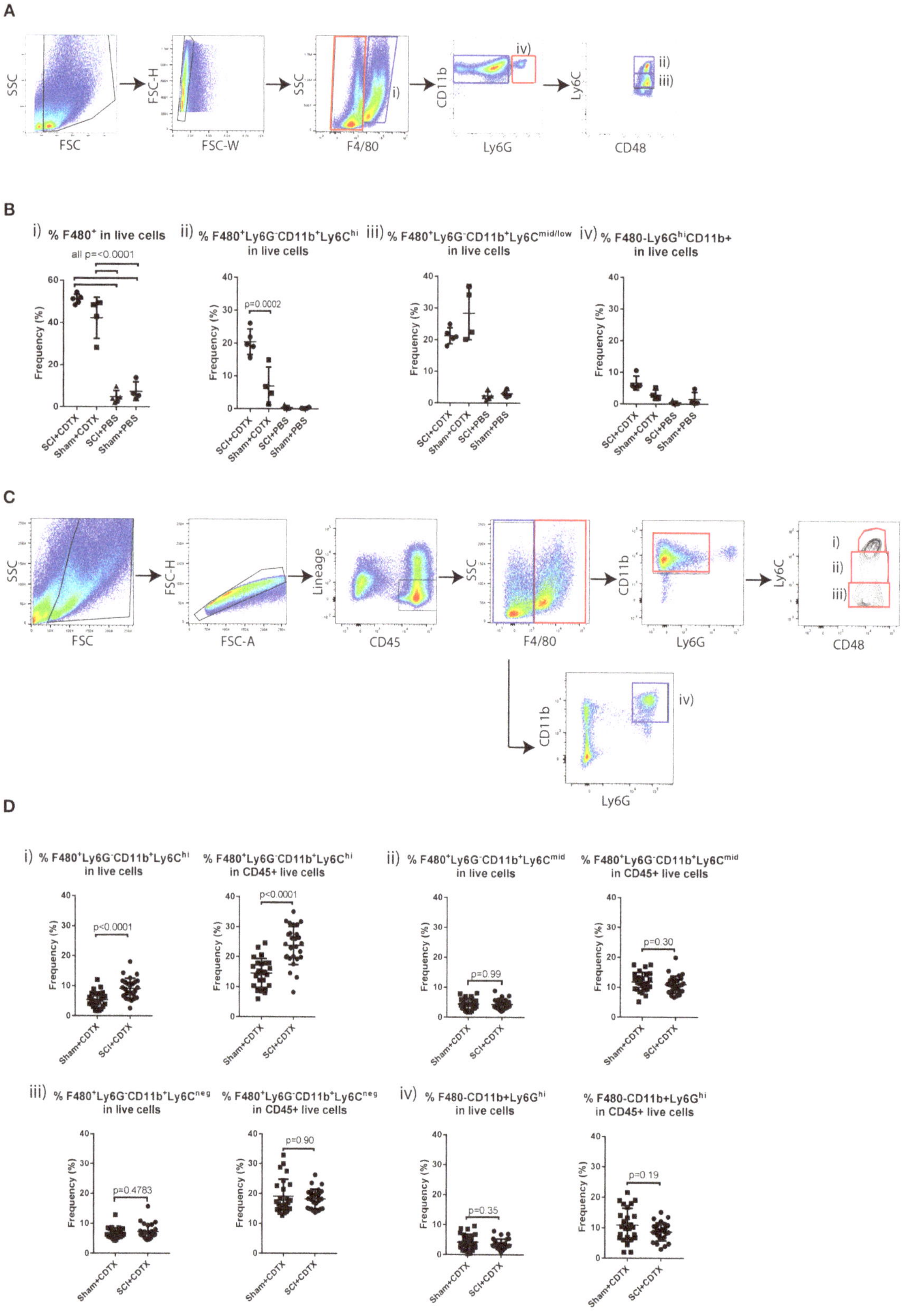

FIGURE 1 | Increased inflammatory monocyte infiltration in injured muscles of mice developing NHO. **(A)** C57BL/6 mice underwent either SCI or Sham surgery followed by an intra muscular injection of CDTX or PBS. Muscle leukocytes were extracted from hamstrings at day 4 post-surgery and isolated into four subsets

(Continued)

FIGURE 1 | based on forward scatter, side scatter as well as zombie aqua negativity (viable cells), F4/80, Ly6G, CD11b, and Ly6C expression. **(B)** Frequencies of each leukocyte population relative to total live muscle cells using the gating strategy outlined: (i) "Total F4/80$^+$ cells" (CD11b$^+$F4/80$^+$, blue gates in **A**), (ii) "Ly6C^{hi} inflammatory monocytes" (F4/80$^+$CD11b$^+$Ly6G$^-$ CD48$^+$Ly6C^{hi}, blue gates in **A**), (iii) "Ly6C$^{mid/lo}$ monocytes/macrophages" (F4/80$^+$ CD11b$^+$ Ly6G$^-$CD48$^+$ Ly6C$^{mid/lo}$, blue gates in **A**), and (iv) "granulocytes" (F4/80$^-$CD11b$^+$Ly6G$^+$, red gates in **A**). The frequency of Ly6C^{hi} inflammatory monocytes (relative to total live muscle cells) in mice developing NHO (SCI+CDTX), compared to all other treatment groups was significantly higher ($p = 0.0002$ ANOVA n = 3–5/group). Each dot represents an individual mouse. Bars represent as mean ± SD. **(C)** Muscle leukocytes were extracted from hamstrings at day 4 post surgery, and 4 separate leukocyte populations were identified by flow cytometry using the following gating strategy: (i) "Ly6C^{hi} inflammatory monocytes" as CD45$^+$ lineage (Ter119,CD3ε,B220)-negative F4/80$^+$ CD11b$^+$ Ly6G$^-$ CD48$^+$Ly6C^{hi}, red gates, (ii) "Ly6C^{mid} monocytes/macrophages" CD45$^+$ Lin$^-$ F4/80$^+$ CD11b$^+$ Ly6G$^-$CD48$^+$ Ly6C^{mid}, red gates, (iii) "Ly6C^{neg} monocytes" CD45$^+$ Lin$^-$ F4/80$^+$ CD11b$^+$ Ly6G$^-$ CD48$^+$ Ly6C^{neg} red gates, and (iv) "granulocytes" CD45$^+$ Lin$^-$ F4/80^{neg} CD11b$^+$ Ly6G$^+$, blue gates. **(D)** Frequencies of each myeloid subset relative to total live muscle cells and to total live CD45$^+$ muscle leukocytes. There was a significant increase in frequency of Ly6C^{hi} monocytes relative to total live muscle cells (Di, $p < 0.0001$ Mann-Whitney test) and to CD45$^+$ live muscle leukocytes (Di, $p < 0.0001$ Mann-Whitney test) after SCI+CDTX compared to Sham+CDTX. Each dot represents an individual mouse, n = 25–27/treatment group. Bars represent mean ± SD.

granulocytes (CD11b$^+$F4/80$^-$Ly6G^{hi}) **(Figure 1Biv),** albeit with lower frequencies compared to monocyte/macrophage subsets. In view of these preliminary results, we focused our subsequent analysis on leukocyte populations infiltrating the CDTX-injured muscles in SCI+CDTX and SHAM+CDTX groups in a larger cohort of mice to achieve higher statistical power. Leukocytes were isolated into 4 separate populations based on forward scatter, side scatter as well as 7-actinomycin D-negativity (7AAD$^-$ viable cells), CD45, lineage (Ter119, CD3ε, B220), F4/80, Ly6G, CD11b, Ly6C expression (**Figure 1C**). Although we initially wanted to incorporate antibodies specific for CD169, Mer tyrosine kinase and VCAM-1 which clearly identifies macrophages from monocytes (31), preliminary experiments on bone marrow cells where macrophages and monocytes are abundant confirmed this was not possible as these antigens are cleaved from the cell surface by the protease cocktail used to extract leukocytes from skeletal muscles (data not shown). Despite this limitation, we again observed that the frequency of "Ly6C^{hi} inflammatory monocytes/macrophages" (CD45$^+$Lin$^-$CD11b$^+$F4/80$^+$Ly6G$^-$Ly6C^{hi}) in live muscle cells was significantly higher in mice that develop NHO (SCI+CDTX) mice compared to SHAM+CDTX mice (**Figure 1Di**, left panel $p < 0.0001$). When the frequency of Ly6C^{hi} monocytes was calculated relative to all CD45$^+$ leukocytes present, the frequency of these inflammatory monocytes was also significantly increased (**Figure 1Di**, right panel $p < 0.0001$). The frequencies of other monocyte/macrophage subsets identified as CD45$^+$Lin$^-$CD11b$^+$F4/80$^+$Ly6G$^-$Ly6C^{mid} monocytes (**Figure 1Dii**), CD45$^+$Lin$^-$CD11b$^+$F4/80$^+$Ly6G$^-$Ly6C^{neg} monocytes (**Figure 1Diii**), as well as CD45$^+$Lin$^-$CD11b$^+$F4/80$^-$Ly6G$^+$ neutrophils (**Figure 1Div**) were not significantly different in SCI+CDTX compared to SHAM+CDTX mice.

Expression of OSM and OSMR in Muscle Cell Populations

We have previously confirmed by qRT-PCR, that *Osm* mRNA is significantly upregulated in the whole muscles of mice developing NHO (15). As there is no commercial monoclonal antibody specific for mouse OSMR that works by flow cytometry, we isolated RNA from the sorted myeloid populations described in **Figure 1D** at 4 days post-surgery, as well as whole skeletal muscle from naïve mice and mouse muscle progenitor cell populations; CD45$^-$Ter119$^-$CD31$^-$CD34$^+$Sca1$^-$ satellite cells and CD45$^-$Ter119$^-$CD31$^-$CD34$^+$Sca1$^+$ interstitial cells [also known as fibro-adipogenic progenitors or FAP (32)] freshly sorted from naïve skeletal muscle, to establish which cell types express *Osm* and *Osmr* mRNA. *Osm* mRNA was detected in all myeloid populations infiltrating the SCI+CDTX-injured muscle with the highest abundance in granulocytes (**Figure 2A**), whereas no *Osm* was detected in whole naïve skeletal muscle. These results are consistent with the tissue expression profile of mouse *Osm* mRNA in the BioGPS database (http://biogps.org). In sharp contrast, *Osmr* mRNA was undetectable in myeloid populations in the muscle but was expressed by both muscle satellite cells and interstitial cells (**Figure 2B**). This suggests that OSM can act directly on muscle progenitor cells that express its receptor OSMR rather than indirectly via infiltrating myeloid cells.

OSM Induces STAT3 Y705 Phosphorylation in Cultured Mouse Muscle Cells

Given that both muscle satellite cells and interstitial cells expressed *Osmr* mRNA, we further investigated OSM/OSMR signaling in these cells. The OSMR/gp130 receptor complex is known to activate both JAK1 and JAK2 tyrosine kinases following OSM binding (23, 24). Once activated, JAK1 and JAK2 tyrosine phosphorylate STAT1 and STAT3 (23) which enable their nuclear translocation to initiate transcription of OSM responsive genes. In preliminary experiments, we were unable to detect phosphorylated JAK1 and JAK2 by immunoprecipitation and western-blot of whole muscle lysates because the very low levels of total JAK1 and JAK2 proteins (data not shown). Instead, we measured the tyrosine phosphorylation status of the JAK1/2 substrate STAT3 in response to recombinant mouse OSM in satellite and interstitial cells sorted from the muscles of naïve mice. The mouse mesenchymal progenitor cell line Kusa4b10 (29, 30) was used as a positive control. By flow cytometry with a mAb specific for STAT3 phosphorylation on tyrosine 705 (pSTAT3 Y705), we confirmed that recombinant mouse OSM caused a rapid phosphorylation of STAT3 Y705 on all cell types tested (**Figure 2C**), confirming that OSMR is functional on mouse muscle satellite and interstitial cells. To confirm that STAT3 Y705 phosphorylation was mediated by JAK1/2, we also preincubated cells for 30 min with the small synthetic JAK1/2 inhibitor ruxolitinib (27, 28). Ruxolitinib completely inhibited phosphorylation of STAT3 Y705 in response to mouse OSM in all three cell types (**Figure 2C**). Together these results suggest that OSMR expressed by satellite and interstitial cells are able

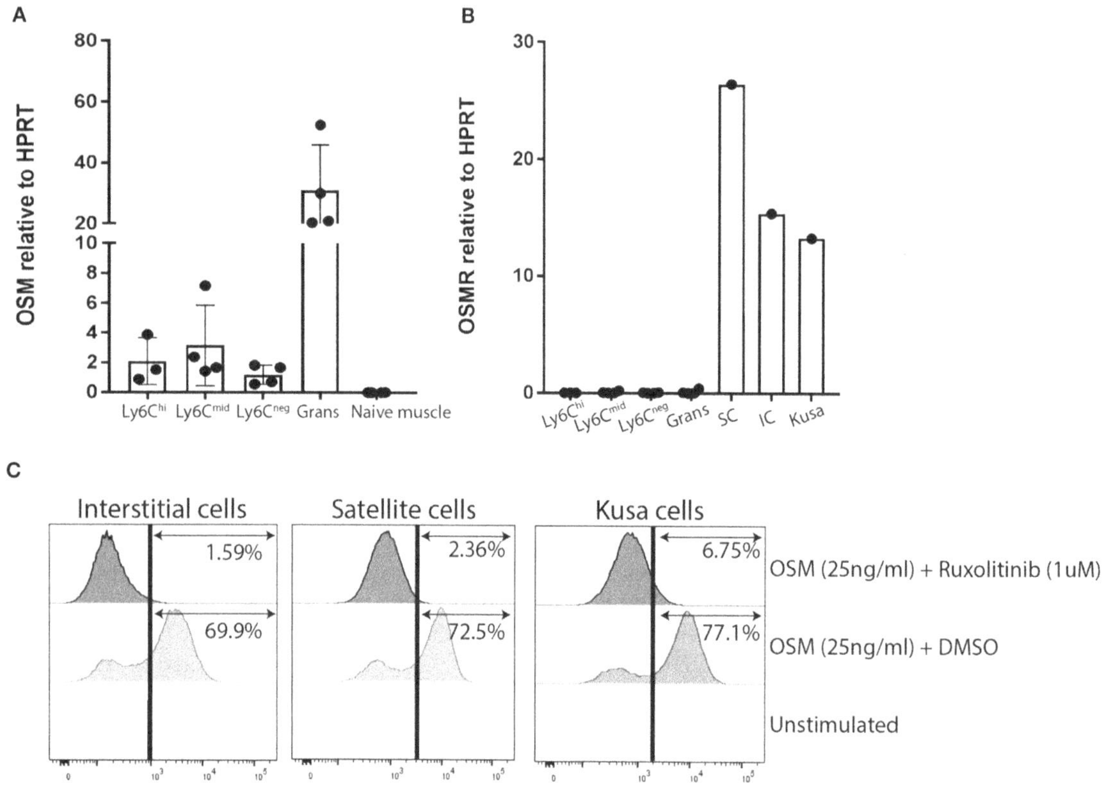

FIGURE 2 | OSM and OSMR expression and signaling in muscle cells. **(A)** *Osm* mRNA expression by qRT-PCR. *Osm* is expressed by all sorted infiltrating myeloid populations but absent in whole naïve skeletal muscle. Each dot represents an individual mouse ($n = 3$–4/group). Bars represent mean ± SD. **(B)** *Osmr* mRNA expression is only present in sorted mouse muscle satellite and interstitial cells, not in any sorted myeloid population infiltrating the injured muscle **(C)** Phos-flow of pSTAT3 Y705 phosphorylation in cultured $CD45^-Ter119^-CD31^-CD34^+Sca1^+$ muscle interstitial cells (IC), $CD45^-Ter119^-CD31^-CD34^+Sca1^-$ muscle satellite cells (SC), and Kusa4b10 cells. Cells were incubated for 10 min at 37°C with medium alone (unstimulated), or 25 ng/ml recombinant mouse OSM plus DMSO or of 25 ng/ml OSM plus 1 μM ruxolitinib. Cell were then fixed and permeabilized before staining with AlexaFluor647-conjugated mouse mAb anti-pSTAT3 (Y705) and analyzed by flow cytometry. Representative figures were one of two independent experiments.

to respond to upregulated OSM in muscle and activate downstream JAK1/2-STAT3 signaling pathway.

Persistence of STAT3 Tyrosine Phosphorylation in the Injured Muscle Following SCI

Next, we examined STAT3 Y705 phosphorylation in the muscles of mice developing NHO. Western blots for pSTAT3 Y705 and total STAT3 were performed using whole muscle lysates from hamstrings of mice that underwent either (1) SCI+CDTX, (2) SCI+PBS, (3) SHAM+CDTX, or (4) SHAM+PBS at day 4, 7, and 14 days post-surgery. At 4 days post-surgery there was a clear increase in STAT3 Y705 phosphorylation in muscle injured with CDTX (**Figure 3A**). Importantly the ratio of pSTAT3 Y705 vs. total STAT3 normalized to the pSTAT3/STAT3 ratio measured in control mice (SHAM+PBS), was significantly higher in SCI+CDTX mice compared to SHAM+CDTX mice (**Figure 3A**). Seven days post-injury, STAT3 Y705 phosphorylation persisted in the injured muscles from the SCI+CDTX group while it was resolving in the SHAM+CDTX group (**Figure 3B**). This pattern of persistent STAT3 Y705 phosphorylation in the injured muscles of the SCI+CDTX group that developed NHO was noted up to 14 days post-surgery (**Figure 3C**) whereas in SHAM+CDTX, pSTAT3 Y705 had returned to levels not significantly different from those observed in controls without muscle injury as expected from previous reports showing that without a SCI, CDTX-injured muscles are mostly repaired 14 post-injury (33). These data establish that the combination of SCI with muscle injury, compared to all other control treatments, caused enhanced STAT3 signaling in the injured muscle which persisted for an extended period of time after the initial injury. Overall these data establish that in the context of a SCI, STAT3 phosphorylation is exaggerated and persists over a longer period of time in injured muscles developing NHO.

JAK1/2 Inhibition Significantly Reduced NHO Development Following SCI

From this we hypothesized that exaggerated and persistent STAT3 tyrosine phosphorylation and activation by JAK1/2 in injured muscles of SCI mice is functionally important in NHO pathogenesis. To test this, we treated mice that underwent

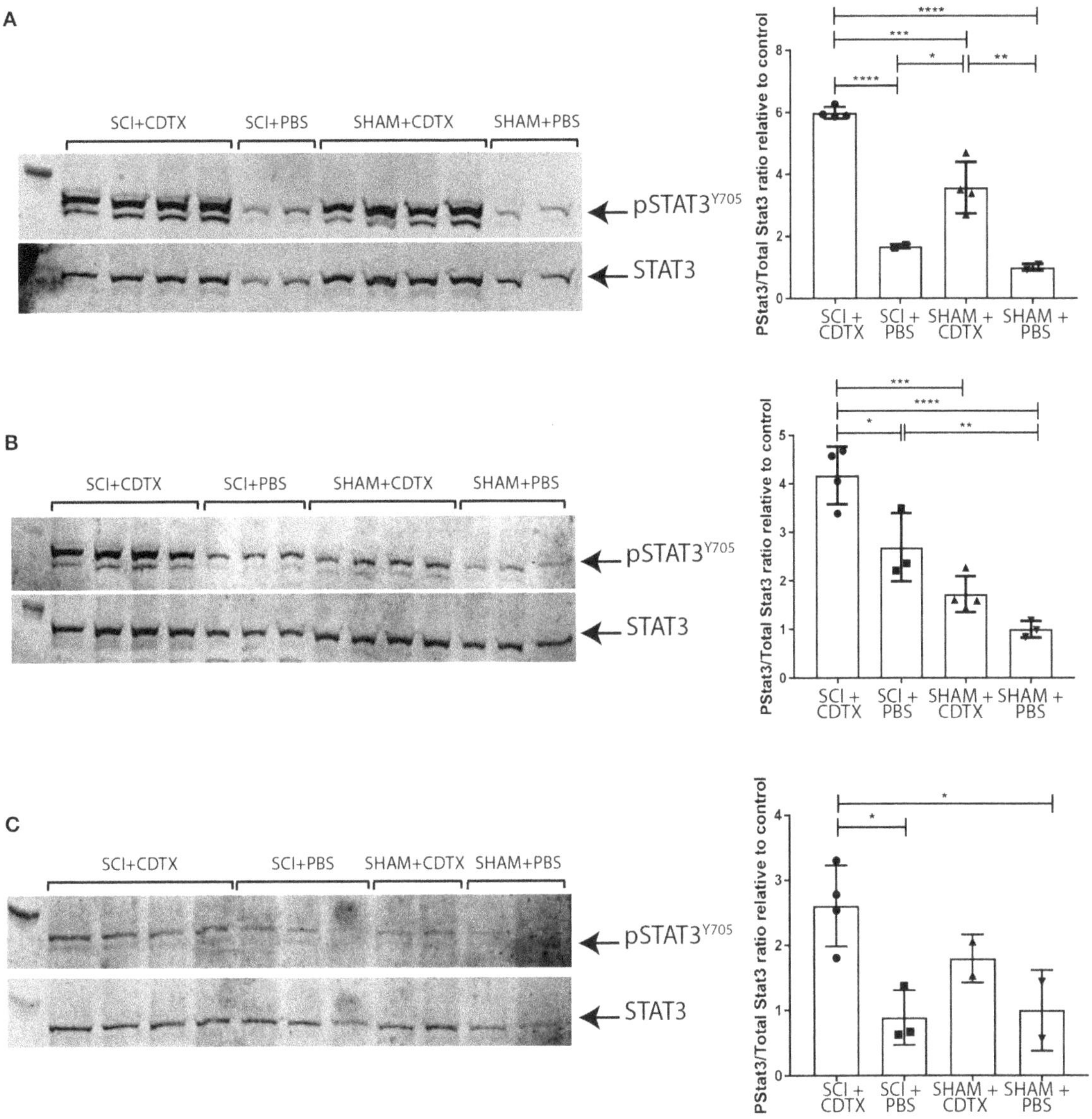

FIGURE 3 | Persistence of STAT3 tyrosine phosphorylation in injured muscles following spinal cord injury. Western-blots of whole muscle lysates collected from mice that underwent either SCI or SHAM surgery together with an intramuscular injection of either CDTX or PBS. Western blot of whole muscle lysates from individual mice taken on day 4 **(A)**, 7 **(B),** or 14 **(C)** post-injury. Each membrane was probed with rabbit anti-pSTAT3 Y705 mAb, stripped and then re-probed with rabbit anti-total STAT3 mAb. Band fluorescence intensity was quantified and ratio of signal intensity of pSTAT3 vs. total STAT3 calculated for each individual mouse and normalized relative to the average pSTAT3/STAT3 ratio in control mice (SHAM+PBS) at each time-point. Each lane and each dot represents a separate mouse, $n = 2$–4 mice/treatment/time-point. Bars represent mean ± SD. *P* values were calculated by ANOVA, $^{*}p < 0.05$, $^{**}p < 0.01$, $^{***}p < 0.001$, $^{****}p < 0.0001$.

SCI+CDTX with ruxolitinib bi-daily for the first 7 days post-surgery. Ruxolitinib treatment significantly reduced STAT3 Y705 phosphorylation at 7 days post-surgery (**Figure 4A** $^{*}p = 0.03$). Micro CT (μCT) confirmed a significant reduction in NHO bone volume at day 7, 14, and 23 post surgery in mice treated with ruxolitinib for the first 7 days post-injury (**Figure 4Bi**,ii $^{**}p = 0.0076$, $^{*}p = 0.031$, and $^{*}p = 0.015$). Visual representation of collagen^{+} NHO by Masson's trichrome staining at 3 weeks post-surgery was consistent with μCT quantification and confirmed the presence of collagen^{+} NHO foci in the muscles of vehicle treated SCI+CDTX mice (**Figure 4C,** crosshatches). Collagen^{+} NHO foci were reduced after ruxolitinib treatment. As previously described by us (13, 15) and others (33), in SHAM+CDTX mice at 3 weeks post-surgery, no NHO and little collagen deposition was observed, with reformation of muscle fibers confirming that in the absence of SCI, the CDTX-injured muscle repairs within 7–14 days post-injury (33). Immunohistochemistry with anti-collagen type I or anti-osterix/SP7 antibodies were consistent with both μCT and Masson's trichrome staining and confirmed that in vehicle treated SCI+CDTX mice the

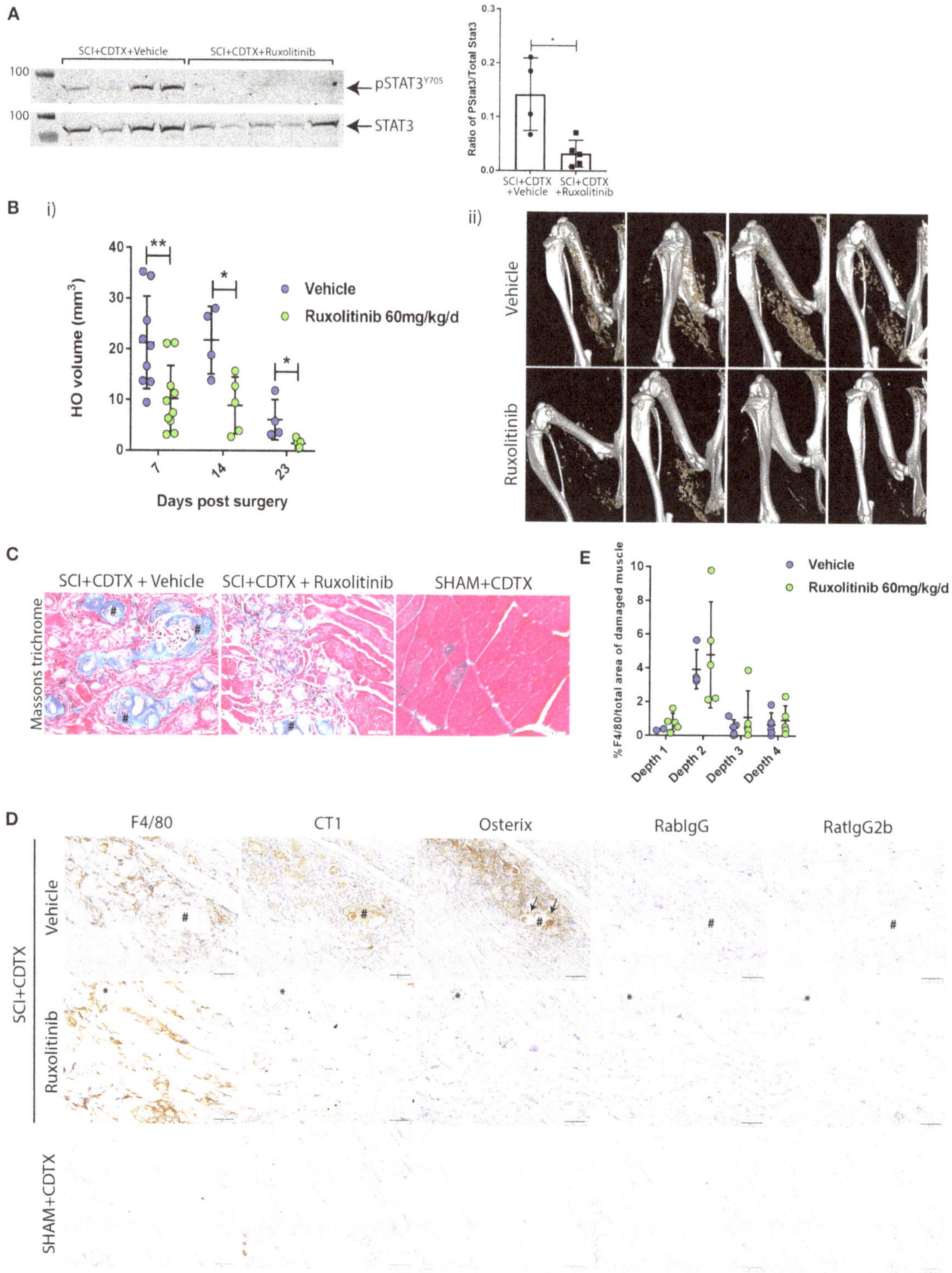

FIGURE 4 | Inhibition of JAK1/2 kinases with ruxolitinib reduces NHO development after SCI *in vivo*. **(A)** Western-blots of whole muscle lysates collected at day 7 from SCI+CDTX mice that were treated with either vehicle control or ruxolitinib (60 mg/kg bi-daily) from day 0–7 post surgery. Western-blots of whole muscle lysates were probed with rabbit anti-pSTAT3 Y705 mAb, and rabbit anti-total STAT3 mAb, then band fluorescence was quantified and ratio of signal intensity of pSTAT3 versus total STAT3 calculated for each individual mouse. Each lane and each dot represents a separate mouse, $n = 4$–5/treatment group. Data represented as mean ± SD, $^{*}p = 0.03$ by Mann-Whitney test. **(B)** Measurement of NHO volume by micro CT (μCT) in mice which received SCI+CDTX and treated with either vehicle control or ruxolitinib (60 mg/kg bi-daily) from day 0–7 post surgery. (i) NHO volumes were quantified *in vivo* by μCT at indicated time points post-surgery illustrating the

(Continued)

FIGURE 4 | reduction in NHO development. Each dot represents a separate mouse, $n = 4$–10 mice/treatment/time point. Data represented as mean ± SD, $^{**}p = 0.0076$, $^{*}p = 0.031$, and $p = 0.015$ respectively by Mann-Whitney test. (ii) Representative μCT images at 7 days post-surgery **(C)** Masson's trichrome staining 3 weeks post-surgery confirming the development of multiple NHO bone and collagen+ foci (crosshatches) within the muscle in vehicle treated mice, which are reduced after ruxolitinib treatment, and absent in control mice (SHAM+CDTX) **(D)** Immunohistochemistry staining of serial sections from SCI+CDTX mice 3 weeks post-surgery (top and middle panels). Mice were treated with vehicle or ruxolitinib (60 mg/kg bi-daily) from day 0–7 post surgery. Stains were performed with either rat anti-F4/80 mAb, rabbit anti-collagen I (CT1), or anti-osterix antibodies. Isotype control (rat IgG2b for F4/80; Rabbit IgG for CT1, and Osterix) are also shown to confirm specificity of staining. In vehicle treated mice CT1$^+$ NHO foci are present within the damaged muscle (crosshatch), these foci are surrounded by F4/80$^+$ macrophages and have Osterix$^+$ cells lining the NHO foci surface (arrows). After ruxolitinib treatment there are still F4/80$^+$ macrophages within the damaged muscle, however there are less CT1$^+$ NHO foci with Osterix$^+$ cells lining the surface. *symbols denote the same anatomical landmark in each image. NHO development is absent in SHAM+CDTX mice 3 weeks post-surgery, with no CT1, and Osterix expression (bottom panel). **(E)** Quantification of F4/80 expression via IHC confirmed that ruxolitinib treatment did not change F4/80$^+$ macrophage expression within the hamstrings of vehicle vs. ruxolitinib treated mice, 7 days post-surgery. Each dot represents a separate mouse, $n = 2$–5/treatment group/sectional depth. Four different depths were analyzed for each sample with at least 50 μm between each depth. Data represented as mean ± SD. All images taken at 40X magnification, scale bar represents 50 μm.

collagen type I$^+$ NHO foci were lined with osterix$^+$ osteo-lineage cells (**Figure 4D,** top panel, arrows). Reduced osterix-positive osteo-lineage cells and type 1 collagen deposition was noted after ruxolitinib treatment (**Figure 4D,** middle panel). In SHAM+CDTX mice there was little expression of collagen type I and osterix (**Figure 4D,** bottom panel). Ruxolitinib treatment had minimal impact on the density of F4/80$^+$ macrophages within the injured muscles 7 days post-surgery (**Figure 4E**).

DISCUSSION

The inflammatory component that frequently accompanies severe trauma of the central nervous system and the spine has been suggested to be a key factor in NHO development (5, 34, 35). We have previously established in a mouse model of SCI-induced NHO in which macrophages infiltrate the damaged muscles was critical for NHO development (13–15). Our current study demonstrates that SCI causes an increased infiltration of Ly6C^{hi} inflammatory monocytes/macrophages into injured muscles. Furthermore, we show that myeloid cells infiltrating the injured muscle express the pro-inflammatory cytokine OSM. Binding of OSM to OSMR, which is expressed by satellite cells and interstitial cells isolated from muscle, activates JAK1/2 tyrosine kinases with subsequent STAT3 tyrosine phosphorylation and activation *in vitro. In vivo* we established that SCI with accompanying muscle injury caused an increase in STAT3 phosphorylation in injured muscles which persisted for up to 2 weeks only in the muscles that develop NHO. Finally, *in vivo* inhibition of JAK1/2 with ruxolitinib reduced STAT3 phosphorylation in injured muscles and most importantly reduced NHO volume subsequent to SCI combined with muscle injury.

OSM has been recently reported to induce muscle satellite cell quiescence *in vivo*, and conditional deletion of the *Osmr* gene specifically in satellite cells led to reduced myofiber regeneration in response to injury (36). In agreement with this, STAT3, which is activated by JAK1/2 immediately downstream of the OSMR:gp130 complex, has been implicated in controlling satellite cell expansion and muscle repair after muscle injury (37). In addition, STAT3 knock-down or conditional *Stat3* gene deletion in satellite cells increased satellite cell proliferation following muscle injury but impaired muscle repair, suggesting that STAT3 activation is required for accelerated muscle repair (37, 38). In contrast, OSM is known to promote osteogenic differentiation of mesenchymal stromal cells *in vitro* (18, 39) and osteoblast differentiation and bone formation *in vivo* (16, 17, 19). Therefore, OSM plays an important role in both muscle repair and osteogenic differentiation and activity. This is consistent with our observations that (1) OSMR is expressed in skeletal muscles by both satellite cells, which regenerate myoblasts following muscle injury (40), and by interstitial cells which are of mesenchymal origin (32), and (2) that OSM causes STAT3 phosphorylation in both cell types *in vitro.* A limitation of our study is that we were unable to demonstrate STAT3 phosphorylation specifically in muscle satellite cells or interstitial cells *in vivo.* The extended enzymatic digestion of muscles at 37°C required to obtain single cell suspension amenable for flow cytometry, removes OSM protein from the extracellular milieu thus disrupting OSMR ligation on satellite and interstitial cells and downstream JAK/STAT signaling. Further immunohistological experiments using reporter mice in which muscle satellite cells or mesenchymal cells are specifically labeled with a fluorescent reporter will be required to definitively prove STAT3 activation *in vivo* in these two cell types.

It is also important to note that in our experiments, ruxolitinib may also block STAT activation in additional cell types particularly myeloid cells that infiltrate the injured muscle. Indeed, these myeloid cells express receptors for other inflammatory cytokines such as IL-6 (41), granulocyte colony-stimulating factor (G-CSF) (42) and granulocyte macrophage colony-stimulating factors (GM-CSF) (43) which also activate STATs via JAK1/2. Although it remains to be determined whether IL-6, G-CSF, and GM-CSF contribute to NHO pathogenesis (44), the ruxolitinib-mediated inhibition of JAK1/2 in both muscle progenitor cells and infiltrating myeloid cells may also contribute to the overall inhibition of NHO in our model.

Intriguingly, while STAT3 inhibition has been reported to improve muscle repair in mice without SCI (37, 38), we did not note improved muscle repair following JAK1/2 inhibitor administration in mice that underwent SCI as macrophage infiltration and collagen deposits remained in the injured muscles even after ruxolitinib treatment. A few hypotheses can be formulated to explain this divergent outcome in terms of muscle repair. Firstly, the SCI may cause a dramatic change in the function of macrophages orchestrating muscle repair (33) and in muscle satellite and interstitial cells, such that inhibition of either

STAT3 or JAK1/2 is not sufficient to re-establish coordinated muscle regeneration. A second possibility is that the JAK1/2 inhibitor used in our study also inhibits the activation of other STAT proteins such as STAT1 and STAT5 which may be activated in response to OSM (16) as well as STAT activation in response to other cytokines such IL-6, IL-12, G-CSF, or GM-CSF in muscle cells and macrophages which orchestrate muscle regeneration as discussed above.

It is also important to note that despite the significant effect of ruxolinitib in reducing STAT3 phosphorylation in muscles of mice developing NHO, and the reduction in NHO volume after ruxolitinib treatment, while pronounced was only partial (**Figure 4**). Herein we find that SCI and muscle injury caused an exaggerated infiltration of Ly6C^{hi} inflammatory monocytes into the injured muscles consistent with our previous observation that *in vivo* depletion of phagocytes with clodronate-loaded liposomes markedly inhibited NHO formation (13). Because of this increased inflammatory monocyte infiltration, it is likely that other pro-inflammatory cytokines and mediators are released within the injured muscle and participate to NHO development. For instance we have previously reported in this model of SCI-induced NHO that substance P may contribute to NHO development (13). Others have reported in a rat model of multi-trauma, that the retinoic acid receptor-γ agonist Palovarotene also partially decreased heterotopic ossification (45). In a similar rat model of multi-trauma, rapamycin was also found to partially decrease heterotopic ossification, suggesting that mammalian targets of rapamycin (mTOR) may also play an important role (46). Altogether these findings suggest that many other pathways could be abnormally activated in injured muscles in the context of a SCI. Indeed since NHO is driven by two different insults, it is unlikely that the pathogenesis converges to a single pathway. Therefore, a highly effective therapy is likely to require a combined approach. We are currently undertaking transcriptome analyses on injured muscles with and without SCI to elucidate the molecular pathways that could potentially promote NHO development.

Although ruxolitinib caused a pronounced but still partial reduction in NHO development, inhibitors of JAK1/2 or STAT3 may represent a new therapeutic approach to decrease NHO development in patients or perhaps to avoid NHO re-occurrence after surgical resection, which is observed in 6% of NHO patients (2, 9, 12). However, the roles of STAT3 and JAK1/2 in spinal cord recovery will need to be carefully evaluated. In a rat model of SCI, treatment with a STAT3 inhibitor post-surgery promoted neural stem cell differentiation (47). In other studies, augmentation of IL-6 after SCI resulted in enhanced infiltration of neutrophils and macrophages with a subsequent increase in lesion size and reduction in axonal growth, suggesting that balanced IL-6 signaling is required for efficient repair after SCI (48). However, other studies have demonstrated that conditional deletion of STAT3 in reactive astrocytes leads to the limited migration of astrocytes, higher infiltration of inflammatory cells, demyelination, and more severe loss of motor function following SCI (49, 50). The SCI-NHO model used in our studies involves a complete spinal cord transection and further analysis on neurological recovery was not possible in this model. Therefore, further studies in a SCI-NHO model where neurological recovery is achievable are necessary to effectively determine whether ruxolitinib treatment to reduce NHO development has any beneficial or negative impact on neurological recovery following SCI.

In conclusion our experiments suggest that STAT3 activation persists in the muscles of mice that are developing NHO following SCI and that targeting STAT3 activation via transient JAK1/2 inhibition immediately following SCI may be a possible therapeutic approach to reduce NHO development in patients.

AUTHOR CONTRIBUTIONS

KA, H-WT, WF, BJ, MS, IK, and SM performed the experiments. KA, H-WT, and J-PL conceived the experiments and the work. KA, H-WT, and J-PL wrote the manuscript. KA, H-WT, FG, ARP, and J-PL edited the manuscript.

FUNDING

This research was supported by Project Grant 1101620 from the National Health and Medical Research Council of Australia (NHMRC) to J-PL, ARP and FG, and award W81XWH-15-1-0606 from the Congressionally Approved Spinal Cord Injury Research Program of the US Department of Defense to J-PL, ARP, and FG, and by funds from the Mater Foundation. J-PL is supported by Research Fellowship 1136130 from the NHMRC. ARP is supported by an Australian Research Council Future Fellowship ARP FT150500335. The Translational Research Institute is partly funded by the Federal Government of Australia.

ACKNOWLEDGMENTS

The authors also acknowledge the scientific and technical assistance of the UQ biological resources TRI facility, histology facility, flow cytometry facility, microscopy facility, and the preclinical Imaging Facility, Translational Research Institute, which is supported by Therapeutic Innovation Australia (TIA). TIA is supported by the Australian Government through the National Collaborative Research Infrastructure Strategy (NCRIS) program.

REFERENCES

1. Ohlmeier M, Suero EM, Aach M, Meindl R, Schildhauer TA, Citak M. Muscle localization of heterotopic ossification following spinal cord injury. *Spine J.* (2017) 17:1519–22. doi: 10.1016/j.spinee.2017.04.021
2. Genet F, Jourdan C, Schnitzler A, Lautridou C, Guillemot D, Judet T, et al. Troublesome heterotopic ossification after central nervous system damage: a survey of 570 surgeries. *PLoS ONE.* (2011) 6:e16632. doi: 10.1371/journal.pone.0016632
3. Dizdar D, Tiftik T, Kara M, Tunc H, Ersoz M, Akkus S. Risk factors for developing heterotopic ossification in patients with traumatic brain injury. *Brain Inj.* (2013) 27:807–11. doi: 10.3109/02699052.2013.775490
4. Reznik JE, Biros E, Marshall R, Jelbart M, Milanese S, Gordon S, et al. Prevalence and risk-factors of neurogenic heterotopic ossification in traumatic spinal cord and traumatic brain injured patients admitted to specialised units in Australia. *J Musculoskelet Neuronal Interact.* (2014) 14:19–28.
5. Brady RD, Shultz SR, McDonald SJ, O'Brien TJ. Neurological heterotopic ossification: current understanding and future directions. *Bone.* (2018) 109:35–42. doi: 10.1016/j.bone.2017.05.015
6. Forsberg JA, Pepek JM, Wagner S, Wilson K, Flint J, Andersen RC, et al. Heterotopic ossification in high-energy wartime extremity injuries: prevalence and risk factors. *J Bone Joint Surg Am.* (2009) 91:1084–91. doi: 10.2106/JBJS.H.00792
7. Vanden Bossche L, Vanderstraeten G. Heterotopic ossification: a review. *J Rehabil Med.* (2005) 37:129–36. doi: 10.1080/16501970510027628
8. Salga M, Jourdan C, Durand MC, Hangard C, Denormandie P, Carlier RY, et al. Sciatic nerve compression by neurogenic heterotopic ossification: use of CT to determine surgical indications. *Skeletal Radiol.* (2015) 44:233–40. doi: 10.1007/s00256-014-2003-6
9. Genet F, Chehensse C, Jourdan C, Lautridou C, Denormandie P, Schnitzler A. Impact of the operative delay and the degree of neurologic sequelae on recurrence of excised heterotopic ossification in patients with traumatic brain injury. *J Head Trauma Rehabil.* (2012) 27:443–8. doi: 10.1097/HTR.0b013e31822b54ba
10. Genet F, Marmorat JL, Lautridou C, Schnitzler A, Mailhan L, Denormandie P. Impact of late surgical intervention on heterotopic ossification of the hip after traumatic neurological injury. *J Bone Joint Surg Br.* (2009) 91:1493–8. doi: 10.1302/0301-620X.91B11.22305
11. Genêt F, Denormandie P, Keenan MA. Orthopaedic surgery for patients with central nervous system lesions: concepts and techniques. *Ann Phys Rehabil Med.* (2018) doi: 10.1016/j.rehab.2018.09.004
12. Genet F, Jourdan C, Lautridou C, Chehensse C, Minooee K, Denormandie P, et al. The impact of preoperative hip heterotopic ossification extent on recurrence in patients with head and spinal cord injury: a case control study. *PLoS ONE.* (2011) 6:e23129. doi: 10.1371/journal.pone.0023129
13. Genet F, Kulina I, Vaquette C, Torossian F, Millard S, Pettit AR, et al. Neurological heterotopic ossification following spinal cord injury is triggered by macrophage-mediated inflammation in muscle. *J Pathol.* (2015) 236:229–40. doi: 10.1002/path.4519
14. Levesque J-P, Sims NA, Pettit AR, Alexander KA, Tseng H-W, Torossian F, et al. Macrophages driving heterotopic ossification: convergence of genetically-driven and trauma-driven mechanisms. *J Bone Miner Res.* (2018) 33:365–6. doi: 10.1002/jbmr.3346
15. Torossian F, Guerton B, Anginot A, Alexander KA, Desterke C, Soave S, et al. Macrophage-derived oncostatin M contributes to human and mouse neurogenic heterotopic ossifications. *JCI Insight.* (2017) 2:e96034. doi: 10.1172/jci.insight.96034
16. Walker EC, McGregor NE, Poulton IJ, Solano M, Pompolo S, Fernandes TJ, et al. Oncostatin M promotes bone formation independently of resorption when signaling through leukemia inhibitory factor receptor in mice. *J Clin Invest.* (2010) 120:582–92. doi: 10.1172/JCI40568
17. Sims NA, Quinn JM. Osteoimmunology: oncostatin M as a pleiotropic regulator of bone formation and resorption in health and disease. *Bonekey Rep.* (2014) 3:527. doi: 10.1038/bonekey.2014.22
18. Guihard P, Danger Y, Brounais B, David E, Brion R, Delecrin J, et al. Induction of osteogenesis in mesenchymal stem cells by activated monocytes/macrophages depends on oncostatin M signaling. *Stem Cells.* (2012) 30:762–72. doi: 10.1002/stem.1040
19. Guihard P, Boutet MA, Brounais-Le Royer B, Gamblin AL, Amiaud J, Renaud A, et al. Oncostatin M, an inflammatory cytokine produced by macrophages, supports intramembranous bone healing in a mouse model of tibia injury. *Am J Pathol.* (2015) 185:765–75. doi: 10.1016/j.ajpath.2014.11.008
20. Gerhartz C, Heesel B, Sasse J, Hemmann U, Landgraf C, Schneider-Mergener J, et al. Differential activation of acute phase response factor/STAT3 and STAT1 via the cytoplasmic domain of the interleukin 6 signal transducer gp130: I. Definition of a novel phosphotyrosine motif mediating STAT1 activation. *J Biol Chem.* (1996) 271:12991–8. doi: 10.1074/jbc.271.22.12991
21. Heinrich PC, Behrmann I, Muller-Newen G, Schaper F, Graeve L. Interleukin-6-type cytokine signalling through the gp130/Jak/STAT pathway. *Biochem J.* (1998) 334:297–314. doi: 10.1042/bj3340297
22. Ichihara M, Hara T, Kim H, Murate T, Miyajima A. Oncostatin M and leukemia inhibitory factor do not use the same functional receptor in mice. *Blood.* (1997) 90:165–73.
23. Levy JB, Schindler C, Raz R, Levy DE, Baron R, Horowitz MC. Activation of the JAK-STAT signal transduction pathway by oncostatin-M cultured human and mouse osteoblastic cells. *Endocrinology.* (1996) 137:1159–65. doi: 10.1210/endo.137.4.8625884
24. Hermanns HM, Radtke S, Haan C, Schmitz-Van de Leur H, Tavernier J, Heinrich PC, et al. Contributions of leukemia inhibitory factor receptor and oncostatin M receptor to signal transduction in heterodimeric complexes with glycoprotein 130. *J Immunol.* (1999) 163:6651–8.
25. Magrangeas F, Boisteau O, Denis S, Jacques Y, Minvielle S. Negative regulation of onconstatin M signaling by suppressor of cytokine signaling (SOCS-3). *Eur Cytokine Netw.* (2001) 12:309–15.
26. Ehlting C, Böhmer O, Hahnel MJ, Thomas M, Zanger UM, Gaestel M, et al. Oncostatin M regulates SOCS3 mRNA stability via the MEK–ERK1/2-pathway independent of p38MAPK/MK2. *Cell Signal.* (2015) 27:555–67. doi: 10.1016/j.cellsig.2014.12.016
27. Quintás-Cardama A, Vaddi K, Liu P, Manshouri T, Li J, Scherle PA, et al. Preclinical characterization of the selective JAK1/2 inhibitor INCB018424: therapeutic implications for the treatment of myeloproliferative neoplasms. *Blood.* (2010) 115:3109–17. doi: 10.1182/blood-2009-04-214957
28. Verstovsek S, Mesa RA, Gotlib J, Levy RS, Gupta V, DiPersio JF, et al. A double-blind, placebo-controlled trial of ruxolitinib for myelofibrosis. *N Engl J Med.* (2012) 366:799–807. doi: 10.1056/NEJMoa1110557
29. Allan EH, Häusler KD, Wei T, Gooi JH, Quinn JM, Crimeen-Irwin B, et al. EphrinB2 regulation by PTH and PTHrP revealed by molecular profiling in differentiating osteoblasts. *J Bone Miner Res.* (2008) 23:1170–81. doi: 10.1359/jbmr.080324
30. Allan EH, Ho PWM, Umezawa A, Hata JI, Makishia F, Gillespie MT, et al. Differentiation potential of a mouse bone marrow stromal cell line. *J Cell Biochem.* (2003) 90:158–69. doi: 10.1002/jcb.10614
31. Kaur S, Raggatt LJ, Millard SM, Wu AC, Batoon L, Jacobsen RN, et al. Self-repopulating recipient bone marrow resident macrophages promote long-term hematopoietic stem cell engraftment. *Blood.* (2018) 132:735–49. doi: 10.1182/blood-2018-01-829663
32. Joe AWB, Yi L, Natarajan A, Le Grand F, So L, Wang J, et al. Muscle injury activates resident fibro/adipogenic progenitors that facilitate myogenesis. *Nat Cell Biol.* (2010) 12:153. doi: 10.1038/ncb2015
33. Mounier R, Théret M, Arnold L, Cuvellier S, Bultot L, Göransson O, et al. AMPKα1 regulates macrophage skewing at the time of resolution of inflammation during skeletal muscle regeneration. *Cell Metab.* (2013) 18:251–64. doi: 10.1016/j.cmet.2013.06.017
34. Banovac K, Williams JM, Patrick LD, Haniff YM. Prevention of heterotopic ossification after spinal cord injury with indomethacin. *Spinal Cord.* (2001) 39:370–4. doi: 10.1038/sj.sc.3101166
35. Banovac K, Williams JM, Patrick LD, Levi A. Prevention of heterotopic ossification after spinal cord injury with COX-2 selective inhibitor (rofecoxib). *Spinal Cord.* (2004) 42:707–10. doi: 10.1038/sj.sc.3101628
36. Sampath SC, Sampath SC, Ho ATV, Corbel SY, Millstone JD, Lamb J, et al. Induction of muscle stem cell quiescence by the secreted niche factor Oncostatin M. *Nat Commun.* (2018) 9:1531. doi: 10.1038/s41467-018-03876-8
37. Tierney MT, Aydogdu T, Sala D, Malecova B, Gatto S, Puri PL, et al. STAT3 signaling controls satellite cell expansion and skeletal muscle repair. *Nat Med.* (2014) 20:1182–6. doi: 10.1038/nm.3656

38. Price FD, von Maltzahn J, Bentzinger CF, Dumont NA, Yin H, Chang NC, et al. Inhibition of JAK-STAT signaling stimulates adult satellite cell function. *Nat Med.* (2014) 20:1174–81. doi: 10.1038/nm.3655
39. Song HY, Jeon ES, Kim JI, Jung JS, Kim JH. Oncostatin M promotes osteogenesis and suppresses adipogenic differentiation of human adipose tissue-derived mesenchymal stem cells. *J Cell Biochem.* (2007) 101:1238–51. doi: 10.1002/jcb.21245
40. Sambasivan R, Yao R, Kissenpfennig A, Van Wittenberghe L, Paldi A, Gayraud-Morel B, et al. Pax7-expressing satellite cells are indispensable for adult skeletal muscle regeneration. *Development.* (2011) 138:3647–56. doi: 10.1242/dev.067587
41. Jenkins BJ, Roberts AW, Najdovska M, Grail D, Ernst M. The threshold of gp130-dependent STAT3 signaling is critical for normal regulation of hematopoiesis. *Blood.* (2005) 105:3512–20. doi: 10.1182/blood-2004-09-3751
42. Panopoulos AD, Zhang L, Snow JW, Jones DM, Smith AM, El Kasmi KC, et al. STAT3 governs distinct pathways in emergency granulopoiesis and mature neutrophils. *Blood.* (2006) 108:3682–90. doi: 10.1182/blood-2006-02-003012
43. Mui AL, Wakao H, O'Farrell AM, Harada N, Miyajima A. Interleukin-3, granulocyte-macrophage colony stimulating factor and interleukin-5 transduce signals through two STAT5 homologs. *Embo J.* (1995) 14:1166–75. doi: 10.1002/j.1460-2075.1995.tb07100.x
44. Wright CR, Ward AC, Russell AP. Granulocyte colony-stimulating factor and its potential application for skeletal muscle repair and regeneration. *Mediators Inflamm.* (2017) 2017:7517350. doi: 10.1155/2017/7517350
45. Pavey GJ, Qureshi AT, Tomasino AM, Honnold CL, Bishop DK, Agarwal S, et al. Targeted stimulation of retinoic acid receptor-γ mitigates the formation of heterotopic ossification in an established blast-related traumatic injury model. *Bone.* (2016) 90:159–67. doi: 10.1016/j.bone.2016.06.014
46. Qureshi AT, Dey D, Sanders EM, Seavey JG, Tomasino AM, Moss K, et al. Inhibition of mammalian target of rapamycin signaling with rapamycin prevents trauma-induced heterotopic ossification. *Am J Pathol.* (2017) 187:2536–45. doi: 10.1016/j.ajpath.2017.07.010
47. Cui M, Ma X, Sun J, He J, Shen L, Li F. Effects of STAT3 inhibitors on neural functional recovery after spinal cord injury in rats. *Biosci Trends.* (2017) 10:460–6. doi: 10.5582/bst.2016.01160
48. Lacroix S, Chang L, Rose-John S, Tuszynski MH. Delivery of hyper-interleukin-6 to the injured spinal cord increases neutrophil and macrophage infiltration and inhibits axonal growth. *J Comp Neurol.* (2002) 454:213–28. doi: 10.1002/cne.10407
49. Okada S, Nakamura M, Katoh H, Miyao T, Shimazaki T, Ishii K, et al. Conditional ablation of Stat3 or Socs3 discloses a dual role for reactive astrocytes after spinal cord injury. *Nat Med.* (2006) 12:829–34. doi: 10.1038/nm1425
50. Faulkner JR, Herrmann JE, Woo MJ, Tansey KE, Doan NB, Sofroniew MV. Reactive astrocytes protect tissue and preserve function after spinal cord injury. *J Neurosci.* (2004) 24:2143–55. doi: 10.1523/JNEUROSCI.3547-03.2004

15

IL-33/Vitamin D Crosstalk in Psoriasis-Associated Osteoporsis

Massimo De Martinis[1*], *Lia Ginaldi*[1], *Maria Maddalena Sirufo*[1], *Enrica Maria Bassino*[1], *Francesca De Pietro*[1], *Giovanni Pioggia*[2†] *and Sebastiano Gangemi*[3†]

[1] Department of Life, Health and Environmental Sciences, University of L'Aquila, L'Aquila, Italy, [2] Institute for Biomedical Research and Innovation (IRIB), National Research Council of Italy (CNR), Messina, Italy, [3] School and Operative Unit of Allergy and Clinical Immunology, Department of Clinical and Experimental Medicine, University of Messina, Messina, Italy

***Correspondence:**
Massimo De Martinis
demartinis@cc.univaq.it

†These authors have contributed equally to this work

Patients with psoriasis (Pso) and, in particular, psoriatic arthritis (PsoA) have an increased risk of developing osteoporosis (OP). It has been shown that OP is among the more common pathologies associated with Pso, mainly due to the well-known osteopenizing conditions coexisting in these patients. Pso and OP share common risk factors, such as vitamin D deficiency and chronic inflammation. Interestingly, the interleukin (IL)-33/ST2 axis, together with vitamin D, is closely related to both Pso and OP. Vitamin D and the IL-33/ST2 signaling pathways are closely involved in bone remodeling, as well as in skin barrier pathophysiology. The production of anti-osteoclastogenic cytokines, e.g., IL-4 and IL-10, is promoted by IL-33 and vitamin D, which are stimulators of both regulatory and Th2 cells. IL-33, together with other Th2 cytokines, shifts osteoclast precursor differentiation towards macrophage and dendritic cells and inhibits receptor activator of nuclear factor kappa-B ligand (RANKL)-induced osteoclastogenesis by regulating the expression of anti-osteoclastic genes. However, while the vitamin D protective functions in OP and Pso have been definitively ascertained, the overall effect of IL-33 on bone and skin homeostasis, because of its pleiotropic action, is still controversial. Emerging evidence suggests a functional link between vitamin D and the IL-33/ST2 axis, which acts through hormonal influences and immune-mediated effects, as well as cellular and metabolic functions. Based on the actions of vitamin D and IL-33 in Pso and OP, here, we hypothesize the role of their crosstalk in the pathogenesis of both these pathologies.

Keywords: osteoporosis, psoriasis, IL-33, vitamin D, osteoimmunology, skin, bone, cytokines

INTRODUCTION

Psoriasis (Pso) is a chronic autoimmune multifactorial disease that is associated with systemic inflammation. It presents with skin erythematous plaques, covered by characteristic white silvery scales (1). It is characterized by increased proliferation of keratinocytes, perivascular skin infiltration by cells belonging to both the adaptive and innate immune system, and imbalances in apoptotic and autophagic pathways (2).

Through the production of inflammatory cytokines, activated and autoreactive immune cells play central roles in its pathogenesis (3). In both skin and blood of psoriatic patients, there are increased levels of various cytokines, growth factors, and chemokines (4). Patients suffering from Pso, particularly those with psoriatic arthritis (PsoA) or more severe forms of the disease, develop multiple comorbidities in addition to joint diseases, including cardiovascular and rheumatologic disorders, infections, obesity, and diabetes (5–7). The link between these comorbidities is likely systemic inflammation (8). Recently, osteoporosis (OP) is also considered to be a relevant comorbidity in Pso (9). Therefore, patients with Pso are now recognized to be at increased risk of pathologic fractures and OP, so today, it is commonly believed that Pso patients might benefit from increased screening for OP (10).

OP is defined as a generalized disease of the skeleton, characterized by low bone mineral density (BMD) and altered microarchitecture, leading to increased bone fragility and, as a result, increased risk of fractures (11, 12). In addition to senile and postmenopausal OP, secondary OP may also occur as a consequence of various pathologies, including endocrinopathies, rheumatic and neoplastic diseases, malnutrition, chronic inflammatory conditions, and 1,25-dihydroxyvitamin D (vitamin D) deficiency (13–17). Several potential mechanisms may explain the association between Pso and OP, including a low vitamin D level, chronic inflammation, and drug usage (18–20). In particular, proinflammatory cytokines, such as interleukin (IL)-1, IL-6, IL-11, IL-15, IL-17, and tumor necrosis factor (TNF)-alpha, might accelerate bone loss, whereas other cytokines, mostly of the Th2 profile, e.g., IL-4 and IL-33, are usually considered osteoprotective (21).

IL-33 and vitamin D are emerging pathogenetic factors of both Pso and OP. However, their role in the development of these associated pathologies is complex and not yet fully clarified. Here, we hypothesize a mechanistic link between vitamin D and IL-33 in patients with Pso and associated OP.

PATHOGENIC MECHANISMS LINKING PSO AND OP

Several pathogenetic mechanisms link Pso and OP (**Box 1**). Although there are conflicting results in the literature about this association and its pathogenetic mechanisms, the majority of studies describe a decreased BMD in patients with long-term Pso and PsoA (9, 22, 23). Like Pso, OP can also be considered a systemic pathology (21). Although it is mainly linked to menopause and aging (14, 24), OP can also accompany a wide range of pathologies, in particular, those with an important inflammatory substrate, including dermatological disorders (25–28).

BOX 1 | Main pathogenetic mechanisms in Pso and OP.

Key points:

- Vitamin D deficiency
- Overexpression of IL-33/IL-31 axis
- Chronic systemic inflammation
- Increased production of inflammatory and osteoclastogenic cytokines
- Unbalanced RANKL-RANK-OPG signaling pathway
- Overexpression of IL-23/IL-17 axis
- Impaired Th17/Treg cell balance
- Increased secretion of IL-17 and IL-22 from IL-23-stimulated ILC3

Many cytokines are involved in the regulation of bone turnover, and most of them also underlie the inflammatory background of Pso (4, 21, 29). Vitamin D deficiency is among the main risk factors of both pathologies (29–31). The hypothesized mechanisms underlying the potential association between Pso and OP involves enhanced bone resorption secondary to increased concentrations of osteoclastogenic cytokines, such as TNF-alpha, IL-6, IL-12, IL-23, or IL-17 (31, 32). The central signal pathway in bone resorption is the system of the receptor activator of nuclear factor kappa-B (NF-kB) ligand (RANKL), mainly expressed by osteoblasts, that binds to its receptor RANK on the osteoclast precursor cells, inducing their differentiation into mature osteoclasts and thus leading to bone resorption. Osteoprotegerin (OPG), the decoy receptor of RANKL, prevents bone resorption by inhibiting osteoclastogenesis. In the pathogenesis of OP, the RANKL-RANK-OPG axis is unbalanced (12). Inflammatory cytokines, whose production is increased in Pso, exert osteoclastogenic effects mainly through the enhancement of RANKL expression. In particular, IL-17, produced by T helper type 17 (Th17) cells, plays a pivotal role in the bone loss of inflammatory conditions, including Pso, by enhancing RANKL expression on osteoblasts and synovial fibroblasts. Moreover, IL-17 stimulates the production of other inflammatory and osteoclastogenic cytokines, such as TNF-α, IL-1, and IL-6, which accelerate osteoclastogenesis, further facilitating the development of OP. High surface expression of RANKL on Th17 cells characterizes the so-called osteoclast subsets of T lymphocytes, that strongly enhance bone resorption. On the contrary, T regulatory (Treg) cells inhibit osteoclastogenesis and support bone formation. Therefore, while Th17 cells induce osteoclastogenesis, mainly by secreting IL-17, IL-4 enhanced Treg exert anti-osteoclastogenic activity by producing suppressor cytokines, including IL-10, and transforming growth factor-beta (TGF-β) (21). An impaired Th17/Treg cell balance is central in the inflammatory background of both Pso and OP. Treg cells are responsible for the maintenance of self-tolerance, thus inhibiting autoimmune diseases, including Pso, and are also able to suppress RANKL-induced osteoclastogenesis, whereas pro-inflammatory Th17 cells contribute to the induction and propagation of inflammation. Th17 cells, converted from Foxp3+ Treg in inflamed tissues, such as psoriatic skin lesions, comprise the most potent osteoclastogenic T cell subset in inflammatory bone loss (33). In the complex cytokine network involved in Pso, a crucial role is also exerted by IL-12/Th1 and IL-23/Th17 axis, by linking components of adaptive and innate immunity in an inflammatory crosstalk. In the skin, activated dendritic cells (DCs) trigger Th1 and Th17 cells to differentiate and release IFN-γ and TNF-α, and IL-17 and IL-22, respectively, which promote keratinocyte proliferation. IL-23 is a heterodimeric cytokine composed of two subunits, p19 and p40. The latter subunit is shared by the Th1-inducing cytokine IL-12. Upon skin injury, IL-23 produced by activated DCs, stressed keratinocytes and other non-immune cells directly drives expansion and survival of Th17 lymphocytes, stimulates IL-17 production, and induces downregulation of IL-10, involved in

Treg cell function, thus creating a self-amplifying inflammatory response that drives the development of skin lesions infiltrated with a mixture of inflammatory cell populations. Innate lymphoid cells (ILCs) represent a heterogeneous group of immune cells lacking specific antigen receptors or T/B cell markers. ILC3, which express the transcription factor retinoid-related orphan receptor γt (ROR γt) and are characterized by the ability to produce Th17 and IL-22 cytokines, are increased in Pso. ILC3 constitutively express the IL-23 receptor, thus representing a target for IL-23-mediated IL-17 and IL-22 increased production. The secretion of IL-17 and IL-22 from IL-23-stimulated ILC3 promotes the aberrant keratinocyte differentiation and hyperproliferation, typically observed in Pso (34). IL-12 and IL-23 involved in skin inflammation, are also critical to inflammation-induced bone resorption, *via* a number of direct and indirect effects that modulate osteoclast formation. In the bone, IL-23 upregulates RANK on preosteoclasts and induces Th17 cells to produce IL-17, which acts on osteoblasts to secrete RANKL. Th17 cells also secrete RANKL directly and further induce osteoclast formation and secretion of bone-degrading enzymes leading to bone destruction (35). Many other cytokines involved in bone remodeling have recently been shown to also exert roles in the pathogenesis of Pso, including, in particular, IL-33 (36–39). In addition, some treatments used in Pso might contribute to bone loss, for example, corticosteroids and cyclosporin, particularly when used systemically (18–20), whereas treatments at the systemic level aimed at reducing inflammation, e.g., biologics or methotrexate, could reduce the risk associated with osteoporotic fractures (40). Finally, psoriatic patients, especially those with associated inflammatory arthritis, engage less in physical activities and tend to cover affected body surfaces with consequent decreases in osteoformation and vitamin D synthesis (41, 42). In particular, the lack of sun exposure, which may affect mainly psoriatic patients with extensive skin involvement and/or arthritis through vitamin D deficiency, negatively affects calcium metabolism, further increasing bone resorption and leading to the onset of OP (43). Psoriatic patients of both sexes appear to have a high prevalence of OP and vitamin D deficiency (10, 44). Low levels of vitamin D metabolizing enzymes (CYP27A1 and CYP27B1) within psoriatic lesions have also been documented (9, 45), and vitamin-D treatment in psoriatic patients has been associated with clinical improvement of skin lesions (46, 47).

Pso is related to vitamin D deficiency through both inflammation and a lack of sun exposure (48). Interestingly, vitamin D deficiency and OP are frequently recognized in the great majority of associated Pso comorbidities (21, 49) For example, Pso is frequently associated with metabolic syndrome, increased body mass index, and obesity (50). All of these associated conditions are characterized by both an inflammatory background and increased fat deposits, in which vitamin D tends to accumulate because of its liposolubility, consequently reducing its circulating bioavailable levels. In these patients, vitamin D deficiency is commonly related to hyperglycemia and higher levels of cholesterol, low-density lipoprotein, and triglycerides (51, 52). Therefore, despite the tendency for a higher body mass index in patients with Pso, which might have a protective effect against OP, both vitamin D deficiency and systemic inflammation can still induce BMD loss.

Chronic inflammation itself has been related to low vitamin D levels and decreased BMD (53, 54). Under pathological conditions, the equilibrium between bone formation and resorption, which physiologically ensures skeletal homeostasis, is shifted towards osteoclast-mediated bone resorption. Proinflammatory cytokines, such as TNF-alpha and IL-17, are notoriously associated with osteoclastic bone resorption in inflammatory diseases (21). These cytokines trigger osteoclastogenesis through the activation of a series of transcription factors, such as NF-kappa B. In PsoA, synovial inflammation can further facilitate the onset of local and systemic OP (29). In these patients, an increase in osteoclast progenitors (OCP) correlates with the extent of joint erosions and inflammation markers (41).

The association between Pso and OP is therefore supported by the existence of pathophysiological mechanisms, namely, excessive production of proinflammatory cytokines that are able to activate osteoclastogenesis, and the frequent lack of vitamin D characterizing psoriatic patients (55, 56).

However, studies on OP development and the increased risk of fractures in patients with Pso are still somewhat controversial, because of the complexity of the network of interconnected cytokines and the regulatory factors linking the two pathologies.

THE ROLE OF VITAMIN D

Vitamin D has multiple functions, including hormonal and immunological control (**Box 2**). Vitamin D regulates more than 200 genes involved in cell proliferation and differentiation, the secretion of different hormones, and immune cell activity (54, 57). The lack of vitamin D in Pso is widely recognized as an important factor that contributes to the development of OP (58). Vitamin D regulates calcium and phosphorous metabolism and parathyroid hormone (PTH) secretion and function. For these activities, it has important implications for the maintenance of skeletal integrity. As a consequence of vitamin D deficiency, bone mineralization disorders arise, mainly through an imbalance in the calcium/phosphorus ratio. Vitamin D is indispensable for physiological bone turnover. In particular, in order to prevent OP, supplementation with vitamin D is strongly recommended as a support for anti-osteoporotic therapies (12, 15, 53). Moreover, in

BOX 2 | Vitamin D functions.

Key points:

- Calcium/phosphorous metabolism regulation
- Parathyroid hormone secretion and function control
- Regulation of cutaneous barrier homeostasis
- Keratinocyte proliferation, apoptosis and function control
- Th1/Th2 cell development modulation
- Induction of regulatory T cells
- Down-regulation of Th17 cells
- Down-regulation of nflammatory cytokine production

addition to its effects on bone, vitamin D also exerts important functions in skin homeostasis and its deficiency is linked with Pso development (48, 59). Vitamin D is therefore no longer considered to just be an essential factor for the maintenance of a normal skeletal structure, but its extraskeletal effects, including cell cycle regulation and immune modulation, are becoming increasingly known (60–62).

The epidermis is the natural source of vitamin D synthesis through the action of ultraviolet light (53), and in turn, vitamin D functions as a key regulator of cutaneous barrier homeostasis. The skin therefore acts as the site of vitamin D synthesis and also as the target organ for its biologically active form (47). Keratinocytes contain enzymes needed for the production of the active form of vitamin D, 1,25 (OH)2D, and express its receptor, vitamin D receptor (VDR), thus being able to synthesize and also respond to vitamin D. Through this signaling pathway, vitamin D is involved in regulating epidermal development, keratinocyte proliferation, differentiation and apoptosis (54), and the synthesis of keratins, involucrin, transglutaminase, loricrin, and filaggrin, helping to modulate skin barrier function (63, 64). These control mechanisms are partly due to its ability to increase intracellular calcium by inducing the production of phospholipases and calcium receptors needed for calcium-dependent keratinocyte differentiation. After activation, VDRs interact with retinoid X receptor (RXR) to exert their functions. VDRs, as well as enzymes able to synthesize the active form of the vitamin, namely 1,25-dihydroxy-vitamin D, are expressed in several tissues beyond the kidneys and bones, including the skin and the immune system, suggesting that vitamin D is involved in many other functions besides the metabolic ones (53, 65). An association between Pso susceptibility and VDR polymorphisms, as well as between reduced tight-junction proteins and decreased VDR expression in psoriatic skin, has been described (57). It has been shown that vitamin D also exerts central roles in both humoral and cellular regulation by suppressing T-cell proliferation and Th2 cell development and through the induction of regulatory T cells, cytokine production modulation, and dendritic cell regulation (66–69).

Through the downregulation of IL-12 production, vitamin D suppresses the maturation of Th1 cells, leading to increased Th2 lymphocyte proliferation (47, 70). However, vitamin D also promotes regulatory T cell maturation and increases IL-10 synthesis, exerting inhibitory effects on Th2 immune responses (71).

Moreover, vitamin D inhibits proliferation and induces apoptosis in various cell types (54). Following dysregulation of the cell cycle, autophagy and apoptosis have important roles in inflammatory processes (72) underlying both OP and Pso. This could represent a further mechanism through which vitamin D deficiency contributes to their pathogeneses (73–76). In psoriatic skin inflammation, cytokines and chemokines produced by dysregulated T lymphocytes play key roles (77). As in Pso, in the pathogenesis of OP, these immune-mediated mechanisms are strongly involved (21). By inhibiting the production of Th1 and Th17 cytokines and stimulating T cells to secrete anti-inflammatory Th2 cytokines in both the skin and bone immune systems, vitamin D reduces the production of osteoclastogenic cytokines as well as the psoriatic inflammatory process (64, 78, 79). Moreover, since vitamin D promotes Th2 and Treg differentiation rather than Th1 and Th17 proinflammatory lymphocytes (48) and inhibits B cell differentiation, thus interfering with the production of antibodies by plasma cells (70), its deficiency is also associated with an increased risk of developing autoimmune diseases (80–82), including Pso, which is a Th1-Th17-Th22-based inflammatory disease involving innate and acquired immunity (53). Therefore, despite being historically associated with rickets, osteomalacia, and OP, now considered an inflammatory Th1-mediated disease (83), vitamin D deficiency has recently been recognized as a risk factor for chronic systemic diseases, including diabetes, neoplasia, allergies, infections, autoimmune, cardiovascular, and neurodegenerative diseases (76). Pso is histologically characterized by keratinocyte hyperproliferation, derangement of the epidermal barrier function, and infiltration of the skin by multiple activated inflammatory cells (53). As a key modulator of systemic inflammation, vitamin D normalizes the dysregulated distribution of CD26 and ICAM-1 integrins in the dermal–epidermal junction of psoriatic skin and suppresses the inflammatory profile of monocytes/macrophages (55), down-regulating the production of cytokines, such as IL-1β, IL-6, IL-8, and TNF-alpha (48, 80). All of these cytokines are involved in inflammatory processes leading to Pso and OP (47, 83, 84). Indeed, vitamin D and its analogues suppress the proliferation of keratinocytes and their proinflammatory molecule production, therefore improving psoriatic lesions and contributing to skeletal health by suppressing bone resorption and favoring bone formation.

THE ROLE OF IL-33

IL-33 is a cytokine that can promote Th2 response, but also has broad activities (**Box 3**) including the promotion of activated Th1 and CD8+ cytotoxic cells and also Treg cells that express ST2 receptor (85, 86). As well as vitamin D, also IL-33 is involved in various biological processes, including tissue homeostasis and repair, cell proliferation, and the immune response, and it plays key roles in the pathogenetic mechanisms of several diseases, such as allergic, autoimmune, neoplastic, and cardiovascular diseases. In particular, IL-33 is involved in skin diseases, including Pso (39, 87, 88), and in OP through its role in bone remodeling (89–92). Its receptor complex consists of a primary receptor, ST2, and an accessory IL-1 receptor protein. The ST2 receptor exists in two different forms: a transmembrane isoform acts as a cellular receptor, whereas a soluble form (sST2) plays the role of decoy receptor inhibiting IL-33 activity (93, 94). Interestingly, the IL-33/

BOX 3 | IL-33 functions.

Key points:

- Induction of Th2 responses and Th2 cytokine production
- Promotion of activated Th1 and CD8+ cytotoxic cells
- Activation of Treg cells expressing ST2 receptor
- Gene expression regulation
- Activation of inflammation and tissue ripair upon danger signals
- Mast cell and neutrophil activation in inflamed skin
- Enhancement of TNFα induced secretion of IL-6, VEGF, and MCP-1

ST2 axis is involved in both Th2 and Th1/Th17 responses (88) as well as in the activation of Treg and natural killer (NKT) cells, B and NK lymphocytes, neutrophils, and macrophages (91, 95–98). A regulatory feedback axis exists between stromal cells expressing IL-33 and adipose resident ST2+ Tregs (99, 100). Obesity alters this homeostatic cellular network and promotes the inflammatory response (101, 102). Several immune cells involved in the type 2 immune response express ST2. Among others, examples of such immune cells are the group 2 innate lymphoid cells (ILC2), eosinophils, basophils, and DCs, as well as mast cells and Th2 cells (103). Increased amphiregulin (AREG) levels are associated with vitamin D deficiency. The ILC2-associated marker AREG, whose encoding gene is a target of vitamin D, activates IL-33-responsive ST2 T cells and ILC2s (104), which function as key effectors producing Th2 cytokines, including IL-4, IL-5, IL-9, and IL-13 (105), when released from necrotic and/or apoptotic epithelial cells. On the other hand, TNF-alpha, INF-gamma, and IL-17, major effectors of the Th1/Th17 responses in Pso and OP pathogenesis, stimulate the release of IL-33. Both skin lesions and unaffected skin biopsies of Pso patients (36, 37, 95) express high IL-33 levels (103, 106). The rapid IL-33 release from keratinocytes after skin injury could be a crucial mechanism involved in the pathogenesis of Pso (107–110). Once released in the local microenvironment, IL-33 could activate mast cells and neutrophils as well as Th1/Th17 cells, triggering both innate and adaptive immune responses. Mast cells can activate other innate immune cells, such as eosinophils and neutrophils, and, in turn, can recruit and activate keratinocytes. The above-mentioned interactions are pivotal for the emergence of skin inflammation and Pso lesions (111). Both TNF-alpha and INF-gamma in psoriatic skin increase the expression of IL-33 which, in turn, is able to suppress the actions of other cytokines (38). Also, IL-17 upregulates IL-33 expression in normal human epidermal keratinocyte (NHEK) cultures through the activation of the p38/MAPK, ERK, and JAK/STAT pathways (112). IL-33 reinforces the TNF-alpha induced secretion of IL-6, VEGF, and MCP-1. However, data on IL-33 serum levels in Pso are controversial (113). A large number of studies suggest that a localized, rather than a generalized, IL-33 linked inflammatory pattern is evident in Pso (114). IL-33 serum levels are not always increased in the serum of patients with Pso, notwithstanding the increased levels of this cytokine in inflamed skin (103, 111, 114). It has also been suggested that IL-33 expression in the nuclei of keratinocytes following IL-17 stimulation may represent a regulatory mechanism aimed at attenuating immune reactions (110).

The expression levels of both IL-33 and ST2 are up-regulated in psoriasis, likely as a consequence of keratinocyte damage. IL-33/ST2 signals may subsequently trigger the activation of neutrophils and mast cells, leading to Pso development. This pathogenetic hypothesis assumes interplay between keratinocytes and the immune system (88, 107, 108). IL-33 exerts a dual function. It acts as a cytokine or as a nuclear factor when involved extracellularly or intracellularly, respectively, thus participating in both inflammation processes and gene expression regulation (4). Upon cellular stress and tissue damage, released IL-33 functions as an alarmin and activates innate and adaptive immune cells, inflammation, or tissue repair. IL-33 is considered a key alarmin in both Pso and OP, although it exerts contrasting effects in these pathological conditions (115). Continuous alarmin release promotes polarization toward a Th1 phenotype, and this effect contributes to the initial background of the local hyperinflammatory environment that characterizes Pso (92, 107).

The IL-33/ST2 pathway intervenes in the pathogenesis of Th2-related diseases, such as allergies (103), but could also exert some protective effects in other inflammatory pathologies, such as cardiovascular diseases and OP, mainly depending on genetics, disease duration, and the cytokine microenvironment (116). In particular, the role of IL-33 in OP and Pso is still debated. Some authors have reported IL-33 inhibition of osteoclast formation (117), whereas others described an IL-33-induced reduction in osteoprotegerin expression by osteoblasts and an increase in osteoclastogenic factor release (118), thus suggesting an IL-33 mediated bone resorption induction during inflammation (98). IL-33 stimulates mast cells to produce IL-6 and IL-13 *via* the canonical NF-kB signaling and p38 pathways. The MAPK-activated protein kinases MK2 and MK3, function as sensors of cell injury and exert pivotal roles in IL-33-induced cytokine production by mast cells in inflammatory responses (87, 98, 107). Due to its pleiotropic nature, IL-33 exerts contrasting roles in different diseases (87, 88), i.e., IL-33 can either drive the underlying inflammation or promote its resolution (99, 113) according to the individual inflammatory context. Disease severity and changes in relation to hormonal influences contribute to the bone remodeling effects of IL-33. For example, notwithstanding the decreased serum IL-33 levels in women undergoing menopause with OP, its protective effect on the bone disappears as OP progresses, likely due to the interference of other proinflammatory osteoclastogenic cytokines. In particular, IL-33 has controversial roles in bone remodeling (115, 119, 120). The majority of studies suggest prevalent anti-osteoclastogenic and osteoanabolic functions of IL-33, but the reduced expression of OPG by osteoblasts and the induced production of the osteoclastogenic cytokine IL-31 (97), have also been reported, suggesting that in particular inflammatory conditions, including arthritis and Pso, IL-33 can induce bone resorption. This hypothesis seems to be supported by the finding of periarticular bone erosions and systemic OP in PsoA, in which IL-33 plays a pathogenetically important role.

THE RELATIONSHIP BETWEEN VITAMIN D AND THE IL-33/ST2 AXIS IN PSORIASIS-ASSOCIATED OSTEOPOROSIS

Link Between Vitamin D and IL-33

There is a close relationship between vitamin D and the IL-33/ST2 axis in bone and skin homeostasis. Nonetheless, the exact role of vitamin D in IL-33 activities, which creates vicious circles in the pathogenesis of Pso-associated OP, remains controversial (91, 93). It is likely that vitamin D and IL-33 share some signal pathways and need each other to perform some important immunological and metabolic functions both the skin and bone levels. In particular, there is evidence that, in some biological processes, they act in synergy, while in other cases, they act by controlling and modulating each other (71). Here, we hypothesize a mechanistic link between vitamin D and IL-33 in patients with Pso and associated OP.

Vitamin D and IL-33 Immunological Crosstalk

IL-33 shares many of the immunoregulatory effects of vitamin D, either potentiating or modulating them (**Box 4**). IL-33 is produced by cells regulated by vitamin D, and often their tissue targets and signal pathways are shared. For example, both vitamin D and IL-33 promote the differentiation of Th2 lymphocytes by inhibiting Th1 differentiation and also act as inducers of immunoregulatory cells. Vitamin D can downregulate the production of inflammatory cytokines and chemokines (121). Moreover, vitamin D activity is determined through vitamin D receptors, which are present not only in the skeleton but also in different types of cells, including antigen-presenting-cells, immune cells, and keratinocytes. In particular, DCs, lymphocytes, monocytes/macrophages, neutrophils, and epithelial cells can produce IL-33 and other cytokines involved in both bone remodeling and Pso inflammation, including IL-31, IL-17, and TNF-alpha (29, 62, 107). IL-33 therefore orchestrates the immune cascade of Pso. Moreover, it takes part in the bone remodeling process (115). Vitamin D plays a central role in both bone turnover and immune regulation. In addition, vitamin D is also implicated in skin homeostasis, acting as a potent immune system modulator and suppressing dendritic cell maturation. Serum vitamin D levels are decreased in Pso patients and, in particular, in those with associated OP.

The impact of low vitamin D levels has been widely investigated in both Pso and OP, as has the role of IL-33. Th2-related cytokines, including IL-4, IL-31, and IL-33, have recently been shown to play important roles in bone remodeling as well as in Pso skin inflammation and PsoA (47, 65). IL-33 may act as an alarmin, exerting both repairing and damaging processes and functioning as a nuclear transcription factor. Similarly, the vitamin D receptor, functioning as a ligand-activated transcription factor, regulates the activation or repression of gene transcription (121). Moreover, vitamin D deficiency likely independently contributes to the increased incidence of OP in Pso patients.

The relationship between IL-33 and vitamin D is highly complex and extremely variable. For example, IL-33 contributes to inflammatory reactions involving vitamin D deficiency but could also counteract some of its deleterious effects, mainly depending on the clinical context as well as on the cytokine and hormonal milieu. As a consequence, it is conceivable that although both vitamin D and IL-33 in the bone environment exert protective effects against OP, in inflamed Pso skin and in PsoA, the deleterious effects of vitamin D deficiency and IL-33/ST2 axis activation potentiate each other (85, 100). Decreased vitamin D and increased IL-33 levels are also both associated to Th2 immunity in allergic inflammatory diseases (122), suggesting that they play contrasting roles in allergies (71). Based on these considerations, a potential complex interaction between vitamin D and IL-33 has been hypothesized, not only in allergic diseases but also in other clinical conditions in which their roles have also been demonstrated, including Pso and OP. Vitamin D promotes anti-inflammatory IL-10 synthesis by inducing α-1-antitrypsin expression in CD4+ T cells (123). IL-10, as an immunosuppressive cytokine, directly limits Th2 cell differentiation and survival during allergic airway inflammation (124). On the other hand, IL-33 induces Th2 cytokines, including IL-31, thus exerting a pivotal role in orchestrating the recruitment and activation of effector cells of the allergic response. IL-31 is a cytokine produced by CD4+ T cells which has a potent immunological link with IL-33 and plays important roles in allergic inflammation and atopic dermatitis as well as in Pso (38, 88). A similar close link has been highlighted as being an important factor in the alteration of the bone remodeling process that underlies OP (92). The IL-31 receptor IL-31RA, the oncostatin M receptor, and the IL-33 receptor ST2 are related to the immunopathological mechanisms of Pso and OP. The ST2 receptor of IL-33, which is a critical component of Th2 responses, stimulates the production of IL-31 (88). At the same time, sST2, which is increased in Pso patients and acts as a decoy receptor for IL-33, is a negative modulator of the IL-33/ST2 axis. There is evidence that a perturbation of this axis exerts essential roles in OP (91). Plasma sST2 levels were found to be correlated with decreased cortical BMD and deterioration of the bone microstructure in Pso. Vitamin D enhances the synthesis of the IL-33 inhibitor sST2, counteracting inflammation in psoriatic skin (66). The association between increased sST2 and decreased vitamin D in Pso might synergistically contribute to the effect of inflammatory mediators in inducing compromised bone quality and OP.

Treg activity is influenced by both vitamin D and IL-33. Normal tissue repair, as well as bone and skin homeostasis, requires both vitamin D and IL-33 to locally expand Treg cells. The impact of Foxp3+ Treg cell derangement is involved in the autoimmune inflammatory processes of Pso (125). IL-33 promotes the recruitment of Treg cells into the site of injury, where they suppress inflammation. Through Treg recruitment and inhibition of NF-kB mediated gene transcription, IL-33

BOX 4 | Vitamin D/IL-33 crosstalk.

Key points:

1. *Shared immunoregulatory and homeostatic effects:*
   - Promotion of Th2 lymphocyte differentiation
   - Induction of immunoregulatory cells
   - Downregulation of inflammatory cytokine and chemokine production
   - Regulation of bone remodeling process
   - Modulation of PTH control of bone turnover
2. *Contrasting roles:*
   - Protective role of vitamin D in allergic diseases vs the induction of allergic inflammation by IL-33
   - Enhanced inflammatory osteoclastogenesis by IL-33-induced secretion of IL-31 vs bone protection by vitamin D
   - IL-33 induced and amplified inflammatory circuits vs vitamin D anti-inflammatory activity in Pso

exerts protective effects on bone. Also, vitamin D may exert its immune regulatory properties through the induction of Treg cells. Low levels of vitamin D in Pso patients could dysregulate immunological homeostasis by decreasing the number of circulatory Tregs (46, 80). Vitamin D modulates CD4+ T cell function, reversing the defective induction of IL-10-secreting regulatory T cells. IL-33 induces IL-10-producing regulatory B cells and promotes IL-10 production in macrophages (125, 126).

PTH Regulation by Vitamin D and IL-33

The links between vitamin D and IL-33 are both hormonal and immunological. PTH, the main hormone that regulates bone turnover and whose production is dependent on the levels of calcium and vitamin D in the body, is, in turn, strictly dependent on the IL-33/ST2 axis (127). Calcium metabolism is finely regulated by vitamin D and IL-33 in concert with PTH. The latter elevates calcium levels and reduces phosphorus levels in the blood. Calcium is a major regulator of sequential keratinocyte differentiation through the different layers of the epidermis until the stratum corneum is formed and is involved in signaling pathways that are central to desmosome and tight junction formation. Calcium receptors initiate the intracellular signaling cascade, driving differentiation in response to extracellular calcium. Calcium metabolism is also central to bone turnover. It is an essential component of hydroxyapatite crystals which confer hardness and resistance to the skeleton through deposits in the extracellular bone matrix. Vitamin D deficiency involves modification of calcium–phosphorus metabolism and increased secretion of PTH, which leads to increases in bone resorption and matrix demineralization. However, PTH could also function as an important osteoanabolic factor when administered pharmacologically (120, 128).

IL-33 and its receptors have roles in the PTH control of bone turnover (129). IL-33 mRNA levels in osteoblasts are increased by PTH and M oncostatin (127), and a positive correlation between PTH and IL-33 serum levels in postmenopausal OP has been observed (99). IL-33 production is stimulated by PTH, which contributes to the osteoanabolic effects of such a hormone. Vitamin D deficiency increases PTH secretion (78). As a consequence, IL-33 also increases, thus modulating the effects of PTH on bone remodeling (127). Therefore, the cytokine IL-33 represents a target of PTH and, synergistically with vitamin D, increases bone matrix mineralization by osteoblasts. IL-33 induced expression of the RANKL-encoding gene has been demonstrated in osteoblasts. RANKL, the major osteoclastogenic cytokine, is produced as a transmembrane protein, whose proteolytic processing is promoted by PTH, leading to the release of its soluble form. RANKL secretion, therefore, depends on integrated actions of both IL-33 and PTH (130). Moreover, both vitamin D and PTH control the levels of sST2. Serum sST2 correlates positively with serum phosphorus and negatively with serum calcium. The osteocyte-derived factor FGF-23, which inhibits PTH and promotes renal phosphorus excretion, also antagonizes some vitamin D effects. The IL-33/ST2 axis is, therefore, a PTH target that is able to both promote osteoblastic calcium deposition in the bone matrix and inhibit osteoclastogenesis (36). Increased levels of PTH induce elevation of sST2 (129). These data suggest that sST2 may play important roles in bone metabolism disorders, such as OP, as well as in inflammatory diseases, such as Pso.

THE PARADOX OF THE VITAMIN D AND IL-33 RELATIONSHIP IN PSO-ASSOCIATED OP

Increased bone resorption with consequent appearance of OP is commonly associated with Pso and, in particular, with the more evolutionary forms characterized by systemic inflammation and joint involvement. It has been ascertained that vitamin D exerts protective effects in both Pso and OP (9). On the contrary, IL-33 is considered a pathogenetic cytokine in Pso, whereas its effects on bone are variable. Therefore, the role of IL-33 seems to be contrasting (111). In reality, this apparent contradiction could be explained by the multiplicity of functions of this cytokine which, depending on the type of tissue, the immune environment, and the presence of other associated factors, can have different effects. It could be hypothesized that, notwithstanding increased IL-33 levels, the skeleton is instead more sensitive to a wide range of osteoporotic risk factors that are increased during Pso, including inflammation and vitamin D deficiency, which potentiate each other. Furthermore, most studies have shown compartmentalization of IL-33 in Pso with increased concentrations in skin lesions but not in the serum (114), potentially explaining the lack of protective effects on bone. The final effect of the IL-33/ST2 axis in both Pso and OP therefore depends on the reciprocal relationship between its various components which influence each other through complex regulatory mechanisms and positive and negative feedback circuits (113). For example, the effect of an increase in IL-33 could be counterbalanced by a consensual increase in its decoy receptor sST2 or, on the contrary, it could be enhanced by increased expression of its receptor on different cell types (66). In turn, there are several types of IL-33 target cells, including immune cells, mesenchymal stromal cells, and epithelial cells (85). Therefore, depending on the target cell type, the effect of the cytokine could vary from pro-inflammatory to anti-inflammatory. In the immunopathogenetic processes driving inflammation, the co-operation of IL-33 with IL-17, IL-22, TNF-alpha, IFN-gamma, or other inflammatory factors has been suggested. In this way, the proinflammatory functions of IL-33 could prevail on its immunoregulatory properties, as observed in several autoimmune diseases, including Pso (129).

The bone protective effect of IL-33 could be masked or prevented by concomitant factors characterizing Pso, such as the deficiency of vitamin D and the consequently altered PTH-mediated calcium–phosphorus metabolism, the prevalence of Th1/Th17 systemic inflammation with an increase in osteoclastogenic cytokines, and mechanisms of counter-regulation of IL-33 signaling associated with the inflammatory process (99). On the other hand, IL-33 itself can perform different and contrasting functions: it can act as a pro-inflammatory factor in some pathological conditions but also as an alarmin with protective functions in response to danger signals, cell injury, and tissue damage (37).

Both vitamin D deficiency and increased circulating sST2 decoy receptor in Pso negatively impact the bone, favoring the production of Th1 rather than Th2 cytokines, suppressing the development of Treg cells and the production of regulatory and anti-inflammatory cytokines, thus promoting osteoclastogenesis and bone resorption (88, 94). The frequent of onset of OP during Pso could also be conditioned by the effective variability of effects of IL-33 on bone remodeling, which are dependent on a wide range of other factors (inflammatory microenvironment, influence of other cytokines, hormones, and vitamins) (9). A vitamin D deficiency could somehow nullify the protective effect of IL-33 on bone through mechanisms that are still unclear (121).

Figure 1 summarizes the complex interaction between vitamin D deficiency and increased IL-33/ST2 axis expression leading to increased bone resorption and OP in Pso.

CONCLUSIONS

In summary, there is clinical evidence that Pso, especially if associated with arthritis and a more advanced age, is associated with hypovitaminosis D, inflammation, and OP, and these factors might shift the effect of IL-33 from osteoprotective to proinflammatory and osteoclastogenic (39). The IL-33 levels in subjects with Pso reflect of increased inflammation, driving OP development. Different hypotheses could explain this paradox. For example, it has been recently demonstrated that the production of the soluble decoy receptor sST2 is enhanced by vitamin D (94). Since sST2 neutralizes the effect of IL-33, it is

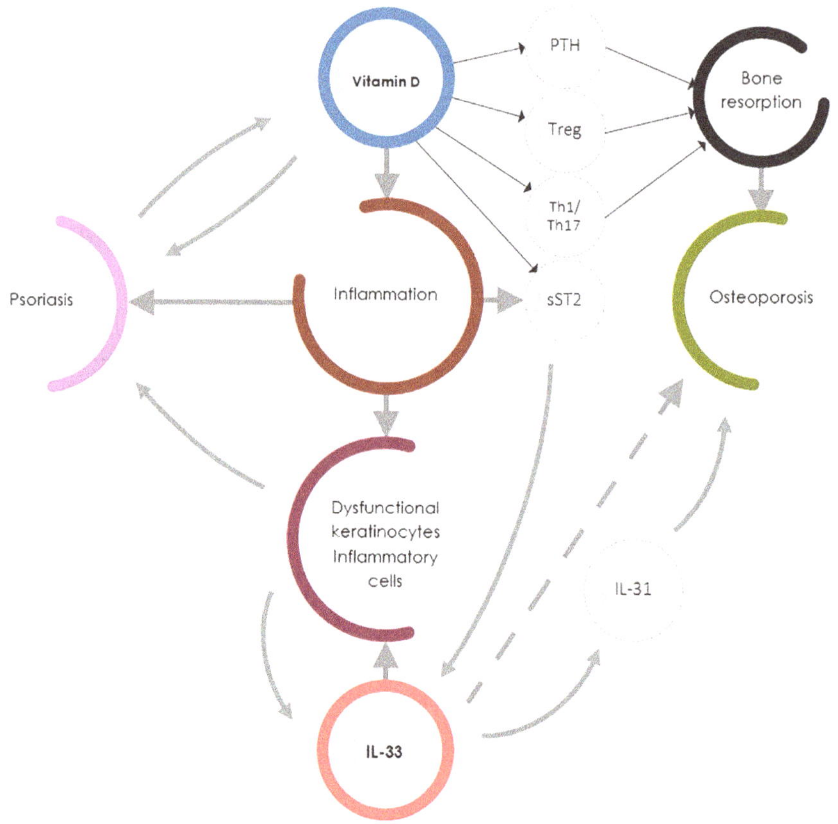

FIGURE 1 | Vitamin D deficiency and increased IL-33/ST2 expression in Pso-associated OP. IL-33 could exert contrasting roles in Pso and OP: it might drive the inflammation underlying Pso by inducing the production of dysfunctional keratinocytes and inflammatory cells but could exert protective effects in OP (dashed arrow). Vitamin D, in synergy with IL-33, regulates bone metabolism through PTH release and function, but also increases the soluble decoy receptor sST2 production, thus regulating IL-33 function. The direct action of vitamin D in inhibiting IL-33 function on bone cells is, however, less important than other vitamin D-mediated osteoprotective mechanisms (e.g., the vitamin D capacity to both inhibit Th1 and Th17 inflammation and induce bone protective Th2-type responses). In Pso-associated OP the complex interaction between vitamin D deficiency and increased IL-33/ST2 expression therefore leads to osteoclastogenesis and bone resorption through several mechanisms: PTH hyperproduction, impaired Treg function, increased Th1 and Th17 inflammatory and osteoclastogenic cytokine production, and decreased sST2 expression by lymphocytes and epithelial cells, resulting in an increase in IL-33 induced skin inflammation. Furthermore, the increase in IL-33 in psoriatic patients leads to an increased production of IL-31 which contributes to the worsening of bone loss.

considered an anti-inflammatory factor in conditions in which IL-33 takes place in the driving inflammatory processes, such as asthma and Pso, and IL-33 neutralization may represent a novel therapeutic approach in these diseases. On the contrary, in the skeleton, the role of IL-33 is likely protective against OP and its sST2 mediated neutralization is detrimental (66). Therefore, in Pso-associated OP, the final effect of vitamin D deficiency and IL-33/ST2 axis overexpression is overall increased bone resorption due to the prevalence of proinflammatory and dysmetabolic processes (9, 66).

AUTHOR CONTRIBUTIONS

All authors contributed to the article and approved the submitted version.

REFERENCES

1. Boehncke WH, Schön MP. Psoriasis. *Lancet* (2015) 386(9997):983–94. doi: 10.1016/S0140-6736(14)61909-7
2. Rendon A, Schäkel K. Psoriasis Pathogenesis and Treatment. *Int J Mol Sci* (2019) 20(6):1475. doi: 10.3390/ijms20061475
3. Veale DJ, Fearon U. The pathogenesis of psoriatic arthritis. *Lancet* (2018) 391(10136):2273–84. doi: 10.1016/S0140-6736(18)30830-4
4. Borsky P, Fiala Z, Andrys C, Beranek M, Hamakova K, Malkova A, et al. Alarmins HMGB1, IL-33, S100A7, and S100A12 in psoriasis vulgaris. *Mediators Inflamm* (2020) 2020:8465083. doi: 10.1155/2020/8465083
5. Boehncke WH. Systemic inflammation and cardiovascular comorbidity in psoriasis patients: causes and consequences. *Front Immunol* (2018) 9:579. doi: 10.3389/fimmu.2018.00579
6. Ciccarelli F, De Martinis M, Sirufo MM, Ginaldi L. Psoriasis Induced by Anti-Tumor Necrosis Factor Alpha Agents: A Comprehensive Review of the Literature. *Acta Dermatovenerol Croat* (2016) 24(3):169–74.
7. Bilal J, Malik SU, Riaz IB, Kurtzman DJB. Psoriasis and psoriatic spectrum disease: a primer for the primary care physician. *Am J Med* (2018) 131 (10):1146–54. doi: 10.1016/j.amjmed.2018.05.013
8. Furue M, Kadono T. Psoriasis: behind the scenes. *J Dermatol* (2016) 43(1):4–8. doi: 10.1111/1346-8138.131865
9. Sirufo MM, De Pietro F, Bassino EM, Ginaldi L, De Martinis M. Osteoporosis in Skin Diseases. *Int J Mol Sci* (2020) 21(13):4749. doi: 10.3390/ijms21134749
10. Lajevardi V, Abedini R, Moghaddasi M, Nassiri S, Goodarzi A. Bone mineral density is lower in male than female patients with plaque-type psoriasis in Iran. *Int J Women's Dermatol* (2017) 3:201–5. doi: 10.1016/j.ijwd.2017.07.007
11. De Martinis M, Sirufo MM, Polsinelli M, Placidi G, Di Silvestre D, Ginaldi L. Gender differences in osteoporosis: A single-center observational study. *WJMH* (2020) 38:e62. doi: 10.5534/wjmh.200099
12. De Martinis M, Sirufo MM, Ginaldi L. Osteoporosis: Current and emerging therapies targeted to immunological checkpoints. *Curr Med Chem* (2020) 27 (37):6356–72. doi: 10.2174/0929867326666190730113123
13. Ginaldi L, Di Benedetto MC, De Martinis M. Osteoporosis, inflammation and ageing. *Immun Ageing* (2005) 2:14. doi: 10.1186/1742-4933-2-14
14. De Martinis M, Di Benedetto MC, Mengoli LP, Ginaldi L. Senile osteoporosis: is it an immune-mediated disease? *Inflammation Res* (2006) 55(10):399–404. doi: 10.1007/s00011-006-6034-x
15. Wacker M, Holick MF. Vitamin D - Effects on skeletal and extraskeletal health and the need for supplementation. *Nutrients* (2013) 5(1):111–48. doi: 10.3390/nu5010111.16
16. Irelli A, Sirufo MM, Scipioni T, De Pietro F, Pancotti A, Ginaldi L, et al. mTOR links tumor immunity and bone metabolism: What are the clinical implications? *Int J Mol Sci* (2019) 20:5841. doi: 10.3390/ijms20235841
17. De Martinis M, Sirufo MM, Nocelli C, Fontanella L, Ginaldi L. Hyperhomocysteinemia is associated with inflammation, bone resorption, vitamin B12 and folate deficiency and MTHFR C677T polymorphism in postmenopausal women with decreased bone mineral density. *Int J Environ Res Public Health* (2020) 17(12):4260. doi: 10.3390/ijerph17124260
18. Kanda J, Izumo N, Furukawa M, Shimakura T, Yamamoto N, Takahashi HE, et al. Effects of the calcineurin inhibitors cyclosporine and tacrolimus on bone metabolism in rats. *BioMed Res* (2018) 39:131–9. doi: 10.2220/biomedres.39.131
19. Ciccarelli F, De Martinis M, Ginaldi L. Glucocorticoids in patients with rheumatic diseases: friends or enemies of bone? *Curr Med Chem* (2015) 22 (5):596–603. doi: 10.2174/0929867321666141106125051
20. Mowad C, Cohen SF, Fussell NF, Martin RE, Ellison CA. Referral patterns to an osteoporosis clinic for dermatology patients undergoing prolonged corticosteroid therapy. *J Am Acad Dermatol* (2018) 78:591–2. doi: 10.1016/j.jaad.2017.01.058
21. Ginaldi L, De Martinis M. Osteoimmunology and Beyond. *Curr Med Chem* (2016) 23(33):3754–74. doi: 10.2174/0929867323666160907162546
22. Ramot Y. Psoriasis and osteoporosis: The debate continues. *Br J Dermatol* (2017) 176:1117–8. doi: 10.1111/bjd.15437
23. Ogdie A, Harter L, Shin D, Baker J, Takeshita J, Choi HK, et al. The risk of fracture among patients with psoriatic arthritis and psoriasis: A population-based study. *Ann Rheum Dis* (2017) 76:882–5. doi: 10.1136/annrheumdis-2016-210441
24. Pedreira PG, Pinheiro MM, Szejnfeld VL. Bone mineral density and body composition in postmenopausal women with psoriasis and psoriatic arthritis. *Arthritis Res* (2011) 13:R16. doi: 10.1186/ar3240
25. Sirufo MM, Suppa M, Ginaldi L, De Martinis M. Does Allergy Break Bones? Osteoporosis and Its Connection to Allergy. *Int J Mol Sci* (2020) 21(3):712. doi: 10.3390/ijms21030712
26. De Martinis M, Ciccarelli F, Sirufo MM, Ginaldi L. An overview of environmental risk factors in systemic sclerosis. *Expert Rev Clin Immunol* (2016) 12(4):465–78. doi: 10.1586/1744666X.2016.1125782
27. Sirufo MM, Ginaldi L, De Martinis M. Successful Treatment With Omalizumab in a Child With Asthma and Urticaria: A Clinical Case Report. *Front Pediatr* (2019) 7:213. doi: 10.3389/fped.2019.00213
28. Sirufo MM, De Martinis M, Ginaldi L. Omalizumab an effective and safe alternative therapy in severe refractory atopic dermatitis: A case report. *Med (Baltimore)* (2018) 97(24):e10897. doi: 10.1097/MD.0000000000010897
29. Raimondo A, Lembo S, Di Caprio R, Donnarumma G, Monfrecola G, Balato N, et al. Psoriatic cutaneous inflammation promotes human monocyte differentiation into active osteoclasts, facilitating bone damage. *Eur J Immunol* (2017) 47:1062–74. doi: 10.1002/eji.201646774
30. Uluçkan Ö, Wagner EF. Chronic systemic inflammation originating from epithelial tissues. *FEBS J* (2017) 284(4):505–16. doi: 10.1111/febs.13904
31. Uluçkan Ö, Wagner EF. Role of IL-17A signalling in psoriasis and associated bone loss. *Clin Exp Rheumatol* (2016) 34(4 Suppl 98):17–20.
32. Mizutani K, Isono K, Matsushima Y, Okada K, Umaoka A, Iida S, et al. Inflammatory skin-derived cytokines accelerate osteoporosis in mice with persistent skin inflammation. *Int J Mol Sci* (2020) 21:3620. doi: 10.3390/ijms21103620
33. Komatsu N, Takayanagi H. Immune-bone interplay in the structural damage in rheumatoid arthritis. *Clin Exp Immunol* (2018) 194(1):1–8. doi: 10.1111/cei.13188
34. Sato Y, Ogawa E, Okuyama R. Role of innate immune cells in psoriasis. *Int J Mol Sci* (2020) 21(18):6604. doi: 10.3390/ijms21186604
35. Michael P, Schön MP, Erpenbeck L. The interleukin-23/interleukin-17 axis links adaptive and innate immunity in psoriasis. *Front Immunol* (2018) 9:1323. doi: 10.3389/fimmu.2018.01323
36. Cannavò SP, Bertino L, Di Salvo E, Papaianni V, Ventura-Spagnolo E, Gangemi S. Possible roles of IL-33 in the innate-adaptive immune crosstalk of psoriasis pathogenesis. *Mediators Inflammation* (2019) 2019:7158014. doi: 10.1155/2019/7158014

37. Sehat M, Talaei R, Dadgostar E, Nikoueinejad H, Akbari H. Evaluating serum levels of IL-33, IL-36, IL-37 and gene expression of IL-37 in patients with psoriasis vulgaris. *Iran J Allergy Asthma Immunol* (2018) 17(2):179–87.
38. Duan Y, Dong Y, Hu H, Wang Q, Guo S, Fu D, et al. IL-33 contributes to disease severity in psoriasis-like models of mouse. *Cytokine* (2019) 119:159–67. doi: 10.1016/j.cyto.2019.02.019
39. Mitsui A, Tada Y, Takahashi T, Shibata S, Kamata M, Miyagaki T, et al. Serum IL-33 levels are increased in patients with psoriasis. *Clin Exp Dermatol* (2016) 41(2):183–9. doi: 10.1111/ced.12670
40. Modalsli EH, Åsvold BO, Romundstad PR, Langhammer A, Hoff M, Forsmo S, et al. Psoriasis, fracture risk and bone mineral density: the HUNT Study, Norway. *Br J Dermatol* (2017) 176(5):1162–9. doi: 10.1111/bjd.15123
41. Kathuria P, Gordon KB, Silverberg JI. Association of psoriasis and psoriatic arthritis with osteoporosis and pathological fractures. *J Am Acad Dermatol* (2017) 76(6):1045–1053.e3. doi: 10.1016/j.jaad.2016.11.046
42. Martinez-Lopez A, Blasco-Morente G, Giron-Prieto MS, Arrabal-Polo MA, Luque-Valenzuela M, Luna-Del Castillo JD, et al. Linking of psoriasis with osteopenia and osteoporosis: A cross-sectional study. *Indian J Dermatol Venereol Leprol* (2019) 85(2):153–9. doi: 10.4103/ijdvl.IJDVL_831_17
43. Attia EA, Khafagy A, Abdel-Raheem S, Fathi S, Saad AA. Assessment of osteoporosis in psoriasis with and without arthritis: correlation with disease severity. *Int J Dermatol* (2011) 50(1):30–5. doi: 10.1111/j.1365-4632.2010.04600.x
44. De Martinis M, Sirufo MM, Suppa M, Di Silvestre D, Ginaldi L. Sex and gender aspects for patient stratification in allergy prevention and treatment. *Int J Mol Sci* (2020) 21(4):1535. doi: 10.3390/ijms21041535
45. Kaukinen A, Pelkonen J, Harvima IT. Mast cells express CYP27A1 and CYP27B1 in epithelial skin cancers and psoriasis. *Eur J Dermatol* (2015) 25 (6):548–55. doi: 10.1684/ejd.2015.2645
46. Zuccotti E, Oliveri M, Girometta C, Ratto D, Di Iorio C, Occhinegro A, et al. Nutritional strategies for psoriasis: current scientific evidence in clinical trials. *Eur Rev Med Pharmacol Sci* (2018) 22(23):8537–51. doi: 10.26355/eurrev-201812-16554
47. Kusuba N, Kitoh A, Dainichi T, Honda T, Otsuka A, Egawa G, et al. Inhibition of IL-17-committed T cells in a murine psoriasis model by a vitamin D analogue. *J Allergy Clin Immunol* (2018) 141(3):972–81.e10. doi: 10.1016/j.jaci.2017.07.033
48. Mattozzi C, Paolino G, Richetta AG, Calvieri S. Psoriasis, vitamin D and the importance of the cutaneous barrier's integrity: An update. *J Dermatol* (2016) 43(5):507–14. doi: 10.1111/1346-8138.13305
49. Takeshita J, Grewal S, Langan SM, Mehta NN, Ogdie A, Van Voorhees AS, et al. Psoriasis and comorbid diseases: Epidemiology. *J Am Acad Dermatol* (2017) 76(3):377–90. doi: 10.1016/j.jaad.2016.07.064
50. Gisondi P, Fostini AC, Fossà I, Girolomoni G, Targher G. Psoriasis and the metabolic syndrome. *Clin Dermatol* (2018) 36(1):21–8. doi: 10.1016/j.clindermatol.2017.09.005
51. Jensen P, Skov L. Psoriasis and obesity. *Dermatology* (2016) 232(6):633–9. doi: 10.1159/000455840
52. Lee SJ, Lee EY, Lee JH, Kim JE, Kim KJ, Rhee Y, et al. Associations of serum 25-hydroxyvitamin D with metabolic syndrome and its components in elderly men and women: the Korean Urban Rural Elderly cohort study. *BMC Geriatr* (2019) 19(1):102. doi: 10.1186/s12877-019-1118-y
53. Barrea L, Savanelli MC, Di Somma C, Napolitano M, Megna M, Colao A, et al. and its role in psoriasis: an overview of the dermatologist and nutritionist. *Rev Endocr Metab Disord* (2017) 18(2):195–205. doi: 10.1007/s11154-017-9411-6
54. Umar M, Sastry KS, Al Ali F, Al-Khulaifi M, Wang E, Chouchane AI. Vitamin D and the pathophysiology of inflammatory skin diseases. *Skin Pharmacol Physiol* (2018) 31(2):74–86. doi: 10.1159/000485132
55. Cubillos S, Krieg N, Norgauer J. Effect of vitamin D on peripheral blood mononuclear cells from patients with psoriasis vulgaris and psoriatic arthritis. *PloS One* (2016) 11(4):e0153094. doi: 10.1371/journal.pone.0153094
56. Kanda N, Hoashi T, Saeki H. Nutrition and psoriasis. *Int J Mol Sci* (2020) 21 (15):E5405. doi: 10.3390/ijms21155405
57. Stefanic M, Rucevic I, Barisic-Drusko V. Meta-analysis of vitamin D receptor polymorphisms and psoriasis risk. *Int J Dermatol* (2013) 52 (6):705–10. doi: 10.1111/j.1365-4632.2012.5813.x
58. Kincse G, Bhattoa PH, Herédi E, Varga J, Szegedi A, Kéri J, et al. Vitamin D3 levels and bone mineral density in patients with psoriasis and/or psoriatic arthritis. *J Dermatol* (2015) 42(7):679–84. doi: 10.1111/1346-8138.12876
59. Hambly R, Kirby B. The relevance of serum vitamin D in psoriasis: a review. *Arch Dermatol Res* (2017) 309(7):499–517. doi: 10.1007/s00403-017-1751-2
60. Morales-Tirado V, Wichlan DG, Leimig TE, Street SE, Kasow KA, Riberdy JM. 1α,25-dihydroxyvitamin D3 (vitamin D3) catalyzes suppressive activity on human natural regulatory T cells, uniquely modulates cell cycle progression, and augments FOXP3. *Clin Immunol* (2011) 138(2):212–21. doi: 10.1016/j.clim.2010.11.003
61. Nair-Shalliker V, Fenech M, Forder PM, Clements MS, Armstrong BK. Sunlight and vitamin D affect DNA damage, cell division and cell death in human lymphocytes: a cross-sectional study in South Australia. *Mutagenesis* (2012) 27(5):609–14. doi: 10.1093/mutage/ges026
62. Janeva-Jovanovska E, Dokic D, Jovkovska-Kaeva B, Breskovska G, Goseva Z, Minov J, et al. Relationship between vitamin D, inflammation and lung function in patients with severe uncontrolled asthma. *Open Access Maced J Med Sci* (2017) 5(7):899–903. doi: 10.3889/oamjms.2017.190
63. Chaiprasongsuk A, Janjetovic Z, Kim TK, Jarrett SG, D'Orazio JA, Holick MF, et al. Protective effects of novel derivatives of vitamin D(3) and lumisterol against UVB-induced damage in human keratinocytes involve activation of Nrf2 and p53 defense mechanisms. *Redox Biol* (2019) 24:101206. doi: 10.1016/j.redox.2019.101206
64. Soleymani T, Hung T, Soung J. The role of vitamin D in psoriasis: a review. *Int J Dermatol* (2015) 54(4):383–92. doi: 10.1111/ijd.12790
65. Gao M, Yao X, Ding J, Hong R, Wu Y, Huang H, et al. Low levels of vitamin D and the relationship between vitamin D and Th2 axis-related cytokines in neuromyelitis optica spectrum disorders. *J Clin Neurosci* (2019) 61:22–7. doi: 10.1016/j.jocn.2018.11.024
66. Pfeffer PE, Chen YH, Woszczek G, Matthews NC, Chevretton E, Gupta A, et al. Vitamin D enhances production of soluble ST2, inhibiting the action of IL-33. *J Allergy Clin Immunol* (2015) 135(3):824–7.e3. doi: 10.1016/j.jaci.2014.09.044
67. Prietl B, Treiber G, Pieber TR, Amrein K, Vitamin D. and immune function. *Nutrients* (2013) 5(7):2502–21. doi: 10.3390/nu5072502
68. Mohammadi-Kordkhayli M, Ahangar-Parvin R, Azizi SV, Nemati M, Shamsizadeh A, Khaksari M, et al. Vitamin D modulates the expression of IL-27 and IL-33 in the central nervous system in experimental autoimmune encephalomyelitis (EAE). *Iran J Immunol* (2015) 12(1):35–49.
69. Jafarzadeh A, Azizi SV, Arabi Z, Ahangar-Parvin R, Mohammadi-Kordkhayli M, Larussa T, et al. Vitamin D down-regulates the expression of some Th17 cell-related cytokines, key inflammatory chemokines, and chemokine receptors in experimental autoimmune encephalomyelitis. *Nutr Neurosci* (2019) 22(10):725–37. doi: 10.1080/1028415X.2018.1436237
70. Skrobot A, Demkow U, Wachowska M. Immunomodulatory role of vitamin D: a review. *Adv Exp Med Biol* (2018) 1108:13–23. doi: 10.1007/5584_2018_246
71. Bonanno A, Gangemi S, La Grutta S, Malizia V, Riccobono L, Colombo P, et al. 25-hydroxyvitamin D, IL-31, and IL-33 in children with allergic disease of the airways. *Mediators Inflammation* (2014) 2014:520241. doi: 10.1155/2014/520241
72. De Martinis M, Franceschi C, Monti D, Ginaldi L. Apoptosis remodeling in immunosenescence: implications for strategies to delay ageing. *Curr Med Chem* (2007) 14(13):1389–97. doi: 10.2174/092986707780831122
73. Guo Y, Zhang X, Wu T, Hu X, Su J, Chen X. Autophagy in skin diseases. *Dermatology* (2019) 235:380–9. doi: 10.1159/000500470
74. Massimini M, Palmieri C, De Maria R, Romanucci M, Malatesta D, De Martinis M, et al. 17-AAG and apoptosis, autophagy, and mitophagy in canine osteosarcoma cell lines. *Vet Pathol* (2014) 54(3):405–12. doi: 10.1177/0300985816681409
75. Sun HQ, Yan D, Wang QN, Meng HZ, Zhang YY, Yin LX, et al. 1,25-Dihydroxyvitamin D3 attenuates disease severity and induces synoviocyte apoptosis in a concentration-dependent manner in rats with adjuvant-induced arthritis by inactivating the NF-κB signaling pathway. *J Bone Miner Metab* (2019) 37(3):430–40. doi: 10.1007/s00774-018-0944-x
76. Marino R, Misra M. Extra-skeletal effects of vitamin D. *Nutrients* (2019) 11 (7):1460. doi: 10.3390/nu110714608-10
77. Deng Y, Chang C, Lu Q. The inflammatory response in psoriasis: a comprehensive review. *Clin Rev Allergy Immunol* (2016) 50(3):377–89. doi: 10.1007/s12016-016-8535-x

78. Goltzman D. Functions of vitamin D in bone. *Histochem Cell Biol* (2018) 149 (4):305–12. doi: 10.1007/s00418-018-1648-y
79. Brembilla NC, Senra L, Boehncke WH. The IL-17 family of cytokines in psoriasis: IL-17A and beyond. *Front Immunol* (2018) 9:1682. doi: 10.3389/fimmu.2018.01682
80. Hau CS, Shimizu T, Tada Y, Kamata M, Takeoka S, Shibata S, et al. The vitamin D(3) analog, maxacalcitol, reduces psoriasiform skin inflammation by inducing regulatory T cells and downregulating IL-23 and IL-17 production. *J Dermatol Sci* (2018) 92(2):117–26. doi: 10.1016/j.jdermsci.2018.08.007
81. Yamamoto EA, Nguyen JK, Liu J, Keller E, Campbell N, Zhang CJ, et al. Low levels of vitamin D promote memory B cells in lupus. *Nutrients* (2020) 12 (2):291. doi: 10.3390/nu12020291
82. Coates LC, FitzGerald O, Helliwell PS, Paul C. Psoriasis, psoriatic arthritis, and rheumatoid arthritis: Is all inflammation the same? *Semin Arthritis Rheumatol* (2016) 46(3):291–304. doi: 10.1016/j.semarthrit.2016.05.012
83. Srivastava RK, Dar HY, Mishra PK. Immunoporosis: immunology of osteoporosis-role of T cells. *Front Immunol* (2018) 9:657. doi: 10.3389/fimmu.2018.00657
84. Zhang J, Fu Q, Ren Z, Wang Y, Wang C, Shen T, et al. Changes of serum cytokines-related Th1/Th2/Th17 concentration in patients with postmenopausal osteoporosis. *Gynecol Endocrinol* (2015) 31(3):183–90. doi: 10.3109/09513590.2014.975683
85. Cayrol C, Girard JP. Interleukin-33 (IL-33): A nuclear cytokine from the IL-1 family. *Immunol Rev* (2018) 281(1):154–68. doi: 10.1111/imr.12619
86. Ding W, Zou GL, Zhang W, Lai XN, Chen HW, Xiong LX. Interleukin-33: its emerging role in allergic diseases. *Molecules* (2018) 23(7):1665. doi: 10.3390/molecules23071665
87. Hueber AJ, Alves-Filho JC, Asquith DL, Michels C, Millar NL, Reilly JH, et al. IL-33 induces skin inflammation with mast cell and neutrophil activation. *Eur J Immunol* (2011) 41(8):2229–37. doi: 10.1002/eji.201041360
88. Vocca L, Di Sano C, Uasuf CG, Sala A, Riccobono L, Gangemi S, et al. IL-33/ST2 axis controls Th2/IL-31 and Th17 immune response in allergic airway diseases. *Immunobiology* (2015) 220(8):954–63. doi: 10.1016/j.imbio.2015.02.005
89. Ginaldi L, De Martinis M, Saitta S, Sirufo MM, Mannucci C, Casciaro M, et al. Interleukin-33 serum levels in postmenopausal women with osteoporosis. *Sci Rep* (2019) 9(1):3786. doi: 10.1038/s41598-019-40212-6
90. Ohori F, Kitaura H, Ogawa S, Shen WR, Qi J, Noguchi T, et al. IL-33 Inhibits TNF-α-Induced Osteoclastogenesis and Bone Resorption. *Int J Mol Sci* (2020) 21(3):1130. doi: 10.3390/ijms21031130
91. De Martinis M, Sirufo MM, Suppa M, Ginaldi L. IL-33/IL-31 Axis in Osteoporosis. *Int J Mol Sci* (2020) 21(4):1239. doi: 10.3390/ijms21041239
92. De Martinis M, Ginaldi L, Sirufo MM, Pioggia G, Calapai G, Gangemi S, et al. Alarmins in Osteoporosis, RAGE, IL-1, and IL-33 Pathways: A Literature Review. *Medicina (Kaunas)* (2020) 56(3):138. doi: 10.3390/medicina56030138
93. Shen J, Shang Q, Wong CK, Li EK, Kun EW, Cheng IT, et al. Carotid plaque and bone density and microarchitecture in psoriatic arthritis: the correlation with soluble ST2. *Sci Rep* (2016) 6:32116. doi: 10.1038/srep32116
94. Haag P, Sharma H, Rauh M, Zimmermann T, Vuorinen T, Papadopoulos NG, et al. Soluble ST2 regulation by rhinovirus and 25(OH)-vitamin D3 in the blood of asthmatic children. *Clin Exp Immunol* (2018) 193(2):207–20. doi: 10.1111/cei.13135
95. Balato A, Di Caprio R, Canta L, Mattii M, Lembo S, Raimondo A, et al. IL-33 is regulated by TNF-α in normal and psoriatic skin. *Arch Dermatol Res* (2014) 306(3):299–304. doi: 10.1007/s00403-014-1447-9
96. Di Salvo E, Ventura-Spagnolo E, Casciaro M, Navarra M, Gangemi S. IL-33/IL-31 Axis: A potential inflammatory pathway. *Mediators Inflammation* (2018) 2018:3858032. doi: 10.1155/2018/3858032
97. Ginaldi L, De Martinis M, Ciccarelli F, Saitta S, Imbesi S, Mannucci C, et al. Increased levels of interleukin 31 (IL-31) in osteoporosis. *BMC Immunol* (2015) 16:60. doi: 10.1186/s12865-015-0125
98. Drube S, Kraft F, Dudeck J, Müller AL, Weber F, Göpfert C, et al. MK2/3 are pivotal for IL-33-induced and mast cell-dependent leukocyte recruitment and the resulting skin inflammation. *J Immunol* (2016) 197(9):3662–8. doi: 10.4049/jimmunol.1600658
99. Spallanzani RG, Zemmour D, Xiao T, Jayewickreme T, Li C, Bryce PJ, et al. Distinct immunocyte-promoting and adipocyte-generating stromal components coordinate adipose tissue immune and metabolic tenors. *Sci Immunol* (2019) 4(35):eaaw3658. doi: 10.1126/sciimmunol.aaw3658
100. Mahlakõiv T, Flamar AL, Johnston LK, Moriyama S, Putzel GG, Bryce PJ, et al. Stromal cells maintain immune cell homeostasis in adipose tissue via production of interleukin-33. *Sci Immunol* (2019) 4(35):eaax0416. doi: 10.1126/sciimmunol.aax0416
101. Dempsey LA. Fat IL-33 sources. *Nat Immunol* (2019) 20:776. doi: 10.1038/s41590-019-0439-5
102. Duffen J, Zhang M, Masek-Hammerman K, Nunez A, Brennan A, Jones JEC, et al. Modulation of the IL-33/IL-13 Axis in Obesity by IL-13Rα2. *J Immunol* (2018) 200(4):1347–59. doi: 10.4049/jimmunol.1701256
103. Murdaca G, Greco M, Tonacci A, Negrini S, Borro M, Puppo F, et al. IL-33/IL-31 axis in immune-mediated and allergic diseases. *Int J Mol Sci* (2019) 20 (23):5856. doi: 10.3390/ijms20235856
104. Wang L, Tang J, Yang X, Zanvit P, Cui K, Ku WL, et al. TGF-β induces ST2 and programs ILC2 development. *Nat Commun* (2020) 11(1):35. doi: 10.1038/s41467-019-13734-w
105. Halvorsen EC, Franks SE, Wadsworth BJ, Harbourne BT, Cederberg RA, Steer CA, et al. IL-33 increases ST2(+) Tregs and promotes metastatic tumour growth in the lungs in an amphiregulin-dependent manner. *Oncoimmunology* (2018) 8 (2):e1527497. doi: 10.1080/2162402X.2018.1527497
106. Li J, Liu L, Rui W, Li X, Xuan D, Zheng S, et al. New interleukins in psoriasis and psoriatic arthritis patients: the possible roles of interleukin-33 to interleukin-38 in disease activities and bone erosions. *Dermatology* (2017) 233(1):37–46. doi: 10.1159/000471798
107. Balato A, Lembo S, Mattii M, Schiattarella M, Marino R, De Paulis A, et al. IL-33 is secreted by psoriatic keratinocytes and induces pro-inflammatory cytokines via keratinocyte and mast cell activation. *Exp Dermatol* (2012) 21 (11):892–4. doi: 10.1111/exd.12027
108. Oshio T, Komine M, Tsuda H, Tominaga SI, Saito H, Nakae S, et al. Nuclear expression of IL-33 in epidermal keratinocytes promotes wound healing in mice. *J Dermatol Sci* (2017) 85(2):106–14. doi: 10.1016/j.jdermsci.2016.10.008
109. Shlomovitz I, Erlich Z, Speir M, Zargarian S, Baram N, Engler M, et al. Necroptosis directly induces the release of full-length biologically active IL-33 in vitro and in an inflammatory disease model. *FEBS J* (2019) 286(3):507–22. doi: 10.1111/febs.14738
110. Nygaard U, van den Bogaard EH, Niehues H, Hvid M, Deleuran M, Johansen C, et al. The "Alarmins" HMBG1 and IL-33 downregulate structural skin barrier proteins and impair epidermal growth. *Acta Derm Venereol* (2017) 97(3):305–12. doi: 10.2340/00015555-2552
111. Meephansan J, Komine M, Tsuda H, Karakawa M, Tominaga S, Ohtsuki M. Expression of IL-33 in the epidermis: The mechanism of induction by IL-17. *J Dermatol Sci* (2013) 71(2):107–14. doi: 10.1016/j.jdermsci.2013.04.014
112. Gruber JV, Holtz R. In vitro expression of NLRP inflammasome-induced active Caspase-1 expression in normal human epidermal keratinocytes (NHEK) by various exogenous threats and subsequent inhibition by naturally derived ingredient blends. *J Inflammation Res* (2019) 12:219–30. doi: 10.2147/JIR.S215776
113. Allegra A, Innao V, Tartarisco G, Pioggia G, Casciaro M, Musolino C, et al. The ST2/Interleukin-33 axis in hematologic malignancies: the IL-33 paradox. *Int J Mol Sci* (2019) 20(20):5226. doi: 10.3390/ijms20205226
114. Talabot-Ayer D, McKee T, Gindre P, Bas S, Baeten DL, Gabay C, et al. Distinct serum and synovial fluid interleukin (IL)-33 levels in rheumatoid arthritis, psoriatic arthritis and osteoarthritis. *Joint Bone Spine* (2012) 79 (1):32–7. doi: 10.1016/j.jbspin.2011.02.011
115. Schulze J, Bickert T, Beil FT, Zaiss MM, Albers J, Wintges K, et al. Interleukin-33 is expressed in differentiated osteoblasts and blocks osteoclast formation from bone marrow precursor cells. *J Bone Miner Res* (2011) 26(4):704–17. doi: 10.1002/jbmr.269
116. Aimo A, Migliorini P, Vergaro G, Franzini M, Passino C, Maisel A, et al. The IL-33/ST2 pathway, inflammation and atherosclerosis: Trigger and target? *Int J Cardiol* (2018) 267:188–92. doi: 10.1016/j.ijcard.2018.05.056
117. Kiyomiya H, Ariyoshi W, Okinaga T, Kaneuji T, Mitsugi S, Sakurai T, et al. IL-33 inhibits RANKL-induced osteoclast formation through the regulation of Blimp-1 and IRF-8 expression. *Biochem Biophys Res Commun* (2015) 460 (2):320–6. doi: 10.1016/j.bbrc.2015.03.033

118. Malcolm J, Awang RA, Oliver-Bell J, Butcher JP, Campbell L, Adrados Planell A, et al. IL-33 exacerbates periodontal disease through Induction of RANKL. *J Dent Res* (2015) 94(7):968–75. doi: 10.1177/0022034515577815
119. Okragly AJ, Hamang MJ, Pena EA, Baker HE, Bullock HA, Lucchesi J, et al. Elevated levels of interleukin (IL)-33 induce bone pathology but absence of IL-33 does not negatively impact normal bone homeostasis. *Cytokine* (2016) 79:66–73. doi: 10.1016/j.cyto.2015.12.011
120. Lima IL, Macari S, Madeira MF, Rodrigues LF, Colavite PM, Garlet GP, et al. Osteoprotective effects of IL-33/ST2 link to osteoclast apoptosis. *Am J Pathol* (2015) 185(12):3338–48. doi: 10.1016/j.ajpath.2015.08.013
121. Annalora AJ, Jozic M, Marcus CB, Iversen PL. Alternative splicing of the vitamin D receptor modulates target gene expression and promotes ligand-independent functions. *Toxicol Appl Pharmacol* (2019) 364:55–67. doi: 10.1016/j.taap.2018.12.009
122. De Martinis M, Sirufo MM, Ginaldi L. Allergy and Aging: An Old/New Emerging Health Issue. *Aging Dis* (2017) 8(2):162–75. doi: 10.14336/AD.2016.0831
123. Dimeloe S, Rice LV, Chen H, Cheadle C, Raynes J, Pfeffer P, et al. Vitamin D (1,25(OH)(2)D3) induces α-1-antitrypsin synthesis by CD4(+) T cells, which is required for 1,25(OH)(2)D3-driven IL-10. *J Steroid Biochem Mol Biol* (2019) 189:1–9. doi: 10.1016/j.jsbmb.2019.01.014
124. Coomes SM, Kannan Y, Pelly VS, Entwistle LJ, Guidi R, Perez-Lloret J, et al. CD4+ Th2 cells are directly regulated by IL-10 during allergic airway inflammation. *Mucosal Immunol* (2017) 10(1):150–61. doi: 10.1038/mi.2016.47
125. Zhang L, Li Y, Yang X, Wei J, Zhou S, Zhao Z, et al. Characterization of Th17 and FoxP3(+) Treg Cells in Paediatric Psoriasis Patients. *Scand J Immunol* (2016) 83(3):174–80. doi: 10.1111/sji.12404
126. Sattler S, Ling GS, Xu D, Hussaarts L, Romaine A, Zhao H, et al. IL-10-producing regulatory B cells induced by IL-33 (Breg(IL-33)) effectively attenuate mucosal inflammatory responses in the gut. *J Autoimmun* (2014) 50(100):107–22. doi: 10.1016/j.jaut.2014.01.032
127. Saleh H, Eeles D, Hodge JM, Nicholson GC, Gu R, Pompolo S, et al. Interleukin-33, a target of parathyroid hormone and oncostatin m, increases osteoblastic matrix mineral deposition and inhibits osteoclast formation in vitro. *Endocrinology* (2011) 152(5):1911–22. doi: 10.1210/en.2010-1268
128. Gruson D, Ferracin B, Ahn SA, Rousseau MF. Soluble ST2, the vitamin D/PTH axis and the heart: new interactions in the air? *Int J Cardiol* (2016) 12:292–4. doi: 10.1016/j.ijcard.2016.03.063
129. Liew FY, Girard JP, Turnquist HR. Interleukin-33 in health and disease. *Nat Rev Immunol* (2016) 16(11):676–89. doi: 10.1038/nri.2016.95
130. Heckt T, Keller J, Peters S, Streichert T, Chalaris A, Rose-John S, et al. Parathyroid hormone induces expression and proteolytic processing of Rankl in primary murine osteoblasts. *Bone* (2016) 92:85–93. doi: 10.1016/j.bone.2016.08.016

16

Immunoporsis: Role of Innate Immune Cells in Osteoporsis

Yogesh Saxena[†], *Sanjeev Routh*[†] *and Arunika Mukhopadhaya*[*]

Department of Biological Sciences, Indian Institute of Science Education and Research Mohali, Mohali, India

***Correspondence:**
Arunika Mukhopadhaya
arunika@iisermohali.ac.in

[†]These authors have contributed equally to this work

Osteoporosis or porous bone disorder is the result of an imbalance in an otherwise highly balanced physiological process known as 'bone remodeling'. The immune system is intricately involved in bone physiology as well as pathologies. Inflammatory diseases are often correlated with osteoporosis. Inflammatory mediators such as reactive oxygen species (ROS), and pro-inflammatory cytokines and chemokines directly or indirectly act on the bone cells and play a role in the pathogenesis of osteoporosis. Recently, Srivastava et al. (Srivastava RK, Dar HY, Mishra PK. Immunoporosis: Immunology of Osteoporosis-Role of T Cells. Frontiers in immunology. 2018;9:657) have coined the term "immunoporosis" to emphasize the role of immune cells in the pathology of osteoporosis. Accumulated pieces of evidence suggest both innate and adaptive immune cells contribute to osteoporosis. However, innate cells are the major effectors of inflammation. They sense various triggers to inflammation such as pathogen-associated molecular patterns (PAMPs), damage-associated molecular patterns (DAMPs), cellular stress, *etc.*, thus producing pro-inflammatory mediators that play a critical role in the pathogenesis of osteoporosis. In this review, we have discussed the role of the innate immune cells in great detail and divided these cells into different sections in a systemic manner. In the beginning, we talked about cells of the myeloid lineage, including macrophages, monocytes, and dendritic cells. This group of cells explicitly influences the skeletal system by the action of production of pro-inflammatory cytokines and can transdifferentiate into osteoclast. Other cells of the myeloid lineage, such as neutrophils, eosinophils, and mast cells, largely impact osteoporosis *via* the production of pro-inflammatory cytokines. Further, we talked about the cells of the lymphoid lineage, including natural killer cells and innate lymphoid cells, which share innate-like properties and play a role in osteoporosis. In addition to various innate immune cells, we also discussed the impact of classical pro-inflammatory cytokines on osteoporosis. We also highlighted the studies regarding the impact of physiological and metabolic changes in the body, which results in chronic inflammatory conditions such as ageing, ultimately triggering osteoporosis.

Keywords: immunoporosis, inflammation, innate immune cells, proinflammatory cytokines, ROS - reactive oxygen species, osteoporosis

INTRODUCTION

A typical bone is composed of collagen, matrix proteins, calcium hydroxyapatite crystals, and cellular components. Different cellular components of a bone are osteoblasts (OBs), osteoclasts (OCs), osteocytes (OYs), stromal cells, mesenchymal stem cells (MSCs), hematopoietic stem cells (HSCs), *etc.* Among these, OBs and OCs play a major role in maintenance. OBs are of mesenchymal origin and have bone anabolic activity. They produce type-I collagen, matrix proteins (e.g., osteonectin and osteocalcin) to help calcium deposition in the form of calcium hydroxyapatite crystals. On the other hand, OCs, giant multinucleated cells of HSCs origin, demineralize the bone by releasing substances like hydrochloric acid and proteolytic enzymes, thus keep in check the anabolic activity of OBs (1). The antagonistic activity of OBs and OCs results in continuous formation and resorption of bone, a process called bone remodeling, which is necessary for maintaining calcium levels in the blood. Bone remodeling occurs in several specific spaces in the bone called bone remodeling compartments (BRC) (2). In a healthy bone, the bone homeostasis is regulated by sophisticated coordination among components of BRC's through RANK (receptor activator of nuclear factor-κB), RANKL (ligand for a RANK receptor), and OPG (osteoprotegerin) interactions. OPG is a decoy receptor of RANKL. RANKL secreted by OBs interacts with RANK and triggers differentiation of precursor-osteoclast into bigger multinucleated active OCs. However, to keep bone resorption in check, OBs also secrete OPG, which competitively inhibits RANKL-RANK interaction (1–3). Any imbalance in the homeostasis can lead to bone anomalies such as osteopenia, osteoporosis, osteopetrosis, *etc.* In osteoporosis, there is an increase in the activity of osteoclast, leading to net bone loss (**Figure 1**).

Many different health conditions and medical procedures are correlated with osteoporosis, such as endocrine disorders (e.g., hyperparathyroidism, diabetes, premature menopause and low levels of testosterone and estrogen in men and women respectively, *etc.*), autoimmune disorders (e.g., rheumatoid arthritis or RA, lupus, multiple sclerosis, *etc.*), prostate cancer, thalassemia, liver dysfunction, organ transplant, *etc.* (4). Not only disease conditions, the later phase of life, aging, is also correlated with osteoporosis (1). During aging, epigenetic-metabolic changes in physiology drive chronic inflammation in the body resulting in osteoporosis (5). Hence, a diverse array of factors seems to be involved as the causative agents of osteoporosis. Though initially, it was thought that hormonal imbalance was the leading cause of osteoporosis, later in the 1970s, the role of the immune system first came to light (6, 7). Researchers observed that supernatant from the human PBMCs increased osteoclastic activity in fetal rat bone culture (6). In the past two decades, even more promising reports have emerged indicating firm involvement of immune cells in bone remodeling (8, 9). Age-driven changes in the status of immune cells explain the presence of chronic inflammation resulting in osteoporosis (10). The study of this intricate relationship between the immune system and skeletal system led to the establishment of a new field called "osteoimmunology" (11). Recently, Srivastava et al. have coined the term "immunoporosis" to emphasize the role of immune cells as a cause of osteoporosis (12). Another review by the same group has summarized the role of innate and adaptive immune cells in osteoporosis (13). In this review, we focus on the role of the innate immune cells in osteoporosis in a more detailed manner.

Cells of innate immunity are known to act immediately to various challenges to the body and cause 'inflammation', which has been observed as one of the major triggers of various bone disorders (13–15). According to a recent hypothesis published, inflammatory cell death, 'pyroptosis' of osteoblast, is critical in osteoporosis (16). Various signals that induce inflammation in the body include exogenous signals, such as PAMPs (Pathogen Associated Molecular Patterns) or endogenous signals, DAMPs (Death/Damage Associated Molecular Pattern), which abruptly challenge the immune system and results in acute inflammatory diseases. In addition, metabolic changes, tissue malfunctions or prolonged infections usually result in chronic inflammatory diseases. Therefore, inflammatory mediators produced in such cases play a key role in the co-morbidity of osteoporosis (17–20). 'Focal infection theory' is an old concept that assumes the foci of infection could cause systemic inflammatory diseases (as observed in periodontitis, psoriatic arthritis), resulting in osteoporosis (19, 20).

Innate immune cells are major producers of pro-inflammatory mediators. However, some of them share a common developmental niche with skeletal cells. Various reports suggest that the immune system is highly linked to the skeletal system and actively involved in the manifestation of the disease. In addition to the major producers of pro-inflammatory mediators, macrophages, monocytes, and DCs can act as precursors of osteoclasts (21, 22). Apart from macrophages, monocytes and DCs, other pro-inflammatory innate immune cells of myeloid origin, contribute to osteoporosis are neutrophils, eosinophils and mast cells (23–25). Innate cells of lymphoid lineage, such as NK cells and innate lymphoid cells (ILCs), also contribute to the manifestation of osteoporosis, majorly as producers of pro-inflammatory mediators (26, 27). Among the pro-inflammatory mediators that play a major role in osteoporosis, IL-6, TNF-α, IFN-γ, IL-1β, and ROS are worth mentioning. In this review, we will discuss the role and contribution of different types of innate immune cells and inflammatory mediators in osteoporosis (**Tables 1** and **2**).

CELLS OF THE MYELOID LINEAGE

Macrophages

Macrophages, one of the most potent inflammatory cells also act as the major sentinel cells. They are present in the tissues and can readily sense infection by various pathogens like bacteria, viruses, parasites, *etc.*, and provide a defense to the host system. They have the potential for phagocytosis as well as the induction of inflammatory responses. This ability comes from the presence of a broad range of pattern recognition receptors (PRRs) such as toll-like receptors (TLRs), nod-like receptors (NLRs), *etc.*, as well

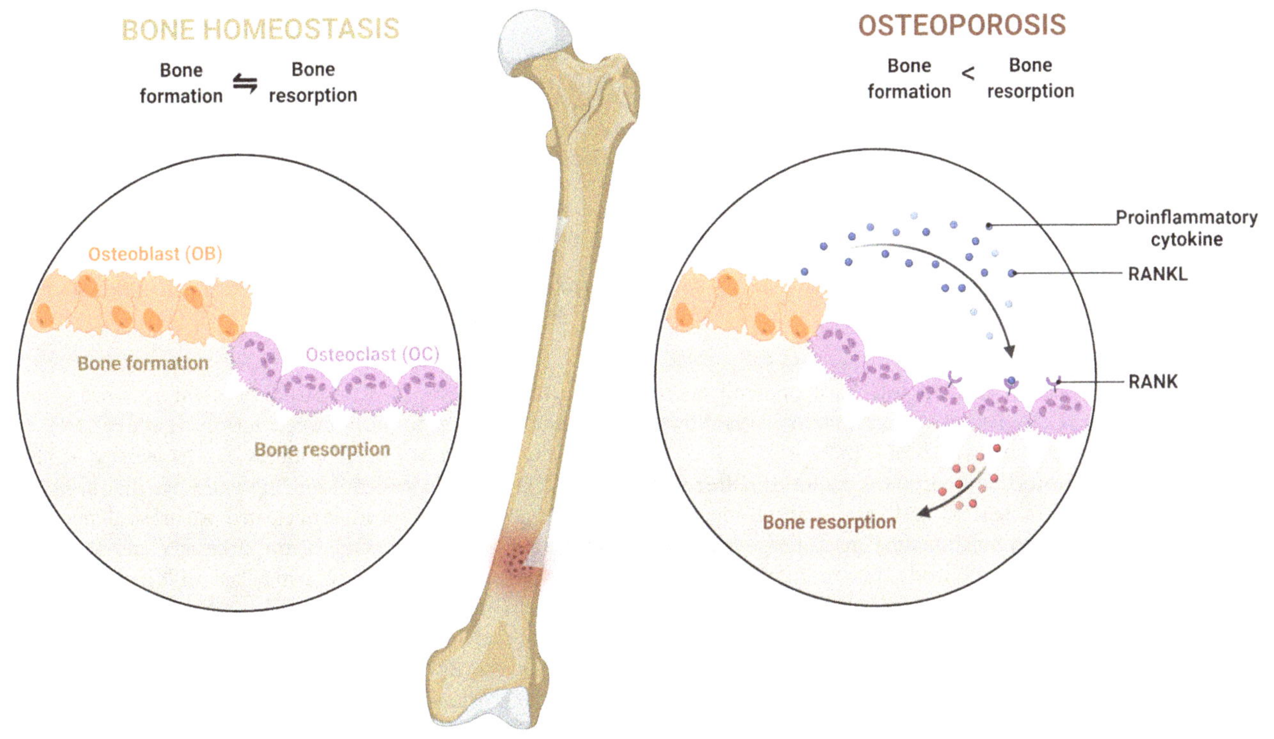

FIGURE 1 | An imbalance in a dynamic equilibrium of bone remodeling leads to osteoporosis. Bone homeostasis is maintained by an equal amount of bone formation, and bone resorption carried out by osteoblast (OB) and osteoclast (OC). Under the influence of various mediators and cellular components, the equilibrium shifts towards greater bone resorption due to exacerbated osteoclast activity. This leads to a decrease in bone mineral density and causes osteoporosis.

as scavenger receptors (SRs) (57). Similar sets of PRRs have been reported to modulate bone metabolism (58–61).

Macrophages are either tissue-resident or differentiated from blood monocytes in response to an inflammatory signal. The tissue-resident macrophages are present in different organs of the body and are known by different names, such as microglia in the brain and kupffer cells in the liver, *etc.* They are adapted uniquely to their location. The bone also possesses different kinds of macrophage populations: bone marrow macrophages (BMMs), OCs, and osteal macrophages or "osteomacs" (62).

TABLE 1 | Function of different innate immune cell types and their role in osteoimmunology.

Cell type	Physiological role	Role in bone biology
Macrophage	Inflammation, phagocytosis, tissue repair	M1 macrophage promotes bone resorption *via* osteoclastogenesis (21, 28); M2 macrophage majorly promotes bone formation by stimulating differentiation of precursor cells into mature OBs (29, 30). However, in the absence of estrogen M2 macrophages can get differentiated in OCs (31). Osteal macrophages help in efficient bone mineralization (32).
Monocyte	Inflammation	Serves as a precursor to OCs, macrophages, and DCs (33). Helps in the recruitment of immune cells to the bone remodeling sites by producing chemokines (34).
Dendritic cell	Inflammation, antigen presentation	Can transdifferentiate to osteoclasts in the inflammatory milieu (35).
Neutrophils	Inflammation, phagocytosis	Promotes bone resorption by increased expression of mRANKL (36).
Eosinophils	Inflammation, allergic response	Found to be increased in number in vitamin D deficiency (37); Source of IL-31 and IL-31 found to be associated in postmenopausal osteoporosis (38)
Mast cell	Allergic response, inflammation	Triggers osteoclastogenesis by producing pro-inflammatory mediators such as, histamine, TNF-α & IL-6 (39, 40).
NK cell	Cellular cytotoxicity, ADCC, inflammation	Promotes osteoclastogenesis by producing RANKL & MCSF (26). Coculture with monocyte in the presence of IL-15 also promotes osteoclast formation (26).
ILCs	Tissue homeostasis, regulation of innate and adaptive immunity	Different subtypes of ILCs produce various factors like RANKL, GMCSF, IL-17 which are involved in multiple bone disorders (27, 41, 42).

TABLE 2 | The role of classical pro-inflammatory cytokines in osteoimmunology.

Pro-inflammatory cytokines	Cellular sources	Role in bone biology
IL-6	OBs, OCs, Stromal cells, OYs, DCs, ILCs Macrophages, *etc.*	RANK-L mediated OCs activation, OCs transmigration (43, 44)
TNF-α	Osteoblast, T cells, B cells, macrophages, monocytes, NK cells, *etc.*	Increases RANK expression on the macrophage (45), increases RANKL production by the stromal cell (45), induces sclerostin in OYs (46), expand OCP pool (47), inhibiting differentiation, proliferation, and activities of osteoblast (48–50), degradation of osterix (48), inhibits differentiation of MSCs (50)
IFN-γ	T cells, NK cells, B cells, ILC1, Neutrophils, Monocytes, Macrophages, MSCs, *etc.*	Fusion of OCs, T cell activation (51)
IL-1β	Osteoblast, T cells, B cells, Macrophages, *etc.*	OCs migration and activation (52–54) Plasminogen cathepsin-B and collagenase secretion (55), Downregulation ALP (56)

Osteal macrophages help in efficient osteoblast mineralization and bone formation (32). Depletion of osteal macrophages shows a decrease in bone mineral density (BMD) (32).

Different tissue microenvironment defines different phenotypes for tissue-resident as well as monocyte-derived macrophages. In addition to inflammation macrophage helps in tissue repair following injury and also maintains tissue homeostasis. To aid these activities (63), they show a great degree of plasticity and hence can undergo a transition between M1 and M2 phenotype depending on the microenvironment (64). M1 is classically activated macrophages (inflammatory phenotype), and M2 is alternatively activated macrophages (reparative phenotype). Macrophage polarization drives bone remodeling activities. Pro-inflammatory cytokines such as, TNF-α and IL-6 can stimulate M1 polarization, whereas anti-inflammatory cytokines such as, IL-4 and IL-13 can stimulate M2 polarization (65), which are generally associated with bone catabolic and anabolic activities, respectively. However, an exciting study by Huang et al. reported that RANKL-induced M1 polarized macrophages display distinct properties compared to LPS and IFN-γ stimulated M1 macrophages (66). In a pathological scenario, it was observed that RANKL-induced M1 macrophages induce bone formation and help in increasing the osteogenic ability of MSC by increasing the expression of osteogenic genes such as *OPN, RUNX2, etc.*, while LPS and IFN-γ induced M1 macrophages shows bone destructive activity (66).

Numerous studies suggested a role of M2 macrophages in osteogenesis. Two groups have demonstrated that M2 polarized macrophages can stimulate MSCs, the precursor of OB cells, into mature OBs and increase bone mineralization *in vitro* (29, 30). Further, it has been observed that the co-culture of pre-osteoblastic cells with macrophage increased the osteogenic ability of pro-osteoblastic cells, and this attribute was enhanced by macrophage transition from M1 to M2 type (67). Based on this observation, it was suggested that a transient inflammatory phase is crucial for enhanced bone formation.

M1 macrophage serves as a precursor of osteoclast (28). Researchers had observed that the osteo-inductive mediators, such as bone morphogenetic protein (BMP) 2 and 6, were reduced when macrophages were stimulated by a known M1-phenotype inducer (68). M1 inducer, such as LPS induces a massive production of pro-inflammatory cytokines and triggers osteoclastogenesis in RANKL-dependent or -independent manner leading to bone destruction (**Figure 2A**) (21). Multinucleation of macrophages is driven by RANKL-dependent or -independent signaling pathways that bring about the changes essential for multinucleated osteoclast differentiation and formation (68–70). One of the necessary and key changes observed in macrophage to osteoclast differentiation is the changes in energy metabolism. A report using RAW 264.7 murine macrophage cell line and bone marrow-derived macrophages (BMDMs) suggested that lysine promotes M1 & M2 activation, whereas tyrosine and phenylalanine have opposite effects (71). Another report indicated that differentiated osteoclasts are rich in lysine degrading proteins and show enhanced biosynthesis of tyrosine and phenylalanine (72). These two reports suggested that inhibition of polarization of macrophage enhances osteoclast differentiation. Additionally, there is an increase in mitochondrial biogenesis in RANKL-induced osteoclastogenesis (73). Consequently, the increase in oxidative phosphorylation allows increasing bone resorption by osteoclasts. In another report, it is observed that there is an increase in GLUT1 and other glycolytic enzymes during osteoclast differentiation (73). Both glycolysis and oxidative phosphorylation thus play an important role in osteoclastogenesis. Recent evidence suggested that glucose transporter expression depends on RANKL (74). It explains why macrophage to osteoclast differentiation and bone resorption is associated with an increase in energy metabolism (75).

A study suggested that, M1/M2 macrophage ratio increases in the bone-marrow of ovariectomized (OVX) osteoporotic mice. In the absence of estrogen, M2 macrophages differentiate into osteoclast upon stimulation with RANKL (**Figure 2A**) (31). Thus, estrogen protects M2 macrophages from RANKL stimulation. Therefore, M1/M2 ratio and estrogen are related to the pathogenesis of postmenopausal osteoporosis.

It is well accepted that macrophages play an essential role in the pathogenesis of inflammatory disease rheumatoid arthritis (RA) by producing pro-inflammatory cytokines like TNF-α, IL-1β, IL-6 that can drive osteoclastogenesis and bone destruction. Similar contributions by macrophages were also observed in osteoarthritis (OA) and peri-implant osteolysis (76). The role of macrophages in RA and OA has been elaborately discussed in other reviews (77, 78).

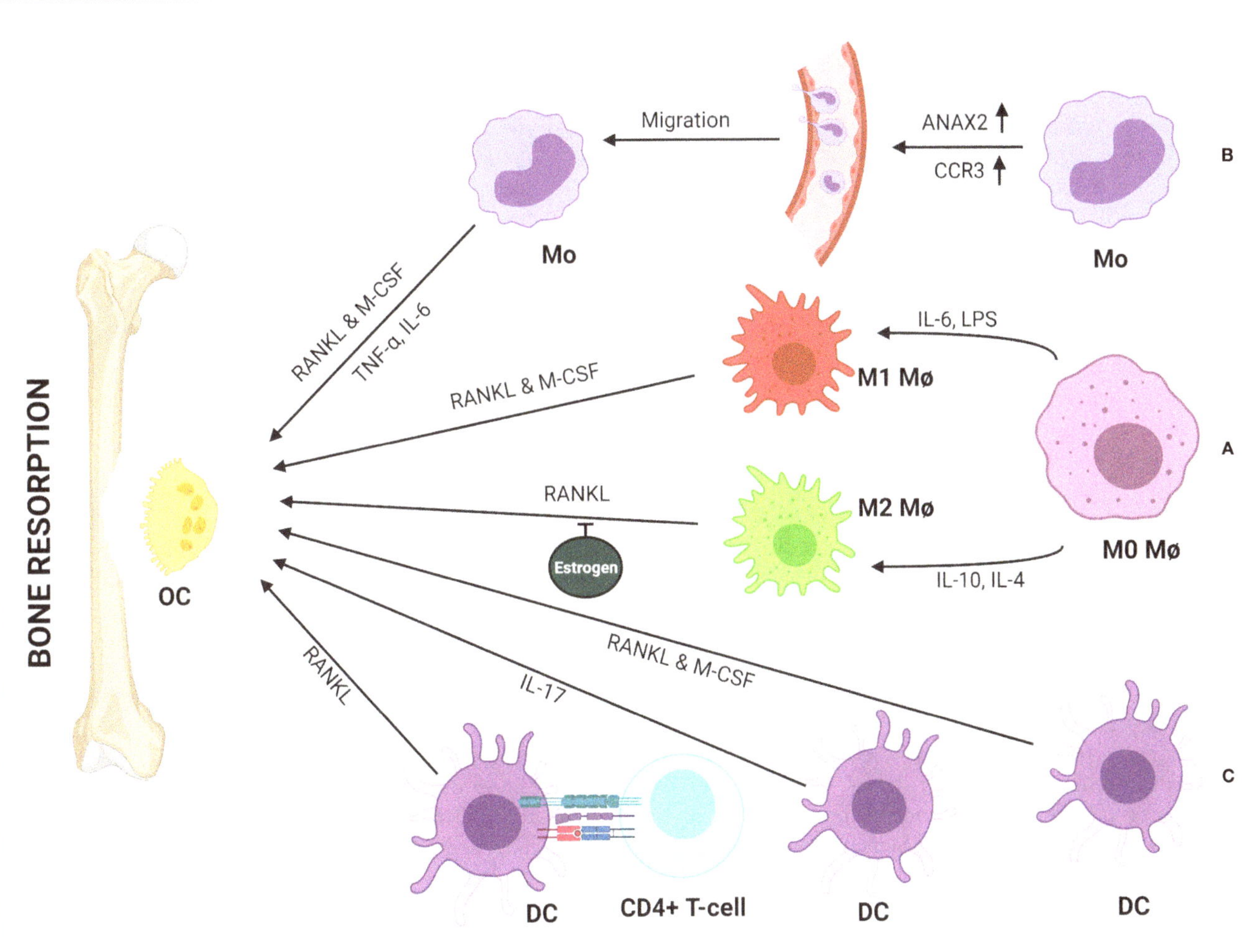

FIGURE 2 | Monocytes (Mo), macrophages (Mφ), and dendritic cells (DCs) can be directly involved in bone resorption by differentiating into osteoclast (OC). **(A)** Both M1 and M2 subtypes of Mφ differentiate into OCs in presence of RANKL & M-CSF or RANKL respectively. Estrogen inhibits RANKL-mediated M2 differentiation to OCs. **(B)** Upregulation of ANAX2 & CCR3 help circulating Mo in trans-endothelial migration and recruitment to the bone remodeling site, where Mo to OC differentiation happens either in the presence of RANKL & M-CSF or TNF-α and IL-6. **(C)** DCs can transdifferentiate into OCs in presence of RANKL & M-CSF or IL-17. Further, immune interaction between CD4+ T-cells and DCs can form OCs in a RANKL/RANK-dependent manner.

Inhibitor studies have helped to elucidate the signaling pathways involved in the RANKL-mediated osteoclastogenesis. Researchers have observed that a Chinese herb, Bergapten inhibits RANKL-induced osteoclastogenesis by suppressing the degradation of IκBα (inhibitor of NF-κB) (79). IκBα keep NF-κB in the cytoplasm by binding to it; degradation of IκB is necessary for translocation of NF-κB to the nucleus and perform its functions. Researchers have also observed that Bergapten attenuates JNK phosphorylation (79). Icariin (ICA) inhibits RANKL-induced osteoclast formation by downregulating signaling mediator TRAF6 (adaptor molecule associated with RANK complex) and further affecting the NF-κB pathway (80). Additionally, it was also observed that ICA inhibits ERK phosphorylation which subsequently leads to a decrease in NFATc expression, which is also a crucial transcription factor for osteoclastogenesis (80). Sappanone A was shown to inhibit RANKL-induced osteoclastogenesis by inhibiting the phosphorylation of AKT and subsequently suppressing the activation of NFATc1 and other osteoclastogenic markers (81). It is interesting to note that RANKL stimulation induces activation of all the three major MAPKs (ERK, JNK, p38); however, only the p38 signaling pathway plays a crucial role in RANKL-mediated differentiation of macrophage to OCs (82). So far no natural inhibitors have been found to inhibit p38 signaling pathway in osteoclastogenesis.

(82, 84)With aging macrophages show an array of dysfunction, including defect in autophagy, morphological changes, and dysregulation of pro-inflammatory cytokine production resulting in age-related altered immune function (10, 83). A study shows significant increase in M1-polarised macrophages in aged mice (84). Aged macrophage shows amplified production of inflammatory mediators (85, 86). Therefore, in macrophage from older people displays an activated phenotype and increased basal level inflammation (86). It is also reported that macrophage polarization dysfunction is related to impaired bone healing in aged mice and rat populations (86–88). Altogether, macrophage dysregulation contributes to a chronic low-grade inflammation during aging, called Inflammaging, which often correlates with osteoporosis.

Apart from inflammatory responses, recent studies have recognized new regulatory mechanisms of macrophages in osteoporosis. A microarray study on RANKL and CSF1 treated *vs.* non-treated BMMs identified differentially expressed circular RNAs (circRNAs) and found that circRNA_28313 was significantly induced in treated cells. Further, it was observed that knockdown of circRNA_28313 significantly inhibited macrophage differentiation to OCs *in vitro* and OVX-induced bone resorption *in vivo* in mice. Bioinformatic analyses revealed that mir-195a microRNA interacts with 3'UTR of CSF1 in non-treated cells (89). However, circRNA_28313 relieves miR-195a-mediated suppression on CSF1 *via* acting as a competing endogenous RNA (ceRNA), modulating the osteoclast differentiation in BMM cells (89). Another miRNA, miR-128, regulates osteoclastogenesis of BMMs through miR-128/SIRT1/NF-kB signaling axis (90). The overexpression or inhibition of miR-128 can increase or decrease macrophage-derived OCs (90). Further reports suggested that miR-506-3p can selectively inhibit NFATc1 in RANKL-induced activated BMMs in rats and minimize the release of bone resorption enzymes (91). The heterogeneity and plasticity of macrophages make them a critical player in bone homeostasis. A more in-depth study is required to understand the role of macrophages in immunoporosis. Modulation of macrophage phenotype could be a potential therapeutic target in dealing with osteoporosis.

Monocytes

Monocytes constitute 10% of total leukocytes in humans and 2-4% in mice (92). The precursors of monocyte arise from HSC in the bone marrow and finally undergo subsequent differentiation to become a committed monocyte progenitor (cMoP) (92). Similar to macrophages, monocytes also exist as different subsets exhibiting different phenotypes and functions. Different subsets of monocyte show distinct functions during steady-state and inflammation. The inflammatory monocytes show high levels of C-C chemokine receptor 2 (CCR2) and low levels of CXC3 chemokine receptor 1 (CX3CR1), whereas the patrolling monocytes show the reverse expression (93). Their recruitment to the inflammatory site is predominantly CCR2 dependent (94). Traditionally, it is considered that monocyte extravasate from blood vessels to the site of inflammation and differentiates into macrophages or dendritic cells, and contributes to the inflammatory process and repair (95). However, a study demonstrated that CCR2-expressing pro-inflammatory monocyte transitioned into CX3CR1-expressing reparative monocyte (96). However, Jakubzick et al., in their study, reported that monocytes can retain their markers or their identity without differentiating into macrophages and DCs while moving through tissues (97). These studies suggest that the monocyte can participate in the inflammatory process directly apart from acting as precursors only. Accordingly, circulating monocyte plays some crucial role by serving as osteoclast precursor and participating in bone remodeling by producing cytokines (33, 34). Recent reports indicate that erythromyeloid progenitor-derived monocytes (EMP-monocyte) also contribute to this pool of circulating monocytes apart from major contributor HSCs-monocytes (98–100). Interestingly, EMP-monocytes, which reside in the adult spleen postnatally, transmigrate to the bone marrow where they differentiate into functional OCs along with HSCs derived OCs and helps in bone repair in fracture scenarios (98). Similar to macrophages, monocytes also undergo metabolic changes like, increase in glucose uptake, oxidative phosphorylation etc. during differentiating into osteoclast (101). Different environmental cues drive different metabolic changes and as a result, monocyte responds differently. The three phenotypic forms of circulating monocyte in human peripheral blood are Classical ($CD14^{++}$ $CD16^{-}$), intermediate ($CD14^{++}$ $CD16^{+}$), and non-classical ($CD14^{+}CD16^{++}$), which differentiate into osteoclast with different order of resorbing ability, that is, normal, high, and non-absorbing, respectively (75). Reports suggest that non classical human monocyte expresses respiratory chain metabolism whereas classical monocyte depends on carbohydrate metabolism and primed more towards anaerobic energy production (102).

In an infection scenario, intermediate monocytes take the lead to become high bone absorbing osteoclast and may result in bone weakening (74), indicating monocytes could also play a critical role in bone disorders (75). Researchers have made some observations towards it. The Association of monocyte with post-menopausal osteoporosis in Caucasian women was shown by Zhang et al. (29, 102, 103). Network-based proteomics analysis of peripheral blood monocytes (PBM) showed significant downregulation of proteins encoded by four genes, namely, *LOC654188, PPIA, TAGLN2, YWHAB* whereas, upregulation of proteins encoded by three genes, namely *LMNB1, ANXA2P2, ANXA2*, in extremely low- *versus* high-BMD subjects (103). Proteomics analysis of PBM of low-BMD subjects showed upregulation of the ANXA2 protein (104). Cellular studies revealed that ANXA2 is important in monocyte migration across the endothelial barrier. Thus, the elevation of ANXA2 probably stimulates the higher migration rate of monocyte from blood to the bone tissue and then differentiate to OCs and contribute to bone-resorbing activity (**Figure 2B**) (104).

Additionally, a microarray study on circulating monocytes in humans suggested that three genes, *CCR3* (C-C chemokine receptor type 3), *HDC* (histidine decarboxylase, a histamine synthesis enzyme), and *GCR* (glucocorticoid receptor), might contribute to bone metabolism and homeostasis. These three genes are found to be upregulated in subjects with low BMD (105). These genes mediate monocyte chemotaxis, which can lead to monocyte infiltration in bone tissue, histamine production, which induces local inflammation and can mediate OC formation, and glucocorticoid sensitivity which promotes OC formation (105). *In vivo* gene expression profiling in human monocyte suggested upregulation of STAT1 and IFN pathway genes in low BMD groups (106). Based on additional observations, the researchers proposed that probably in peripheral blood, IFN-mediated by *STAT1* stimulates circulating monocytes to produce cytokines (such as IL-1, TNF, CXCL10, and IL-15) that increase the bone resorption function of osteoclast. Daswani et al. provided further insight into monocyte proteomics, which revealed the involvement of phosphorylated heat-shock protein 27 (HSP27) in low BMD subjects (107). They have observed elevation of total phosphorylated HSP27 (pHSP27) in monocyte of low BMD subjects and validated that pHSP27, not a chemoattractant itself but acts as an actin reorganizer, facilitating migration (107). As Hsp27 inhibits stress-induced apoptosis, and since osteoclast formation involves ROS generation, the anti-apoptotic activity of pHSP27 may foster monocyte survival and hence more precursor for osteoclastogenesis (107). Transcriptome study identified the downregulation of two apoptosis-inducing genes, death-associated protein 6 (DAXX) and polo-like kinase 3 (PLK3), in low BMD subjects (108). This report supported the fact that due to monocyte survival, more precursors are available to augment osteoclastogenesis and hence osteoporosis.

It was observed that the *SBDS* gene, which is responsible for the disease SDS (Shwachman-Diamond Syndrome showing skeletal defects), plays a role in monocyte migration and fusion before osteoclastogenesis (109). Sbds mutant showed a decrease in Rac2 (GTPase required in cytoskeletal remodeling for migration) and RANKL-mediated DC-STAMP (required for fusion of osteoclast precursor) levels. This fusion defect reduces osteoclastogenesis. Reduced osteoclastogenesis expects osteopetrosis phenotype. Surprisingly, SDS patients show an osteoporotic phenotype. The potential explanation for this phenomenon is that since a reduced number of TRAP-positive multinucleated OCs are still present, there is no complete uncoupling of bone remodeling homeostasis, which probably triggers a shift of MSCs towards adipocyte cell lineage instead of osteoblast. Other observations supporting this phenomenon have been reported earlier by the same group (110).

Dendritic Cells

Dendritic cells are majorly antigen-presenting cells (APCs) endowed with abilities to activate the adaptive immune response. They express high levels of MHC class II and co-stimulatory molecules such as CD80 and CD86 which are required for antigen presentation. DCs are distributed throughout the body and survey for external and internal dangers using a broad range of PRRs such as TLRs, CLRs, NLRs, *etc.* Dendritic cells can be divided into three subgroups: plasmacytoid DCs (pDCs) derived from lymphoid progenitors, classical or conventional DCs (cDCs) derived from both lymphoid or myeloid progenitors, and monocyte-derived DCs (moDCs). pDCs function against viral infections by secreting type I IFNs (111). In addition to pDCs, cDCs and moDCs play a role in providing defense against other microbes.

However, the profound effect of DCs on bone metabolism has been widely recognized recently. DCs contribute to inflammation-mediated osteoclastogenesis and take part in inflammatory bone disease. Using an *in vivo* model, Maitra et al. reported the osteolytic potential of DCs (112). They observed that dendritic cells recruit to bone inflammatory sites and participate in bone resorption (112). In addition, DCs can activate T-cells by acting as APCs, and the activated T-cells produce cytokines and soluble factors that drive bone remodeling (113). It was also observed that DCs directly interact with T-cells to form aggregates which play a role in bone pathologies like synovitis and periodontitis (114, 115). In a recent study, the role of DCs in manifesting osteoporosis in OVX mice was reported (116). Estrogen is known to regulate the number of DCs that express IL-7 and IL-15. In the absence of estrogen, the DCs sustains for long and express more IL-7 and IL-15, which, together, induces a subset of memory T-cell to produce IL-17A and TNF-α in an antigen-independent manner. The cytokines so produced drive inflammation-mediated bone loss (116). There are also reports suggesting a more direct role of DCs in osteoclastogenesis. It has been observed that the DCs can potentially trans-differentiate and fuse to form OCs, and this fusion is faster and efficient than monocyte fusion. There is downregulation in the expression of 3997 genes for differentiation from monocytes to OCs, while there is upregulation in the expression of 3821 genes. However, when immature dendritic cells differentiate into OCs, there is downregulation of only 2107 genes and upregulation of 1966 genes suggesting that DCs are more closely related to osteoclast than monocytes (117). The newly formed OCs can summon more DCs by inducing chemotaxis of DCs, and the OC-DC loop continues to increase bone destruction (117).

Studies showed that DCs can trans-differentiate to OCs in the presence of RANKL and macrophage colony-stimulating factor (M-CSF) (**Figure 2C**) (35, 118). Another study suggested that activated DCs (bone-marrow-derived and splenic CD11c$^+$ cells) upon interaction with T helper-cells (CD4$^+$ T cells or Th) can develop into functional OCs (TRAP$^+$CT-R$^+$cathepsin-k$^+$) in RANKL/RANK-dependent manner (**Figure 2C**) (119). In a report, Th17 cells were shown to play a role in the trans-differentiation of DC to OCs (120). It has been observed in RA patients that inflammatory milieu can recruit Th17 cells, which produce a huge amount of IL-17 to stimulate RANKL production by bone stromal cells and promotes nuclear fusion of immature DCs *via* IL-17R (IL-17 receptor) (**Figure 2C**) (117). T-cells not only augment trans-differentiation of DCs to OCs but also can inhibit it by producing cytokines like IFN-γ. T-cell-derived IFN-γ can inhibit RANKL signaling by blocking TRAF6 to inhibit osteoclast maturation and activation (8). Hence, T-cells could act as a balance switch in mediating DC-OC trans-differentiation. Moreover, in specific conditions, DCs are known to produce TGF-β which is a potent anti-osteoporotic molecule (121–123). This indicates a potential alternative role of DCs in osteoporosis. A more in-depth study is required to understand the full potential of DCs in the induction of immunoporosis.

Neutrophils

Neutrophils are the polymorphonuclear (PMN) phagocytic cells and the first leukocyte to be recruited at the site of inflammation (124). They make up 40-60% of leukocytes in the human blood. Neutrophils contain different granules, which are a source of several anti-microbial molecules. They continuously monitor for microbial infections and kill the pathogen by various mechanisms that include phagocytosis, production of ROS, and molecules like granzyme-B and perforins (125, 126). In addition, neutrophils also exhibit a unique strategy of immobilizing and killing microorganisms by extruding a meshwork of chromatin fibers covered with granule-derived antimicrobial peptides and enzymes. These are called neutrophils extracellular traps (NET), and the mode of killing is termed as NETosis (127).

Current research has emphasized the diverse role of neutrophils beyond killing pathogens. Neutrophils respond to different signals in the inflammatory milieu by producing cytokines and chemokines, which can regulate inflammation and other pro-inflammatory cells (128, 129). In contradiction to the old belief as short-lived innate effector cells, recent evidence suggested the role of neutrophils in regulating adaptive immune response (130). Thus, neutrophils interact with both innate and adaptive arms of the immune system and differentially respond depending on the context.

Neutrophils are also involved in the pathophysiology of various diseases, including inflammation-mediated bone loss (131). Moreover, neutrophils can produce chemokines and recruit pro-osteoporotic cells such as Th17 (12, 131). A strong correlation was indicated between an increase in RANKL positive neutrophils with inflammatory disease conditions and a decrease in BMD (23). A report demonstrated that neutrophils from the blood of a healthy individual express membrane-associated RANKL (mRANKL) while RANK expression depends on IL-4 and TNF-α stimulation (**Figure 3A**) (132). Interestingly, it was observed that synovial fluid (SF) neutrophils from RA patients express both mRANKL and RANK and also secrete OPG (131, 132). This observation that inflammatory neutrophils impetuously express RANK whereas healthy blood neutrophils express only after stimulation gives an insight into the involvement of neutrophils in bone remodeling. The evidence of inflammatory neutrophils expressing RANK could be related partly to acquiring a dendritic cell phenotype and further activating T-cells in RA condition (133). A study reported that mRANKL of TLR4-activated neutrophils induce osteoclastic bone resorption (**Figure 3A**) (36). The mRANKL of activated neutrophils act on both OCs and their mononuclear precursors, converting them into mature and functional OCs that contribute to bone resorption. Interestingly, they have demonstrated that the membrane fraction of activated neutrophils can augment the osteoclastogenic effect but not the culture supernatant, suggesting the importance of the involvement of mRANKL (22, 36). Another study reported that there is an increase in RANKL positive neutrophil in the blood of chronic obstructive pulmonary disease (COPD) patients compared to smokers and healthy controls, and it is related to low BMD (24).

Neutrophils can augment bone loss; however, some reports suggested that neutrophils play a to reduce bone loss by maintaining a homeostatic condition. The defective neutrophil recruitment in leukocyte adhesion deficiency type I (LAD-I) disorder results in IL-17 driven inflammatory bone loss (134). There is a defect in the expression or function of β2 integrin or related adhesion molecule in LAD-I disorder. Due to this defect, there is an impairment in neutrophil extravasation to the inflammatory site. The absence of neutrophils results in unrestrained production of IL-23 from macrophages, which in turn triggers IL-17 production from T-cells and can drive IL-17-mediated inflammatory bone loss. Another report supported the role of neutrophils in preventing inflammation-mediated bone loss. Gif1 is a molecule in HSC development, and a defect in *Gif1* causes severe neutropenia (135). This condition can induce osteoporosis depending on pathogen load and systemic inflammation (135). Hence, neutrophils can be a very critical player in the regulation and manifestation of osteoporosis.

Eosinophils

Eosinophils are known to be involved in the pathogenesis of various allergic and inflammatory diseases (136). However, recently reported association of Vitamin D (VD) deficiency with an increased number of blood eosinophils indicates potential role of eosinophils in bone biology. Moreover, VD, which is a well-known osteoprotective molecule, decreases production of IgE as well as, release of peroxidase from eosinophil and while increases the production of the osteoprotective cytokine IL-10 (37, 137, 138). Eosinophils play a role in the manifestation of various inflammatory diseases (138), including chronic obstructive pulmonary disease (COPD), eosinophilic esophagitis (EoE), *etc.* (139, 140). Literature indicates a strong correlation between COPD and osteoporosis (141). However, the reason identified for the co-morbidity of osteoporosis is the use of a steroid-based treatment regime. Steroid-based treatments are frequently used to manage symptoms in COPD and EoE. Although, the role of eosinophils with steroid-induced osteoporosis is under scrutiny and not fully understood yet (141, 142).

Eosinophils carry out allergic responses by producing inflammatory mediators such as ROS, cysteinyl leukotrienes, and various cytokines and chemokines (143). Transcription factors such as NF-κB mounts such allergic inflammatory responses. However, such transcription factors can also induce osteoclastogenesis in an inflammatory condition. Interestingly, eosinophils are the source of IL-31 in an inflammatory skin condition called Bullous pemphigoid (BP) (144). IL-31 is a pro-inflammatory cytokine that serves as a biomarker for allergic disease. It is involved in the regulation of cell proliferation and tissue remodeling (145). It is reported to be involved in the regulation of the transcription factors and cytokines that are associated with osteoporosis. It is also observed that there is an increase in serum IL-31 level in post-menopausal women with a decrease in BMD, correlating with age (38). Association of eosinophil with IL-31 suggests that eosinophil may play a role in the manifestation of osteoporosis in an exacerbated allergic and autoimmune inflammatory disease condition. However, more studies are required to understand the contribution of eosinophil towards osteoporosis.

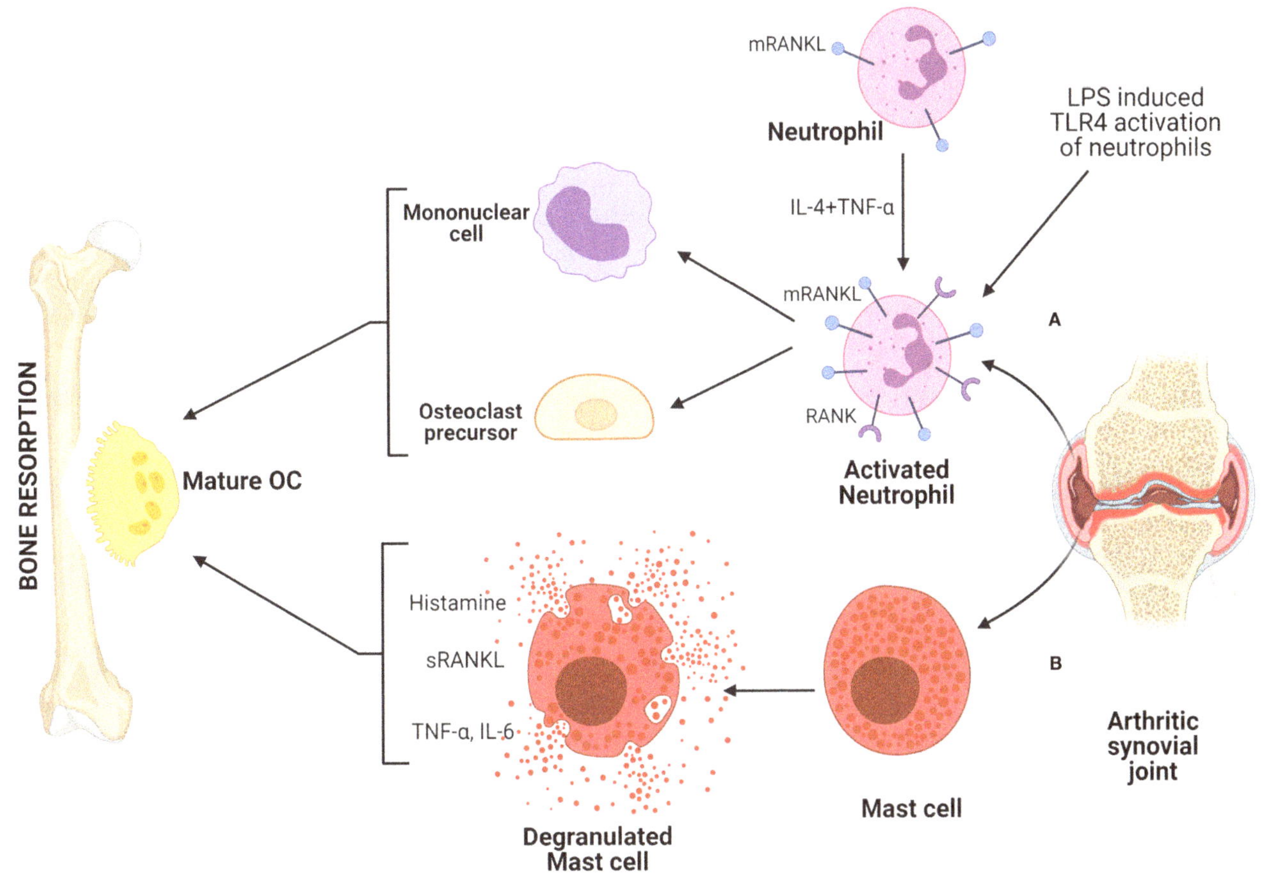

FIGURE 3 | Neutrophils and mast cells are involved in bone resorption by producing factors that can drive osteoclastogenesis. **(A)** Activated neutrophils, either stimulated with TLR agonist or derived from patients with inflammatory disease, such as, from SF (synovial fluid) of RA (rheumatoid arthritis) patient, express higher membrane bound RANKL (mRANKL) and act on OC precursors or mononuclear cells to form mature and functional OCs, resulting in bone resorption. **(B)** Mast cells derived from SF of arthritic patient produces mediators like histamine, TNF-α, IL-6 that drive osteoclastogenesis and further bone resorption.

Mast Cells

Mast cells are the tissue-resident immune cells that originated from pluripotent progenitor cells of bone marrow. Mast cell progenitors migrate into the tissue, where they differentiate and mature (146). Though they are best known for fostering allergic responses, they are also involved in numerous physiological functions and pathophysiology of various diseases (147). Mast cells are the first cells to respond to invading foreign entities as they are present at the tissue boundaries. They can be activated by PAMPs *via* PRRs such as TLRs or complement systems. Mast cells store a wide variety of preformed inflammatory mediators, including histamine, TNF-α, IL-6 as well as proteases in their secretory granules (148). As these inflammatory mediators are known to regulate bone homeostasis and involved in pathogenesis of various bone disorders, mast cells could be a probable candidate associated with bone disorder. Indeed, few reports suggested that there was increase in number of mast cells in the patient with reduced bone density and associated with post-menopausal osteoporosis (149, 150). Experimental evidences suggested that in OVX-induced estrogen depletion there was an increase in numbers of mast cells as well as osteoclasts (151, 152). These observations indicated that mast cells probably promote osteoclast formation in estrogen-deficient conditions. Treatment with calcium and promethazine (a blocker of the histamine H1 receptor) to post-menopausal women helped increase BMD in comparison to calcium alone. The observation that H1 receptor blocking resulted in the termination of osteoclast formation by mast cell supernatant suggested that the histamine, one of the main preformed mediators of mast cell, has a role in the reduction of BMD (153). Other reports indicated that estrogen affects mast cells and the release of its mediators, suggesting estrogen has an inhibitory effect on the osteoclast-inducing potential of mast cells (148). However, there are contradicting reports which indicated that estrogen could induce degranulation of mast cells since estrogen did not stimulate degranulation in ERα (estrogen receptor) knockout mice (154).

Mast cells have been suggested to be involved in the RA disease condition. Similar to other immune cells, mast cells are also abundantly found in inflamed synovial joints of RA patients. Mast cell mediators such as histamine and tryptase were found to be increased in SF (39, 40). Mast cells also contribute to the inflammatory milieu of SF as activated mast cells can produce mediators like TNF-α, IL-6, etc., which have the ability to induce osteoclastogenesis (**Figure 3B**). Even increased levels of RANKL found in the synovial tissue of RA patients could be contributed by mast cells as activated mast cells secrete RANKL (155). In a mice model of CIA (collagen-induced arthritis), reduction in T-cell numbers (both $CD4^+$ and $CD8^+$) along with reduced IFN-γ and IL-17 were observed upon depletion of mast cells (156). This indicated that mast cells might be involved in regulating T-cell expansion and Th1 and Th17 polarization, which is further involved in T-cell-driven arthritis. Various reports suggested that mast cells also play a role in OA. This could be due to mast cell-driven increased pro-inflammatory responses. An increase in the number of mast cells, as well as histamine or tryptase levels, were observed in SF of OA patients (157–159). It has been observed that in OA, mast cells are activated *via* IgE/FcεRI receptor axis (158). Another report showed that synovial mast cells from OA patients produce TNF-α upon stimulation *via* high-affinity receptor of IgG (160). The link between mast cells and bone was also exemplified by the presence of mast cells during fracture healing. A gradual increase in mast cell numbers was observed in periosteal fracture callus, followed by a decrease during callus remodeling (161). The highest number of mast cells was also found in the vicinity of OCs and bone resorption sites during callus remodeling, indicating that mast cells could be involved in regulating osteoclast activity (162). Further investigation is required to understand the mechanism of action of mast cells in the physiology of bone turnover and bone disorders.

CELLS OF THE LYMPHOID LINEAGE

NK Cells

Natural killer (NK) cells are developed from HSCs in the bone marrow. However, recent evidence suggested that they can also develop and mature in secondary lymphoid tissues (SLTs) and show some adaptive features such as memory generation (163). In the 1970s, NK cells were described as large granular lymphocytes with the ability of "natural cytotoxicity" against various tumor cells. In recent times, it is now appreciated that apart from cytotoxicity against tumor cells, it is also capable of showing cytotoxicity against virus-infected and stressed cells (164, 165). NK cell surveillance system consists of various cell surface activating and inhibitory receptors that help identify and kill target cells (166). Additionally, they can perform antibody-mediated cell cytotoxicity (ADCC), making it a potent effector cell of the humoral response. They also exhibit cytokine-producing effector function. Upon engagement with target cells, they can secrete various pro-inflammatory cytokines and chemokines and, thus, regulate other immune cells' functionality by modulating the local milieu (167). NK cells also play a crucial role in maintaining homeostasis and immunoregulation *via* control of T-cells activity.

Since NK cells are well poised to carry out inflammatory processes and cytotoxicity, they are involved in the manifestation of inflammatory diseases. There are reports which displayed the presence of NK cells in inflamed synovial tissues at an early stage of RA (168, 169). Such NK cells express M-CSF and RANKL, potent activators of osteoclastogenesis (**Figure 4A**). These molecules are further upregulated by IL-15, which is abundantly present in the synovium of RA patients (170). Soderstrom et al. showed that NK cells from SF of RA patients trigger efficient formation OCs from monocyte (**Figure 4A**) (26). They had also demonstrated that OCs formed from monocyte when co-cultured with NK cells were capable of eroding bone in the presence of IL-15 but not in the absence of it (26). In the CIA mice model, many synovial NK cells express RANKL suggesting the role of NK cells in bone erosion, and it was observed that depletion of NK cells prevents bone erosion in CIA.

A study suggested that IL-15 activated NK cells can kill OCs (**Figure 4A**). In the presence of IL-15, it seems that NK cells' action is contradictory to the report mentioned above (171). IL-15 upregulate leucocyte function-associated antigen-1 (LFA-1) and DNAX accessory molecule-1 (DNAM-1) on NK cells. These are ligands of ICAM-1 and CD155 (PVR) receptors, respectively. These receptors are present on OCs, and they are essential for their development, function, and interaction with stromal cells (172). Receptor blocking studies between OCs and NK cells has displayed restoration of bone resorption. Thus, IL-15 activated NK cells kill OC *via* LFA-1 and DNAM-1 (171). Therefore, NK cell-mediated inhibition of osteoclast is contact-dependent, although IL-15-activated NK cells produce soluble factors like IFN-γ that can be anti-osteoclastogenic. Thus, NK cells can control or augment osteoporosis depending on the tissue microenvironment. More in-depth study is required to understand the NK cell-mediated regulation of bone remodeling and osteoporosis.

ILCs

Innate lymphoid-like cells or ILCs are the heterogeneous populations of cells that arise from the lymphoid lineage (173). Although they lack antigen-specific receptors, upon tissue damage or pathogen invasion, they can sense changes in the local milieu by cytokine receptors and modulate subsequent antigen-specific lymphocyte responses. ILCs are mainly tissue-resident cells, especially present at the mucosal surface of the intestine and lungs (174). Based on cytokine signature and transcription factors, ILCs can be divided into four groups: ILC1, ILC2, ILC3, and regulatory ILC (ILCreg). ILC1 functions highly overlap with NK cells as both produce IFN-γ, enhancing the ability of macrophages and DCs to remove intracellular pathogens. ILC2s are the innate counterpart of Th2 cells that produce IL-5 and IL-13 and helps in the expulsion of helminths. Notably, type-2 cytokines produced by ILC2s have tissue repair and anti-inflammatory function post-infection (175, 176). ILC3s are the innate counterpart of Th17 cells as they produce IL-17 and IL-22 in response to IL-1β and IL-23. IL-22 can stimulate the secretion of anti-microbial peptides from intestinal cells and provides a barrier in the intestine, whereas IL-17 induces granulopoiesis (177, 178). IL-17 also drives inflammatory response by recruiting cells to the site of inflammation (179).

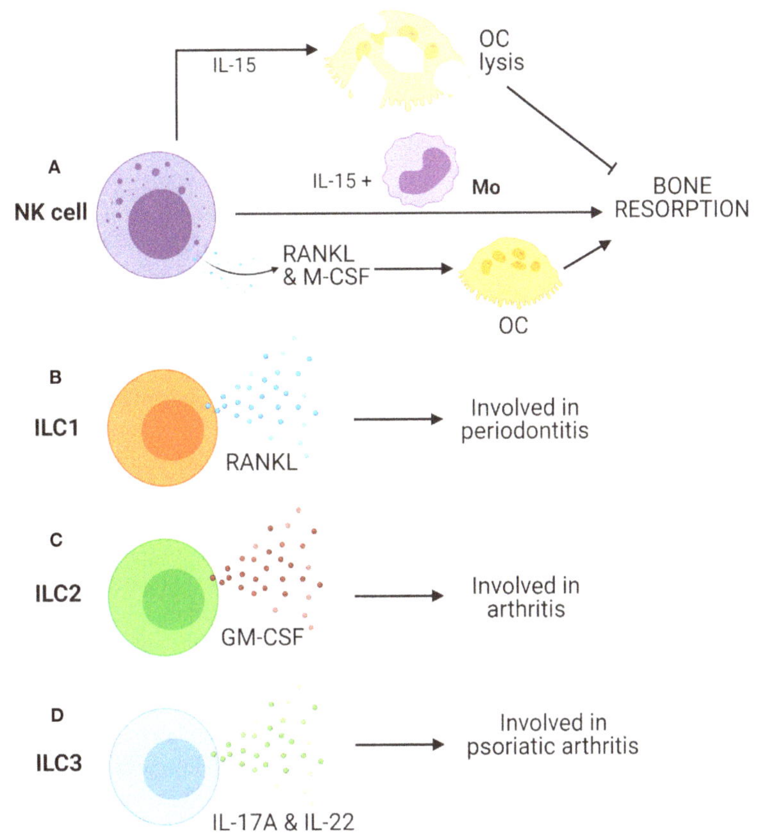

FIGURE 4 | Innate cells from lymphoid lineages, such as Natural killer (NK) cells and Innate lymphoid cells (ILCs) can contribute to bone resorption. **(A)** IL-15 activated NK cells can induce OC lysis and inhibits bone resorption. However, co-culture of NK cells with monocytes (Mo) triggers bone resorption in presence of IL-15. Further, NK cell-mediated production of RANKL & M-CSF can drive osteoclastogenesis. **(B)** ILC1 produces RANKL and is associated with periodontitis. **(C)** ILC2 produces GM-CSF and is associated with arthritis. **(D)** ILC3 produces IL-17A & IL-22 and is associated with psoriatic arthritis.

There are key evidences that suggested the involvement of ILCs in inflammatory bone diseases such as spondylarthritis (SA) (180). It is reported that there is an enrichment in the number of ILC3s in SF of patients with psoriatic arthritis (181). Enrichment of ILC3 is also found in the gut, in the peripheral blood, bone marrow, and SF of patients with ankylosing spondylitis. A recent study has shown that CCR6 positive ILC3s ($ILC3^{CCR6+}$) are enriched in inflamed joints of CIA mice and RA patients and show high IL-17A and IL-22 in arthritic mice (**Figure 4D**) (27). These reports suggested a critical role of ILC3s in the development of all these diseases, probably due to their highly pro-inflammatory nature.

Hirota et al. have reported that GM-CSF-producing ILC2s have a pathogenic role in augmenting arthritis (**Figure 4C**) (41). However, recent studies demonstrated the protective role of ILC2s. They can reduce inflammatory arthritis and prevents bone loss in mice (182). Another study by Omata et al. supported the immune-regulatory role of ILC2s (183). IL-4 and IL-13 secretion from ILC2 trigger STAT6 activation in myeloid cells, resulting in suppression of OC formation, thus preventing OVX-induced bone loss (183). Therefore, ILC2s exert regulatory function on bone homeostasis by impairing osteoclastogenesis. Additionally, ILC2s can have a regulatory effect on bone *via* Treg cells, which are inhibitors of OC formation.

ILC1s are known contributors of IFN-γ and are enriched in many chronic inflammatory diseases. ILC1 is the more predominant ILCs in SF of RA patients (180). ILC1 is the primary subtype of ILCs in gingivitis and periodontitis, and they express RANKL (**Figure 4B**) (42). More descriptive studies on ILC1s expressing RANKL are required to understand their role in bone remodeling.

Recently, a study has recognized a new subset of IL-10 producing ILCs named regulatory ILCs (ILCreg). These are $Lin^{-}CD45^{+}CD127^{+}$ $IL\text{-}10^{+}$ cells and are mostly present in gut tissue (184). In inflammatory conditions, ILCreg can be stimulated in the intestine and acts on other ILCs such as ILC1 and ILC3 to suppress their activation *via* IL-10. Additionally, ILCreg can also produce TGF-β that acts in an autocrine manner for its expansion in inflammatory conditions. Interestingly, IL-10 is a potent anti-inflammatory cytokine that can downregulate the synthesis of pro-inflammatory cytokines such as IL-6, TNF-α, *etc.*, preventing inflammatory-driven osteoclastogenesis and bone resorption (185). Since ILCreg produces IL-10 and suppresses intestinal inflammation, it may also play a role in suppressing inflammatory bone loss. The role of TGF-β in osteoclastogenesis is very complex and controversial, but TGF-β enhances osteoblast proliferation and survival (186). Thus, TGF-β produced by ILCreg may enhance bone formation. Moreover, detailed studies are required to understand the contribution of ILCreg in the suppression of inflammatory disease conditions such as osteoporosis.

INFLAMMATORY MEDIATORS AND OSTEOPOROSIS

Some of the key pro-inflammatory mediators secreted by innate immune cells are IL-6, TNF-α, IL-1β, ROS, and IFN-γ (1–3, 187, 188).

IL-6 is prominently involved in osteoporosis. An increase in IL-6 in the body induces an increase in osteoclastogenesis *via* the induction of RANKL production from osteoblasts (43). IL-6 upregulates S1PR2 [Sphingosine-1-phosphate (S1P)] receptor on the surface of osteoclast precursor and helps in its transmigration from the bone marrow to the blood and thus play a crucial role in the hallmark systemic bone loss (44). Moreover, two of the inflammatory chemokines CXCL8 and CCL20, enhance osteoblast-induced osteoclastic activity *via* IL-6 production (189).

TNF-α is an important molecule in osteoporotic disorders, especially in post-menopausal osteoporosis (190–193). It acts as pro-osteoporotic either by acting as pro-osteoclastogenic or by impairing osteoblast function. It directly acts on macrophages to increase RANK expression and acts on stromal cells to increase RANKL production (45). TNF-α triggers osteoclastogenesis by synergistically acting with RANKL and M-CSF *via* NF-κB and PI3k/AKT pathway (193). This intensifies the osteoclastic activity by many folds comparing RANKL alone (193). Moreover, another report suggests that TNF-α priming sensitizes M-CSF-induced M2 macrophages to pro-inflammatory M1 macrophage polarization in RelB dependent manner, resulting in expanding osteoclast precursor pool with higher osteoclastic potential (47). TNF-α also induces sclerostin (SOST) expression, which triggers RANKL expression in osteocytes and further enhances osteoclastogenesis (46). Together with IL-6, TNF-α can actively cause osteoclastogenesis independent of RANKL (194).

TNF-α acts as anti-osteogenic by inhibiting differentiation, proliferation, and activities of osteoblast. It upregulates CHIP-ubiquitin ligase protein, which results in the degradation of osterix (pro-osteoblastic transcription factor) (48). TNF-α also inhibits expression of BMP-induced 'special AT-rich sequence binding protein 2' (SATB2), which is another pro-osteoblastic transcription factor, by triggering NF-κB binding to SATB2 promoter (49). Further, TNF-α induces upregulation of purinoreceptor P2Y2 through ERK and JNK signaling pathways and hinder the differentiation of MSCs (48, 50). The Canonical WNT/β-catenin pathway is known to regulate bone homeostasis and development. Both IL-6 and TNF-α hamper the pro-osteoblastic WNT/β-catenin pathway by upregulating its antagonists, Dickkopf-related protein 1 (DKK1) and SOST, which prevent osteoblast differentiation (46, 195).

IFN-γ, a type-II interferon, affects later phases of maturation of osteoclasts. An active osteoclast must fuse to form a functional multinucleated osteoclast. This fusion is aided by a transmembrane protein called DC-STAMP, which is expressed by IFN-γ-induced-transcription factors NFATc1 and c-FOS (51). Moreover, IFN-γ-induced upregulation of MHC-II on APCs helps in T-Cell activation. The activated T-Cells produce more TNF-α and RANKL, which further help in the differentiation and maturation of OCs (51).

IL-1β, another highly pro-inflammatory cytokine, promotes RANKL dependent osteoclast differentiation *via* activation of transcription factors NF-κB and AP-1. IL-1β also increases CCR7, which promotes osteoclast migration and activation (52). IL-1β is a prerequisite for the C5a (complement protein)-induced osteoclast activation (53, 54). IL-1β has also been reported to enhance proteolytic enzymes like plasminogen, collagenases, and cathepsin-B, which break down bone matrix proteins resulting in bone loss (55). In addition, it has also been shown to downregulate osteoblastic activities by inhibiting alkaline phosphatase (ALP), which is required for bone mineralization and collagen synthesis activities *via* modulating STATs and SMAD pathways (56).

Reactive oxygen species or ROS, especially hydrogen peroxide and superoxide ions, has been recently shown critical in osteoclast development. ROS has been shown to increase osteoclastic activities and bone loss (196). It has been reported to induce apoptosis in osteoblasts. ROS-activated FOXOs, a subclass of forkhead proteins involved in cell cycle arrest, hinders the WNT/β-catenin pathway in MSCs, thus impairs osteoblastogenesis (197). Moreover, ROS is critical in maintaining body homeostasis, it would be interesting to understand more about the role of ROS in context of osteoporosis.

CONCLUSION AND FUTURE PERSPECTIVE

Bone is a complex and dynamic tissue. Bone health depends on multiple factors like diet, age, hormonal, and the inflammatory status of the body. In addition to these factors, osteoporosis is also correlated with age-driven complications in the senile population. A considerable impact of aging has been reported on the immune system and associated pathologies (1, 5). Macrophages, which are the major contributor to initiation and resolution of inflammation, sense the age-related metabolic epigenetic changes and with a constitutive change to M1-type play a major role in 'Inflammaging': chronic low-grade inflammation in aged people (10, 83). Thus, our immune system is capable of sensing different stimulus as well as different phases of life and results in pathologies like osteoporosis.

In the past 20 years, the field of osteoimmunology allowed us to appreciate the underlying mechanisms of different bone pathologies by integrating the knowledge from the immune system and bone biology. Such studies have provided new insights into how both the system functions in a concerted manner to carry out a complex process of bone modeling and remodeling. The advent of the new field of "immunoporosis" emphasizes the role of immune system players in the pathophysiology of osteoporosis. As discussed in the review, several innate immune cells have emerged as key regulators of immunoporosis. These innate immune cells modulate osteoporosis by producing several pro-inflammatory mediators and *via* modulation of cells important for causing osteoporosis largely by affecting the RANK/RANKL/OPG axis. Net bone destructive activity of osteoclasts seemingly is the decisive factor manifesting in bone status. Moreover, the fact that OCs and some major innate immune cells share a common origin as well as developmental niche, allow them to carry various overlapping features such as expression of common array of PRRs, production of various pro-inflammatory cytokines and their receptors, creating an efficient nexus of information between skeletal and immune system. That is how immune system senses the physiological status of the body and controls the skeletal system. Therefore, research towards this can allow us to find more therapeutic molecular targets to tackle osteoporosis. In addition to the innate immune cells discussed above, inflammation-mediated by intestinal epithelial cells, B1 cells, $\gamma\delta$ T cells could play an important role in osteoporosis, and further study on these cells could be intriguing.

Additionally, in the past few years, there has been increasing evidence linking gut microbiota with bone health. It is now known that the gut controls several inflammatory diseases by the cross-talk between the innate immune cells and gut-microbiota (198, 199). Further, studying the cross talk between gut microbiota and ILCs and intestinal cells could be important in immunoporosis and of great clinical value.

AUTHOR CONTRIBUTIONS

YS and SR wrote the manuscript, and prepared the figures and table. AM conceived the idea, organized the overall design of the manuscript, and wrote the manuscript. All authors contributed to the article and approved the submitted version.

FUNDING

Funding from Indian Institute of Science Education and Research Mohali.

ACKNOWLEDGMENTS

Figures were prepared with Biorender (Biorender.com).

REFERENCES

1. Clowes JA, Riggs BL, Khosla S. The Role of the Immune System in the Pathophysiology of Osteoporosis. *Immunol Rev* (2005) 208:207–27. doi: 10.1111/j.0105-2896.2005.00334.x
2. Okman-Kilic T. *Estrogen Deficiency and Osteoporosis. Advances in Osteoporosis. Yannis Dionyssiotis*. IntechOpen (2015). doi: 10.5772/59407
3. Walsh MC, Takegahara N, Kim H, Choi Y. Updating Osteoimmunology: Regulation of Bone Cells by Innate and Adaptive Immunity. *Nat Rev Rheumatol* (2018) 14(3):146–56. doi: 10.1038/nrrheum.2017.213
4. Tsukasaki M, Takayanagi H. Osteoimmunology: Evolving Concepts in Bone-Immune Interactions in Health and Disease. *Nat Rev Immunol* (2019) 19(10):626–42. doi: 10.1038/s41577-019-0178-8
5. Ferrucci L, Fabbri E. Inflammageing: Chronic Inflammation in Ageing, Cardiovascular Disease, and Frailty. *Nat Rev Cardiol* (2018) 15(9):505–22. doi: 10.1038/s41569-018-0064-2
6. Horton JE, Raisz LG, Simmons HA, Oppenheim JJ, Mergenhagen SE. Bone Resorbing Activity in Supernatant Fluid From Cultured Human Peripheral Blood Leukocytes. *Science* (1972) 177(4051):793–5. doi: 10.1126/science.177.4051.793
7. Mundy GR, Luben RA, Raisz LG, Oppenheim JJ, Buell DN. Bone-Resorbing Activity in Supernatants From Lymphoid Cell Lines. *New Engl J Med* (1974) 290(16):867–71. doi: 10.1056/NEJM197404182901601
8. Takayanagi H, Ogasawara K, Hida S, Chiba T, Murata S, Sato K, et al. T-Cell-Mediated Regulation of Osteoclastogenesis by Signalling Cross-Talk Between RANKL and IFN-Gamma. *Nature* (2000) 408(6812):600–5. doi: 10.1038/35046102
9. Wong BR, Josien R, Choi Y. TRANCE is a TNF Family Member That Regulates Dendritic Cell and Osteoclast Function. *J Leukocyte Biol* (1999) 65 (6):715–24. doi: 10.1002/jlb.65.6.715
10. Yarbro JR, Emmons RS, Pence BD. Macrophage Immunometabolism and Inflammaging: Roles of Mitochondrial Dysfunction, Cellular Senescence, CD38, and NAD. *Immunometabolism* (2020) 2(3):e200026. doi: 10.20900/immunometab20200026
11. Arron JR, Choi Y. Bone *Versus* Immune System. *Nature* (2000) 408 (6812):535–6. doi: 10.1038/35046196
12. Srivastava RK, Dar HY, Mishra PK. Immunoporosis: Immunology of Osteoporosis-Role of T Cells. *Front Immunol* (2018) 9:657. doi: 10.3389/fimmu.2018.00657
13. Sapra L, Azam Z, Rani L, Saini C, Bhardwaj A, Shokeen N, et al. "Immunoporosis": Immunology of Osteoporosis. *Proc Natl Acad Sci India Section B: Biol Sci* (2021) 1–9. doi: 10.1007/s40011-021-01238-x
14. Hardy R, Cooper MS. Bone Loss in Inflammatory Disorders. *J Endocrinol* (2009) 201(3):309–20. doi: 10.1677/JOE-08-0568
15. Hato T, Dagher PC. How the Innate Immune System Senses Trouble and Causes Trouble. *Clin J Am Soc Nephrology: CJASN* (2015) 10(8):1459–69. doi: 10.2215/CJN.04680514
16. Tao Z, Wang J, Wen K, Yao R, Da W, Zhou S, et al. Pyroptosis in Osteoblasts: A Novel Hypothesis Underlying the Pathogenesis of Osteoporosis. *Front Endocrinol* (2020) 11:548812. doi: 10.3389/fendo.2020.548812
17. Adami G, Saag KG. Osteoporosis Pathophysiology, Epidemiology, and Screening in Rheumatoid Arthritis. *Curr Rheumatol Rep* (2019) 21(7):34. doi: 10.1007/s11926-019-0836-7
18. Cobo G, Lindholm B, Stenvinkel P. *Chronic Inflammation in End-Stage Renal Disease and Dialysis* Vol. 33. Nephrology, dialysis, transplantation: official publication of the European Dialysis and Transplant Association - European Renal Association (2018) p. iii35–40. doi: 10.1093/ndt/gfy175
19. Munoz-Torres M, Aguado P, Dauden E, Carrascosa JM, Rivera R. Osteoporosis and Psoriasis. *Actas dermo-sifiliograficas* (2019) 110(8):642–52. doi: 10.1016/j.ad.2019.02.005
20. Wang CJ, McCauley LK. Osteoporosis and Periodontitis. *Curr Osteoporosis Rep* (2016) 14(6):284–91. doi: 10.1007/s11914-016-0330-3
21. Ponzetti M, Rucci N. Updates on Osteoimmunology: What's New on the Cross-Talk Between Bone and Immune System. *Front Endocrinol* (2019) 10:236. doi: 10.3389/fendo.2019.00236
22. Quinn JM, Neale S, Fujikawa Y, McGee JO, Athanasou NA. Human Osteoclast Formation From Blood Monocytes, Peritoneal Macrophages,

and Bone Marrow Cells. *Calcified Tissue Int* (1998) 62(6):527–31. doi: 10.1007/s002239900473

23. Yu XY, Li XS, Li Y, Liu T, Wang RT. Neutrophil-Lymphocyte Ratio Is Associated With Arterial Stiffness in Postmenopausal Women With Osteoporosis. *Arch GerontoL Geriatrics* (2015) 61(1):76–80. doi: 10.1016/j.archger.2015.03.011
24. Hu X, Sun Y, Xu W, Lin T, Zeng H. Expression of RANKL by Peripheral Neutrophils and its Association With Bone Mineral Density in COPD. *Respirology* (2017) 22(1):126–32. doi: 10.1111/resp.12878
25. Ragipoglu D, Dudeck A, Haffner-Luntzer M, Voss M, Kroner J, Ignatius A, et al. The Role of Mast Cells in Bone Metabolism and Bone Disorders. *Front Immunol* (2020) 11:163. doi: 10.3389/fimmu.2020.00163
26. Soderstrom K, Stein E, Colmenero P, Purath U, Muller-Ladner U, de Matos CT, et al. Natural Killer Cells Trigger Osteoclastogenesis and Bone Destruction in Arthritis. *Proc Natl Acad Sci USA* (2010) 107(29):13028–33. doi: 10.1073/pnas.1000546107
27. Takaki-Kuwahara A, Arinobu Y, Miyawaki K, Yamada H, Tsuzuki H, Irino K, et al. CCR6+ Group 3 Innate Lymphoid Cells Accumulate in Inflamed Joints in Rheumatoid Arthritis and Produce Th17 Cytokines. *Arthritis Res Ther* (2019) 21(1):198. doi: 10.1186/s13075-019-1984-x
28. Lassus J, Salo J, Jiranek WA, Santavirta S, Nevalainen J, Matucci-Cerinic M, et al. Macrophage Activation Results in Bone Resorption. *Clin Orthopaedics Related Res* (1998) 352):7–15. doi: 10.1097/00003086-199807000-00003
29. Gong L, Zhao Y, Zhang Y, Ruan Z. The Macrophage Polarization Regulates MSC Osteoblast Differentiation *In Vitro*. *Ann Clin Lab Sci* (2016) 46(1):65–71.
30. Zhang Y, Bose T, Unger RE, Jansen JA, Kirkpatrick CJ, van den Beucken J. Macrophage Type Modulates Osteogenic Differentiation of Adipose Tissue MSCs. *Cell Tissue Res* (2017) 369(2):273–86. doi: 10.1007/s00441-017-2598-8
31. Dou C, Ding N, Zhao C, Hou T, Kang F, Cao Z, et al. Estrogen Deficiency-Mediated M2 Macrophage Osteoclastogenesis Contributes to M1/M2 Ratio Alteration in Ovariectomized Osteoporotic Mice. *J Bone Mineral Research: Off J Am Soc Bone Mineral Res* (2018) 33(5):899–908. doi: 10.1002/jbmr.3364
32. Chang MK, Raggatt LJ, Alexander KA, Kuliwaba JS, Fazzalari NL, Schroder K, et al. Osteal Tissue Macrophages are Intercalated Throughout Human and Mouse Bone Lining Tissues and Regulate Osteoblast Function *In Vitro* and *In Vivo*. *J Immunol* (2008) 181(2):1232–44. doi: 10.4049/jimmunol.181.2.1232
33. Sprangers S, de Vries TJ, Everts V. Monocyte Heterogeneity: Consequences for Monocyte-Derived Immune Cells. *J Immunol Res* (2016) 2016:1475435. doi: 10.1155/2016/1475435
34. Gebraad A, Kornilov R, Kaur S, Miettinen S, Haimi S, Peltoniemi H, et al. Monocyte-Derived Extracellular Vesicles Stimulate Cytokine Secretion and Gene Expression of Matrix Metalloproteinases by Mesenchymal Stem/Stromal Cells. *FEBS J* (2018) 285(12):2337–59. doi: 10.1111/febs.14485
35. Rivollier A, Mazzorana M, Tebib J, Piperno M, Aitsiselmi T, Rabourdin-Combe C, et al. Immature Dendritic Cell Transdifferentiation Into Osteoclasts: A Novel Pathway Sustained by the Rheumatoid Arthritis Microenvironment. *Blood* (2004) 104(13):4029–37. doi: 10.1182/blood-2004-01-0041
36. Chakravarti A, Raquil MA, Tessier P, Poubelle PE. Surface RANKL of Toll-Like Receptor 4-Stimulated Human Neutrophils Activates Osteoclastic Bone Resorption. *Blood* (2009) 114(8):1633–44. doi: 10.1182/blood-2008-09-178301
37. Sirufo MM, Suppa M, Ginaldi L, De Martinis M. Does Allergy Break Bones? Osteoporosis and Its Connection to Allergy. *Int J Mol Sci* (2020) 21(3):712. doi: 10.3390/ijms21030712
38. Ginaldi L, De Martinis M, Ciccarelli F, Saitta S, Imbesi S, Mannucci C, et al. Increased Levels of Interleukin 31 (IL-31) in Osteoporosis. *BMC Immunol* (2015) 16:60. doi: 10.1186/s12865-015-0125-9
39. Buckley MG, Walters C, Wong WM, Cawley MI, Ren S, Schwartz LB, et al. Mast Cell Activation in Arthritis: Detection of Alpha- and Beta-Tryptase, Histamine and Eosinophil Cationic Protein in Synovial Fluid. *Clin Sci* (1997) 93(4):363–70. doi: 10.1042/cs0930363
40. Malone DG, Irani AM, Schwartz LB, Barrett KE, Metcalfe DD. Mast Cell Numbers and Histamine Levels in Synovial Fluids From Patients With Diverse Arthritides. *Arthritis Rheum* (1986) 29(8):956–63. doi: 10.1002/art.1780290803
41. Hirota K, Hashimoto M, Ito Y, Matsuura M, Ito H, Tanaka M, et al. Autoimmune Th17 Cells Induced Synovial Stromal and Innate Lymphoid Cell Secretion of the Cytokine GM-CSF to Initiate and Augment Autoimmune Arthritis. *Immunity* (2018) 48(6):1220–32.e5. doi: 10.1016/j.immuni.2018.04.009
42. Kindstedt E, Koskinen Holm C, Palmqvist P, Sjostrom M, Lejon K, Lundberg P. Innate Lymphoid Cells are Present in Gingivitis and Periodontitis. *J Periodontol* (2019) 90(2):200–7. doi: 10.1002/JPER.17-0750
43. Wang T, He C. TNF-Alpha and IL-6: The Link Between Immune and Bone System. *Curr Drug Targets* (2020) 21(3):213–27. doi: 10.2174/1389450120666190821161259
44. Tanaka K, Hashizume M, Mihara M, Yoshida H, Suzuki M, Matsumoto Y. Anti-Interleukin-6 Receptor Antibody Prevents Systemic Bone Mass Loss *via* Reducing the Number of Osteoclast Precursors in Bone Marrow in a Collagen-Induced Arthritis Model. *Clin Exp Immunol* (2014) 175(2):172–80. doi: 10.1111/cei.12201
45. Luo G, Li F, Li X, Wang ZG, Zhang B. TNFalpha and RANKL Promote Osteoclastogenesis by Upregulating RANK *via* the NFkappaB Pathway. *Mol Med Rep* (2018) 17(5):6605–11. doi: 10.3892/mmr.2018.8698
46. Ohori F, Kitaura H, Marahleh A, Kishikawa A, Ogawa S, Qi J, et al. Effect of TNF-Alpha-Induced Sclerostin on Osteocytes During Orthodontic Tooth Movement. *J Immunol Res* (2019) 2019:9716758. doi: 10.1155/2019/9716758
47. Zhao Z, Hou X, Yin X, Li Y, Duan R, Boyce BF, et al. TNF Induction of NF-kappaB RelB Enhances RANKL-Induced Osteoclastogenesis by Promoting Inflammatory Macrophage Differentiation But Also Limits It Through Suppression of NFATc1 Expression. *PloS One* (2015) 10(8):e0135728. doi: 10.1371/journal.pone.0135728
48. Xie J, Gu J. Identification of C-Terminal Hsp70-Interacting Protein as a Mediator of Tumour Necrosis Factor Action in Osteoblast Differentiation by Targeting Osterix for Degradation. *J Cell Mol Med* (2015) 19(8):1814–24. doi: 10.1111/jcmm.12553
49. Zuo C, Zhao X, Shi Y, Wu W, Zhang N, Xu J, et al. TNF-Alpha Inhibits SATB2 Expression and Osteoblast Differentiation Through NF-kappaB and MAPK Pathways. *Oncotarget* (2018) 9(4):4833–50. doi: 10.18632/oncotarget.23373
50. Du D, Zhou Z, Zhu L, Hu X, Lu J, Shi C, et al. TNF-Alpha Suppresses Osteogenic Differentiation of MSCs by Accelerating P2Y2 Receptor in Estrogen-Deficiency Induced Osteoporosis. *Bone* (2018) 117:161–70. doi: 10.1016/j.bone.2018.09.012
51. Tang M, Tian L, Luo G, Yu X. Interferon-Gamma-Mediated Osteoimmunology. *Front Immunol* (2018) 9:1508. doi: 10.3389/fimmu.2018.01508
52. Lee J, Park C, Kim HJ, Lee YD, Lee ZH, Song YW, et al. Stimulation of Osteoclast Migration and Bone Resorption by C-C Chemokine Ligands 19 and 21. *Exp Mol Med* (2017) 49(7):e358. doi: 10.1038/emm.2017.100
53. Ignatius A, Schoengraf P, Kreja L, Liedert A, Recknagel S, Kandert S, et al. Complement C3a and C5a Modulate Osteoclast Formation and Inflammatory Response of Osteoblasts in Synergism With IL-1beta. *J Cell Biochem* (2011) 112(9):2594–605. doi: 10.1002/jcb.23186
54. Pobanz JM, Reinhardt RA, Koka S, Sanderson SD. C5a Modulation of Interleukin-1 Beta-Induced Interleukin-6 Production by Human Osteoblast-Like Cells. *J Periodontal Res* (2000) 35(3):137–45. doi: 10.1034/j.1600-0765.2000.035003137.x
55. Panagakos FS, Jandinski JJ, Feder L, Kumar S. Effects of Plasminogen and Interleukin-1 Beta on Bone Resorption *In Vitro*. *Biochimie* (1994) 76 (5):394–7. doi: 10.1016/0300-9084(94)90114-7
56. Ruscitti P, Cipriani P, Carubbi F, Liakouli V, Zazzeroni F, Di Benedetto P, et al. The Role of IL-1beta in the Bone Loss During Rheumatic Diseases. *Mediators Inflamm* (2015) 2015:782382. doi: 10.1155/2015/782382
57. Mukhopadhyay S, Pluddemann A, Gordon S. Macrophage Pattern Recognition Receptors in Immunity, Homeostasis and Self Tolerance. *Adv Exp Med Biol* (2009) 653:1–14. doi: 10.1007/978-1-4419-0901-5_1
58. Alonso-Perez A, Franco-Trepat E, Guillan-Fresco M, Jorge-Mora A, Lopez V, Pino J, et al. Role of Toll-Like Receptor 4 on Osteoblast Metabolism and Function. *Front Physiol* (2018) 9:504. doi: 10.3389/fphys.2018.00504
59. Kassem A, Lindholm C, Lerner UH. Toll-Like Receptor 2 Stimulation of Osteoblasts Mediates Staphylococcus Aureus Induced Bone Resorption and Osteoclastogenesis Through Enhanced RANKL. *PloS One* (2016) 11(6): e0156708. doi: 10.1371/journal.pone.0156708
60. Koduru SV, Sun BH, Walker JM, Zhu M, Simpson C, Dhodapkar M, et al. The Contribution of Cross-Talk Between the Cell-Surface Proteins CD36

and CD47-TSP-1 in Osteoclast Formation and Function. *J Biol Chem* (2018) 293(39):15055–69. doi: 10.1074/jbc.RA117.000633
61. Li X, Wang X, Hu Z, Chen Z, Li H, Liu X, et al. Possible Involvement of the oxLDL/LOX-1 System in the Pathogenesis and Progression of Human Intervertebral Disc Degeneration or Herniation. *Sci Rep* (2017) 7(1):7403. doi: 10.1038/s41598-017-07780-x
62. Michalski MN, McCauley LK. Macrophages and Skeletal Health. *Pharmacol Ther* (2017) 174:43–54. doi: 10.1016/j.pharmthera.2017.02.017
63. Sica A, Mantovani A. Macrophage Plasticity and Polarization: *In Vivo* Veritas. *J Clin Invest* (2012) 122(3):787–95. doi: 10.1172/JCI59643
64. Liu H, Wu X, Gang N, Wang S, Deng W, Zan L, et al. Macrophage Functional Phenotype can be Consecutively and Reversibly Shifted to Adapt to Microenvironmental Changes. *Int J Clin Exp Med* (2015) 8(2):3044–53.
65. Murray PJ. Macrophage Polarization. *Annu Rev Physiol* (2017) 79:541–66. doi: 10.1146/annurev-physiol-022516-034339
66. Huang R, Wang X, Zhou Y, Xiao Y. RANKL-Induced M1 Macrophages are Involved in Bone Formation. *Bone Res* (2017) 5:17019. doi: 10.1038/boneres.2017.19
67. Loi F, Cordova LA, Zhang R, Pajarinen J, Lin TH, Goodman SB, et al. The Effects of Immunomodulation by Macrophage Subsets on Osteogenesis *In Vitro*. *Stem Cell Res Ther* (2016) 7:15. doi: 10.1186/s13287-016-0276-5
68. Champagne CM, Takebe J, Offenbacher S, Cooper LF. Macrophage Cell Lines Produce Osteoinductive Signals That Include Bone Morphogenetic Protein-2. *Bone* (2002) 30(1):26–31. doi: 10.1016/S8756-3282(01)00638-X
69. Takito J, Nakamura M. Heterogeneity and Actin Cytoskeleton in Osteoclast and Macrophage Multinucleation. *Int J Mol Sci* (2020) 21(18):6629. doi: 10.3390/ijms21186629
70. Feng W, Guo J, Li M. RANKL-Independent Modulation of Osteoclastogenesis. *J Oral Biosci* (2019) 61(1):16–21. doi: 10.1016/j.job.2019.01.001
71. Bordbar A, Mo ML, Nakayasu ES, Schrimpe-Rutledge AC, Kim YM, Metz TO, et al. Model-Driven Multi-Omic Data Analysis Elucidates Metabolic Immunomodulators of Macrophage Activation. *Mol Syst Biol* (2012) 8:558. doi: 10.1038/msb.2012.21
72. An E, Narayanan M, Manes NP, Nita-Lazar A. Characterization of Functional Reprogramming During Osteoclast Development Using Quantitative Proteomics and mRNA Profiling. *Mol Cell Proteomics: MCP* (2014) 13(10):2687–704. doi: 10.1074/mcp.M113.034371
73. Park-Min KH. Metabolic Reprogramming in Osteoclasts. *Semin Immunopathol* (2019) 41(5):565–72. doi: 10.1007/s00281-019-00757-0
74. Kim JM, Jeong D, Kang HK, Jung SY, Kang SS, Min BM. Osteoclast Precursors Display Dynamic Metabolic Shifts Toward Accelerated Glucose Metabolism at an Early Stage of RANKL-Stimulated Osteoclast Differentiation. *Cell Physiol Biochem: Int J Exp Cell Physiol Biochem Pharmacol* (2007) 20(6):935–46. doi: 10.1159/000110454
75. Yao Y, Cai X, Ren F, Ye Y, Wang F, Zheng C, et al. The Macrophage-Osteoclast Axis in Osteoimmunity and Osteo-Related Diseases. *Front Immunol* (2021) 12:664871. doi: 10.3389/fimmu.2021.664871
76. Gu Q, Yang H, Shi Q. Macrophages and Bone Inflammation. *J Orthopaedic Transl* (2017) 10:86–93. doi: 10.1016/j.jot.2017.05.002
77. Yang X, Chang Y, Wei W. Emerging Role of Targeting Macrophages in Rheumatoid Arthritis: Focus on Polarization, Metabolism and Apoptosis. *Cell Prolif* (2020) 53(7):e12854. doi: 10.1111/cpr.12854
78. Wu CL, Harasymowicz NS, Klimak MA, Collins KH, Guilak F. The Role of Macrophages in Osteoarthritis and Cartilage Repair. *Osteoarthritis Cartilage* (2020) 28(5):544–54. doi: 10.1016/j.joca.2019.12.007
79. Chen G, Xu Q, Dai M, Liu X. Bergapten Suppresses RANKL-Induced Osteoclastogenesis and Ovariectomy-Induced Osteoporosis *via* Suppression of NF-kappaB and JNK Signaling Pathways. *Biochem Biophys Res Commun* (2019) 509(2):329–34. doi: 10.1016/j.bbrc.2018.12.112
80. Kim B, Lee KY, Park B. Icariin Abrogates Osteoclast Formation Through the Regulation of the RANKL-Mediated TRAF6/NF-Kappab/ERK Signaling Pathway in Raw264.7 Cells. *Phytomedicine: Int J Phytother Phytopharmacol* (2018) 51:181–90. doi: 10.1016/j.phymed.2018.06.020
81. Choo YY, Tran PT, Min BS, Kim O, Nguyen HD, Kwon SH, et al. Sappanone A Inhibits RANKL-Induced Osteoclastogenesis in BMMs and Prevents Inflammation-Mediated Bone Loss. *Int Immunopharmacol* (2017) 52:230–7. doi: 10.1016/j.intimp.2017.09.018
82. Matsumoto M, Sudo T, Saito T, Osada H, Tsujimoto M. Involvement of P38 Mitogen-Activated Protein Kinase Signaling Pathway in Osteoclastogenesis Mediated by Receptor Activator of NF-kappa B Ligand (RANKL). *J Biol Chem* (2000) 275(40):31155–61. doi: 10.1074/jbc.M001229200
83. Stahl EC, Haschak MJ, Popovic B, Brown BN. Macrophages in the Aging Liver and Age-Related Liver Disease. *Front Immunol* (2018) 9:2795. doi: 10.3389/fimmu.2018.02795
84. Kim OH, Kim H, Kang J, Yang D, Kang YH, Lee DH, et al. Impaired Phagocytosis of Apoptotic Cells Causes Accumulation of Bone Marrow-Derived Macrophages in Aged Mice. *BMB Rep* (2017) 50(1):43–8. doi: 10.5483/BMBRep.2017.50.1.167
85. Barrett JP, Costello DA, O'Sullivan J, Cowley TR, Lynch MA. Bone Marrow-Derived Macrophages From Aged Rats are More Responsive to Inflammatory Stimuli. *J Neuroinflamm* (2015) 12:67. doi: 10.1186/s12974-015-0287-7
86. Smallwood HS, Lopez-Ferrer D, Squier TC. Aging Enhances the Production of Reactive Oxygen Species and Bactericidal Activity in Peritoneal Macrophages by Upregulating Classical Activation Pathways. *Biochemistry* (2011) 50(45):9911–22. doi: 10.1021/bi2011866
87. Clark D, Brazina S, Yang F, Hu D, Hsieh CL, Niemi EC, et al. Age-Related Changes to Macrophages Are Detrimental to Fracture Healing in Mice. *Aging Cell* (2020) 19(3):e13112. doi: 10.1111/acel.13112
88. Gibon E, Loi F, Cordova LA, Pajarinen J, Lin T, Lu L, et al. Aging Affects Bone Marrow Macrophage Polarization: Relevance to Bone Healing. *Regenerative Eng Trans Med* (2016) 2(2):98–104. doi: 10.1007/s40883-016-0016-5
89. Chen X, Ouyang Z, Shen Y, Liu B, Zhang Q, Wan L, et al. CircRNA_28313/miR-195a/CSF1 Axis Modulates Osteoclast Differentiation to Affect OVX-Induced Bone Absorption in Mice. *RNA Biol* (2019) 16(9):1249–62. doi: 10.1080/15476286.2019.1624470
90. Shen G, Ren H, Shang Q, Zhang Z, Zhao W, Yu X, et al. miR-128 Plays a Critical Role in Murine Osteoclastogenesis and Estrogen Deficiency-Induced Bone Loss. *Theranostics* (2020) 10(10):4334–48. doi: 10.7150/thno.42982
91. Dinesh P, Kalaiselvan S, Sujitha S, Rasool M. miR-506-3p Alleviates Uncontrolled Osteoclastogenesis *via* Repression of RANKL/NFATc1 Signaling Pathway. *J Cell Physiol* (2020) 235(12):9497–509. doi: 10.1002/jcp.29757
92. Italiani P, Boraschi D. From Monocytes to M1/M2 Macrophages: Phenotypical vs. Functional Differentiation. *Front Immunol* (2014) 5:514. doi: 10.3389/fimmu.2014.00514
93. Auffray C, Fogg D, Garfa M, Elain G, Join-Lambert O, Kayal S, et al. Monitoring of Blood Vessels and Tissues by a Population of Monocytes With Patrolling Behavior. *Science* (2007) 317(5838):666–70. doi: 10.1126/science.1142883
94. Tsou CL, Peters W, Si Y, Slaymaker S, Aslanian AM, Weisberg SP, et al. Critical Roles for CCR2 and MCP-3 in Monocyte Mobilization From Bone Marrow and Recruitment to Inflammatory Sites. *J Clin Invest* (2007) 117 (4):902–9. doi: 10.1172/JCI29919
95. Auffray C, Sieweke MH, Geissmann F. Blood Monocytes: Development, Heterogeneity, and Relationship With Dendritic Cells. *Annu Rev Immunol* (2009) 27:669–92. doi: 10.1146/annurev.immunol.021908.132557
96. Kratofil RM, Kubes P, Deniset JF. Monocyte Conversion During Inflammation and Injury. *Arteriosc Thromb Vasc Biol* (2017) 37(1):35–42. doi: 10.1161/ATVBAHA.116.308198
97. Jakubzick C, Gautier EL, Gibbings SL, Sojka DK, Schlitzer A, Johnson TE, et al. Minimal Differentiation of Classical Monocytes as They Survey Steady-State Tissues and Transport Antigen to Lymph Nodes. *Immunity* (2013) 39 (3):599–610. doi: 10.1016/j.immuni.2013.08.007
98. Yahara Y, Barrientos T, Tang YJ, Puviindran V, Nadesan P, Zhang H, et al. Erythromyeloid Progenitors Give Rise to a Population of Osteoclasts That Contribute to Bone Homeostasis and Repair. *Nat Cell Biol* (2020) 22(1):49–59. doi: 10.1038/s41556-019-0437-8
99. Yahara Y, Ma X, Gracia L, Alman BA. Monocyte/Macrophage Lineage Cells From Fetal Erythromyeloid Progenitors Orchestrate Bone Remodeling and Repair. *Front Cell Dev Biol* (2021) 9(123):1–16. doi: 10.3389/fcell.2021.622035
100. Jacome-Galarza CE, Percin GI, Muller JT, Mass E, Lazarov T, Eitler J, et al. Developmental Origin, Functional Maintenance and Genetic Rescue of Osteoclasts. *Nature* (2019) 568(7753):541–5. doi: 10.1038/s41586-019-1105-7

101. Da W, Tao L, Zhu Y. The Role of Osteoclast Energy Metabolism in the Occurrence and Development of Osteoporosis. *Front Endocrinol* (2021) 12 (556):1–18. doi: 10.3389/fendo.2021.675385
102. Schmidl C, Renner K, Peter K, Eder R, Lassmann T, Balwierz PJ, et al. Transcription and Enhancer Profiling in Human Monocyte Subsets. *Blood* (2014) 123(17):e90–9. doi: 10.1182/blood-2013-02-484188
103. Zhang L, Liu YZ, Zeng Y, Zhu W, Zhao YC, Zhang JG, et al. Network-Based Proteomic Analysis for Postmenopausal Osteoporosis in Caucasian Females. *Proteomics* (2016) 16(1):12–28. doi: 10.1002/pmic.201500005
104. Deng FY, Lei SF, Zhang Y, Zhang YL, Zheng YP, Zhang LS, et al. Peripheral Blood Monocyte-Expressed ANXA2 Gene is Involved in Pathogenesis of Osteoporosis in Humans. *Mol Cell Proteomics: MCP* (2011) 10(11):M111 011700. doi: 10.1074/mcp.M111.011700
105. Liu YZ, Dvornyk V, Lu Y, Shen H, Lappe JM, Recker RR, et al. A Novel Pathophysiological Mechanism for Osteoporosis Suggested by an *In Vivo* Gene Expression Study of Circulating Monocytes. *J Biol Chem* (2005) 280 (32):29011–6. doi: 10.1074/jbc.M501164200
106. Chen XD, Xiao P, Lei SF, Liu YZ, Guo YF, Deng FY, et al. Gene Expression Profiling in Monocytes and SNP Association Suggest the Importance of the STAT1 Gene for Osteoporosis in Both Chinese and Caucasians. *J Bone Mineral Research: Off J Am Soc Bone Mineral Res* (2010) 25(2):339–55. doi: 10.1359/jbmr.090724
107. Daswani B, Gupta MK, Gavali S, Desai M, Sathe GJ, Patil A, et al. Monocyte Proteomics Reveals Involvement of Phosphorylated HSP27 in the Pathogenesis of Osteoporosis. *Dis Markers* (2015) 2015:196589. doi: 10.1155/2015/196589
108. Liu YZ, Zhou Y, Zhang L, Li J, Tian Q, Zhang JG, et al. Attenuated Monocyte Apoptosis, a New Mechanism for Osteoporosis Suggested by a Transcriptome-Wide Expression Study of Monocytes. *PloS One* (2015) 10 (2):e0116792. doi: 10.1371/journal.pone.0116792
109. Leung R, Cuddy K, Wang Y, Rommens J, Glogauer M. Sbds is Required for Rac2-Mediated Monocyte Migration and Signaling Downstream of RANK During Osteoclastogenesis. *Blood* (2011) 117(6):2044–53. doi: 10.1182/blood-2010-05-282574
110. Leung R, Wang Y, Cuddy K, Sun C, Magalhaes J, Grynpas M, et al. Filamin A Regulates Monocyte Migration Through Rho Small GTPases During Osteoclastogenesis. *J Bone Mineral Res* (2010) 25(5):1077–91. doi: 10.1359/jbmr.091114
111. Swiecki M, Colonna M. The Multifaceted Biology of Plasmacytoid Dendritic Cells. *Nat Rev Immunol* (2015) 15(8):471–85. doi: 10.1038/nri3865
112. Maitra R, Follenzi A, Yaghoobian A, Montagna C, Merlin S, Cannizzo ES, et al. Dendritic Cell-Mediated *In Vivo* Bone Resorption. *J Immunol* (2010) 185(3):1485–91. doi: 10.4049/jimmunol.0903560
113. Gillespie MT. Impact of Cytokines and T Lymphocytes Upon Osteoclast Differentiation and Function. *Arthritis Res Ther* (2007) 9(2):103. doi: 10.1186/ar2141
114. Sarkar S, Fox DA. Dendritic Cells in Rheumatoid Arthritis. *Front Biosci: J Virtual Library* (2005) 10:656–65. doi: 10.2741/1560
115. Teng YT. Protective and Destructive Immunity in the Periodontium: Part 2–T-Cell-Mediated Immunity in the Periodontium. *J Dental Res* (2006) 85 (3):209–19. doi: 10.1177/154405910608500302
116. Cline-Smith A, Axelbaum A, Shashkova E, Chakraborty M, Sanford J, Panesar P, et al. Ovariectomy Activates Chronic Low-Grade Inflammation Mediated by Memory T Cells, Which Promotes Osteoporosis in Mice. *J Bone Mineral Research: Off J Am Soc Bone Mineral Res* (2020) 35(6):1174–87. doi: 10.1002/jbmr.3966
117. Wang B, Dong Y, Tian Z, Chen Y, Dong S. The Role of Dendritic Cells Derived Osteoclasts in Bone Destruction Diseases. *Genes Dis* (2020) 8 (4):401–11. doi: 10.1016/j.gendis.2020.03.009
118. Narisawa M, Kubo S, Okada Y, Yamagata K, Nakayamada S, Sakata K, et al. Human Dendritic Cell-Derived Osteoclasts With High Bone Resorption Capacity and T Cell Stimulation Ability. *Bone* (2021) 142:115616. doi: 10.1016/j.bone.2020.115616
119. Alnaeeli M, Penninger JM, Teng YT. Immune Interactions With CD4+ T Cells Promote the Development of Functional Osteoclasts From Murine CD11c+ Dendritic Cells. *J Immunol* (2006) 177(5):3314–26. doi: 10.4049/jimmunol.177.5.3314
120. Ono T, Takayanagi H. Osteoimmunology in Bone Fracture Healing. *Curr Osteoporosis Rep* (2017) 15(4):367–75. doi: 10.1007/s11914-017-0381-0
121. Jin Y, Wi HJ, Choi M-H, Hong S-T, Bae YM. Regulation of Anti-Inflammatory Cytokines IL-10 and TGF-β in Mouse Dendritic Cells Through Treatment With Clonorchis Sinensis Crude Antigen. *Exp Mol Med* (2014) 46(1):e74–e. doi: 10.1038/emm.2013.144
122. Dumitriu IE, Dunbar DR, Howie SE, Sethi T, Gregory CD. Human Dendritic Cells Produce TGF-β1 Under the Influence of Lung Carcinoma Cells and Prime the Differentiation of CD4+CD25+Foxp3+ Regulatory T Cells. *J Immunol* (2009) 182(5):2795–807. doi: 10.4049/jimmunol.0712671
123. Hughes DE, Dai A, Tiffee JC, Li HH, Mundy GR, Boyce BF. Estrogen Promotes Apoptosis of Murine Osteoclasts Mediated by TGF-β. *Nat Med* (1996) 2(10):1132–6. doi: 10.1038/nm1096-1132
124. Nathan C. Neutrophils and Immunity: Challenges and Opportunities. *Nat Rev Immunol* (2006) 6(3):173–82. doi: 10.1038/nri1785
125. Selders GS, Fetz AE, Radic MZ, Bowlin GL. An Overview of the Role of Neutrophils in Innate Immunity, Inflammation and Host-Biomaterial Integration. *Regenerative Biomaterials* (2017) 4(1):55–68. doi: 10.1093/rb/rbw041
126. Wagner C, Iking-Konert C, Denefleh B, Stegmaier S, Hug F, Hansch GM. Granzyme B and Perforin: Constitutive Expression in Human Polymorphonuclear Neutrophils. *Blood* (2004) 103(3):1099–104. doi: 10.1182/blood-2003-04-1069
127. Kaplan MJ, Radic M. Neutrophil Extracellular Traps: Double-Edged Swords of Innate Immunity. *J Immunol* (2012) 189(6):2689–95. doi: 10.4049/jimmunol.1201719
128. Nauseef WM, Borregaard N. Neutrophils at Work. *Nat Immunol* (2014) 15 (7):602–11. doi: 10.1038/ni.2921
129. Scapini P, Cassatella MA. Social Networking of Human Neutrophils Within the Immune System. *Blood* (2014) 124(5):710–9. doi: 10.1182/blood-2014-03-453217
130. Mantovani A, Cassatella MA, Costantini C, Jaillon S. Neutrophils in the Activation and Regulation of Innate and Adaptive Immunity. *Nat Rev Immunol* (2011) 11(8):519–31. doi: 10.1038/nri3024
131. Hajishengallis G, Moutsopoulos NM, Hajishengallis E, Chavakis T. Immune and Regulatory Functions of Neutrophils in Inflammatory Bone Loss. *Semin Immunol* (2016) 28(2):146–58. doi: 10.1016/j.smim.2016.02.002
132. Poubelle PE, Chakravarti A, Fernandes MJ, Doiron K, Marceau AA. Differential Expression of RANK, RANK-L, and Osteoprotegerin by Synovial Fluid Neutrophils From Patients With Rheumatoid Arthritis and by Healthy Human Blood Neutrophils. *Arthritis Res Ther* (2007) 9(2):R25. doi: 10.1186/ar2137
133. Iking-Konert C, Ostendorf B, Sander O, Jost M, Wagner C, Joosten L, et al. Transdifferentiation of Polymorphonuclear Neutrophils to Dendritic-Like Cells at the Site of Inflammation in Rheumatoid Arthritis: Evidence for Activation by T Cells. *Ann Rheum Dis* (2005) 64(10):1436–42. doi: 10.1136/ard.2004.034132
134. Moutsopoulos NM, Konkel J, Sarmadi M, Eskan MA, Wild T, Dutzan N, et al. Defective Neutrophil Recruitment in Leukocyte Adhesion Deficiency Type I Disease Causes Local IL-17-Driven Inflammatory Bone Loss. *Sci Trans Med* (2014) 6(229):229ra40. doi: 10.1126/scitranslmed.3007696
135. Geissler S, Textor M, Stumpp S, Seitz S, Lekaj A, Brunk S, et al. Loss of Murine Gfi1 Causes Neutropenia and Induces Osteoporosis Depending on the Pathogen Load and Systemic Inflammation. *PloS One* (2018) 13(6): e0198510. doi: 10.1371/journal.pone.0198510
136. Fulkerson PC, Rothenberg ME. Targeting Eosinophils in Allergy, Inflammation and Beyond. *Nat Rev Drug Discov* (2013) 12(2):117–29. doi: 10.1038/nrd3838
137. Arshi S, Ghalehbaghi B, Kamrava S-K, Aminlou M. Vitamin D Serum Levels in Allergic Rhinitis: Any Difference From Normal Population? *Asia Pacif Allergy* (2012) 2(1):45–8. doi: 10.5415/apallergy.2012.2.1.45
138. Azimi A, Ghajarzadeh M, Sahraian MA, Mohammadifar M, Roostaei B, Samani SMV, et al. Effects of Vitamin D Supplements on IL-10 and INFgamma Levels in Patients With Multiple Sclerosis: A Systematic Review and Meta-Analysis. *Maedica* (2019) 14(4):413–7. doi: 10.26574/maedica.2019.14.4.413
139. Rossetti D, Isoldi S, Oliva S. Eosinophilic Esophagitis: Update on Diagnosis and Treatment in Pediatric Patients. *Pediatr Drugs* (2020) 22(4):343–56. doi: 10.1007/s40272-020-00398-z

140. Saha S, Brightling CE. Eosinophilic Airway Inflammation in COPD. *Int J Chronic Obstructive Pulmonary Dis* (2006) 1(1):39–47. doi: 10.2147/copd.2006.1.1.39
141. Loke YK, Cavallazzi R, Singh S. Risk of Fractures With Inhaled Corticosteroids in COPD: Systematic Review and Meta-Analysis of Randomised Controlled Trials and Observational Studies. *Thorax* (2011) 66(8):699–708. doi: 10.1136/thx.2011.160028
142. Otaki F, Daniel W, Geno DM, Tholen C, Alexander JA. Interval Bone Density in Patients With Eosinophilic Esophagitis on Steroids: 368. *Off J Am Coll Gastroenterol | ACG* (2017) 112:S197. doi: 10.14309/00000434-201710001-00368
143. Nagata M, Nakagome K, Soma T. Mechanisms of Eosinophilic Inflammation. *Asia Pacif Allergy* (2020) 10(2):e14. doi: 10.5415/apallergy.2020.10.e14
144. Amber KT, Valdebran M, Kridin K, Grando SA. The Role of Eosinophils in Bullous Pemphigoid: A Developing Model of Eosinophil Pathogenicity in Mucocutaneous Disease. *Front Med* (2018) 5:201. doi: 10.3389/fmed.2018.00201
145. Murdaca G, Greco M, Tonacci A, Negrini S, Borro M, Puppo F, et al. IL-33/IL-31 Axis in Immune-Mediated and Allergic Diseases. *Int J Mol Sci* (2019) 20(23):5856. doi: 10.3390/ijms20235856
146. Krystel-Whittemore M, Dileepan KN, Wood JG. Mast Cell: A Multi-Functional Master Cell. *Front Immunol* (2015) 6:620. doi: 10.3389/fimmu.2015.00620
147. Galli SJ, Tsai M. IgE and Mast Cells in Allergic Disease. *Nat Med* (2012) 18 (5):693–704. doi: 10.1038/nm.2755
148. Kroner J, Kovtun A, Kemmler J, Messmann JJ, Strauss G, Seitz S, et al. Mast Cells Are Critical Regulators of Bone Fracture-Induced Inflammation and Osteoclast Formation and Activity. *J Bone Mineral Research: Off J Am Soc Bone Mineral Res* (2017) 32(12):2431–44. doi: 10.1002/jbmr.3234
149. Fallon MD, Whyte MP, Craig RB Jr, Teitelbaum SL. Mast-Cell Proliferation in Postmenopausal Osteoporosis. *Calcified Tissue Int* (1983) 35(1):29–31. doi: 10.1007/BF02405002
150. McKenna MJ. Histomorphometric Study of Mast Cells in Normal Bone, Osteoporosis and Mastocytosis Using a New Stain. *Calcified Tissue Int* (1994) 55(4):257–9. doi: 10.1007/BF00310402
151. Lesclous P, Guez D, Llorens A, Saffar JL. Time-Course of Mast Cell Accumulation in Rat Bone Marrow After Ovariectomy. *Calcified Tissue Int* (2001) 68(5):297–303. doi: 10.1007/BF02390837
152. Lesclous P, Saffar JL. Mast Cells Accumulate in Rat Bone Marrow After Ovariectomy. *Cells Tissues Organs* (1999) 164(1):23–9. doi: 10.1159/000016639
153. Tyan ML. Effect of Promethazine on Lumbar Vertebral Bone Mass in Postmenopausal Women. *J Internal Med* (1993) 234(2):143–8. doi: 10.1111/j.1365-2796.1993.tb00723.x
154. Zaitsu M, Narita S, Lambert KC, Grady JJ, Estes DM, Curran EM, et al. Estradiol Activates Mast Cells *via* a Non-Genomic Estrogen Receptor-Alpha and Calcium Influx. *Mol Immunol* (2007) 44(8):1977–85. doi: 10.1016/j.molimm.2006.09.030
155. Rivellese F, Nerviani A, Rossi FW, Marone G, Matucci-Cerinic M, de Paulis A, et al. Mast Cells in Rheumatoid Arthritis: Friends or Foes? *Autoimmun Rev* (2017) 16(6):557–63. doi: 10.1016/j.autrev.2017.04.001
156. Feyerabend TB, Weiser A, Tietz A, Stassen M, Harris N, Kopf M, et al. Cre-Mediated Cell Ablation Contests Mast Cell Contribution in Models of Antibody- and T Cell-Mediated Autoimmunity. *Immunity* (2011) 35 (5):832–44. doi: 10.1016/j.immuni.2011.09.015
157. de Lange-Brokaar BJ, Kloppenburg M, Andersen SN, Dorjee AL, Yusuf E, Herb-van Toorn L, et al. Characterization of Synovial Mast Cells in Knee Osteoarthritis: Association With Clinical Parameters. *Osteoarthritis Cartilage* (2016) 24(4):664–71. doi: 10.1016/j.joca.2015.11.011
158. Wang Q, Lepus CM, Raghu H, Reber LL, Tsai MM, Wong HH, et al. IgE-Mediated Mast Cell Activation Promotes Inflammation and Cartilage Destruction in Osteoarthritis. *eLife* (2019) 8:1–23. doi: 10.7554/eLife.39905
159. Nakano S, Mishiro T, Takahara S, Yokoi H, Hamada D, Yukata K, et al. Distinct Expression of Mast Cell Tryptase and Protease Activated Receptor-2 in Synovia of Rheumatoid Arthritis and Osteoarthritis. *Clin Rheumatol* (2007) 26(8):1284–92. doi: 10.1007/s10067-006-0495-8
160. Lee H, Kashiwakura J, Matsuda A, Watanabe Y, Sakamoto-Sasaki T, Matsumoto K, et al. Activation of Human Synovial Mast Cells From Rheumatoid Arthritis or Osteoarthritis Patients in Response to Aggregated IgG Through Fcgamma Receptor I and Fcgamma Receptor II. *Arthritis Rheum* (2013) 65(1):109–19. doi: 10.1002/art.37741
161. Lindholm R, Lindholm S, Liukko P. Fracture Healing and Mast Cells. I. The Periosteal Callus in Rats. *Acta Orthopaedica Scand* (1967) 38(2):115–22. doi: 10.3109/17453676708989624
162. Banovac K, Renfree K, Makowski AL, Latta LL, Altman RD. Fracture Healing and Mast Cells. *J Orthopaedic Trauma* (1995) 9(6):482–90. doi: 10.1097/00005131-199509060-00005
163. Scoville SD, Freud AG, Caligiuri MA. Modeling Human Natural Killer Cell Development in the Era of Innate Lymphoid Cells. *Front Immunol* (2017) 8:360. doi: 10.3389/fimmu.2017.00360
164. Brandstadter JD, Yang Y. Natural Killer Cell Responses to Viral Infection. *J Innate Immun* (2011) 3(3):274–9. doi: 10.1159/000324176
165. Trinchieri G. Biology of Natural Killer Cells. *Adv Immunol* (1989) 47:187–376. doi: 10.1016/S0065-2776(08)60664-1
166. Parham P. MHC Class I Molecules and KIRs in Human History, Health and Survival. *Nat Rev Immunol* (2005) 5(3):201–14. doi: 10.1038/nri1570
167. Fauriat C, Long EO, Ljunggren HG, Bryceson YT. Regulation of Human NK-Cell Cytokine and Chemokine Production by Target Cell Recognition. *Blood* (2010) 115(11):2167–76. doi: 10.1182/blood-2009-08-238469
168. de Matos CT, Berg L, Michaelsson J, Fellander-Tsai L, Karre K, Soderstrom K. Activating and Inhibitory Receptors on Synovial Fluid Natural Killer Cells of Arthritis Patients: Role of CD94/NKG2A in Control of Cytokine Secretion. *Immunology* (2007) 122(2):291–301. doi: 10.1111/j.1365-2567.2007.02638.x
169. Tak PP, Kummer JA, Hack CE, Daha MR, Smeets TJ, Erkelens GW, et al. Granzyme-Positive Cytotoxic Cells are Specifically Increased in Early Rheumatoid Synovial Tissue. *Arthritis Rheum* (1994) 37(12):1735–43. doi: 10.1002/art.1780371205
170. McInnes IB, Leung BP, Sturrock RD, Field M, Liew FY. Interleukin-15 Mediates T Cell-Dependent Regulation of Tumor Necrosis Factor-Alpha Production in Rheumatoid Arthritis. *Nat Med* (1997) 3(2):189–95. doi: 10.1038/nm0297-189
171. Feng S, Madsen SH, Viller NN, Neutzsky-Wulff AV, Geisler C, Karlsson L, et al. Interleukin-15-Activated Natural Killer Cells Kill Autologous Osteoclasts *via* LFA-1, DNAM-1 and TRAIL, and Inhibit Osteoclast-Mediated Bone Erosion *In Vitro*. *Immunology* (2015) 145(3):367–79. doi: 10.1111/imm.12449
172. Kurachi T, Morita I, Murota S. Involvement of Adhesion Molecules LFA-1 and ICAM-1 in Osteoclast Development. *Biochim Biophys Acta* (1993) 1178 (3):259–66. doi: 10.1016/0167-4889(93)90202-Z
173. Colonna M. Innate Lymphoid Cells: Diversity, Plasticity, and Unique Functions in Immunity. *Immunity* (2018) 48(6):1104–17. doi: 10.1016/j.immuni.2018.05.013
174. Mjosberg J, Spits H. Human Innate Lymphoid Cells. *J Allergy Clin Immunol* (2016) 138(5):1265–76. doi: 10.1016/j.jaci.2016.09.009
175. Monticelli LA, Sonnenberg GF, Abt MC, Alenghat T, Ziegler CG, Doering TA, et al. Innate Lymphoid Cells Promote Lung-Tissue Homeostasis After Infection With Influenza Virus. *Nat Immunol* (2011) 12(11):1045–54. doi: 10.1038/ni.2131
176. Turner JE, Morrison PJ, Wilhelm C, Wilson M, Ahlfors H, Renauld JC, et al. IL-9-Mediated Survival of Type 2 Innate Lymphoid Cells Promotes Damage Control in Helminth-Induced Lung Inflammation. *J Exp Med* (2013) 210 (13):2951–65. doi: 10.1084/jem.20130071
177. Stark MA, Huo Y, Burcin TL, Morris MA, Olson TS, Ley K. Phagocytosis of Apoptotic Neutrophils Regulates Granulopoiesis *via* IL-23 and IL-17. *Immunity* (2005) 22(3):285–94. doi: 10.1016/j.immuni.2005.01.011
178. Zheng Y, Valdez PA, Danilenko DM, Hu Y, Sa SM, Gong Q, et al. Interleukin-22 Mediates Early Host Defense Against Attaching and Effacing Bacterial Pathogens. *Nat Med* (2008) 14(3):282–9. doi: 10.1038/nm1720
179. Kuwabara T, Ishikawa F, Kondo M, Kakiuchi T. The Role of IL-17 and Related Cytokines in Inflammatory Autoimmune Diseases. *Mediators Inflamm* (2017) 2017:3908061. doi: 10.1155/2017/3908061

180. Fang W, Zhang Y, Chen Z. Innate Lymphoid Cells in Inflammatory Arthritis. *Arthritis Res Ther* (2020) 22(1):25. doi: 10.1186/s13075-020-2115-4
181. Leijten EF, van Kempen TS, Boes M, Michels-van Amelsfort JM, Hijnen D, Hartgring SA, et al. Brief Report: Enrichment of Activated Group 3 Innate Lymphoid Cells in Psoriatic Arthritis Synovial Fluid. *Arthritis Rheumatol* (2015) 67(10):2673–8. doi: 10.1002/art.39261
182. Omata Y, Frech M, Primbs T, Lucas S, Andreev D, Scholtysek C, et al. Group 2 Innate Lymphoid Cells Attenuate Inflammatory Arthritis and Protect From Bone Destruction in Mice. *Cell Rep* (2018) 24(1):169–80. doi: 10.1016/j.celrep.2018.06.005
183. Omata Y, Frech M, Lucas S, Primbs T, Knipfer L, Wirtz S, et al. Type 2 Innate Lymphoid Cells Inhibit the Differentiation of Osteoclasts and Protect From Ovariectomy-Induced Bone Loss. *Bone* (2020) 136:115335. doi: 10.1016/j.bone.2020.115335
184. Wang S, Xia P, Chen Y, Qu Y, Xiong Z, Ye B, et al. Regulatory Innate Lymphoid Cells Control Innate Intestinal Inflammation. *Cell* (2017) 171 (1):201–16.e18. doi: 10.1016/j.cell.2017.07.027
185. Zhang Q, Chen B, Yan F, Guo J, Zhu X, Ma S, et al. Interleukin-10 Inhibits Bone Resorption: A Potential Therapeutic Strategy in Periodontitis and Other Bone Loss Diseases. *BioMed Res Int* (2014) 2014:284836. doi: 10.1155/2014/284836
186. Kasagi S, Chen W. TGF-Beta1 on Osteoimmunology and the Bone Component Cells. *Cell Biosci* (2013) 3(1):4. doi: 10.1186/2045-3701-3-4
187. Di Munno O, Ferro F. The Effect of Biologic Agents on Bone Homeostasis in Chronic Inflammatory Rheumatic Diseases. *Clin Exp Rheumatol* (2019) 37 (3):502–7.
188. Kaji H. Effects of Myokines on Bone. *BoneKEy Rep* (2016) 5:826. doi: 10.1038/bonekey.2016.48
189. Pathak JL, Bakker AD, Verschueren P, Lems WF, Luyten FP, Klein-Nulend J, et al. CXCL8 and CCL20 Enhance Osteoclastogenesis *via* Modulation of Cytokine Production by Human Primary Osteoblasts. *PloS One* (2015) 10(6): e0131041. doi: 10.1371/journal.pone.0131041
190. Fu SC, Wang P, Qi MX, Peng JP, Lin XQ, Zhang CY, et al. The Associations of TNF-Alpha Gene Polymorphisms With Bone Mineral Density and Risk of Osteoporosis: A Meta-Analysis. *Int J Rheum Dis* (2019) 22(9):1619–29. doi: 10.1111/1756-185X.13647
191. Kotrych D, Dziedziejko V, Safranow K, Sroczynski T, Staniszewska M, Juzyszyn Z, et al. TNF-Alpha and IL10 Gene Polymorphisms in Women With Postmenopausal Osteoporosis. *Eur J Obstet Gynecol Reprod Biol* (2016) 199:92–5. doi: 10.1016/j.ejogrb.2016.01.037
192. Weitzmann MN. Bone and the Immune System. *ToxicoL Pathol* (2017) 45 (7):911–24. doi: 10.1177/0192623317735316
193. Zha L, He L, Liang Y, Qin H, Yu B, Chang L, et al. TNF-Alpha Contributes to Postmenopausal Osteoporosis by Synergistically Promoting RANKL-Induced Osteoclast Formation. *Biomedicine Pharmacother = Biomedecine Pharmacother* (2018) 102:369–74. doi: 10.1016/j.biopha.2018.03.080
194. O'Brien W, Fissel BM, Maeda Y, Yan J, Ge X, Gravallese EM, et al. RANK-Independent Osteoclast Formation and Bone Erosion in Inflammatory Arthritis. *Arthritis Rheumatol* (2016) 68(12):2889–900. doi: 10.1002/art.39837
195. Li S, Yin Y, Yao L, Lin Z, Sun S, Zhang J, et al. TNFalpha Treatment Increases DKK1 Protein Levels in Primary Osteoblasts *via* Upregulation of DKK1 mRNA Levels and Downregulation of Mir3355p. *Mol Med Rep* (2020) 22 (2):1017–25. doi: 10.3892/mmr.2020.11152
196. Callaway DA, Jiang JX. Reactive Oxygen Species and Oxidative Stress in Osteoclastogenesis, Skeletal Aging and Bone Diseases. *J Bone Mineral Metab* (2015) 33(4):359–70. doi: 10.1007/s00774-015-0656-4
197. Manolagas SC. From Estrogen-Centric to Aging and Oxidative Stress: A Revised Perspective of the Pathogenesis of Osteoporosis. *Endocrine Rev* (2010) 31(3):266–300. doi: 10.1210/er.2009-0024
198. Locantore P, Del Gatto V, Gelli S, Paragliola RM, Pontecorvi A. The Interplay Between Immune System and Microbiota in Osteoporosis. *Mediators Inflamm* (2020) 2020:3686749. doi: 10.1155/2020/3686749
199. Pacifici R. Bone Remodeling and the Microbiome. *Cold Spring Harbor Perspect Med* (2018) 8(4):1–20. doi: 10.1101/cshperspect.a031203

17

T Cell Protein Tyrosine Phosphatase in Osteoimmunology

Ya-nan Wang[1,2,3†], *Shiyue Liu*[2,3,4†], *Tingting Jia*[1,2,3], *Yao Feng*[1,2,3], *Wenjing Zhang*[1,2,3], *Xin Xu*[1,2,3] *and Dongjiao Zhang*[1,2,3*]

[1] Department of Implantology, School and Hospital of Stomatology, Cheeloo College of Medicine, Shandong University, Jinan, China, [2] Shandong Key Laboratory of Oral Tissue Regeneration, Jinan, China, [3] Shandong Engineering Laboratory for Dental Materials and Oral Tissue Regeneration, Jinan, China, [4] Department of Periodontology, School and Hospital of Stomatology, Cheeloo College of Medicine, Shandong University, Jinan, China

***Correspondence:**
Dongjiao Zhang
djzhang1109@163.com

†These authors have contributed equally to this work

Osteoimmunology highlights the two-way communication between bone and immune cells. T cell protein tyrosine phosphatase (TCPTP), also known as protein-tyrosine phosphatase non-receptor 2 (PTPN2), is an intracellular protein tyrosine phosphatase (PTP) essential in regulating immune responses and bone metabolism *via* dephosphorylating target proteins. *Tcptp* knockout in systemic or specific immune cells can seriously damage the immune function, resulting in bone metabolism disorders. This review provided fresh insights into the potential role of TCPTP in osteoimmunology. Overall, the regulation of osteoimmunology by TCPTP is extremely complicated. TCPTP negatively regulates macrophages activation and inflammatory factors secretion to inhibit bone resorption. TCPTP regulates T lymphocytes differentiation and T lymphocytes-related cytokines signaling to maintain bone homeostasis. TCPTP is also expected to regulate bone metabolism by targeting B lymphocytes under certain time and conditions. This review offers a comprehensive update on the roles of TCPTP in osteoimmunology, which can be a promising target for the prevention and treatment of inflammatory bone loss.

Keywords: T cell protein tyrosine phosphatase (TCPTP), Protein tyrosine phosphatase non-receptor 2 (PTPN2), osteoimmunology, macrophages, T cell, B cell

INTRODUCTION

Inflammatory bone diseases characterized by severe bone loss, such as osteoarthritis, rheumatoid arthritis, and periodontitis, are a manifestation of imbalance between the skeletal and immune systems (1–3). Their interactions, known as osteoimmunology, were firstly proposed by Choi and Aaron in 2000, which highlights the two-way communication between bone and immune cells (4). With a comprehensive and profound acknowledgment of osteoimmunology, targeting regulatory proteins involved in osteoimmune responses can be a feasible means against inflammatory bone diseases. T-cell protein tyrosine phosphatase (TCPTP), one of the protein tyrosine phosphatases (PTPs) family, was identified by Cool et al. using T-cell-based cDNA library screening (5). There is growing evidence that TCPTP is a critical regulator in immune responses and bone metabolism. Nevertheless, the potential effect of TCPTP in the field of osteoimmunology is less explored. As a result, we intended to offer a comprehensive update on the known and potential roles of TCPTP in osteoimmunology in this review. Our study will lay a theoretical foundation for further basic researches of TCPTP in the field of osteoimmunology and provide references for treatment strategies of inflammatory bone diseases.

OSTEOIMMUNOLOGY

During osteoimmune responses, different immune cells and bone cells interact reciprocally to maintain the homeostasis between the immune and skeletal systems (**Figure 1**). The two-way communication may influence either immune or bone cells *via* cytokine activities in the immune-bone interface. The proposal of screening new targets interfering with osteoimmunology may be feasible for identifying critical targets suppressing immune hyperactivity in inflammatory bone loss diseases.

Influence of Immune Cells on Bone Cells

Immune cells, such as T lymphocytes (Th1, Th2, Treg, and Th17 cells), B lymphocytes, dendritic cells, and macrophages, actively regulate the homeostasis of bone metabolism. Th1 cells secrete interferon-γ (IFN-γ) that has been found to exert controversial

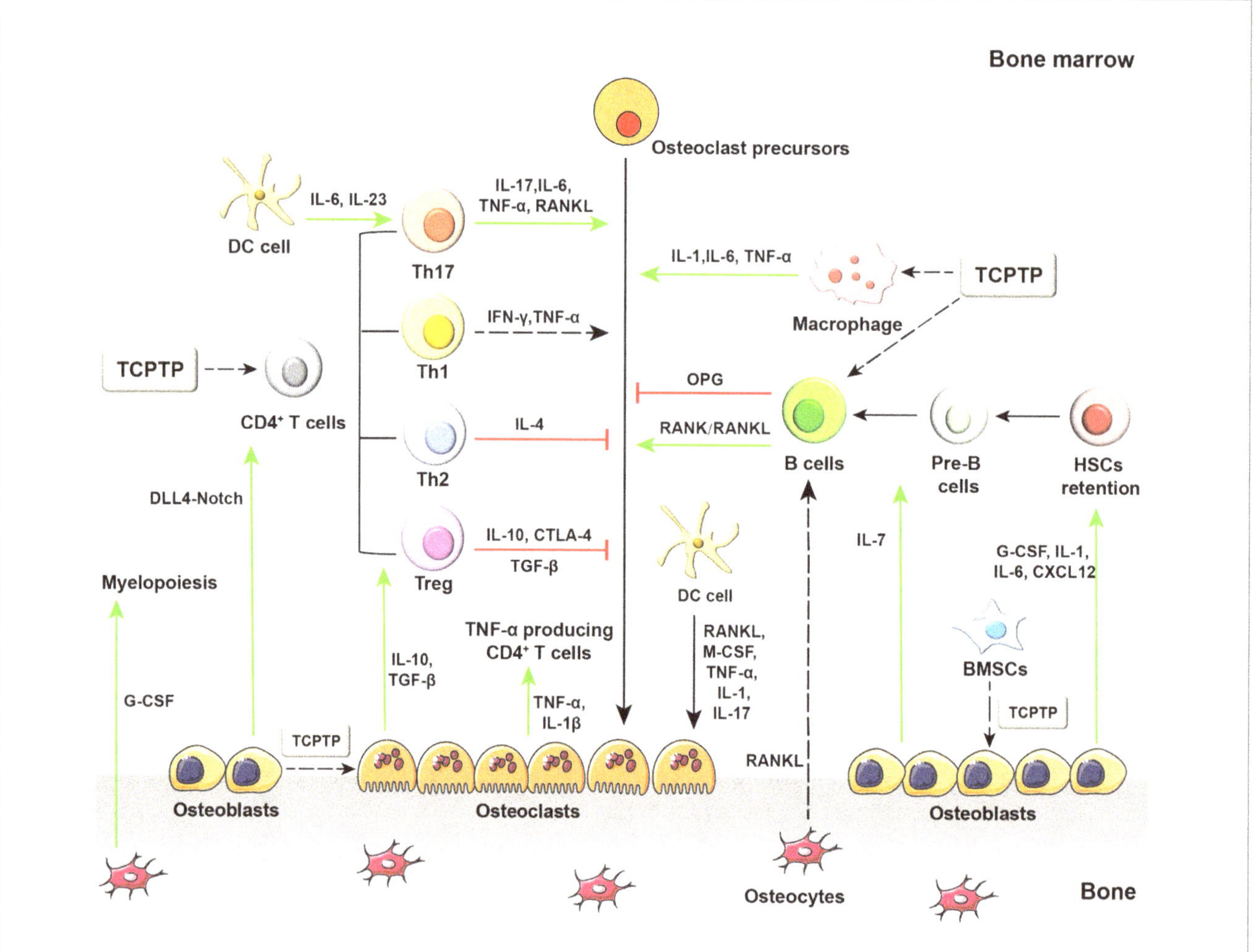

FIGURE 1 | Diagram of osteoimmunology and potential regulatory sites of TCPTP. Regarding the regulation of bone-related cells by immune cells, some CD4⁺ T cell subsets can produce osteoclastogenic cytokines (e.g., TNF-α from Th1 cells and IL-17 from Th17 cells), while other subsets secrete anti-osteoclastogenic cytokines (e.g., IL-4 from Th2 cells, IL-10 and CTLA4 from Treg cells). IFN-γ released by Th1 cells may exert both pro- and anti-osteoclastogenic effects as reported by previous studies. B cells physiologically inhibit osteoclastogenesis but stimulate osteoclastogenesis through activating the RANK/RANKL axis in the pathological state. Different stages of dendritic cells exhibit distinct properties in immune responses: immature dendritic cells differentiate into osteoclasts in response to M-CSF, RANKL, TNF-α, IL-1, and IL-17, while mature ones drive the activation and expansion of Th17 cells. Macrophages are essential to bone loss with the involvement of TNF-α, IL-1, and IL-6 released by themselves. On the other hand, bone-related cells also provide feedback to immune cells. Osteoblasts secrete G-CSF, IL-1, IL-6, IL-7, and CXCL12, which are required for HSCs maintenance. In addition, osteoblasts secrete IL-7 to support B lymphopoiesis and regulate DLL4-Notch signaling pathway to support T lymphopoiesis. Osteocytes are supposed to mobilize HSCs and are involved in myelopoiesis. Osteocyte-derived RANKL participates in estrogen deficiency-induced bone loss by indirect regulation of B cell development. Osteoclasts are also involved in antigen presentation and T cell activation. Osteoclasts secrete tolerogenic cytokines (e.g., IL-10, TGF-β) and activate regulatory T cells in physiological conditions, while in pathological conditions, osteoclasts secrete inflammatory cytokines (e.g., TNFα, IL-1β) and activate TNF-α producing CD4⁺ T cells. Generally, TCPTP regulates bone metabolism mainly by changing the biofunction of macrophages, T cells, and B cells. TCPTP, T cell protein tyrosine phosphatase; DC cell, dendritic cell; IL-6, interleukin-6; IL-23, interleukin-23; IL-17, interleukin-17; TNF-α, tumor necrosis factor-α; RANK, receptor activator of nuclear factor–κB; RANKL, receptor activator of nuclear factor–κB ligand; IL-1, interleukin-1; IL-4, interleukin-4; IL-10, interleukin-10; CTLA4, cytotoxic T lymphocyte protein 4; OPG, osteoprotegerin; Th17, T helper 17 cells; Th1, T helper 1 cells; Th2, T helper 2 cells; Treg, regulatory T cells; G-CSF, granulocyte colony-stimulating factor; M-CSF, macrophage colony-stimulating factor; TGF-β, transforming growth factor β; DLL4, Delta-like protein 4; IL-1β, interleukin-1β; IL-7, interleukin-7; CXCL12, CXC-motif chemokine 12; HSCs, hematopoietic stem cells.

effects in bone metabolism (6, 7). Sato et al. demonstrated that Th1 cells generated amounts of IFN-γ and mediated osteoclastogenesis inhibition *in vitro* (8). However, another study reported that IFN-γ could promote osteoclast maturation in the late period of osteoclastogenesis (9). Th1 cells are found to induce orthodontic tooth movement and bone resorption indirectly by upregulating the tumor necrosis factor-alpha (TNF-α) secretion and promoting osteoclastogenesis (10, 11). Th2 cells secrete interleukin-4 (IL-4), interleukin-5 (IL-5), and interleukin-13 (IL-13) leading to the osteoclastogenesis inhibition in a signal transducer and activator of transcription 6 (STAT6)-dependent pathway (12). Cytotoxic T-lymphocyte antigen 4 (CTLA4) secreted by Treg cells can promote apoptosis of osteoclasts *via* binding to CD80/CD86 on osteoclast precursors (13). Besides, Treg cells not only inhibit osteoclastogenesis directly *via* suppressing receptor activator of nuclear factor-κB ligand (RANKL) generation (14) but also suppress osteoclast differentiation and bone resorption by secreting interleukin-10 (IL-10) and transforming growth factor-β (TGF-β) (15). Th17 cells are one of the osteoclastogenic subsets of T cells that participate in various inflammatory diseases, such as rheumatoid arthritis, osteoporosis, inflammatory bowel disease, and periodontal disease (16–18). In the process of osteoclastogenesis and bone loss, higher amounts of osteoclastogenic cytokines, including interleukin-17 (IL-17), interleukin-6 (IL-6), interleukin-1 (IL-1), and TNF-α, are released from Th17 cells (19, 20). Among these cytokines, IL-17 stimulates the synthesis of cyclooxygenase-2 dependent prostaglandin E2 and the gene transcription of osteoclast differentiation factor (ODF) in osteoblasts to induce osteoclastogenesis (21). B cells inhibit osteoclastogenesis *via* secreting osteoprotegerin in the physiological state but stimulate osteoclastogenesis through activating the receptor activator of nuclear factor–κB (RANK)/RANKL axis in the pathological state (22, 23). Human immature dendritic cells differentiate into osteoclasts in response to macrophage colony-stimulating factor (M-CSF), RANKL, TNF-α, IL-1, and IL-17 (24–26), while mature dendritic cells can drive the activation of Th17 cells that produce IL-17, thereby enhancing osteoclastogenesis (27). Macrophages are reported to secrete different proinflammatory cytokines (e.g., TNF-α, IL-1, and IL-6) to enhance bone loss (28).

Influence of Bone Cells on Immune Cells

Bone-related cells (e.g., osteoblasts, osteocytes, osteoclasts) could also regulate the immune system. In this process, numerous cytokines (e.g., granulocyte colony-stimulating factor [G–CSF], IL–1, IL–6, IL–7, and CXC-motif chemokine 12 [CXCL12]) are secreted from osteoblasts for hematopoietic stem cell (HSC) maintenance, lymphoid progenitor cell maintenance, as well as the balance of T cell or B cell generation (29–31). Zhu et al. reported that osteoblasts support all stages of B lymphopoiesis *via* locally secreting interleukin-7 (IL-7) and stromal cell derived factor-1 (SDF-1) (32, 33). Osteoblasts-specific knockout of osteocalcin results in a marked reduction in mature T cells through disrupting the delta-like protein 4-notch signaling (34). Osteocytes are supposed to mobilize hematopoietic stem cells (HSCs) and might also be involved in myelopoiesis. In mice with targeted ablation of osteocytes, the mobilization of HSCs was suppressed in bone marrow (35). Besides, deficiency of the G -protein subunit GSα in osteocytes results in increased G–CSF production and dramatic expansion of myeloid lineage cells (36). RANKL generated by osteocytes participates in estrogen deficiency-induced bone loss by regulating B cell development indirectly (37). Several studies reported that osteoclasts could promote the mobilization of hematopoietic progenitor cells (38), while others revealed that they were dispensable for HSC maintenance and mobilization (39). Osteoclasts are also involved in antigen presentation and T cell activation. In the physiological conditions, osteoclasts secrete tolerogenic cytokines (such as IL-10 and TGF-β) and activate $CD4^+$ and $CD8^+$ regulatory T cells, while in the pathological conditions, osteoclasts activate TNF-α producing $CD4^+$ T cells *via* unleashing myriads of inflammatory cytokines (e.g., TNF-α and IL-1) (26, 40, 41).

TCPTP

Overview of TCPTP

TCPTP is a tyrosine-specific phosphatase that is firstly identified by Cool et al. (5). There are two splice variants of TCPTP: TC45 (45 kDa) which is located in nuclear and TC48 (48 kDa) which is located in the endoplasmic reticulum (42). TC45 is a widely expressed form in various species, including humans and mice, and TC48 is human-specific. In most species, TC45 shuttles between the nucleus and cytoplasm in response to cytokine stimulation (43).

TCPTP regulates diverse signaling pathways related to glucose metabolism, inflammation control, cancer progress, and other biological processes *via* dephosphorylation of distinct substrates (44–50). Experiments *in vitro* and *in vivo* have confirmed that TCPTP could regulate several cytokine signaling pathways by inhibiting Janus activated kinase (JAK)/signal transducer and activator of transcription (STAT) predominantly (51–54). The direct substrates have been recognized as JAK1, JAK3, STAT1, STAT3, and STAT5 (55–59). Some members of the tyrosine kinase receptor (RTK) family, comprising insulin receptors (IRs) (60, 61), epidermal growth factor receptors (EGFRs) (62, 63), vascular endothelial growth factor receptors (VEGFRs) (64), platelet-derived growth factor receptors (PDGFRs) (65, 66) and colony-stimulating factor-1 receptors (CSF-1Rs) are also the specific dephosphorylating substrates of TCPTP (67).

TCPTP and Immunomodulation

Growing evidence has indicated that TCPTP is a key player in regulating innate and acquired immune responses. GWA studies found single nucleotide polymorphisms (SNPs) of TCPTP are associated with the onset of several inflammatory diseases and autoimmunology disorders, such as inflammatory bowel disease (68, 69), ocular Behcet's disease (70), rheumatoid arthritis (53), and juvenile inflammatory arthritis (71). *Tcptp* knockout in the systemic or specific cells can seriously jeopardize immune reactions.

Mice null for *Tcptp* ($Tcptp^{-/-}$) showed a smaller body size, decreased mobility, severe anemia, and diarrhea followed by death at three to 5 weeks of age (72). From the perspective of histology, *Tcptp*$^{-/-}$ mice showed mononuclear cell infiltration in the salivary gland and gastric mucosa at 1 week of age (72). Dramatic increases in TNF-α and inducible nitric oxide synthase (iNOS) were also detected at 3 weeks of age in *Tcptp*$^{-/-}$ mice (73).

Loss of PTPN2 in T cells (TCPTP-CD4Cre) not only led to increased intestinal inflammation risk but also resulted in T-lymphocyte infiltration in the liver, kidney, and skin (74, 75). This may be caused by the enhanced induction of Th1 cells, Th17 cells, and effector and memory CD8^{+} T cells, but the impaired induction of Tregs after T cell-specific knockout of *Tcptp*. Myeloid cell-specific loss of TCPTP (TCPTP-LysMCre) also enhanced susceptibility to colitis and serum IL-1β levels in mice (76). Spalinger et al. reported that TCPTP loss in macrophages compromises epithelial cell-macrophage interactions and reduces epithelial barrier integrity (77). Furthermore, TCPTP knockdown in THP-1 cells elevated the IFN-γ-induced secretion of the proinflammatory cytokines IL-6 (78). TCPTP silencing in rheumatoid arthritis synovial fibroblasts could also increase IL-6 production (53).

TCPTP and Hematopoiesis

Although ubiquitously expressed, TCPTP is pronouncedly expressed in hematopoietic tissues and plays a significant role in the development of hematopoietic lineages (5).

TCPTP and Hematopoiesis: Stem Cells

Hematopoietic stem cells (HSCs) are one of the adult stem cells and can differentiate into various mature blood cells (79). Compared with the control group, *Tcptp* knockout resulted in a nine-fold increase of the HSC number in the bone marrow (80). Lymphoid and myeloid precursors were also more abundant in *Tcptp*$^{-/-}$ mice compared with the wide type controls (45). Bourdeau et al. also demonstrated that this effect could be reproduced by TCPTP inhibiting agents and interleukin-18 (IL-18) signaling pathway involved in this process (80). The above results implicated that TCPTP plays an important role in the regulation of HSC proliferation.

TCPTP and Hematopoiesis: Myeloid Cells

Tcptp$^{-/-}$ mice exhibited increased splenic macrophage populations and yielded four times of the macrophage colony-forming unit (CFU-M) number (67). TCPTP is also involved in myeloid progenitor development. *Tcptp*$^{-/-}$ mice had 4 times of the granulocyte/macrophage precursors (GMPs) compared with wildtype mice and CSF-1/CSF-1R signaling may involve in this process (67).

Tcptp$^{-/-}$ mice were reported to suffer from severe anemia which could contribute to their early lethality. You-Ten et al. reported a failure to initiate hematopoietic function in the bone marrow of *Tcptp*$^{-/-}$ animals after 2–3 weeks (72). What's more, the deficiency of bone marrow stromal cell numbers, the impairment of remaining stromal cells, and the inadequate cytokines production by the bone marrow microenvironment could be the possible explanations for the defective hematopoiesis in *Tcptp*$^{-/-}$ mice (72).

TCPTP and Hematopoiesis: Lymphocytes

Tcptp$^{-/-}$ mice exhibited specific defects of B cell lymphopoiesis in the bone marrow, however, T cell development in the thymus was not significantly affected (72). The defects of B cell lymphopoiesis were characterized by fewer pre-B cell colonies and impaired transition to the immature B-cell stage (81). Bourdeau et al. have found that bone marrow stromal cells from *Tcptp*$^{-/-}$ mice could secrete higher levels of IFN-γ resulting in a 2-fold reduction in the mitotic index on IL-7 stimulation of *Tcptp*$^{-/-}$ pre-B cells (81).

TCPTP and Bone Metabolism

Recent studies using gene knockout mice have emphasized the importance of TCPTP in bone metabolism. *Tcptp*$^{-/-}$ BALB/c mice showed significantly reduced femoral length and width, as reflected by the large volume of unabsorbed cartilage at the epiphysis by 14 days of age (82); however the latter was no longer evident at 21 days of age (82). Besides, *Tcptp*$^{-/-}$ mice have a higher incidence of synovitis in the knee joint (83). Loh et al. found that the runted body of neuronal cell-specific *Tcptp* knockout mice is associated with decreased circulating growth hormone (84). However, the precise mechanisms that underlie the bone development in *Tcptp*$^{-/-}$ mice still need further investigation.

Insulin signaling in osteoblast inhibits the expression of osteoprotegerin (OPG), an osteoclastogenesis inhibitory factor (85). TCPTP expressed in osteoblasts regulates insulin receptor phosphorylation, thus activating insulin signaling (86). A classical coculture assay revealed that osteoblasts lacking TCPTP induced more tartrate-resistant acid phosphatase (TRAP) positive osteoclasts than wild-type osteoblasts did (86). Accordingly, osteoclast activity was increased in osteoblasts-specific *Tcptp*$^{-/-}$ mice which was proved by increased serum levels of CTx, a marker of bone resorption (86).

TCPTP IN OSTEOIMMUNOLOGY

As shown in **Figure 1**, TCPTP could influence bone metabolism by regulating the biofunction of macrophages, T cells, and B cells. Besides, TCPTP in osteoblasts and bone marrow stem cells also regulates bone metabolism. The potential roles of TCPTP in osteoimmunology are discussed below.

TCPTP and Macrophages in Osteoimmunology

Macrophages, a significant component of the non-specific immunity, are crucial regulators in bone metabolism and can be regulated by TCPTP (77, 87, 88). The potential influences of TCPTP on osteoimmunology through macrophages can be expounded from four aspects. Firstly, TCPTP negatively regulates macrophages development (45). *Tcptp*$^{-/-}$ animals exhibited significantly impaired bone marrow microenvironment (including impairment of erythropoiesis, the decline of pre-B and mature B cells, and reduced stromal cells) and increased macrophage numbers (89). Secondly, TCPTP participates in the process of macrophage polarization. M1 and M2 macrophages, the two major phenotypes of macrophages, are pro-inflammatory and anti-inflammatory respectively. A previous study reported that the increased M1/M2 ratio finally promoted osteoclastogenesis (90), and TCPTP could reverse diabetes-mediated high M1/M2 polarization in mice (91). This can be attributed to the fact that macrophages from *Tcptp*$^{-/-}$ mice are inherently hypersensitive to lipopolysaccharide and IFN-γ stimulation, which are two main cytokines that induce M1 differentiation (73, 92). Thirdly, the colony-stimulating factor 1 (CSF-1)/colony-stimulating factor 1 receptor (CSF-1R) signaling has been proven to be downregulated by TCPTP in macrophages. After CSF-1 stimulation, tyrosine phosphorylation of the CSF-1R markedly increased, and the activation of extracellular regulated protein kinases (ERK) was enhanced in *Tcptp*$^{-/-}$ macrophages (67). Zhang et al. ascertained that TCPTP inhibited alveolar bone resorption in diabetic periodontitis *via* dephosphorylating CSF-1R at the Y807 site, thereby prohibiting osteoclast differentiation (93). Fourthly, the dephosphorylating of c-Jun N-terminal kinase (JNK) in macrophages is another means how TCPTP protects against inflammatory response and bone loss caused by inflammasome-mediated interleukin-1β secretion (76). These studies suggest that TCPTP may be a potential treatment target against inflammatory bone loss induced by macrophage-related disorders, for example, periodontitis and synovitis (**Figure 2A**).

TCPTP and T Cells in Osteoimmunology

Undoubtedly, T cells play a critical role in bone homeostasis, wherein the effects of TCPTP on T cell function cannot be neglected (**Figure 2C**). TCPTP negatively regulates T cell activation (94, 95). *Tcptp*$^{-/-}$ T cells show enhanced cell activity *via* the reduction of T cell receptor (TCR) threshold and hyperphosphorylation of the activated tyrosine residue of Lck (75). Furthermore, TCPTP regulates T cell differentiation (91, 96, 97). TCPTP regulated the activation and differentiation of T cells in colonic inflammation (96). Wiede et al. showed that TCPTP attenuates the activity of the STAT5 signaling to regulate αβ TCR versus γδ TCR T cell development (97). Li et al. reported that TCPTP overexpression reversed the high Th1/Treg and Th17/Treg ratios in epididymal white adipose tissue of diabetic mice (91). Spalinger et al. showed that *Tcptp*$^{-/-}$ CD4^{+} T cell reinfusion led to a nearly 3-fold increase in the frequency of Th1 cells, a 2-fold increase in the frequency of Th17 cells, and by contrast, a 3-fold decrease in the frequency of Tregs in colitis animal models (74). In addition, the inhibition of the interleukin-2 (IL-2)/IL-2 receptor pathway mediated by JAK1, JAK3, and STAT5 dephosphorylation was found to be the mechanism of how TCPTP drives Treg differentiation possibly (98). As illustrated above, various cytokines (e.g., IFN-γ and IL-6 from Th1 cells) released from stimulated T cells bridge the two-way communications in osteoimmune responses. These two cytokines, which are closely associated with osteoimmunology, can be regulated by TCPTP. Therefore, the interactions between the two cytokines and TCPTP in bone metabolism were discussed in detail below.

TCPTP and IFN-γ

IFN-γ is a classical cytokine secreted from Th1 cells. On the one hand, IFN-γ promotes osteoclastogenesis *via* promoting the fusion of mononucleated pre-osteoclasts in the late period of osteoclastogenesis directly and stimulating the secretion of osteoclastic factors (such as RANKL and TNF-α)indirectly (9, 99, 100). By contrast, IFN-γ can also intensively suppress osteoclastogenesis by degrading tumor necrosis factor receptor-associated factor 6 and inhibiting the RANK/RANKL signaling pathway (6). TCPTP downregulates the IFN-γ signaling through JAK1, STAT1, and STAT3 dephosphorylation (52, 55, 59, 92). So, a rational thread of targeting TCPTP to suppress IFN-γ activity is expected to regulate osteoclastogenesis, and this hypothesis still needs more validations.

TCPTP and IL-6

IL-6 is an inflammatory cytokine that exerts pathological effects on inflammatory bone loss (101, 102), directly supporting osteoclast formation, stimulating osteoclast differentiation, and accelerating bone resorption (103, 104). IL-6 is associated with Th17 cell differentiation (105), and abnormalities in the IL-6 signaling can disturb the Th17/Treg balance and influence bone homeostasis indirectly (106). Concerning the regulation of IL-6 by TCPTP, TCPTP curbs both IL-6 secretion and signaling. Aradi et al. confirmed that TCPTP silencing significantly increased IL-6 secretion from synovial fibroblasts in rheumatoid arthritis animals (53). TCPTP also dephosphorylate STAT3 at the Y705 site, thereby suppressing IL-6 signaling (107, 108). Besides, TCPTP inhibits the IL-6-driven pathogenic loss of Foxp3 after Tregs have acquired RORγt expression through dephosphorylation of STAT3 (109). Therefore, TCPTP can be expected to inhibit bone resorption through inhibiting IL-6 generation and IL-6 signaling directly or reversing IL-6-induced Th17/Treg imbalance indirectly.

TCPTP and B Cells in Osteoimmunology

B lymphocytes play an extremely vital role in both immune responses and bone metabolism, but the detailed relationship between B lymphocytes and osteoclastogenesis remains some points for debate. Physiologically, B cells produce osteoprotegerin to inhibit osteoclastogenesis but stimulate osteoclastogenesis *via* the RANK/RANKL axis in the pathological state (22, 23, 110). Recently, increasing evidence tended to support that B cell development and proliferation were crucially affected by TCPTP (**Figure 2B**). An impaired transition from pre-B to immature B cell was found in *Tcptp*$^{-/-}$ mice (45, 89), which might be associated with the abnormally increased release of IFN-γ and enhanced STAT1 phosphorylation in the pre-B cell compartment (81). With interleukin-21-induced hyperactivity of the STAT-3 signaling in *Tcptp*$^{-/-}$ mice, B cell proliferation was simultaneously boosted (111). These results ascertain TCPTP as an important regulator of B cells in bone homeostasis. However, concerning the complexity of the two-way effect between B lymphocytes and bone homeostasis or between TCPTP and B lymphocytes, the specific effect and the mechanisms behind each regulation should be confirmed in further explorations.

TCPTP and Bone-Related Cells in Osteoimmunology

TCPTP that is expressed in osteoblasts and bone marrow stem cells participates in the regulation of bone metabolism

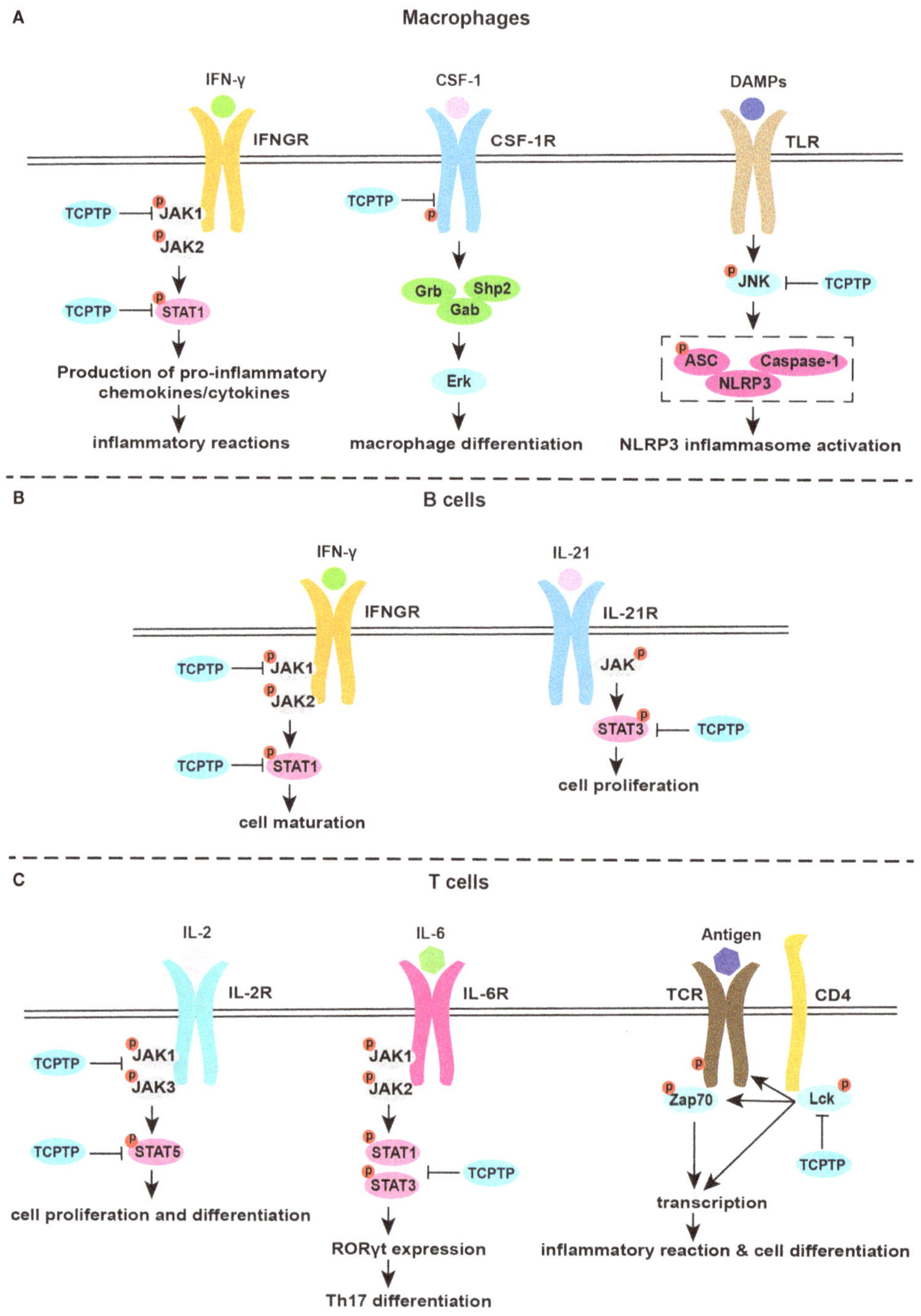

FIGURE 2 | TCPTP-related signaling pathways in macrophages, B cells, and T cells. **(A)** TCPTP downregulates the IFN-γ signaling, the CSF-1/CSF-1R signaling, and inflammasome activation in macrophages. **(B)** TCPTP drives B cell maturation *via* suppressing the IFN-γ signaling and prohibits B cell proliferation by downregulating the IL-21 signaling. **(C)** TCPTP inhibits IL-6-driven pathogenic loss of Foxp3 after Tregs have acquired RORγt expression through dephosphorylation of STAT3. TCPTP negatively regulates the IL-2 receptor signaling by JAK1, JAK3, and STAT5 dephosphorylation, which is an important way related to Treg differentiation. TCPTP inhibits TCR activation and hyperphosphorylation of Lck to inhibit inflammatory reactions and cell differentiation. TCPTP, T cell protein tyrosine phosphatase; JAK1, Janus activated kinase 1; JAK2, Janus activated kinase 2; JAK3, Janus activated kinase 3; STAT1, signal transducer and activator of transcription1; STAT3, signal transducer and activator of transcription3; STAT5, signal transducer and activator of transcription5; IFN-γ, interferon-γ; IFNGR, interferon-γ receptor; CSF-1, colony-stimulating factor 1; CSF-1R, colony-stimulating factor 1 receptor; DAMPs, damage-associated molecular pattern molecules; TLR, toll-like receptor; JNK, c-Jun N-terminal kinase; IL-21, interleukin-21; IL-21R, interleukin-21R; IL-6, interleukin-6; IL-6R, interleukin-6R; TCR, T cell receptor.

(**Figure 1**). Zee et al. demonstrated that TCPTP deficiency in osteoblasts enhanced the activity of osteoclasts by activating insulin signaling and inhibiting the expression of OPG *in vitro* (86). Our previous study found that TCPTP improved the osteogenic differentiation ability *via* ERK dephosphorylation in rat bone marrow stem cells in high glucose conditions (112). However, to our knowledge, no specific studies have reported the impacts of TCPTP in bone-related cells on immune cells which may be a novel aspect in the future, and the underlying mechanism also needs further exploration.

THERAPEUTIC ASPECTS FROM "TCPTP AND OSTEOIMMUNOLOGY" PERSPECTIVE

TCPTP exerts an anti-inflammatory role in innate and adaptive immunity (113). As described in Section *TCPTP and Immunomodulation*, *Tcptp* knockout in systemic or specific immune cells brings about serious immune disorders. TCPTP deficiency also leads to subchondral bone loss and spontaneous synovitis mediated by excessive inflammatory cytokines (83). Loss-of-function variants of TCPTP increase the risk of rheumatoid arthritis due to Treg cell dysfunction (114). Therefore, using TCPTP agonists to overexpress or activate TCPTP seems to be a rational strategy against inflammatory bone resorption. This proposal can be supported by other studies. Zhang P. et al. found that TCPTP alleviated inflammatory responses and bone resorption in periodontal tissues *via* the JAK/STAT pathway in human oral keratinocytes and type 2 diabetes mellitus (T2DM) *db*/*db* mice (115). Zhang D.J. et al. demonstrated that TCPTP inhibited alveolar bone resorption in T2DM C57BL/6 wild-type mice *via* dephosphorylating CSF1 receptor (93). Consistently, our previous study series ascertained that TCPTP improves implant osseointegration in T2DM rats *via* ERK dephosphorylation (112). It is obvious that TCPTP could work as an effective potential target for preventing and treating inflammatory bone resorption. However, concerning the ubiquitous distribution and wide regulation of TCPTP related to glucose metabolism, immunoregulation, oncogenesis, and other various life processes in a cell or tissue-specific way, designing specific agents targeting TCPTP in specific cells, tissues or organs is a promising research direction and a novel aspect of osteoimmunology in the future.

CONCLUSION

TCPTP bridges the two-way communication between immune cells and bone cells and it could work as a potential target for the prevention and treatment of inflammatory bone diseases, such as periodontitis, synovitis, and osteoarthritis. The proposal of identifying whether TCPTP can be used as an independent therapeutic target is feasible for the development of TCPTP agonists binding to a target of interest. This review provides clear insights into the potential roles of TCPTP in osteoimmunology, which may pave the way for further bone studies on osteoimmunological aspects.

AUTHOR CONTRIBUTIONS

Y-NW, SL, TJ, YF, and DZ made substantial contributions to conception, design, and acquisition of data. Y-NW, SL, WZ, and XX drafted the initial manuscript. XX and DZ critically reviewed it for important intellectual content. All authors contributed to the article and approved the submitted version.

FUNDING

This work was supported by the National Natural Science Foundation of China (no. 82071148; no. 82001055), the Construction Engineering Special Fund of Taishan Scholars (TS201511106), the Key Project of Chinese National Programs for Research and Development (2016YFC1102705), the Shandong Provincial Natural Science Foundation (ZR2020QH158), the Fundamental Research Funds of Shandong University (2018GN024), the China Postdoctoral Science Foundation (2019M662371), and the Youth scientific research funds of School of Stomatology, Shandong University (2019QNJJ03).

REFERENCES

1. Orsolini G, Bertoldi I, Rossini M. Osteoimmunology in rheumatoid and psoriatic arthritis: potential effects of tofacitinib on bone involvement. *Clin Rheumatol* (2020) 39:727–36. doi: 10.1007/s10067-020-04930-x
2. Gruber R. Osteoimmunology: Inflammatory osteolysis and regeneration of the alveolar bone. *J Clin Periodontol* (2019) 46 Suppl 21:52–69. doi: 10.1111/jcpe.13056
3. Chen Z, Bozec A, Ramming A, Schett G. Anti-inflammatory and immune-regulatory cytokines in rheumatoid arthritis. *Nat Rev Rheumatol* (2019) 15:9–17. doi: 10.1038/s41584-018-0109-2
4. Arron JR, Choi Y. Bone versus immune system. *Nature* (2000) 408:535–6. doi: 10.1038/35046196
5. Cool DE, Tonks NK, Charbonneau H, Walsh KA, Fischer EH, Krebs EG. cDNA isolated from a human T-cell library encodes a member of the protein-tyrosine-phosphatase family. *Proc Natl Acad Sci USA* (1989) 86:5257–61. doi: 10.1073/pnas.86.14.5257
6. Takayanagi H, Ogasawara K, Hida S, Chiba T, Murata S, Sato K, et al. T-cell-mediated regulation of osteoclastogenesis by signalling cross-talk between RANKL and IFN-gamma. *Nature* (2000) 408:600–5. doi: 10.1038/35046102
7. Tang M, Tian L, Luo G, Yu X. Interferon-Gamma-Mediated Osteoimmunology. *Front Immunol* (2018) 9:1508:1508. doi: 10.3389/fimmu.2018.01508
8. Sato K, Suematsu A, Okamoto K, Yamaguchi A, Morishita Y, Kadono Y, et al. Th17 functions as an osteoclastogenic helper T cell subset that links T cell activation and bone destruction. *J Exp Med* (2006) 203:2673–82. doi: 10.1084/jem.20061775
9. Kim JW, Lee MS, Lee CH, Kim HY, Chae SU, Kwak HB, et al. Effect of interferon-γ on the fusion of mononuclear osteoclasts into bone-resorbing osteoclasts. *BMB Rep* (2012) 45:281–6. doi: 10.5483/bmbrep.2012.45.5.281

10. Yan Y, Liu F, Kou X, Liu D, Yang R, Wang X, et al. T Cells Are Required for Orthodontic Tooth Movement. *J Dent Res* (2015) 94:1463–70. doi: 10.1177/0022034515595003
11. Marahleh A, Kitaura H, Ohori F, Kishikawa A, Ogawa S, Shen WR, et al. TNF-α Directly Enhances Osteocyte RANKL Expression and Promotes Osteoclast Formation. *Front Immunol* (2019) 10:2925:2925. doi: 10.3389/fimmu.2019.02925
12. Palmqvist P, Lundberg P, Persson E, Johansson A, Lundgren I, Lie A, et al. Inhibition of hormone and cytokine-stimulated osteoclastogenesis and bone resorption by interleukin-4 and interleukin-13 is associated with increased osteoprotegerin and decreased RANKL and RANK in a STAT6-dependent pathway. *J Biol Chem* (2006) 281:2414–29. doi: 10.1074/jbc.M510160200
13. Wing K, Yamaguchi T, Sakaguchi S. Cell-autonomous and -non-autonomous roles of CTLA-4 in immune regulation. *Trends Immunol* (2011) 32:428–33. doi: 10.1016/j.it.2011.06.002
14. Wang J, Jiang H, Qiu Y, Wang Y, Sun G, Zhao J. Effector memory regulatory T cells were most effective at suppressing RANKL but their frequency was downregulated in tibial fracture patients with delayed union. *Immunol Lett* (2019) 209:21–7. doi: 10.1016/j.imlet.2019.03.018
15. Luo CY, Wang L, Sun C, Li DJ. Estrogen enhances the functions of CD4(+) CD25(+)Foxp3(+) regulatory T cells that suppress osteoclast differentiation and bone resorption in vitro. *Cell Mol Immunol* (2011) 8:50–8. doi: 10.1038/cmi.2010.54
16. Miossec P, Korn T, Kuchroo VK. Interleukin-17 and type 17 helper T cells. *N Engl J Med* (2009) 361:888–98. doi: 10.1056/NEJMra0707449
17. Yasuda K, Takeuchi Y, Hirota K. The pathogenicity of Th17 cells in autoimmune diseases. *Semin Immunopathol* (2019) 41:283–97. doi: 10.1007/s00281-019-00733-8
18. Dey I, Bishayi B. Role of Th17 and Treg cells in septic arthritis and the impact of the Th17/Treg -derived cytokines in the pathogenesis of S. aureus induced septic arthritis in mice. *Microb Pathog* (2017) 113:248–64. doi: 10.1016/j.micpath.2017.10.033
19. Samuel RO, Ervolino E, de Azevedo Queiroz ÍO, Azuma MM, Ferreira GT, Cintra LTA. Th1/Th2/Th17/Treg Balance in Apical Periodontitis of Normoglycemic and Diabetic Rats. *J Endod* (2019) 45:1009–15. doi: 10.1016/j.joen.2019.05.003
20. Li JY, Yu M, Tyagi AM, Vaccaro C, Hsu E, Adams J, et al. IL-17 Receptor Signaling in Osteoblasts/Osteocytes Mediates PTH-Induced Bone Loss and Enhances Osteocytic RANKL Production. *J Bone Miner Res* (2019) 34:349–60. doi: 10.1002/jbmr.3600
21. Kotake S, Udagawa N, Takahashi N, Matsuzaki K, Itoh K, Ishiyama S, et al. IL-17 in synovial fluids from patients with rheumatoid arthritis is a potent stimulator of osteoclastogenesis. *J Clin Invest* (1999) 103:1345–52. doi: 10.1172/jci5703
22. Li Y, Toraldo G, Li A, Yang X, Zhang H, Qian WP, et al. B cells and T cells are critical for the preservation of bone homeostasis and attainment of peak bone mass in vivo. *Blood* (2007) 109:3839–48. doi: 10.1182/blood-2006-07-037994
23. Weitzmann MN. T-cells and B-cells in osteoporosis. *Curr Opin Endocrinol Diabetes Obes* (2014) 21:461–7. doi: 10.1097/med.0000000000000103
24. Rivollier A, Mazzorana M, Tebib J, Piperno M, Aitsiselmi T, Rabourdin-Combe C, et al. Immature dendritic cell transdifferentiation into osteoclasts: a novel pathway sustained by the rheumatoid arthritis microenvironment. *Blood* (2004) 104:4029–37. doi: 10.1182/blood-2004-01-0041
25. Speziani C, Rivollier A, Gallois A, Coury F, Mazzorana M, Azocar O, et al. Murine dendritic cell transdifferentiation into osteoclasts is differentially regulated by innate and adaptive cytokines. *Eur J Immunol* (2007) 37:747–57. doi: 10.1002/eji.200636534
26. Madel MB, Ibáñez L, Wakkach A, de Vries TJ, Teti A, Apparailly F, et al. Immune Function and Diversity of Osteoclasts in Normal and Pathological Conditions. *Front Immunol* (2019) 10:1408:1408. doi: 10.3389/fimmu.2019.01408
27. Dhodapkar KM, Barbuto S, Matthews P, Kukreja A, Mazumder A, Vesole D, et al. Dendritic cells mediate the induction of polyfunctional human IL17-producing cells (Th17-1 cells) enriched in the bone marrow of patients with myeloma. *Blood* (2008) 112:2878–85. doi: 10.1182/blood-2008-03-143222
28. Kwan Tat S, Padrines M, Théoleyre S, Heymann D, Fortun Y. IL-6, RANKL, TNF-alpha/IL-1: interrelations in bone resorption pathophysiology. *Cytokine Growth Factor Rev* (2004) 15:49–60. doi: 10.1016/j.cytogfr.2003.10.005
29. Mercier FE, Ragu C, Scadden DT. The bone marrow at the crossroads of blood and immunity. *Nat Rev Immunol* (2011) 12:49–60. doi: 10.1038/nri3132
30. Taichman RS, Emerson SG. Human osteoblasts support hematopoiesis through the production of granulocyte colony-stimulating factor. *J Exp Med* (1994) 179:1677–82. doi: 10.1084/jem.179.5.1677
31. Nakamura Y, Arai F, Iwasaki H, Hosokawa K, Kobayashi I, Gomei Y, et al. Isolation and characterization of endosteal niche cell populations that regulate hematopoietic stem cells. *Blood* (2010) 116:1422–32. doi: 10.1182/blood-2009-08-239194
32. Zhu J, Garrett R, Jung Y, Zhang Y, Kim N, Wang J, et al. Osteoblasts support B-lymphocyte commitment and differentiation from hematopoietic stem cells. *Blood* (2007) 109:3706–12. doi: 10.1182/blood-2006-08-041384
33. Wu JY, Purton LE, Rodda SJ, Chen M, Weinstein LS, McMahon AP, et al. Osteoblastic regulation of B lymphopoiesis is mediated by Gs{alpha}-dependent signaling pathways. *Proc Natl Acad Sci USA* (2008) 105:16976–81. doi: 10.1073/pnas.0802898105
34. Yu VW, Saez B, Cook C, Lotinun S, Pardo-Saganta A, Wang YH, et al. Specific bone cells produce DLL4 to generate thymus-seeding progenitors from bone marrow. *J Exp Med* (2015) 212:759–74. doi: 10.1084/jem.20141843
35. Asada N, Katayama Y, Sato M, Minagawa K, Wakahashi K, Kawano H, et al. Matrix-embedded osteocytes regulate mobilization of hematopoietic stem/progenitor cells. *Cell Stem Cell* (2013) 12:737–47. doi: 10.1016/j.stem.2013.05.001
36. Azab E, Chandler KB, Uda Y, Sun N, Hussein A, Shuwaikan R, et al. Osteocytes control myeloid cell proliferation and differentiation through Gsα-dependent and -independent mechanisms. *FASEB J* (2020) 34:10191–211. doi: 10.1096/fj.202000366R
37. Fujiwara Y, Piemontese M, Liu Y, Thostenson JD, Xiong J, O'Brien CA. RANKL (Receptor Activator of NFκB Ligand) Produced by Osteocytes Is Required for the Increase in B Cells and Bone Loss Caused by Estrogen Deficiency in Mice. *J Biol Chem* (2016) 291:24838–50. doi: 10.1074/jbc.M116.742452
38. Kollet O, Dar A, Shivtiel S, Kalinkovich A, Lapid K, Sztainberg Y, et al. Osteoclasts degrade endosteal components and promote mobilization of hematopoietic progenitor cells. *Nat Med* (2006) 12:657–64. doi: 10.1038/nm1417
39. Miyamoto K, Yoshida S, Kawasumi M, Hashimoto K, Kimura T, Sato Y, et al. Osteoclasts are dispensable for hematopoietic stem cell maintenance and mobilization. *J Exp Med* (2011) 208:2175–81. doi: 10.1084/jem.20101890
40. Kiesel JR, Buchwald ZS, Aurora R. Cross-presentation by osteoclasts induces FoxP3 in CD8+ T cells. *J Immunol* (2009) 182:5477–87. doi: 10.4049/jimmunol.0803897
41. Ibáñez L, Abou-Ezzi G, Ciucci T, Amiot V, Belaïd N, Obino D, et al. Inflammatory Osteoclasts Prime TNFα-Producing CD4(+) T Cells and Express CX(3) CR1. *J Bone Miner Res* (2016) 31:1899–908. doi: 10.1002/jbmr.2868
42. Bussieres-Marmen S, Hutchins AP, Schirbel A, Rebert N, Tiganis T, Fiocchi C, et al. Characterization of PTPN2 and its use as a biomarker. *Methods* (2014) 65:239–46. doi: 10.1016/j.ymeth.2013.08.020
43. Tiganis T, Kemp BE, Tonks NK. The protein-tyrosine phosphatase TCPTP regulates epidermal growth factor receptor-mediated and phosphatidylinositol 3-kinase-dependent signaling. *J Biol Chem* (1999) 274:27768–75. doi: 10.1074/jbc.274.39.27768
44. Sharp RC, Abdulrahim M, Naser ES, Naser SA. Genetic Variations of PTPN2 and PTPN22: Role in the Pathogenesis of Type 1 Diabetes and Crohn's Disease. *Front Cell Infect Microbiol* (2015) 5:95. doi: 10.3389/fcimb.2015.00095
45. Doody KM, Bourdeau A, Tremblay ML. T-cell protein tyrosine phosphatase is a key regulator in immune cell signaling: lessons from the knockout mouse model and implications in human disease. *Immunol Rev* (2009) 228:325–41. doi: 10.1111/j.1600-065X.2008.00743.x
46. Stuible M, Doody KM, Tremblay ML. PTP1B and TC-PTP: regulators of transformation and tumorigenesis. *Cancer Metastasis Rev* (2008) 27:215–30. doi: 10.1007/s10555-008-9115-1
47. LaFleur MW, Nguyen TH. PTPN2 regulates the generation of exhausted CD8(+) T cell subpopulations and restrains tumor immunity. *Nat Immunol* (2019) 20:1335–47. doi: 10.1038/s41590-019-0480-4

48. Manguso RT, Pope HW, Zimmer MD, Brown FD, Yates KB, Miller BC, et al. In vivo CRISPR screening identifies Ptpn2 as a cancer immunotherapy target. *Nature* (2017) 547:413–18. doi: 10.1038/nature23270
49. Wiede F, Lu K-H, Du X, Liang S, Hochheiser K, Dodd GT, et al. PTPN2 phosphatase deletion in T cells promotes anti-tumour immunity and CAR T-cell efficacy in solid tumours. *EMBO J* (2020) 39:e103637–e37. doi: 10.15252/embj.2019103637
50. Wiede F, Brodnicki TC. T-Cell-Specific PTPN2 Deficiency in NOD Mice Accelerates the Development of Type 1 Diabetes and Autoimmune Comorbidities. *Diabetes* (2019) 68:1251–66. doi: 10.2337/db18-1362
51. Scharl M, McCole DF, Weber A, Vavricka SR, Frei P, Kellermeier S, et al. Protein tyrosine phosphatase N2 regulates TNFalpha-induced signalling and cytokine secretion in human intestinal epithelial cells. *Gut* (2011) 60:189–97. doi: 10.1136/gut.2010.216606
52. Scharl M, Hruz P, McCole DF. Protein tyrosine phosphatase non-receptor Type 2 regulates IFN-gamma-induced cytokine signaling in THP-1 monocytes. *Inflammation Bowel Dis* (2010) 16:2055–64. doi: 10.1002/ibd.21325
53. Aradi B, Kato M, Filkova M, Karouzakis E, Klein K, Scharl M, et al. Protein tyrosine phosphatase nonreceptor type 2: an important regulator of Interleukin-6 production in rheumatoid arthritis synovial fibroblasts. *Arthritis Rheumatol* (2015) 67:2624–33. doi: 10.1002/art.39256
54. Parlato M, Nian Q, Charbit-Henrion F, Ruemmele FM, Rodrigues-Lima F, Cerf-Bensussan N. Loss-of-Function Mutation in PTPN2 Causes Aberrant Activation of JAK Signaling Via STAT and Very Early Onset Intestinal Inflammation. *Gastroenterology* (2020) 159:1968–71. doi: 10.1053/j.gastro.2020.07.040
55. Simoncic PD, Lee-Loy A, Barber DL, Tremblay ML, McGlade CJ. The T cell protein tyrosine phosphatase is a negative regulator of janus family kinases 1 and 3. *Curr Biol* (2002) 12:446–53. doi: 10.1016/s0960-9822(02)00697-8
56. Krishnan M, McCole DF. T cell protein tyrosine phosphatase prevents STAT1 induction of claudin-2 expression in intestinal epithelial cells. *Ann New Y Acad Sci* (2017) 1405:116–30. doi: 10.1111/nyas.13439
57. Fukushima A, Loh K, Galic S, Fam B, Shields B, Wiede F, et al. T-cell protein tyrosine phosphatase attenuates STAT3 and insulin signaling in the liver to regulate gluconeogenesis. *Diabetes* (2010) 59:1906–14. doi: 10.2337/db09-1365
58. Gurzov EN, Tran M, Fernandez-Rojo MA, Merry TL, Zhang X, Xu Y, et al. Hepatic oxidative stress promotes insulin-STAT-5 signaling and obesity by inactivating protein tyrosine phosphatase N2. *Cell Metab* (2014) 20:85–102. doi: 10.1016/j.cmet.2014.05.011
59. ten Hoeve J, de Jesus Ibarra-Sanchez M, Fu Y, Zhu W, Tremblay M, David M, et al. Identification of a nuclear Stat1 protein tyrosine phosphatase. *Mol Cell Biol* (2002) 22:5662–68. doi: 10.1128/mcb.22.16.5662-5668.2002
60. Galic S, Klingler-Hoffmann M, Fodero-Tavoletti MT, Puryer MA, Meng TC, Tonks NK, et al. Regulation of insulin receptor signaling by the protein tyrosine phosphatase TCPTP. *Mol Cell Biol* (2003) 23:2096–108. doi: 10.1128/mcb.23.6.2096-2108.2003
61. Dodd GT, Lee-Young RS, Bruning JC, Tiganis T. TCPTP Regulates Insulin Signaling in AgRP Neurons to Coordinate Glucose Metabolism With Feeding. *Diabetes* (2018) 67:1246–57. doi: 10.2337/db17-1485
62. Tiganis T, Bennett AM, Ravichandran KS, Tonks NK. Epidermal growth factor receptor and the adaptor protein p52Shc are specific substrates of T-cell protein tyrosine phosphatase. *Mol Cell Biol* (1998) 18:1622–34. doi: 10.1128/mcb.18.3.1622
63. Stanoev A, Mhamane A, Schuermann KC, Grecco HE, Stallaert W, Baumdick M, et al. and Phosphatases Spatially Established by Vesicular Dynamics Generates a Growth Factor Sensing and Responding Network. *Cell Syst* (2018) 7:295–309.e11. doi: 10.1016/j.cels.2018.06.006
64. Mattila E, Auvinen K, Salmi M, Ivaska J. The protein tyrosine phosphatase TCPTP controls VEGFR2 signalling. *J Cell Sci* (2008) 121:3570–80. doi: 10.1242/jcs.031898
65. Persson C, Sävenhed C, Bourdeau A, Tremblay ML, Markova B, Böhmer FD, et al. Site-selective regulation of platelet-derived growth factor beta receptor tyrosine phosphorylation by T-cell protein tyrosine phosphatase. *Mol Cell Biol* (2004) 24:2190–201. doi: 10.1128/mcb.24.5.2190-2201.2004
66. Kramer F, Dernedde J, Mezheyeuski A, Tauber R, Micke P, Kappert K. Platelet-derived growth factor receptor β activation and regulation in murine myelofibrosis. *Haematologica* (2020) 105:2083–94. doi: 10.3324/haematol.2019.226332
67. Simoncic PD, Bourdeau A, Lee-Loy A, Rohrschneider LR, Tremblay ML, Stanley ER, et al. T-cell protein tyrosine phosphatase (Tcptp) is a negative regulator of colony-stimulating factor 1 signaling and macrophage differentiation. *Mol Cell Biol* (2006) 26:4149–60. doi: 10.1128/MCB.01932-05
68. Lees CW, Barrett JC, Parkes M, Satsangi J. New IBD genetics: common pathways with other diseases. *Gut* (2011) 60:1739–53. doi: 10.1136/gut.2009.199679
69. Marcil V, Mack DR, Kumar V, Faure C, Carlson CS, Beaulieu P, et al. Association between the PTPN2 gene and Crohn's disease: dissection of potential causal variants. *Inflammation Bowel Dis* (2013) 19:1149–55. doi: 10.1097/MIB.0b013e318280b181
70. Zhang Q, Li H, Hou S, Yu H, Su G, Deng B, et al. Association of genetic variations in PTPN2 and CD122 with ocular Behcet's disease. *Br J Ophthalmol* (2018) 102:996–1002. doi: 10.1136/bjophthalmol-2017-310820
71. Killock D. Genetics: Etiological insight into the genetic association of TCPTP with RA and JIA? *Nat Rev Rheumatol* (2011) 7:683. doi: 10.1038/nrrheum.2011.167
72. You-Ten KE, Muise ES, Itié A, Michaliszyn E, Wagner J, Jothy S, et al. Impaired bone marrow microenvironment and immune function in T cell protein tyrosine phosphatase-deficient mice. *J Exp Med* (1997) 186:683–93. doi: 10.1084/jem.186.5.683
73. Heinonen KM, Nestel FP, Newell EW, Charette G, Seemayer TA, Tremblay ML, et al. T-cell protein tyrosine phosphatase deletion results in progressive systemic inflammatory disease. *Blood* (2004) 103:3457–64. doi: 10.1182/blood-2003-09-3153
74. Spalinger MR, Kasper S, Chassard C, Raselli T, Frey-Wagner I, Gottier C, et al. PTPN2 controls differentiation of CD4(+) T cells and limits intestinal inflammation and intestinal dysbiosis. *Mucosal Immunol* (2015) 8:918–29. doi: 10.1038/mi.2014.122
75. Wiede F, Shields BJ, Chew SH, Kyparissoudis K, van Vliet C, Galic S, et al. T cell protein tyrosine phosphatase attenuates T cell signaling to maintain tolerance in mice. *J Clin Invest* (2011) 121:4758–74. doi: 10.1172/JCI59492
76. Spalinger MR, Manzini R, Hering L, Riggs JB, Gottier C, Lang S, et al. PTPN2 Regulates Inflammasome Activation and Controls Onset of Intestinal Inflammation and Colon Cancer. *Cell Rep* (2018) 22:1835–48. doi: 10.1016/j.celrep.2018.01.052
77. Spalinger MR, Sayoc-Becerra A, Santos AN, Shawki A, Canale V, Krishnan M, et al. PTPN2 Regulates Interactions Between Macrophages and Intestinal Epithelial Cells to Promote Intestinal Barrier Function. *Gastroenterology* (2020) 159:1763–77. doi: 10.1053/j.gastro.2020.07.004
78. Zheng L, Zhang W, Li A, Liu Y, Yi B, Nakhoul F, et al. PTPN2 Downregulation Is Associated with Albuminuria and Vitamin D Receptor Deficiency in Type 2 Diabetes Mellitus. *J Diabetes Res* (2018) 2018:3984797. doi: 10.1155/2018/3984797
79. Dzierzak E, Bigas A. Blood Development: Hematopoietic Stem Cell Dependence and Independence. *Cell Stem Cell* (2018) 22:639–51. doi: 10.1016/j.stem.2018.04.015
80. Bourdeau A, Trop S, Doody KM, Dumont DJ, Tremblay ML. Inhibition of T cell protein tyrosine phosphatase enhances interleukin-18-dependent hematopoietic stem cell expansion. *Stem Cells* (2013) 31:293–304. doi: 10.1002/stem.1276
81. Bourdeau A, Dube N, Heinonen KM, Theberge JF, Doody KM, Tremblay ML. TC-PTP-deficient bone marrow stromal cells fail to support normal B lymphopoiesis due to abnormal secretion of interferon-{gamma}. *Blood* (2007) 109:4220–8. doi: 10.1182/blood-2006-08-044370
82. Wiede F, Chew SH, van Vliet C, Poulton IJ, Kyparissoudis K, Sasmono T, et al. Strain-dependent differences in bone development, myeloid hyperplasia, morbidity and mortality in ptpn2-deficient mice. *PloS One* (2012) 7:e36703. doi: 10.1371/journal.pone.0036703
83. Doody KM, Bussières-Marmen S, Li A, Paquet M, Henderson JE, Tremblay ML. T cell protein tyrosine phosphatase deficiency results in spontaneous synovitis and subchondral bone resorption in mice. *Arthritis Rheumatism* (2012) 64:752–61. doi: 10.1002/art.33399
84. Loh K, Fukushima A, Zhang X, Galic S, Briggs D, Enriori Pablo J, et al. Elevated Hypothalamic TCPTP in Obesity Contributes to Cellular Leptin Resistance. *Cell Metab* (2011) 14:684–99. doi: 10.1016/j.cmet.2011.09.011

85. Ferron M, Wei J, Yoshizawa T, Del Fattore A, DePinho RA, Teti A, et al. Insulin signaling in osteoblasts integrates bone remodeling and energy metabolism. *Cell* (2010) 142:296–308. doi: 10.1016/j.cell.2010.06.003
86. Zee T, Settembre C, Levine RL. Karsenty G. T-cell protein tyrosine phosphatase regulates bone resorption and whole-body insulin sensitivity through its expression in osteoblasts. *Mol Cell Biol* (2012) 32:1080–88. doi: 10.1128/MCB.06279-11
87. Sinder BP, Pettit AR, McCauley LK. Macrophages: Their Emerging Roles in Bone. *J Bone Miner Res* (2015) 30:2140–9. doi: 10.1002/jbmr.2735
88. Spalinger MR, Sayoc-Becerra A, Ordookhanian C, Canale V, Santos AN, King SJ, et al. The JAK inhibitor tofacitinib rescues intestinal barrier defects caused by disrupted epithelial-macrophage interactions. *J Crohns Colitis* (2020) jjaa182. doi: 10.1093/ecco-jcc/jjaa182
89. You-Ten KE, Muise ES, Itié A, Michaliszyn E, Wagner J, Jothy S, et al. Impaired bone marrow microenvironment and immune function in T cell protein tyrosine phosphatase-deficient mice. *J Exp Med* (1997) 186:683–93. doi: 10.1084/jem.186.5.683
90. He D, Kou X, Luo Q, Yang R, Liu D, Wang X, et al. Enhanced M1/M2 macrophage ratio promotes orthodontic root resorption. *J Dent Res* (2015) 94:129–39. doi: 10.1177/0022034514553817
91. Li Y, Zhou HM, Wang F, Han L, Liu MH, Li YH, et al. Overexpression of PTPN2 in Visceral Adipose Tissue Ameliorated Atherosclerosis via T Cells Polarization Shift in Diabetic Apoe(-/-) Mice. *Cell Physiol Biochem* (2018) 46:118–32. doi: 10.1159/000488415
92. Heinonen KM, Bourdeau A, Doody KM, Tremblay ML. Protein tyrosine phosphatases PTP-1B and TC-PTP play nonredundant roles in macrophage development and IFN-gamma signaling. *Proc Natl Acad Sci USA* (2009) 106:9368–72. doi: 10.1073/pnas.0812109106
93. Zhang D, Jiang Y, Song D, Zhu Z, Zhou C, Dai L, et al. Tyrosine-protein phosphatase non-receptor type 2 inhibits alveolar bone resorption in diabetic periodontitis via dephosphorylating CSF1 receptor. *J Cell Mol Med* (2019) 23:6690–99. doi: 10.1111/jcmm.14545
94. Rhee I, Veillette A. Protein tyrosine phosphatases in lymphocyte activation and autoimmunity. *Nat Immunol* (2012) 13:439–47. doi: 10.1038/ni.2246
95. Flosbach M, Oberle SG, Scherer S, Zecha J, von Hoesslin M, Wiede F, et al. PTPN2 Deficiency Enhances Programmed T Cell Expansion and Survival Capacity of Activated T Cells. *Cell Rep* (2020) 32:107957. doi: 10.1016/j.celrep.2020.107957
96. Pike KA, Tremblay ML. Protein Tyrosine Phosphatases: Regulators of CD4 T Cells in Inflammatory Bowel Disease. *Front Immunol* (2018) 9:2504:2504. doi: 10.3389/fimmu.2018.02504
97. Wiede F, Dudakov JA, Lu K-H, Dodd GT, Butt T, Godfrey DI, et al. PTPN2 regulates T cell lineage commitment and αβ versus γδ specification. *J Exp Med* (2017) 214:2733–58. doi: 10.1084/jem.20161903
98. Yi Z, Lin WW, Stunz LL, Bishop GA. The adaptor TRAF3 restrains the lineage determination of thymic regulatory T cells by modulating signaling via the receptor for IL-2. *Nat Immunol* (2014) 15:866–74. doi: 10.1038/ni.2944
99. Cenci S, Toraldo G, Weitzmann MN, Roggia C, Gao Y, Qian WP, et al. Estrogen deficiency induces bone loss by increasing T cell proliferation and lifespan through IFN-gamma-induced class II transactivator. *Proc Natl Acad Sci USA* (2003) 100:10405–10. doi: 10.1073/pnas.1533207100
100. Gao Y, Grassi F, Ryan MR, Terauchi M, Page K, Yang X, et al. IFN-gamma stimulates osteoclast formation and bone loss in vivo via antigen-driven T cell activation. *J Clin Invest* (2007) 117:122–32. doi: 10.1172/jci30074
101. Lazzaro L, Tonkin BA, Poulton IJ, McGregor NE, Ferlin W, Sims NA. IL-6 trans-signalling mediates trabecular, but not cortical, bone loss after ovariectomy. *Bone* (2018) 112:120–27. doi: 10.1016/j.bone.2018.04.015
102. Kuroyanagi G, Adapala NS, Yamaguchi R, Kamiya N, Deng Z, Aruwajoye O, et al. Interleukin-6 deletion stimulates revascularization and new bone formation following ischemic osteonecrosis in a murine model. *Bone* (2018) 116:221–31. doi: 10.1016/j.bone.2018.08.011
103. Udagawa N, Takahashi N, Katagiri T, Tamura T, Wada S, Findlay DM, et al. Interleukin (IL)-6 induction of osteoclast differentiation depends on IL-6 receptors expressed on osteoblastic cells but not on osteoclast progenitors. *J Exp Med* (1995) 182:1461 8. doi: 10.1084/jem.182.5.1461
104. Wu Q, Zhou X, Huang D, Ji Y, Kang F. IL-6 Enhances Osteocyte-Mediated Osteoclastogenesis by Promoting JAK2 and RANKL Activity In Vitro. *Cell Physiol Biochem* (2017) 41:1360–69. doi: 10.1159/000465455
105. Yamashita T, Iwakura T, Matsui K, Kawaguchi H, Obana M, Hayama A, et al. IL-6-mediated Th17 differentiation through RORγt is essential for the initiation of experimental autoimmune myocarditis. *Cardiovasc Res* (2011) 91:640–8. doi: 10.1093/cvr/cvr148
106. Aqel SI, Kraus EE, Jena N, Kumari V, Granitto MC, Mao L, et al. Novel small molecule IL-6 inhibitor suppresses autoreactive Th17 development and promotes T(reg) development. *Clin Exp Immunol* (2019) 196:215–25. doi: 10.1111/cei.13258
107. Zhang Y, Ding H, Wang X, Ye SD. Modulation of STAT3 phosphorylation by PTPN2 inhibits naive pluripotency of embryonic stem cells. *FEBS Lett* (2018) 592:2227–37. doi: 10.1002/1873-3468.13112
108. Yamamoto T, Sekine Y, Kashima K, Kubota A, Sato N, Aoki N, et al. The nuclear isoform of protein-tyrosine phosphatase TC-PTP regulates interleukin-6-mediated signaling pathway through STAT3 dephosphorylation. *Biochem Biophys Res Commun* (2002) 297:811–7. doi: 10.1016/s0006-291x(02)02291-x
109. Svensson MN, Doody KM, Schmiedel BJ, Bhattacharyya S, Panwar B, Wiede F, et al. Reduced expression of phosphatase PTPN2 promotes pathogenic conversion of Tregs in autoimmunity. *J Clin Invest* (2019) 129:1193–210. doi: 10.1172/JCI123267
110. Onal M, Xiong J, Chen X, Thostenson JD, Almeida M, Manolagas SC, et al. Receptor activator of nuclear factor κB ligand (RANKL) protein expression by B lymphocytes contributes to ovariectomy-induced bone loss. *J Biol Chem* (2012) 287:29851–60. doi: 10.1074/jbc.M112.377945
111. Wiede F, Sacirbegovic F, Leong YA, Yu D, Tiganis T. PTPN2-deficiency exacerbates T follicular helper cell and B cell responses and promotes the development of autoimmunity. *J Autoimmun* (2017) 76:85–100. doi: 10.1016/j.jaut.2016.09.004
112. Wang YN, Jia T, Zhang J, Lan J, Zhang D, Xu X. PTPN2 improves implant osseointegration in T2DM via inducing the dephosphorylation of ERK. *Exp Biol Med (Maywood)* (2019) 244:1493–503. doi: 10.1177/1535370219883419
113. Niechcial A, Butter M, Manz S, Obialo N, Bäbler K, van der Lely L, et al. Presence of PTPN2 SNP rs1893217 Enhances the Anti-inflammatory Effect of Spermidine. *Inflammation Bowel Dis* (2020) 26:1038–49. doi: 10.1093/ibd/izaa013
114. Hsieh WC, Svensson MN, Zoccheddu M, Tremblay ML, Sakaguchi S, Stanford SM, et al. PTPN2 links colonic and joint inflammation in experimental autoimmune arthritis. *JCI Insight* (2020) 5:e141868. doi: 10.1172/jci.insight.141868
115. Zhang P, Zhang W, Zhang D, Wang M, Aprecio R, Ji N, et al. 25-Hydroxyvitamin D3 -enhanced PTPN2 positively regulates periodontal inflammation through the JAK/STAT pathway in human oral keratinocytes and a mouse model of type 2 diabetes mellitus. *J Periodontal Res* (2018) 53:467–77. doi: 10.1111/jre.12535

Permissions

All chapters in this book were first published in CPO, by Frontiers; hereby published with permission under the Creative Commons Attribution License or equivalent. Every chapter published in this book has been scrutinized by our experts. Their significance has been extensively debated. The topics covered herein carry significant findings which will fuel the growth of the discipline. They may even be implemented as practical applications or may be referred to as a beginning point for another development.

The contributors of this book come from diverse backgrounds, making this book a truly international effort. This book will bring forth new frontiers with its revolutionizing research information and detailed analysis of the nascent developments around the world.

We would like to thank all the contributing authors for lending their expertise to make the book truly unique. They have played a crucial role in the development of this book. Without their invaluable contributions this book wouldn't have been possible. They have made vital efforts to compile up to date information on the varied aspects of this subject to make this book a valuable addition to the collection of many professionals and students.

This book was conceptualized with the vision of imparting up-to-date information and advanced data in this field. To ensure the same, a matchless editorial board was set up. Every individual on the board went through rigorous rounds of assessment to prove their worth. After which they invested a large part of their time researching and compiling the most relevant data for our readers.

The editorial board has been involved in producing this book since its inception. They have spent rigorous hours researching and exploring the diverse topics which have resulted in the successful publishing of this book. They have passed on their knowledge of decades through this book. To expedite this challenging task, the publisher supported the team at every step. A small team of assistant editors was also appointed to further simplify the editing procedure and attain best results for the readers.

Apart from the editorial board, the designing team has also invested a significant amount of their time inunderstanding the subject and creating the most relevant covers. They scrutinized every image to scout for the most suitable representation of the subject and create an appropriate cover for the book.

The publishing team has been an ardent support to the editorial, designing and production team. Their endless efforts to recruit the best for this project, has resulted in the accomplishment of this book. They are a veteran in the field of academics and their pool of knowledge is as vast as their experience in printing. Their expertise and guidance has proved useful at every step. Their uncompromising quality standards have made this book an exceptional effort. Their encouragement from time to time has been an inspiration for everyone.

The publisher and the editorial board hope that this book will prove to be a valuable piece of knowledge forresearchers, students, practitioners and scholars across the globe.

List of Contributors

Marco Ponzetti and Nadia Rucci
Department of Biotechnological and Applied Clinical Sciences, University of L'Aquila, L'Aquila, Italy

S. Anand Narayanan
Department of Medical Physiology, Texas A&M Health Science Center, Bryan, TX, United States

Teun J. de Vries, Ismail el Bakkali and Ineke D. C. Jansen
Department of Periodontology, Academic Centre for Dentistry Amsterdam (ACTA), University of Amsterdam and Vrije Universiteit Amsterdam, Amsterdam, Netherlands

Thomas Kamradt
Institute of Immunology, Universitätsklinikum Jena, Jena, Germany

Georg Schett
Department of Internal Medicine III, Friedrich-Alexander University Erlangen-Nürnberg and Universitatsklinikum Erlangen, Erlangen, Germany

Patrizia D'Amelio
Gerontology and Bone Metabolic Diseases Division, Department of Medical Science, University of Turin, Turin, Italy

Noymar Luque-Campos, Rafael A. Contreras-López, María Jose Paredes-Martínez and Patricia Luz-Crawford
Laboratorio de Inmunología Celular y Molecular, Centro de Investigación Biomédica, Facultad de Medicina, Universidad de los Andes, Santiago, Chile

Maria Jose Torres
Escuela de Ingeniería Bioquímica, Pontificia Universidad Católica de Valparaíso, Valparaíso, Chile

Sarah Bahraoui and Farida Djouad
IRMB, INSERM, Univ Montpellier, Montpellier, France

Mingxing Wei
Cellvax, SAS, Parc BIOCITECH, Romainville, France

Francisco Espinoza
Cells for Cells, Universidad de los Andes, Santiago, Chile

Roberto Javier Elizondo-Vega
Laboratorio de Biología Celular, Departamento de Biología Celular, Facultad de Ciencias Biológicas, Universidad de Concepción, Concepción, Chile

Kylie A. Alexander, Hsu-Wen Tseng, Whitney Fleming, Beulah Jose, Irina Kulina, Susan M. Millard, Allison R. Pettit and Jean-Pierre Levesque
Mater Research Institute – The University of Queensland, Translational Research Institute, Woolloongabba, QLD, Australia

Marjorie Salga
Mater Research Institute – The University of Queensland, Translational Research Institute, Woolloongabba, QLD, Australia
CIC-IT 1429, Service de Médecine Physique et de Réadaptation, Raymond Poincaré University Hospital, AP-HP, Garches, France

François Genêt
CIC-IT 1429, Service de Médecine Physique et de Réadaptation, Raymond Poincaré University Hospital, AP-HP, Garches, France
Université de Versailles Saint Quentin en Yvelines, END:ICAP Inserm U1179, Montigny le Bretonneux, France

Trias Thireou
Laboratory of Genetics, Department of Biotechnology, Agricultural University of Athens, Athens, Greece

Maria Papadaki, Vagelis Rinotas, Foteini Violitzi and Eleni Douni
Laboratory of Genetics, Department of Biotechnology, Agricultural University of Athens, Athens, Greece
Division of Immunology, Biomedical Sciences Research Center "Alexander Fleming", Athens, Greece

George Panayotou and Martina Samiotaki
Division of Molecular Oncology, Biomedical Sciences Research Center "Alexander Fleming", Athens, Greece

Ulrike Steffen, Georg Schett and Aline Bozec
Department of Internal Medicine 3, University of Erlangen-Nuremberg, Erlangen, Germany

Tetsuo Hasegawa
Department of Immunology and Cell Biology, Graduate School of Medicine and Frontier Biosciences, Osaka University, Osaka, Japan
Division of Rheumatology, Department of Internal Medicine, Keio University School of Medicine, Tokyo, Japan

Junichi Kikuta and Masaru Ishii
WPI-Immunology Frontier Research Center, Osaka University, Osaka, Japan

Niamh Fahy, Ursula Menzel, Mauro Alini and Martin J. Stoddart
AO Research Institute Davos, Davos, Switzerland

Elisabeth Seebach and Katharina F. Kubatzky
Department of Infectious Diseases, Medical Microbiology and Hygiene, Heidelberg University Hospital, Heidelberg, Germany

Anne Wilson
Department of Oncology, University of Lausanne, Epalinges, Switzerland

He Fu, Mariano Schiffrin, Carine Winkler, Federica Gilardi and Béatrice Desvergne
Faculty of Biology and Medicine, Center for Integrative Genomics, Genopode, University of Lausanne, Lausanne, Switzerland

Meriem Koufany and Jean-Yves Jouzeau
IMoPA, UMR7365 CNRS-Université de Lorraine, Vandoeuvre-lès-Nancy, France

Nicolas Bonnet
Division of Bone Diseases, Department of Internal Medicine Specialties, Faculty of Medicine, Geneva University Hospital, Geneva, Switzerland

François Renevey and Sanjiv A. Luther
Department of Biochemistry, Center for Immunity and Infection, University of Lausanne, Epalinges, Switzerland

David Moulin
IMoPA, UMR7365 CNRS-Université de Lorraine, Vandoeuvre-lès-Nancy, France
CHRU de Nancy, Contrat d'interface, Vandoeuvre-lès-Nancy, France

Isabelle Duroux-Richard and Florence Apparailly
IRMB, Univ Montpellier, INSERM, CHU Montpellier, Montpellier, France

Claire Lozano
IRMB, Univ Montpellier, INSERM, CHU Montpellier, Montpellier, France
Immunology Department, CHU Montpellier, Montpellier, France

Hüseyin Firat and Eric Schordan
Firalis SA, Molecular Diagnostics, Huningue, France

Cristina Sobacchi and Ciro Menale
Milan Unit, Institute for Genetic and Biomedical Research (CNR-IRGB), Milan, Italy
Humanitas Clinical and Research Center IRCCS, Rozzano, Italy

Anna Villa
Milan Unit, Institute for Genetic and Biomedical Research (CNR-IRGB), Milan, Italy
San Raffaele Telethon Institute for Gene Therapy (SR-Tiget), IRCCS San Raffaele Scientific Institute, Milan, Italy

Christian J. Schipp
Julius Wolff Institute and Center for Musculoskeletal Surgery, Charité–Universitätsmedizin Berlin, Berlin, Germany

Sebastian Wendler, Claudia Schlundt, Christian H. Bucher and Katharina Schmidt-Bleek
Julius Wolff Institute and Center for Musculoskeletal Surgery, Charité–Universitätsmedizin Berlin, Berlin, Germany
Berlin-Brandenburg Center for Regenerative Therapies, Charité–Universitätsmedizin Berlin, Berlin, Germany

Jan Birkigt
Department of Isotope Biogeochemistry, Helmholtz Centre for Environmental Research–UFZ, Leipzig, Germany

Hans-Dieter Volk
Berlin-Brandenburg Center for Regenerative Therapies, Charité–Universitätsmedizin Berlin, Berlin, Germany
Institute of Medical Immunology, Charité–Universitätsmedizin Berlin, Berlin, Germany

Georg N. Duda
Julius Wolff Institute and Center for Musculoskeletal Surgery, Charité–Universitätsmedizin Berlin, Berlin, Germany
Berlin-Brandenburg Center for Regenerative Therapies, Charité–Universitätsmedizin Berlin, Berlin, Germany
Berlin Institute of Health Center for Regenerative Therapies, Berlin, Germany

Chen Zhang, Fengjiao Han, Jie Yu, Xiang Hu, Mingqiang Hua, Chaoqin Zhong, Ruiqing Wang, Xueyun Zhao and Daoxin Ma
Department of Hematology, Qilu Hospital of Shandong University, Jinan, China

Yufeng Shi
Institute for Financial Studies and School of Mathematics, Shandong University, Jinan, China

Chunyan Ji
Department of Hematology, Qilu Hospital of Shandong University, Jinan, China
Shandong Provincial Key Laboratory of Immunohematology, Qilu Hospital of Shandong University, Jinan, China

Emma Persson
Department of Molecular Periodontology, Umeå University, Umeå, Sweden

Thais Floriano-Marcelino
Bone Biology Research Group, Department of Physiology and Pathology, School of Dentistry, São Paulo State University (UNESP), Araraquara, Brazil

Pedro P. C. Souza
Bone Biology Research Group, Department of Physiology and Pathology, School of Dentistry, São Paulo State University (UNESP), Araraquara, Brazil
School of Dentistry, Federal University of Goiás, Goiânia, Brazil

Howard Herschel Conaway
Department of Physiology and Biophysics, University of Arkansas for Medical Sciences, Little Rock, AR, United States

Petra Henning and Ulf H. Lerner
Department of Molecular Periodontology, Umeå University, Umeå, Sweden
Department of Internal Medicine and Clinical Nutrition, Centre for Bone and Arthritis Research, Institute for Medicine, Sahlgrenska Academy, University of Gothenburg, Gothenburg, Sweden

Massimo De Martinis, Lia Ginaldi, Maria Maddalena Sirufo, Enrica Maria Bassino and Francesca De Pietro
Department of Life, Health and Environmental Sciences, University of L'Aquila, L'Aquila, Italy

Giovanni Pioggia
Institute for Biomedical Research and Innovation (IRIB), National Research Council of Italy (CNR), Messina, Italy

Sebastiano Gangemi
School and Operative Unit of Allergy and Clinical Immunology, Department of Clinical and Experimental Medicine, University of Messina, Messina, Italy

Yogesh Saxena, Sanjeev Routh and Arunika Mukhopadhaya
Department of Biological Sciences, Indian Institute of Science Education and Research Mohali, Mohali, India

Ya-nan Wang, Tingting Jia, Yao Feng, Wenjing Zhang, Xin Xu and Dongjiao Zhang
Department of Implantology, School and Hospital of Stomatology, Cheeloo College of Medicine, Shandong University, Jinan, China
Shandong Key Laboratory of Oral Tissue Regeneration, Jinan, China
Shandong Engineering Laboratory for Dental Materials and Oral Tissue Regeneration, Jinan, China

Shiyue Liu
Shandong Key Laboratory of Oral Tissue Regeneration, Jinan, China
Shandong Engineering Laboratory for Dental Materials and Oral Tissue Regeneration, Jinan, China
Department of Periodontology, School and Hospital of Stomatology, Cheeloo College of Medicine, Shandong University, Jinan, China

Index

N

O

P

R

S

T

W

www.ingramcontent.com/pod-product-compliance
Lightning Source LLC
LaVergne TN
LVHW060543210926
848485LV00005B/1250